Excision and Reconstruction
in Head and Neck Cancer

For Churchill Livingstone

Publisher: Sheila Khullar
Copy Editors: Jill Whittaker, Paul Singleton
Indexer: Jill Halliday
Design: Design Resources Unit
Production Controller: Mark Sanderson
Sales Promotion Executive: Caroline Boyd

Excision and Reconstruction in Head and Neck Cancer

Edited by

David S. Soutar ChM FRCS(Edin) FRCS(Glas) MB ChB

Consultant Plastic Surgeon, West of Scotland Regional Plastic and Maxillofacial Surgery Unit, Canniesburn Hospital, Glasgow; Honorary Clinical Senior Lecturer, University of Glasgow, UK

Rammohan Tiwari MD MS(Surg) FRCS PhD

Associate Professor, Department of Otolaryngology–Head and Neck Surgery, Division of Surgical Oncology, Reconstructive and Skull Base Surgery, Free University Hospital, Amsterdam, The Netherlands

Foreword by

John M. Loré Jr MD FACS

Medical Director of Head and Neck Oncology Service and Center, Sisters Hospital, Buffalo; Professor and Chairman Emeritus, Department of Otolaryngology, State University of New York at Buffalo, New York, USA

CHURCHILL LIVINGSTONE

EDINBURGH LONDON MADRID MELBOURNE NEW YORK AND TOKYO 1994

CHURCHILL LIVINGSTONE
Medical Division of Longman Group Limited

Distributed in the United States of America by Churchill
Livingstone Inc., 650 Avenue of the Americas, New York, N.Y.
10011, and by associated companies, branches and
representatives throughout the world.

© Longman Group Limited 1994

First published 1994
  Reprinted 1995

ISBN 0 443 04526 7

British Library Cataloguing in Publication Data
A catalogue record for this book is available from the British
Library.

Library of Congress Cataloging in Publication Data
A catalog record for this book is available from the Library of
Congress.

Printed in Hong Kong
LYP/02

Contents

Contributors

Louis C. Argenta MD
Professor and Chairman, Department of Plastic and
Reconstructive Surgery, Bowman Gray Medical School,
Winston-Salem, North Carolina, USA

Shan R. Baker MD FACS
Professor and Chief, Section of Facial Plastic and
Reconstructive Surgery, University of Michigan, Ann
Arbor, Michigan, USA

Andrew G. Batchelor BSc MB FRCS(Plast Surg)
Consultant Plastic Surgeon and Senior Clinical Lecturer,
St James's University Hospital NHS Trust, Leeds, UK

Paul J. Donald MD FRCS(C) FACS
Professor, Department of Otolaryngology–Head and
Neck Surgery; Director, Center for Skull Base Surgery,
University of California, Davis Medical Center,
Sacramento, California, USA

Patricia M. Finlay BDS FDSRCPS
Associate Specialist in Oral and Maxillofacial Surgery,
Canniesburn Hospital, Glasgow; Honorary Clinical
Lecturer, University of Glasgow, UK

Paulo R. Godoy MD
Assistant Surgeon, Head and Neck Service, Hospital
Santa Rita, Porto Alegre, Brazil

Nilton T. Herter MD
Professor and Chief, Head and Neck Service, Hospital
Santa Rita; Professor of Surgery, Federal Medical Science
School, Porto Alegre, Brazil

Ian T. Jackson MB ChB FRCS FACS FRACS(Hon)
Director, Institute of Craniofacial and Reconstructive
Surgery, Providence Hospital, Southfield, Michigan,
USA

Neil Ford Jones MA FRCS
Professor of Plastic and Reconstructive Surgery,
University of California, UCLA Medical Center,
Los Angeles, California, USA

Dennis H. Kraus MD
Assistant Professor, Division of Head and Neck
Surgery, Memorial Sloan-Kettering Cancer Center,
New York, USA

Ricardo Gallicchio Kroef MD
Research Fellow, International Hearing Foundation,
Minneapolis, Minnesota, USA; Assistant Surgeon, Head
and Neck Service, Hospital Santa Rita, Porto Alegre,
Brazil

Robert E. Marx DDS FAAOMS
Professor of Surgery, Director of Tumor and
Reconstructive Surgery, University of Miami School of
Medicine; Consultant to the Surgeon General, United
States Air Force, USA

Alan D. McGregor MD FRCS(Glas) FRCS(Plast Surg)
Consultant Plastic Surgeon, St Lawrence Hospital,
Chepstow, Gwent, UK

Bryan J. Michelow FRCS(Edin) FRCS(Glas)
Clinical and Research Fellow, Paediatric Plastic Surgery,
University of Toronto, Ontario, Canada

Michael R. Morris MD FACS
Otolaryngology–Head and Neck Surgeon, Residency
Program Director, Madigan Army Medical Center,
Tacoma, Washington, USA

William R. Panje MD FACS
Professor of Otolaryngology, Rush Medical School,
University Head and Neck Associates, Chicago, Illinois,
USA

Bruce W. Pearson MD FRCS(C) FACS
Serene M. and Francis C. Durling Professor of
Otolaryngology and Chief, Section of Otolaryngology,
Mayo Clinic, Jacksonville; Chief of Section of
Otolaryngology, St Luke's Hospital, Jacksonville, Florida,
USA

Jeffrey C. Posnick DMD MD FRCS(C) FACS
Chief, Craniomaxillofacial Surgery, Georgetown
University Medical Center, Washington, DC, USA

Dieter Riediger MD DDS
Medical Director, Clinic for Maxillofacial and Plastic
Surgery, Katharinen Teaching Hospital, University of
Tübingen, Stuttgart, Germany

David E. Schuller MD
Professor and Chairman, Department of Otolaryngology;
Director, Comprehensive Cancer Center–Arthur G.
James Cancer Hospital and Research Institute,
Ohio State University, Columbus, Ohio, USA

Jatin P. Shah MD MS(Surg) FACS
Chief, Head and Neck Service, Memorial Sloan-Kettering
Cancer Center, New York; Professor of Surgery, Cornell
University Medical College, New York, USA

David S. Soutar ChM FRCS(Edin) FRCS(Glas) MB ChB
Consultant Plastic Surgeon, West of Scotland Regional
Plastic and Maxillofacial Surgery Unit, Canniesburn
Hospital, Glasgow; Honorary Clinical Senior Lecturer,
University of Glasgow, UK

Mirec F. Stranc FRCS FRCS(C) Dipl.Amer.Board of Plast.Surg.
Professor of Surgery, University of Manitoba, Winnipeg,
Manitoba, Canada

Rammohan Tiwari MD MS(Surg) FRCS PhD
Associate Professor, Department of Otolaryngology–Head
and Neck Surgery, Division of Surgical Oncology,
Reconstructive and Skull Base Surgery, Free University
Hospital, Amsterdam, The Netherlands

Christoph von Ilberg MD
Professor and Head of Department of Ear, Nose and
Throat, University of Frankfurt-am-Main, Germany

Alexander Weber MD
Assistant, ENT Department, University of Frankfurt-am-
Main, Germany

Hilko Weerda MD DMD
Professor, ENT and Plastic Surgery, Medical University
Lübeck, Lübeck, Germany

Keith M. Wilson MD
Head and Neck Oncologic Surgery Fellow, Department
of Otolaryngology, Comprehensive Cancer Center, Ohio
State University, Columbus, Ohio, USA

Ronald M. Zuker MD FRCS(C) FACS
Associate Professor of Surgery, University of Toronto;
Head, Division of Plastic Surgery, The Hospital for Sick
Children, Toronto, Ontario, Canada

Foreword

Both editors, Dr Soutar and Dr Tiwari, have been able to assemble a first-class group of physicians and dentists to contribute to this book, which is an excellent compendium related to ablative and reconstructive surgery for head and neck cancer. These contributing experts in their field include head and neck surgeons with backgrounds in the disciplines of general surgery, plastic and reconstructive surgery and otolaryngology, including dentists and prosthodontists. With the editors representing Scotland in the United Kingdom and Amsterdam in The Netherlands, in addition to contributions from other parts of Europe as well as North and South America, this work is an example of ecumenism in head and neck oncologic surgery at an unusual level. It is hard to imagine such a cross-section of ideas, techniques and experiences.

The list of contents indicates the broad scope of the book, which is divided into 26 chapters. However, there is sufficient overlap by the various authors to enable the reader to obtain different points of view in the overall managements of any one specific histologic neoplasm, as well as location of neoplasm. Although the area of resection may be the same, surgical approaches, as well as methods of reconstruction, are varied. All of this information is well covered in the text but, even more importantly, in photographs of the surgical procedures and often accompanied by line drawings. The photographs are excellent and whether the credit goes to the surgeon who may have taken them himself or to a professional photographer makes little difference. They are good and good operative photographs are difficult to achieve. The publisher should be complimented for the quality of reproduction of both black-and-white and colour photographs.

It would be impossible, in the Foreword, to comment on each surgical procedure, but suffice to say that, in many instances, various approaches and, most importantly, reconstructive techniques are demonstrated. Just about every method is covered – various local and distant flaps, vascularized free flaps, myocutaneous flaps, both with and without osseous components, as well as free bone grafts, tissue expanders, dental implants and gold weights in the upper lid for 7th nerve paralysis.

Along with basic head and neck oncologic surgery, the skull base aspects of the field are well covered, not only in the chapter so named, but also in overlap in other chapters. The historical references are very important in this field since the surgery dates back to the early 1960s and possibly before that, encompassing Dr Alfred Ketchems with craniofacial resections and Dr John Lewis with temporal bone resections. The more recent aspects of middle cranial fossa surgery are included.

The natural history of tumour spread is another phase which is well illustrated, for example, in the chapter on approaches to the mandible; and, speaking of the mandible, especially reconstruction, there are four chapters which address various aspects of this problem besides which there are other methods. This serves to demonstrate that there is no one simple method suitable for all mandibular defects. When a surgeon masters one basic method and is satisfied with the results, it might be best to stay with that procedure. Nevertheless, the broad knowledge covered in the four chapters is very worthwhile to the surgeon's armamentarium.

The various discussions regarding the pros and cons of the use of prosthetic material and devices vs autologous tissue is well presented. Just because a surgeon *can* perform a procedure does not indicate that he *should* perform that procedure. Rather the consequences related to the long-term follow-up relative to both success and failures are most important and so reviewed in a number of chapters with supporting photographs. The old adage 'the proof of the pudding is in the eating' is aptly portrayed.

The bottom line is that this is a work which covers ablative and reconstructive surgery in a comprehensive and excellent fashion, a work which is a significant addition to the head and neck surgeon's library. There are many phases of the field well portrayed and if only one of the many procedures helps the surgeon with one patient, the entire effort is worthwhile both to the authors and to the readers. I'm sure many patients and many head and neck surgeons will glean benefit from this work. Congratulations to the editors, authors and publishers!

J.M.L.

Preface

The management of patients with head and neck cancer demands a multi-disciplinary approach involving a variety of specialties. Although the aim of treatment remains to cure the disease wherever possible, the emphasis has shifted from survival and prolongation of life towards preservation of quality of life and restoration of function. Advances in diagnostic imaging techniques, medicine, anaesthesia, pain control, radiotherapy, prosthodontics, nursing and para-medical services have all contributed to the welfare of patients with head and neck cancer.

Perhaps the single most important contribution relates to the change in excisional and reconstructive surgery techniques. On the one hand, there has been an effort to preserve structures and organs, best illustrated in the sections on surgical management of the mandible, the neck and the larynx. On the other hand, more aggressive excisions have been made possible as a result of advances in craniofacial and skull base surgery. Extensive excisions have become possible because of the wide variety of reconstructive techniques now available.

Head and neck surgery has come a long way to be recognised as a specialty in its own right. A variety of disciplines, namely general surgery, otolaryngology, plastic surgery, maxillofacial surgery, neurosurgery and paediatric surgery have contributed to its development. Although some centres have all these specialties represented, the young head and neck surgeon is not uncommonly required to go out of his parental discipline to seek additional training and knowledge.

In this book, we have attempted to provide the reader with a multi-disciplinary approach by presenting contributions from colleagues who are internationally recognised in the field of head and neck surgery. A wide variety of sites and pathologies have been included and basic philosophies of management, their historical background, techniques involved, advantages and disadvantages of differing approaches, results and complications and future developments have all been addressed in an attempt to present the reader with an up-to-date and comprehensive text.

Excision and reconstruction, like two sides of a coin, are intimately related. It is the advancement of the latter that has made excision bold and effortless. We hope that our philosophy of combining these two aspects of tumour surgery will enrich the knowledge of the reader, stimulate research and development and lead to improvements in the service and care we offer to our patients with head and neck cancer.

Glasgow and
Amsterdam, 1994

D.S.S.
R.T.

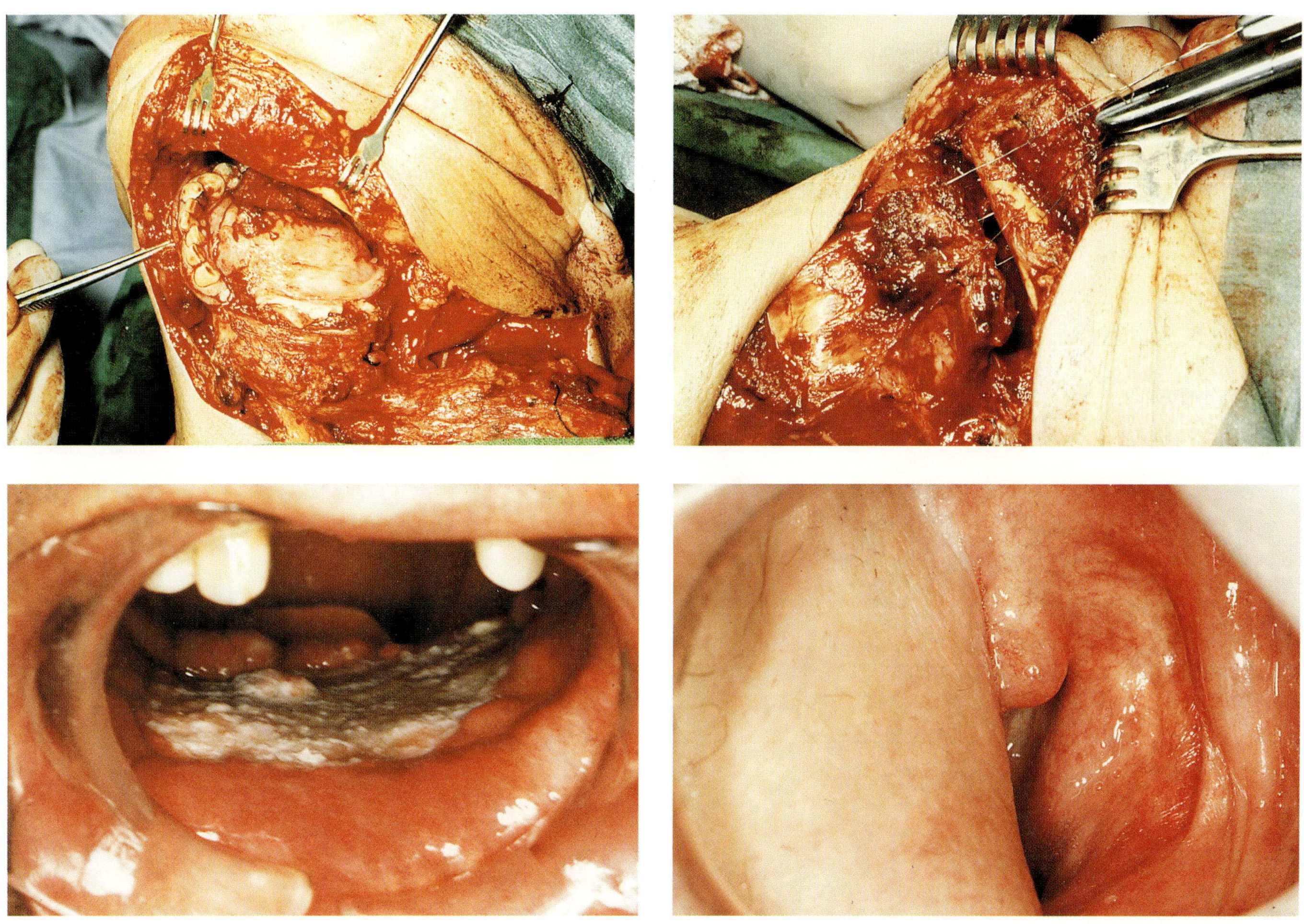

Fig. 10.3 *(top left)* Total glossectomy with marginal mandibular resection. The specimen is being delivered into the neck while the intact mandible is retracted upwards. (See text, p. 123)

Fig. 10.5 *(top right)* Steps in laryngeal suspension. The specimen has been removed. Stainless steel wires for laryngeal suspension are in place. Infralaryngeal muscles have been sectioned, and the larynx and trachea have been mobilized. (See text, p.136–137)

Fig. 10.8 *(bottom left)* Total glossectomy reconstruction with pectoralis major muscle and split skin graft. Note the epiglottis in the background and its high position because of laryngeal suspension. (See text, p. 138)

Fig. 10.9 *(bottom right)* Reconstruction after total glossectomy and segmental mandibular resection with laryngeal preservation. The contralateral floor of the mouth has been used along with the myocutaneous flap from pectoralis major. The epiglottis is not seen. (See text, p.138)

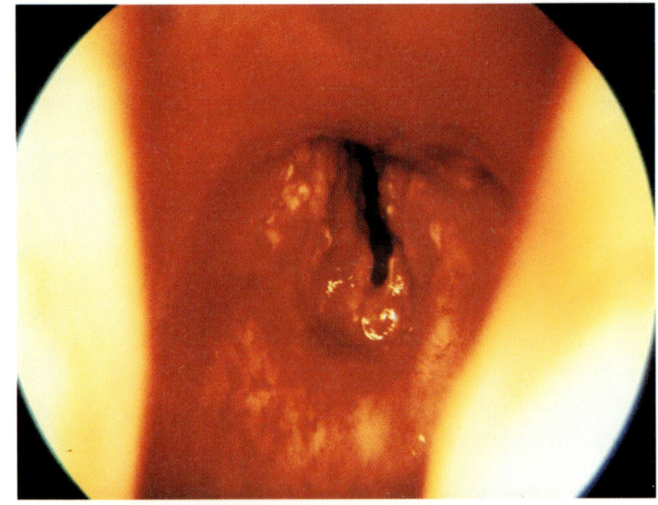

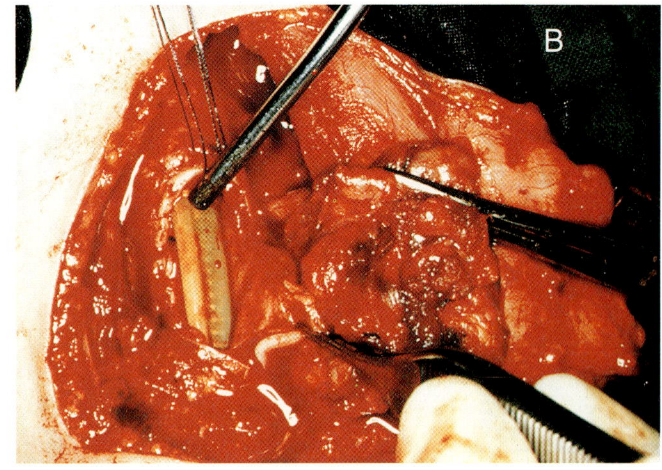

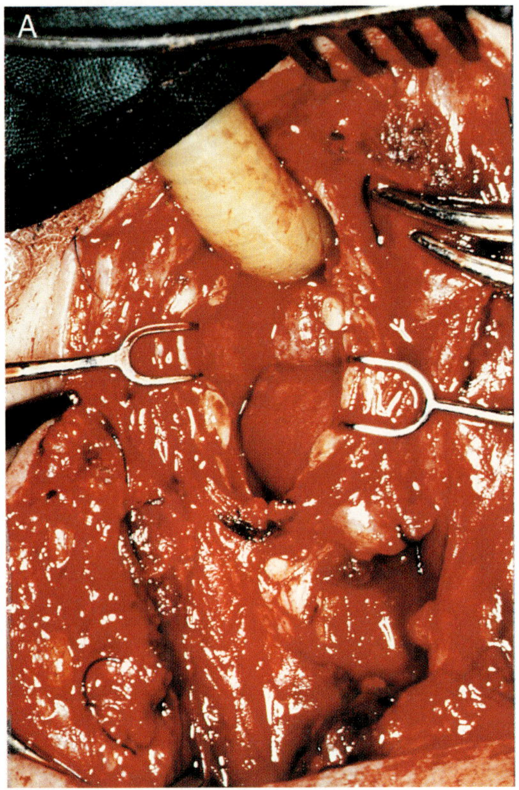

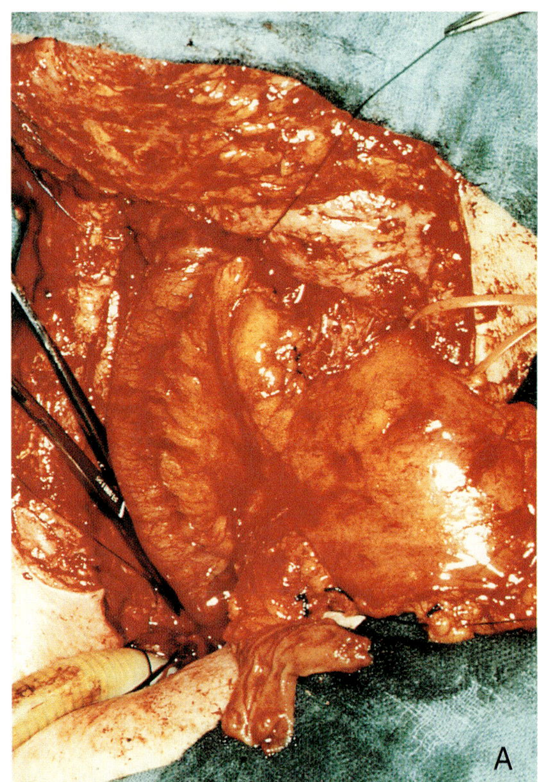

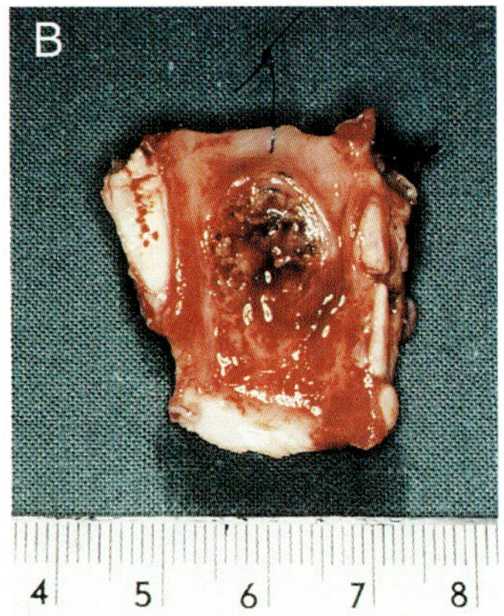

Fig. 15.6 *(top left)* Endoscopic view of a patient with circular growing carcinoma of the upper trachea (0 Optic Storz with Olympus OM2 Camera). (See text, p. 202)

Fig. 15.8B *(top right)* Tracheal segment resection in a 12-year-old girl with rhabdomyosarcoma of the left upper trachea. (See text, p. 203)

Fig. 15.9A and **B** *(middle left and bottom left)* Lateral 'window resection' of the subcricoidal region in a 51-year-old female patient with adenoid cystic carcinoma. (See text, p.204)

Fig. 15.14A *(above)* Reconstruction of the hypopharynx and cervical oesophagus with free jejunum graft. (See text, p.205–206)

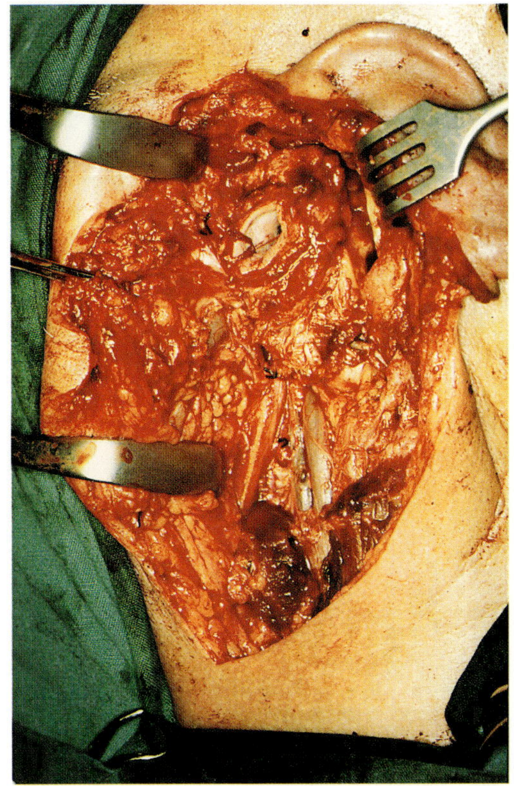

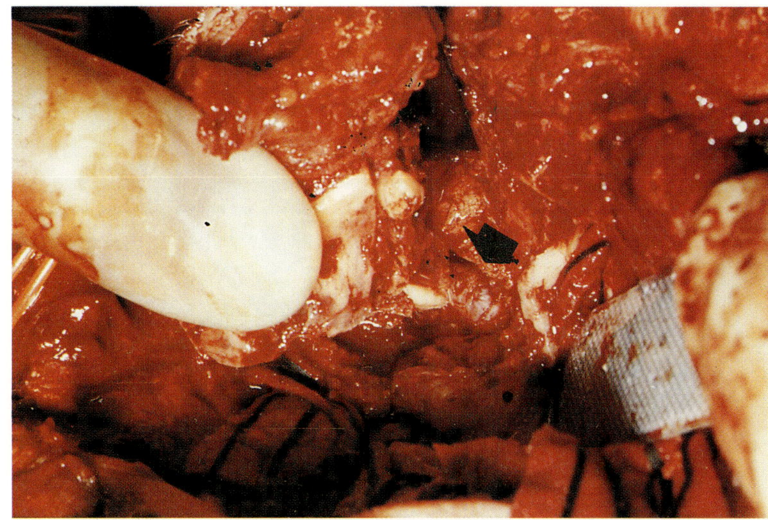

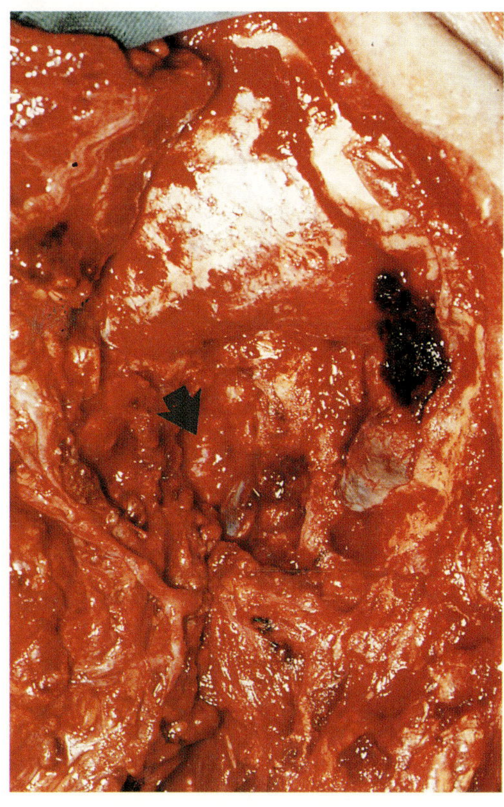

Fig. 17.8 *(top left)* Exposure of the infratemporal region. The ear canal has been transected. The facial nerve is dissected in a retrograde fashion from its marginal branch and divided. The parotid gland can be seen attached to the antero-inferior aspect of the ear canal. The carotid vessels, internal jugular vein and the X, XI and XII nerves have been dissected. (See text, p. 232)

Fig. 17.11 *(top right)* Intra-operative photograph of left temporal bone resection. The specimen is being detached from the petrous apex. The dura is being retracted medially. The internal carotid artery is visible in the carotid canal (arrow). (See text, p. 233)

Fig. 17.17 *(right)* Intra-operative photograph. The specimen has been removed. The sigmoid sinus is visible posteriorly and the jugular bulb slightly anterior to it. The dura is seen superiorly, and the sectioned main strand of the facial nerve with the main trunks is clearly seen on the left. The internal carotid artery is seen medially and slightly superior to the jugular bulb (arrow). (See text, p. 235)

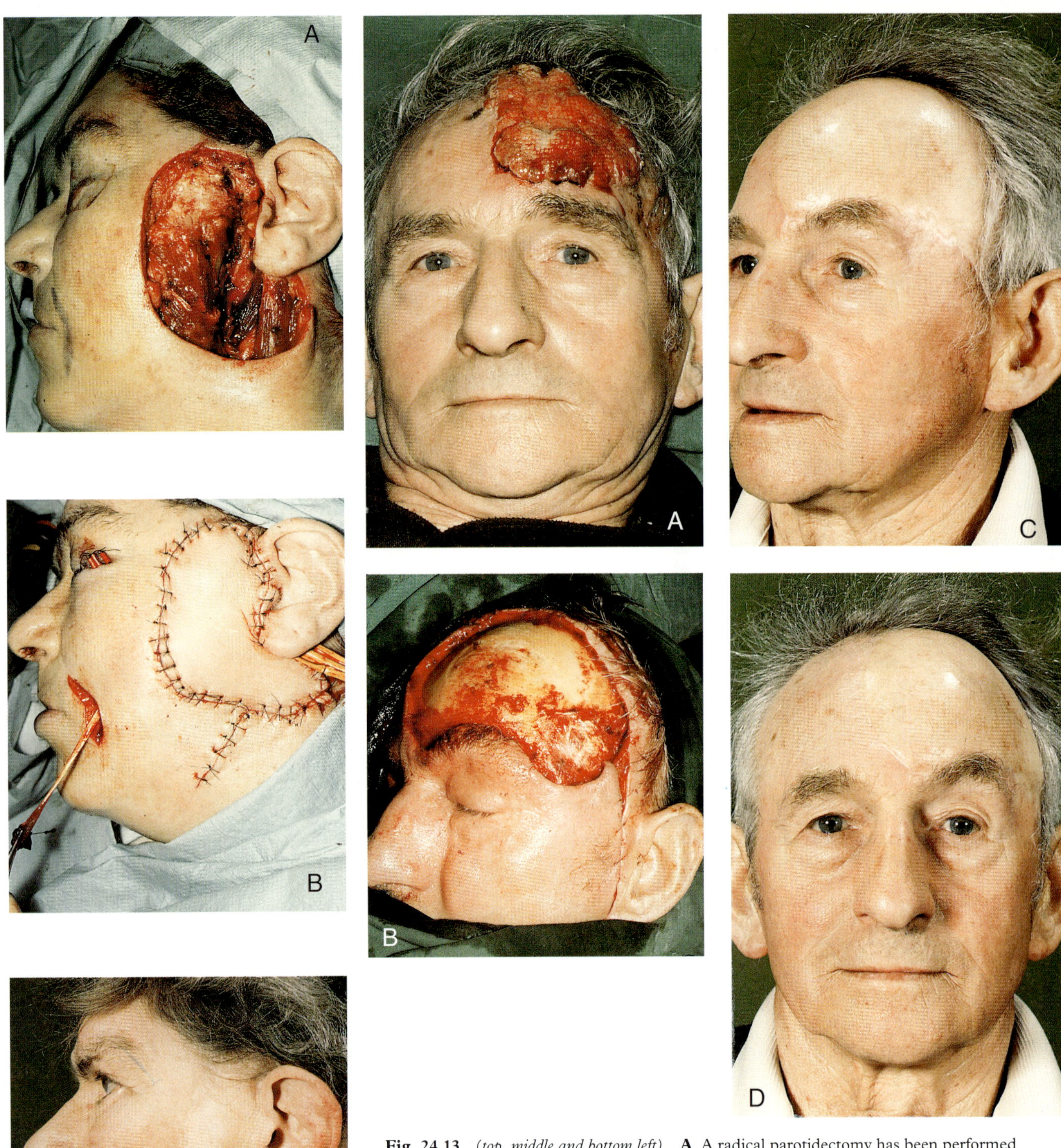

Fig. 24.13 *(top, middle and bottom left)* **A** A radical parotidectomy has been performed including facial musculature and overlying skin. **B** A free radial forearm flap incorporating a vascularized palmaris longus tendon was used for reconstruction. The tendon provided a reconstructive sling for the oral cavity. A lateral tarsorrhaphy has also been performed.

C The patient underwent radical postoperative radiotherapy and the appearance at 5 years postoperatively is shown. The patient remains disease- free at 8 years. The angle of the mouth has been retained in a good position, and oral competence is maintained. (See text, p.384–385)

Fig. 24.14 *(above)* **A** A metatypical basal-cell carcinoma of the forehead in a patient aged over 70 years. **B** Excision involved removal of the periosteum and exposure of bare cranial bone. **C, D** The appearance following reconstruction with a scapular flap which required one thinning procedure. The patient remains alive and free of disease 8 years following surgery. Contour has been satisfactorily achieved, but the colour and texture of the skin are not ideal. (See text, p. 385)

1. Strategies in head and neck cancer

Rammohan Tiwari   David S. Soutar

INTRODUCTION

In the fight against cancer, the last quarter of this century, especially the last decade, has been eventful. Our understanding of the disease process, the diagnostic modalities, as well as therapeutic possibilities have made significant progress. Basic research into genetics, molecular biology, cellular kinetics and cellular pathology and angiogenesis have revealed new facets of the disease process (Weinhouse 1980, Goepfert et al 1984, Klein & Klein 1985, Bishop 1987, Schantz et al 1988, Saranath 1989, Carter 1990, Gunn et al 1977, Folkman et al 1989, Wilson et al 1988). Newer imaging techniques have made visualisation of tumour outline possible as never before making precise therapy easier for the clinician (Grevers et al 1991). The ability of the pathologist to diagnose and subclassify tumours with a high degree of precision has been made possible due to advances in immunohistochemistry and the use of markers (Mukai & Rosai 1980, Hanna et al 1990). Progress in immunology has led to the application of newer therapeutic possibilities such as the use of retinoids (Lippman et al 1988, Hong et al 1990) and Interleukin (Cortesina et al 1988, Boscia et al 1988).

Much effort has been devoted in the last decades to chemotherapy, either alone or in combination with surgery and/or radiotherapy in the management of head and neck cancer. Whilst sporadic reports of improved survivals with chemotherapy appear in the literature, the overall results in squamous cell carcinoma have been disappointing (Green 1978, Hong 1988, Stell 1990, Snow & Vermorken 1989, Eschwege & Lartigau 1990). A few recent studies have reported short-term successes in laryngeal preservation in advanced laryngeal cancer. The value of such approaches with respect to long-term benefits, however, remains to be established (Kaplan et al 1985, Johnson et al 1985, Leitner et al 1985, Synderman et al 1986, Jacobs et al 1986, Bosl et al 1991, Wolf et al 1991, Pai et al 1991). The role of chemotherapy in recurrent cancer remains palliative.

Radiotherapeutic techniques have greatly improved with innovative approaches and the advent of accurate computerised tomography (CT) planning for external beam radiotherapy. Much effort has been placed on fractionation of radiotherapy with the object of improving overall survival results while at the same time minimising local tissue reaction. Local tissue changes and the long-term prospect of radiation-induced tumours have to be weighed against immediate gains (Seagren et al 1979, Harwood & Lawson 1982, Seagren 1982, Vikram et al 1985, Fuks et al 1991, Dische 1989). New regimens such as intraoperative radiotherapy or hyperfractionation of radiotherapy continuous hyperfractionated accelerated radiation therapy (CHART), (Saunders & Dische 1986) have shown initial promise but require further study. In the light of the fact that treatment results with surgery, radiotherapy and chemotherapy have virtually reached a plateau over the last decade, these efforts and developments are praiseworthy and we should look forward to the long-term results.

Surgery has also shown remarkable developments in the last two decades, particularly in the fields of access for tumour excision, the increased radical nature of the surgery, and the vast range of reconstructive techniques now available. Despite forecasts that surgical oncology had reached its zenith, new surgical approaches and advances continue to be made (McCraw et al 1979, Ariyan 1979, Mckee & Berry 1971, Taylor 1982, Soutar et al 1983, Terzis 1987, Robertson 1986, Panje 1987, Hidalgo 1989). Improved reconstructive techniques have now given the excisional surgeon a freedom with regard to excision in the knowledge that the defect can be reconstructed. Many of the new techniques have made a significant impact on our ability to restore the structure and especially the function of the part or the organ involved.

The search for alloplastic materials suitable for reconstruction in head and neck surgery continues and materials such as titanium have added a new dimension to reconstructive techniques. In particular, the advent of osseointegration techniques for fixation of facial prostheses has altered many of our traditional ideas regarding

1

reconstructive surgery (Branemark et al 1975).

Many of these developments have occurred hand in hand with rising standards of living. Patients today are not satisfied just with 'cure' of the disease but expect to return to society and resume all their responsibilities. They therefore expect both efficient and effective treatment. While there is no doubt that major surgical advances have resulted from the pioneering efforts of our predecessors and the continuing dedication of the present generation, changes in public opinion have also undoubtedly served as source of stimulation to this goal.

PRINCIPLES OF SURGICAL MANAGEMENT

Once the decision has been taken to treat a given tumour surgically, several factors need to be considered in the planning of the procedure. The histopathology of the tumour and its stage are two 'tumour factors' to consider since they determine the ultimate behaviour of the tumour process. The clinician and in turn the patient are forewarned as to what is likely to be expected. Some tumours are more aggressive than others, while some may be better treated with modalities other than surgery. The patholigist therefore is a key person in the head and neck team and in this respect the emergence of a group of tumour pathologists who superspecialise in head and neck tumours is a positive development. The surgical oncologist should have a sound knowledge of the behaviour of the various tumours and decide the right treatment. The saying 'a surgeon knows when not to operate' is perhaps never more true than in surgical oncology.

The clinical staging of disease is a key factor in determining surgical treatment. The TNM-staging system lays stress on tumour dimensions rather than tumour volume, which is all-important in treatment. It is not easy to determine exactly the volume of a given tumour but using imaging techniques and measuring the depth of infiltration can provide the necessary information. A T2 glottic carcinoma of the larynx is a good example. Although the TNM classification makes no differentiation between a bulky and a non-bulky T2 glottic cancer, radiotherapists are aware that the bulky T2 cancer sometimes subclassified by them as T2b cancer has a poorer prognosis than the less bulky T2a cancer (Karim et al 1980). Carcinoma of the tongue is another example. While some information as to the infiltrative character of the tumour may be obtained by palpation and by imaging techniques (particularly MRI – magnetic resonance imaging), more precise information is obtained by histopathological assessment of the extent of infiltration. The prognostic significance of this measurement in early tongue carcinoma (T1, T2) is well documented in the literature. Studies have shown that the incidence of cervical nodal metastasis is higher in tumours of deeper infiltration and the subsequent prognosis of these cases is poorer (Spiro et al 1986, Tabatabai et al 1986, Fakih et al 1989, Nathason & Agren 1989).

PRINCIPLES OF EXCISION

The head and neck is an area of functional and aesthetic significance and consequently there is a tendency to be conservative in excision. While conservation may be tempting it is worth bearing in mind that free margins offer the most reasonable chance of a successful outcome. For excision to be a viable treatment option, it must encompass sufficient lateral margins and also adequate depth, increasing T stage being directly proportional to wider and deeper excisions. Residual or recurrent disease reduces the chance of survival. Despite histological verification of negative margins, local recurrence does occur in about 20% of cases. Survival of patients with free margin relates linearly to the T stage of their cancer. A small tumour with free margins is less likely to recur than a large infiltrative growth (Looser et al 1978, Batsakis 1988, Borges et al 1989). An ideal excision is one where the margins and the depth are free with a wide area of healthy tissue around. Should one or more margins on histological examination show incomplete excision then re-excision is the safest course. A retrospective study by Ziekse showed that 8.8% of surgical resections had positive margins. Some 60% of these patients failed to achieve loco-regional control when treated with radiotherapy (Ziekse et al 1986). Frozen section at the time of primary surgery is helpful in ensuring free margins and in addition to mucosal margins, muscle, glandular tissue, lymph nodes and peripheral nerves can be subjected to frozen section. Hard tissue such as cartilage and bone, however, have to await formal fixed histological sections. If in the final histological report there is still evidence of positive margins, then re-excision is the ideal step. It is a sound basic principle, wherever possible, to ensure safe excision margins before embarking on reconstruction. It should be remembered that in surgery on previously irradiated patients, frozen section interpretation may be difficult and may lead to false positive reports (Barney 1970, Bauer 1974, Bauer et al 1975, Holaday & Assor 1974, Dehner & Rosai 1977).

Radiotherapy as primary modality treatment for head and neck cancer is still practised in many centres throughout the world. Although the quality of radiotherapy has improved over the years, radiation fibrosis is still encountered and may make recognition of tissue planes difficult. Unless the surgeon has evaluated the patient himself prior to radiotherapy and/or the tumour extent has been precisely recorded with the margins tattooed, it may be difficult to assess the extent of excision. The importance of proper documentation prior to the institution of any form of therapy cannot be overemphasised.

In the management of large tumours (T3–T4), it is generally agreed that combined modality treatment is superior to single modality and there is evidence that surgery followed by postoperative radiotherapy yields better long-term results (Lawrence et al 1974, Van den Brouck et al 1977, Vikram et al 1980, Robertson et al 1986, Wanebo et al 1992).

Recurrence after previous surgical excision denotes either previous irradical surgery or a tumour with multicentric origin. Occasionally revision of the previous histology may show an incorrect diagnosis of clear margins. Surgery may still have a role to play in the treatment of recurrent tumours. Surgery for recurrent tumours can also be combined with brachytherapy and chemotherapy is still widely used in the palliation of recurrent disease. Advances in laser technology and their application have added greatly to palliation of large tumours. In addition, laser excision of early lesions such as the tongue and vocal cords can preserve function and spare these patients a long and drawn out period of radiation.

The increase in the average life expectancy of patients with head and neck cancer has increased the chances of these patients developing new or second primaries. The incidence of second primary tumours varies from country to country and at various sites in the head and neck and incidences from 3.8 to 38% have been reported. The highest incidence is in relation to hypopharyngeal cancers (De Vries 1990) Oral cavity mucosa is well known to show generalised dysplastic changes in a high percentage of cases with oral cancer and new cancers tend to appear after successful treatment of a previous tumour. Two or three cancers in the same patient over a period of a few years are not uncommon and up to five primaries have been seen by the authors. Surgical management of these cancers is often necessary and many of these patients, particularly those with the hypopharyngeal cancers, have received a full course of radiotherapy. Such patients can, however, be successfully rehabilitated and this is a testimony to modern reconstructive surgery (Vikram et al 1984). Reports on second primary tumours in the lung show that nearly 30% of the second primaries are synchronous and have a better prognosis than metachronous tumours (Atabek et al 1987). Multi-institutional studies targeted at prevention of second primaries with retinoids and other vitamins are presently underway. These studies underline the value of better nutritional standards in the prevention of cancer. It should be remembered, however, that the epidemiology and nature of secondary tumours varies according to the life style in various countries. It may, for instance, be a cancer of the oesophagus in Japan, while in Australia one may have to deal with a variety of skin cancers.

SURGICAL MANAGEMENT OF CERVICAL LYMPH NODES

In any resection of a malignant tumour, the regional nodes must be taken into account (Table 1.1). The prognostic significance of lymph node metastasis in head and neck cancer has long been documented (Martin et al 1951, Cachin et al 1979, Snow et al 1986, Trible & Dias 1964). The questions that need to be answered are:

Table 1.1 Regional lymph nodes – staging after AJC and UICC

The definition of the N categories for all head and neck sites except thyroid gland are:

N	Regional lymph nodes
NX	Regional lymph nodes cannot be assessed
N0	No regional lymph node metastasis
N1	Metastasis in a single ipsilateral lymph node, 3 cm or less in greatest dimension
N2	Metastasis in a single ipsilateral lymph node, more than 3 cm but not more than 6 cm in greatest dimesion, or in multiple ipsilateral lymph nodes, none more than 6 cm in greatest dimension, or in bilateral or contralateral lymph nodes, none more than 6 cm in greatest dimension
N2a	Metastasis in a single ipsilateral lymph node, more than 3 cm but not more than 6 cm in greatest dimension
N2b	Metastasis in multiple ipsilateral lymph nodes, none more than 6 cm in greatest dimension
N2c	Metastasis in bilateral or contralateral lymph nodes, none more than 6 cm in greatest dimension
N3	Metastasis in a lymph node more than 6 cm in greatest dimension

1. Is regional nodal clearance indicated?
2. Should the neck nodes be removed at the same time as the primary tumour or at a later date?
3. Should the nodes be cleared unilaterally or on both sides?
4. What kind of neck dissection will offer the patient the optimum chance of 'cure'?
5. What are the consequences of surgery?
6. Should the neck be treated by radiotherapy instead of surgery?

In early lesions (T1, T2) the site and degree of infiltration undoubtedly are the most important considerations. For example, in a T2 carcinoma of the mobile tongue, an elective neck dissection may well be indicated whether concurrent or at a later date. Continuous en bloc neck dissections give fewer regional recurrences, however, but this may not always be preferable because of the necessary sacrifice of normal tissues (Leemans et al 1991) and discontinuous neck dissection may then be the only alternative. In a N+ neck, the decision to perform a neck dissection is clear. In a N0 neck such a decision is largely influenced by the statistical possibilities of occult metastasis from a given site.

Several studies have in the past reported on this subject and formed the basis of the policies for elective neck dissection (Ali et al 1985, Candela et al 1990). The significantly low incidence of false negative nodes in supraglottic carcinoma in the reports by Ali et al (1985) has led to a policy of wait and watch. Experience over several years has confirmed that this has been a correct approach and these patients have been spared unnecessary neck dissection. A good follow up is, however, essential.

The diagnosis of cervical nodal metastasis has greatly improved with the advent of imaging techniques. Ultrasound – guided fine needle aspiration offers the highest chance (93%) of an accurate diagnosis (Van de Brekel et al

1991). This is a relatively innocuous and inexpensive technique which can be globally adapted. In general when the neck is entered for access or as part of the resection of the primary tumour, it is a sound policy to consider neck node clearance at the same operation. Neck dissection also serves as a staging procedure.

In recent years, there has been a trend to perform limited neck dissections as opposed to the radical or modified radical dissection. These limited neck dissections which excise particular groups of lymph nodes (Fig. 1.1) are termed selective neck dissections (Robbins 1991). The concept of selective neck dissections is not new and has been influenced by the fact that nodes in the posterior triangle are involved in only a small percentage of cases (Skolnik et al 1976). Several types of selective neck dissections are in common practice and these include supraomohyoid neck dissection for anterior tongue and floor of mouth cancers encompassing levels I, II and III and lateral neck dissection including levels II, III and IV for laryngeal cancers. In addition, there is the anterior neck dissection involving levels II, III and IV on both sides for thyroid cancers and the anterolateral dissection including levels I to IV commonly used in intraoral malignancy (Medina 1989).

It must be appreciated that there are additional areas in the neck that require dissection depending on the site of the

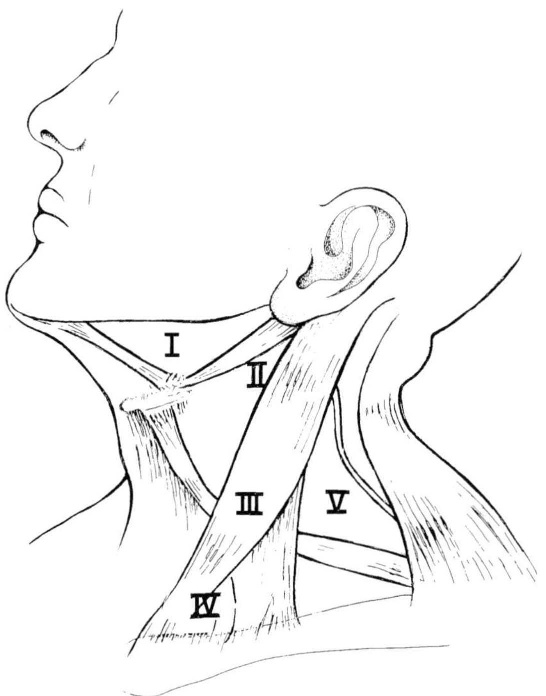

Fig. 1.1 Lymph node groups and zones in the neck as used at the Sloan Kettering Memorial Hospital. The submental and submandibular gions form zone I, the subdigastric group of lymph nodes are designated zone II, the midjugular or jugulo-omohyoid group is zone III, the lower jugular nodes are designated zone IV and the nodes in the posterior triangle form zone V.

primary tumour. There is at present no separate sub-classification of these particular neck dissections and it has been suggested that any additional dissection should be denoted as an extension (Medina 1989). Extensions in a neck dissection therefore would include paratracheal dissection so vital in transglottic and subglottic cancers, extensive posterior triangle dissection for cutaneous malignancy particularly of the posterior scalp, neck dissection which includes superficial parotidectomy as part of the lymphatic drainage and excision of the postauricular mastoid skin when performing a neck dissection for malignancy of the ear.

It is well recognised that lymphatics from the posterior part of the oral cavity, the oropharynx, the soft palate and the posterior aspect of the nose and paranasal sinuses drain into the retropharyngeal group of nodes. These nodes are located one on the body of the vertebra in the midline, and one on either side of the transverse process. Recurrences after treatment of oropharyngeal carcinoma commonly occur behind the ascending ramus of the mandible, suggestive of recurrence in the lateral chain of the retropharyngeal nodes. Dissection of retropharyngeal lymph nodes was suggested by Krespi and Sisson (1982). This aspect of lymph node metastasis is seldom addressed in the literature and dissection of the retropharyngeal nodes is seldom practised. It is, however, good practice to include these nodes in the dissection or in the irradiation field whenever the primary is located in one of the above mentioned sites.

Modified neck dissection with preservation of the accessory nerve was advocated by Skolnik and has been shown to be oncologically safe (Skolnik et al 1967, Jesse et al 1978). The selective neck dissections preserve not only the accessory nerve but also the internal jugular vein and the sternomastoid muscle. The posterior limit of dissection in the supraomohyoid and anterolateral dissections are the roots of the cervical plexus. Undoubtedly much individual variation is to be expected in the quality of these dissections and the long-term results have yet to be evaluated. Spiro reported on a 2-year follow up of 139 supraomohyoid dissections. The results of this study showed a recurrence rate of 5% in N0 necks, 15% in occult metastasis and 29% in N+ necks, despite postoperative radiotherapy (Spiro et al 1988). Bocca, who advocated functional neck dissection (Bocca & Pignataro 1967) reported a recurrence rate of 2.38% for N0 and 30.4% for N+ necks which did not include N3 (Bocca et al 1984). In a recent retrospective study of 494 comprehensive neck dissections with preservation of accessory nerve, Leemans et al (1990) reported a recurrence rate over 5 years of 3% in N0 necks and 10% in N+ necks. These are three relatively large studies from well recognised institutions and reflect the present state of neck dissection. In assessing these results, it should be remembered that selective neck dissections are technically demanding operations requiring significant expertise.

There continues to be debate as to the indications for

postoperative radiotherapy to the neck. While some centres radiate every positive neck on the grounds that this indicates stage II disease, others believe that postoperative radiotherapy should be reserved for more than one positive node and those necks where extra capsular spread of disease has been shown histopathologically. It must be stated that while fears of functional impairment following radiotherapy are genuine, much depends on the quality of the radiotherapy and the techniques that are used.

When it is decided to treat the primary tumour with radiotherapy, neck nodes are as a rule included in the field. After excision of a primary tumour only, elective radiotherapy to the neck may also be considered if the chances of neck node metastasis are higher than 15–20%.

PRINCIPLES OF RECONSTRUCTION

The surgeon carrying out excision must not only be equipped with an understanding of the oncological aspects but also of the reconstructive techniques which can restore the defect. The concept of a two team approach is gradually being replaced by the concept of a group of head and neck surgeons from similar or differing surgical disciplines familiar with both excision and reconstructive techniques. In modern oncological surgery, reconstruction plays a significant role. It is important to realise that reconstruction does not begin after the tumour has been excised but when the very first incision is laid. Primary reconstruction is ideal but a delayed surgical procedure may be chosen in the interests of the patient, depending on the nature of the disease process. In general, where combined modality treatment is planned, then primary reconstruction is the method of choice to enable rapid healing so that the second phase of treatment can commence at an early date. This particularly applies to planned surgery and postoperative radical radiotherapy since for this treatment to be effective as a combined modality treatment, the radiotherapy should be instituted within 6 weeks of surgery. Such aggressive treatment places increased demands on the reconstruction which must be capable of withstanding full dose tumouricidal radiotherapy. Delayed reconstruction or staged methods of

reconstruction are only applicable in cases where there is no urgency either to reconstruct or to give additional treatment.

When vital structures are exposed, such as major vessels or the extension into the cranial cavity, then primary reconstruction is mandatory and can prove to be life saving. Despite the reported increased risk of complications in the elderly (Morgan et al 1982, Barzan et al 1990), excision and primary reconstruction can be performed with minimal complications (Panje & Pitcock 1989). This is a tribute to present day surgery, anaesthesia and nursing, particularly in a population whose average age is increasing.

Modern reconstructive techniques have made excision of large tumours possible with reasonable restoration of external appearance and function. Maxillofacial prosthetics have made giant strides and now play a major role in rehabilitation. Certain procedures such as total glossectomy which were not so long ago associated with severe disability of swallowing and speech can now be performed with preservation of swallowing and speech (Tiwari et al 1993).

Surgical treatment of cancer of the head and neck has passed through a phase of change in the last decade. On the one hand, there have been attempts to conserve function such as speech in lesions of the larynx and piriform sinuses through innovative techniques such as near total laryngectomy (Pearson et al 1980). On the other hand, surgical excision of tumours from the base of skull and infratemporal fossa (Obwegeser 1985) have been described and carried out successfully. While this change concerns advances in surgical technique, it also reflects our understanding of the biology of disease processes, especially our awareness of subclinical cancer and the causes of regional failure. Surgeons must accept that the object of excisional surgery for cancer is not to wipe out each individual cell. When carried out at the appropriate time and in co-ordination with other treatment modalities, surgery offers the patient the possibility of eliminating abnormal cells (Goepfert 1988). Surgeons have now joined hands with radiotherapy and medical oncology colleagues to provide planned and co-ordinated treatment. Our aim is not only to improve survival but also to restore quality of life.

REFERENCES

Ali S, Tiwari R M, Snow G B 1985 False positive and false negative neck nodes. Head and Neck Surgery 8: 78–82
Ariyan S 1979 The pectoralis major myocutaneous flap. A versatile flap for reconstruction in the head and neck. Plastic and Reconstructive Surgery 63: 73–81
Atabek U, Tabatabai M A M, Raina S, Rush J B F, Dasmahapatra K S 1987 Lung cancer in patients with head and neck cancer. Incidence and long term survival. American Journal of Surgery 154: 434–437
Barney P L 1970 Histopathological problems and frozen section diagnosis in diseases of the larynx. Otolaryngological Clinics of North America 3: 493–515
Barzan L, Veronesi A, Caruso G, Serraino D, Margi D, Zagonel V, Tirelli V et al 1990 Head and neck cancer and aging. A retrospective study in 438 patients. Journal of Laryngology and Otology 104: 634

Batsakis J G 1988 Surgical margins in squamous cell carcinomas. Annals of Otology, Rhinology and Laryngology 97: 213–214
Bauer W C 1974 The use of frozen section in otolaryngology. Transactions of American Academy of Ophthalmology and Otolaryngology 78: 88–97
Bauer W C, Lesinkski S G, Ogura J H 1975 The significance of positive margins in hemilaryngectomy specimens. The Laryngoscope 85: 1–13
Bishop J M 1987 The molecular genetics of cancer. Science 235: 305–311
Bocca E, Pignataro O 1967 A conservation technique in radical neck dissection. Annals of Otology, Rhinology and Laryngology 76: 975
Bocca E, Pignataro O, Oldin C, Cappa C 1984 Functional neck dissection: an evaluation and review of 843 cases. Laryngoscope 94: 942
Bosl G J, Strong E, Harrison L, Pfister D G 1991 Chemotherapy and

the management of locally advanced squamous cell carcinoma of the head and neck. Role in larynx preservation. In: Devita Jr V T, Hellman S, Rosenberg S A (eds) Important advances in oncology. J B Lippincott, Philadelphia, 191–203

Borges A M, Shrikhande S S, Ganesh B 1989 Surgical pathology of squamous cell carcinoma of the oral cavity. Its impact on management. Seminars in Surgical Oncology 5: 310–317

Boscia R, Johnson T T, Chen K, Whiteside T L 1988 Evaluation of therapeutic potential of interleukin-2 expanded tumour infiltrating lymphocytes in squamous cell carcinoma of the head and neck. Annals of Otology, Rhinology and Laryngology 97: 414–421

Branemark P, Lindström J, Hallen O, Breine V, Jeppson P H, Ohman A 1975 Reconstruction of the mandible. Scandinavian Journal of Plastic Surgery 9:116–128

Cachin Y, Sancho Garnier H, Micheau C, Marandas P 1979 Nodal metastases from carcinoma of the oropharynx. Otolaryngological Clinics of North America 12: 145–155

Candela F C, Kothari K, Shah J P 1990 Patterns of cervical node metastasis from squamous carcinoma of the oropharynx and hypopharynx. Head and Neck 12: 197–203

Carter R L 1990 Pathology of squamous cell carcinoma of the head and neck. Current Opinion in Oncology 2: 552–556

Cortesina G, De Stefani A, Giovarelli M, Barioglio M G, Careallo G P, Jemma C, Forni G 1988 Treatment of recurrent squamous cell carcinoma of the head and neck with low doses of interleukin-2 injected perilymphatically. Cancer 62: 2482–2485

De Vries N 1990 The magnitude of the problem. In: De Vries N, Gluckman J L (eds). Multiple primary tumours in the head and neck. Thieme Medical Publishers, New York, p 12–19

Dehner L P, Rosai J 1977 Frozen section examination in surgical pathology. Minnesota Medicin 60: 83–94

Dische S, Saunders M I 1989 Continuous hyperfractionated accelerated radiotherapy (CHART). British Journal of Cancer 59: 325–326

Eschwege F, Lartigau E 1990 Radiotherapy and combined chemoradiotherapy in head and neck carcinoma. Current Opinion in Oncology 2: 573–577

Fakih A R, Rao R S, Borges A M, Patel A R 1989 Elective versus therapeutic neck dissection in early carcinoma of the oral tongue. American Journal of Surgery 158: 309–313

Folkman J, Watson K, Ingber D, Hanahan D 1989 Induction of angiogenesis during the transition from hyperplasia to neoplasia. Nature 339: 58–61

Fuks Z, Leibel S A, Kutcher G J, Mohan R, Ling C C 1991 Three dimensional conformal treatment. A new frontier in radiation therapy. In: De Vita Jr V T, Hellman S, Rosenberg S A (eds) Important advances in oncology. J B Lippincott, Philadelphia, p 151–172

Goepfert H 1988 Subclinical cancer. Head and Neck surgery 9: 217–218

Goepfert H, Dichtel W J, Medina J E, Lindberg R D, Luna M D 1984 Perineural invasion in squamous cell carcinoma of the head and neck. American Journal of Surgery 148: 542–547

Green M R 1978 Chemotherapy of head and neck cancer. Head and Neck Surgery 1: 75–86

Grevers G, Assal J, Vogl T, Wilimzig C 1991 Three dimensional magnetic resonance imaging in skull base lesions. American Journal of Otolaryngology 12: 139–145

Gunn J M, Clark M G, Knowles S E et al 1977 Reduced rates of proteolysis in transformed cells. Nature 266: 58–60

Hanna E Y N, Papay F A, Gupta M D, Lavertu P, Tucker H M 1990 Serum tumour markers of head and neck cancer. Head and Neck 12: 50–59

Harwood A R, Lawson V G 1982 Radiation therapy for melanomas of the head and neck. Head and Neck Surgery 4: 468–474

Hidalgo D A 1989 Fibula free flap. A new method of mandibular reconstruction. Plastic and Reconstructive Surgery 84: 71–79

Holaday W J, Assor D 1974 Ten thousand consecutive frozen sections. American Journal of Clinical Pathology 61: 769–777

Hong W K 1988 Induction chemotherapy for advanced head and neck cancer. Head and Neck Surgery 8: 147–149

Hong W K et al 1990 Prevention of second primary tumours with isoretinoin in squamous cell carcinoma of the head and neck. The New England Journal of Medicine 323: 795–801

Jacobs J R, Kish J, Ensley J F, Ahmad K, Weaver K, Crissman J, Alsarraf M 1986 Combined modality therapy utilizing a cisplatin combination for effective chemotherapy in patients with previously untreated head and neck cancer. American Journal of Surgery 152: 451–455

Jesse R H, Ballantyne A J, Larson D 1978 Radical or modified neck dissection. A therapeutic dilemma. American Journal of Surgery 136: 516–519

Johnson J T, Myers E N, Srodes C H, Mayernik D G, Sigler B A, Schramm V L, Nolan T A et al 1985 Maintainance chemotherapy for high risk patients. Archives of Otolaryngology 111: 727–729

Kaplan M J, Hahn S S, Johns M E, Stewart M F, Constable W C, Cantrell E 1985 Mitomycin and flurouracil with concomitant radiotherapy in head and neck cancer. Archives of Otolaryngology 111: 220–222

Karim A B M F, Snow G B, Ruys P N, Bosch H 1980 The heterogenicity of the T2 glottic carcinoma and its local control possibility after radiation therapy. International Journal of Radiation Oncology, Biology and Physics 12: 1653–1657

Klein G, Klein E 1985 Evolution of tumours and the impact of molecular oncology. Nature 315: 190–195

Krespi Y P, Sisson G A 1982 Skull base surgery in composite resection. Archives of Otolaryngology 108: 681–684

Lawrence W Jr, Terz J J, Rogers C, King R E, Wolf J S, King E R 1974 Preoperative radiation for head and neck cancer. A prospective study. Cancer 33: 318

Leemans C R, Tiwari R M, Van der Waal I, Karim A B M F, Nauta J J P, Snow G B 1990 The efficacy of comprehensive neck dissection with or without postoperative radiotherapy in nodal metastases of squamous cell carcinoma of the upper respiratory and digestive tracts. The Laryngoscope 100: 1194–1198

Leemans C R, Tiwari R M, Nauta J J P, Snow G B 1991 Discontinuous versus in continuity neck dissection in carcinoma of the oral cavity. Archives of Otolaryngology Head and Neck Surgery 117: 1003–1006

Leitner S P, Bosl G J, Strong E W, Gerold F P, Spiro R H, Shah J P, Sessions R B et al 1986 A pilot study of cisplatin–vinblastin as the initial treatment of advanced head and neck cancer. Cancer 58: 1014–1017

Lippman S M, Kessler J F, Al–Sarraf M, Alberts D S, Itri L M, Mattox D, Van Hoff D D et al 1988 Treatment of advanced squamous cell carcinoma of the head and neck with isotretinoin. A phase II randomized trial. Investigating New Drugs 6: 51–56

Looser K G, Shah J P, Strong E W 1978. The significance of positive margins in surgically resected epidermoid carcinoma. Head and Neck Surgery 1: 107–111

Martin H, Del Valle B, Ehrlich H, Cahan W G 1951 Neck dissection. Cancer 4: 441–499

McCraw J B, Magee W P, Kalwaic H 1979 Uses of trapezius and sternomastoid myocutaneous flaps in head and neck reconstruction. Plastic and Reconstructive Surgery 63: 49–57

McKee P C R, Berry B F 1971 Pharyngooesophageal reconstruction with revascularised jejunum transplants. American Journal of Surgery 121: 675

Medina J E 1989 A rational classification of neck dissections. Archives of Otolaryngology Head and Neck Surgery 100: 100–169

Morgan R F, Hirata R M, Jaques D A, Hoopes J E 1982 Head and neck surgery in the aged. American Journal of Surgery 144: 449–451

Mukai K, Rosai J 1980 Applications of immunoperioxidase techniques in surgical pathology. In: Gengolio C M, Wolf M (eds) Progress in surgical pathology. Masson Publishing, New York.

Nathason A, Agren K 1989 Evaluation of some prognostic factors in small squamous cell carcinoma of the mobile tongue. A multicentric study in Sweden. Head and Neck 11: 387–392

Obwegeser H L 1985 Temporal approach to the TMJ, the orbit and the retromaxillary infracranial region. Head and Neck Surgery 7: 185–199

Pai V R, Parikh O M, Mazumdar A T 1991 Chemotherapy protocols for advanced oral cancer. In: Rao R S, Desai P B (eds) Oral Cancer. Professional Educational Division, Tata Memorial Hospital, Bombay, p 147

Panje W R, Pitcock J K 1989 Free omental flap reconstruction of complicated head and neck wounds. Archives of Otolaryngology Head and Neck Surgery 100: 88–93

Pearson B W, Woods R W, Hartman D 1980 Extended hemilaryngectomy for T3 glottic carcinoma with preservation of speech and swallowing. The Laryngoscope 90: 1950–1961

Robertson A G, McGregor I A, Soutar D S et al 1986 Postoperative radiotherapy in the management of advanced intraoral tumours. Clinical Radiology 37: 173

Robertson G A 1986 The role of sternum in osteomyocutaneous reconstruction of major mandibular defects. American Journal of Surgery 152: 367-370

Robbins K T, Medina J E, Wolfe G T, Lerine P A, Sessions R B, Pruet C W 1991 Standardizing neck dissection terminology. Archives of Otolaryngology, Head and Neck Surgery 117: 60

Saranath D, Panchal R G, Nai R et al 1989 Oncogene amplication in squamous cell carcinoma of the oral cavity. Japanese Journal of Cancer Research 80: 430–437

Saunders M I, Dische S 1986 Radiotherapy employing three fractions– each day over a continuous period of twelve days. British Journal of Radiology 59: 523

Schantz S P, Weber R S. Carey T E 1988 Growth and promotion of head and neck cancer. A report of the upper aerodigestive cancer task force workshop. Head and Neck Surgery 10: 179–186

Seagren S L, Syed A M N, Byfield J E 1979 Interstitial implant radiotherapy in upper aerodigestive tract malignancy. Head and Neck Surgery 1: 409–416

Seagren S L 1982 Recent advances in radiotherapy of head and neck cancer. Head and Neck Surgery 4: 227–232

Skolnik E M, Tenta L T, Wineinger D M, Tardy M E 1967 Preservation of XI cranial nerve in neck dissection. The Laryngoscope 77: 1304–1314

Skolnik E M, King F Y, Friedman F, Golden T A 1976 The posterior triangle in radical neck surgery. Archives of Otolaryngology 102: 2–4

Snow G B, Balm A J M, Arendse J W, Karim A B M F, Bartelinks H, Van der Waal I, Tiwari R M 1986 Prognostic factors in neck node metastasis. In: Larson D L, Ballantyne A J, Guillamondgui O M (eds) Cancer in the neck – evaluation and treatment. Macmillan, New York, p 53–63

Snow G B, Vermorken J B 1989 Neoadjuvant chemotherapy in head and neck cancer. State of art. Clinical Otolaryngology 14: 371–375

Soutar D S, Scheker L R, Tanner N S B, McGregor I A 1983 The radial forearm flap. A versatile method for intraoral reconstruction. British Journal of Plastic Surgery 36: 1

Spiro J D, Spiro R H, Shah J P, Sessions R, Strong E 1988 Critical assessment of supraomohyoid neck dissection. American Journal of Surgery 156: 288

Spiro R H, Huvos A G,Wong G Y, Spiro J D, Gineco C A, Strong E A 1986 Predictive value of tumour thickness in squamous cell carcinoma confined to the tongue and floor of the mouth. American Journal of Surgery 152: 345–350

Stell P M 1990 Adjuvant chemotherapy in head and neck cancer. Clinical Otolaryngology 15: 193–195

Synderman N L, Wetmore S J, Suen J Y, 1986 Cisplatin sensitization to radiotherapy in stage IV squamous cell carcinoma of the head and neck. Archives of Otolaryngology Head and Neck Surgery 112: 1147–1149

Tabatabai M A M, Sobel H J, Rush B F, Mashberg A 1986 Relation of thickness of floor of mouth stage I and II cancers to regional metastasis. American Journal of Surgery 152: 351-353

Taylor G I 1982 Reconstruction of the mandible with free composite iliac bone grafts. Annals of Plastic Surgery 9: 361

Terzis J K 1987 Vascularised nerve grafts. An experimental and clinical review. Annals of Plastic Surgery 18: 137–146

Tiwari R M, Karim A B M F, Snow G B 1993 Total glossectomy with laryngeal preservation. Archives of Otolaryngology Head and Neck Surgery In press

Trible W M Dias A 1964 Cervical node metastases. Prognosis related to level and distribution. Archives of Otolaryngology 79: 247–249

Van de Brekel M W M, Castelijns J A, Stel H V, Luth W J, Valk J, Van der Waal I, Snow G B 1991 Occult metastatic neck disease. Detection with US and US guided fine needle aspiration cytology. Radiology 180: 457–461

Van den Brouck C, Sancho H, Le Fur R, Richard J M, Cachin Y 1977 Results of randomized clinical trial of preoperative irradiation versus postoperative in treatment of tumour of the hypopharynx. Cancer 39: 1445–1449

Vikram B, Strong E W, Shah J P, Spiro R H 1980 Elective postopera- tive radiotherapy in stages III and IV epidermoid carcinoma of the head and neck. American Journal of Surgery 140: 580–584

Vikram B, Strong E W, Shah J P, Spiro R 1984 Second malignant neoplasms in patients successfully treated with multimodality treatment for advanced head and neck cancer. Head and Neck Surgery 6: 734–737

Vikram B, Strong E W, Shah J P et al 1985 Intraoperative radiotherapy in patients with recurrent head and neck cancer. American Journal of Surgery 150: 485–487

Wanebo H J, Koness J, MacFarlane J K, Eilber F R, Byers R M, Elias E G, Spiro R H 1992 Head and neck sarcoma. Report of the head and neck sarcoma registry. Head and Neck 14: 1–7

Weinhouse S 1980 New dimensions in the biology of cancer. Cancer 45: 2975–2980

Wilson G D, McNally N T, Dische S et al 1988 Cell proliferation in human tumours measured by in-vivo labelling with bromodeoxy- uridine. British Journal of Radiology 61: 419

Wolf G T, Fischer S R, Hong W K et al 1991 Induction chemotherapy plus radiation compared with surgery plus radiation in patients with advanced laryngeal cancer. New England Journal of Medicine 324: 1685–1691

Ziekse L A, Johnson J T, Myers E N, Thearle P B 1986 Squamous cell carcinoma with positive margins. Archives of Otolaryngology Head and Neck Surgery 112: 863–866

2. The lip

Mirek F. Stranc

INTRODUCTION AND HISTORICAL REVIEW

The lips form a circular, fleshy, mobile and sensate curtain which separates the external environment from the intraoral milieu. Though the anatomy and external landmarks of the lips are well known their functions are not often fully appreciated: when intact, the lips are responsible for oral continence and so participate in the creation and maintenance of the intraoral environment. They also serve to assist with eating, facilitate oral access and are essential to interpersonal communication (Fogel & Stranc 1984). Thus conservation of lip function as well as aesthetic considerations must be of major concern when planning lip resection.

Over the years, various methods of reconstruction of extensive full-thickness lip defects have been described. An early champion of lower lip repair, Dieffenbach, outlined his technique in 1834. In this method, the new lip was formed through full thickness medial advancement of cheek tissues either unilaterally or bilaterally, depending on the size of the defect. Advancement of the flap was made possible by a full thickness horizontal cheek incision, which extended laterally from the oral commissure. This technique was later modified by Burow (1855), Szymanowski (1858) and May (1946). A similar approach was developed by Bernard in 1852: he proposed advancing the cheek tissues medially, after excising the triangles of redundant tissue above and below the zone of tissue transfer.

In 1859, von Bruns pioneered the use of full–thickness nasolabial flaps to create a new lower lip. However, this method quickly fell into disrepute as it led to extensive denervation of the muscles of the upper lip. Estlander (1872) and Abbe (1898) popularised the use of residual tissues following resection to reconstruct the lip through 'lip sharing'. The Gillies fan flap represented a further extension of this technique (Gillies & Millard 1957). In 1974, Karapandzic subsequently refined the concept of lip sharing and produced an excellent one-stage method of functional lip reconstruction for defects of not more than one half of the lip. Also in 1974, Johanson and his co-workers described a step technique for lower lip reconstruction. In this method, the conservation of function through anatomical muscle realignment was emphasised.

All of the procedures described above could only be used with defects of up to one half of the lip curtain: their use in larger defects resulted in severe microstomia. The steeple flap (Stranc & Robertson 1983) provided the most satisfactory method of repair that utilised local tissues for lower lip defects affecting in excess of one half of the lip curtain. However, although this method avoided postoperative microstomia. it still resulted in severely impaired lip function.

Surgeons had always been reluctant to use distant tissues: both forehead and neck tissue transfers had been described, as well as even more distant transfers using tubed-pedicle flaps. The multi-stage nature of the process, significant morbidity and poor functional outcome made these procedures unattractive. Recently, the advent of microsurgery has prompted renewed interest in the use of distant tissues. Recent work from Germany (Reidiger et al 1989) emphasises the need to achieve maximal sensory rehabilitation of the lips. Microsurgical techniques have both reduced the number of operative stages and increased the reliability of tissue transfer. One of the major concerns with this method of repair has been the compromised sensation of the reconstructed lip. Using a radial artery flap to repair the defect, and following antebrachial–mental nerve anastomosis, the sensation though imperfect, appeared adequate to prevent drooling. However, the lips themselves functioned as mechanical barriers stemming the flow of saliva, with the lack of orbicularis muscle in the reconstructed lip compensated for, in part, by a palmaris sling (Freedman & Hidalgo 1990, Sadove et al 1991).

SURGICAL ANATOMY

The lips surround the orifice of the mouth. They are formed externally by skin, internally by mucous membrane and extend from the nose above to the chin below with the nasolabial lines marking their lateral limit. A study of lip structure reveals the following layers from without to within: skin and vermilion, subcutaneous fat, muscle, submucous

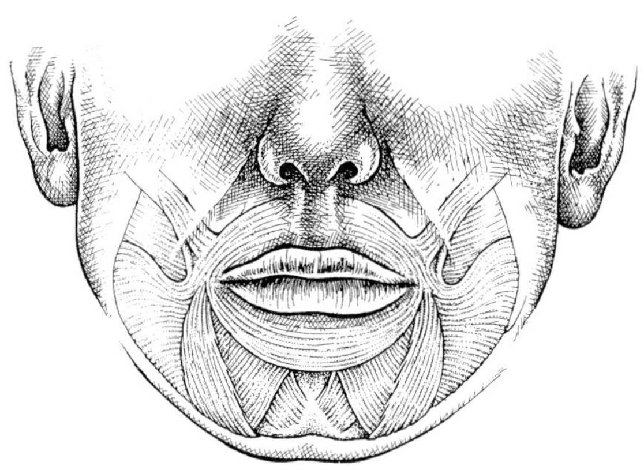

Fig. 2.1   Arrangement of extrinsic and intrinsic lip muscles.

glands and mucosa. Figure 2.1 shows the arrangement of the intrinsic and extrinsic lip muscles. The vermilion is bounded by the vermilion–skin junction and the wet–dry line, which occurs at the zone of contact of the two lips. Fat and submucous glands are absent under the vermilion.

The main neurovascular structures are found in the submucous plane. This is of importance, as it is the sensation of the inner (and not the outer) lip layer which determines the adequacy of the lip seal.

Lymphatic drainage of the lips is directed to the submental and submadibular nodes in the first instance: the central portion of the lower lip drains into the submental nodes, whereas the lateral portions of the lower lip and the whole of the upper lip drain into the submandibular group.

In order to provide an unbiased assessment of function following reconstruction, a knowledge of normal lip parameters is crucial. These can be broadly grouped into the following criteria: intercommissural distance, soft tissue gape, sulcus depth, lip sensitivity and lip strength (Stranc & Fogel 1984).

NORMAL LIP PARAMETERS

A. INTERCOMMISSURAL DISTANCE

This value is determined by measuring the distance between the commissures whilst the subject is swallowing using a nylon tape measure draped over and following the natural curvature of the lips. (The act of swallowing prevents the jaw from being subconsciously postured). In healthy individuals, values for this parameter increase with increasing age until full growth is achieved. The intercommissural distance then remains constant until the seventh decade of life following which it gradually decreases (Fig. 2.2A).

B. SOFT TISSUE GAPE

Unlike the skeletal gape measurement which is determined

by the straight line distance between the upper and lower incisors, soft tissue gape is defined as the straight line distance between the wet–dry line in the centre of the upper lip and the wet–dry line of the centre of the lower lip whilst the mouth is open as widely as possible. In healthy individuals, values for this parameter increase with increasing age until maturity is attained. From that point it gradually declines (Fig. 2.2B).

C. SULCUS DEPTH

This should be determined for both upper and lower lips as it reflects the height of the lip curtain. It is measured by draping a tape measure over the lip at a point adjacent to the frenulum and recording the distance between the bottom of the labio–gingival sulcus and the wet–dry line of the vermilion.

D. LIP SENSITIVITY

Sensation is assessed using the two–point discrimination test in all four lip quadrants. In healthy individuals, values for this parameter increase as age increases and as sensitivity decreases (Fig. 2.2C).

E. SPHINCTERIC POWER

The maximum strength of the orbicularis oris is measured using the pommeter (peri-oral-muscularmeter). With the mouth and pommeter held in the horizontal plane, and after the teeth or dentures are placed in normal occlusion, the subject is asked to grip the mouthpiece with the lips alone and to exert as much sphincteric power as possible. The pommeter is then gradually withdrawn against the resistance of the contracting lips and the lip strength is registered on the dial. In healthy individuals, values for this parameter dramatically increase after the pubertal growth spurt and start to decline following the fifth decade (Fig. 2.2D).

Intercommissural distance, both at rest and during maximal lateral retraction (whilst grinning), as well as soft tissue gape are useful predictors for the ultimate motor function for the reconstructed lip: a soft tissue gape of less than 2.5 cm or significant reduction of the intercommissural distance will not permit adequate oral hygiene or normal eating habits. Conservation of normal, or near normal, lip sensation and orbicularis strength also play major roles in the provision of a satisfactory lip seal (Stranc & Fogel 1984, Stranc et al 1987). Other factors, such as the height of the reconstructed lip, are of lesser importance except in those individuals where the lack of lip height is so severe that mouth closure is impossible.

PATHOLOGY

By far the commonest tumour involving the lips is squamous

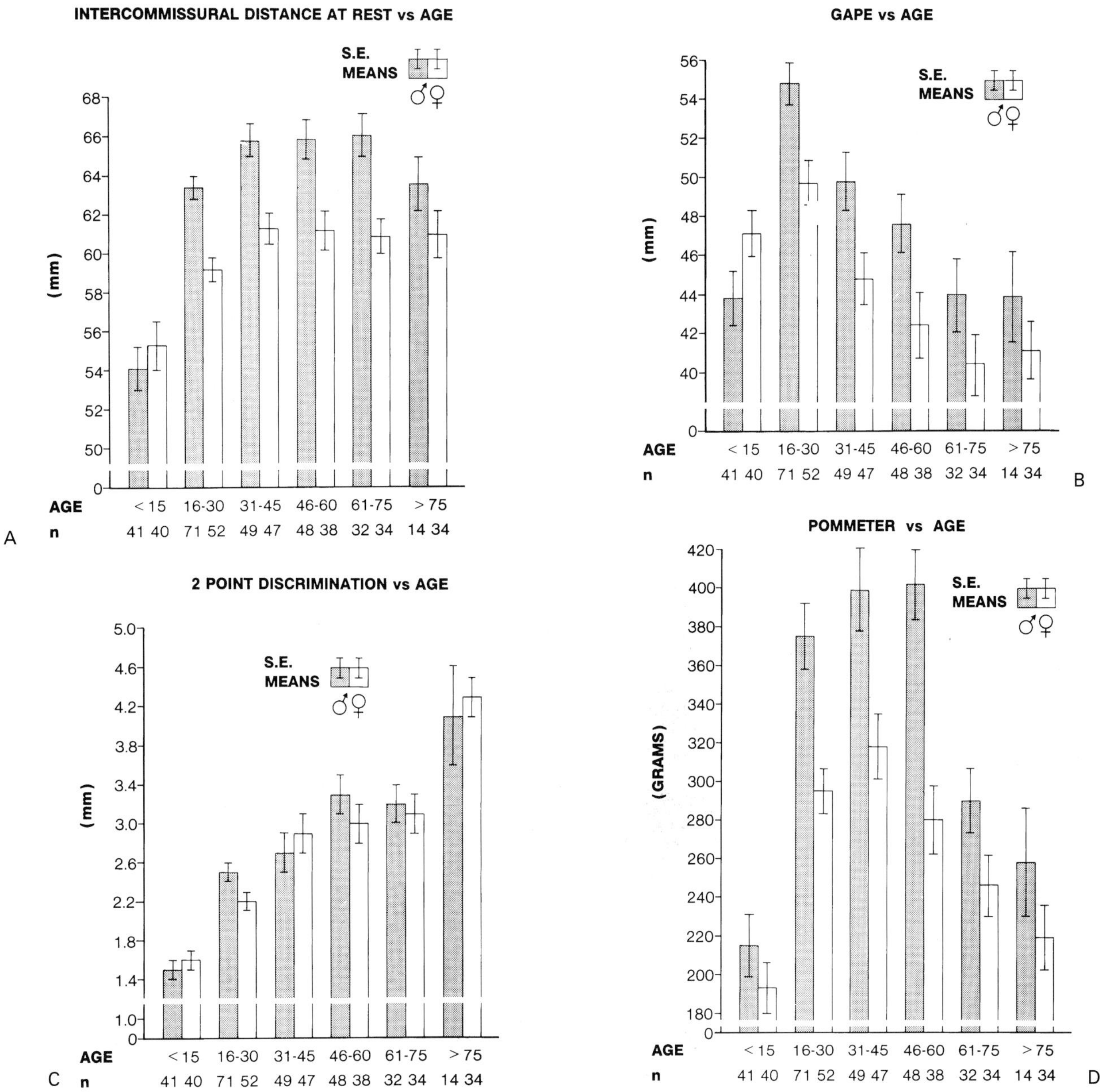

Fig. 2.2 **A** Normal values for intercommissural distance. **B** Normal values for soft tissue gaps. **C** Normal values for lip sensitivity – two-point discrimination. **D** Normal pommeter values for orbicularis oris.

cell carcinoma, though basal cell cancer of the skin of the lip is not rare. Other malignant tumours such as melanoma, malignant mixed salivary tumour and sarcoma are very uncommon and will not be considered further. Squamous cell carcinoma is a multifactorial entity; its development and natural history are controlled by both environmental and host factors (Kwa et al 1992). Among host factors the patient's age, skin pigmentation, immune status and the presence of certain genetic disorders (such as xeroderma pigmentosum) should be considered. The most important environmental factor is long-term sun exposure (specifically to UVB radiation 290–320 nm) which induces actinic damage to the skin. Other agents such as chemical carcinogens, X–ray radiation and chronic irritants are less important. Suppression of the immune response, as is found in transplant patients, may significantly increase the incidence of cutaneous squamous cell carcinoma; rates as high as 42% have been reported (Penn 1980).

The metastatic potential of squamous cell carcinoma depends on many factors: in squamous cell carcinoma of the lip, the average time from diagnosis to metastasis is 1 year (Frierson & Cooper 1986). Reports on the frequency of metastasis vary from 3–29% (Kwa et al 1992). Lesions arising from the mucosa appear to be more aggressive.

The size of the tumour has a definite impact on its metastatic potential: the average diameter for metastasising squamous cell carcinoma of the lip is 3.7 cm compared with 2 cm or less for non-metastasising lesions. Lesions under 1 cm in diameter have a metastatic rate of 3% (Kwa et al 1992). Tumour thickness too is of prognostic significance: lesions 2–6 mm in thickness showed a 4.5% rate of metastasis. Lesions 6 mm or more had a 15% incidence of distant spread. Histological grading indicates that the more differentiated the tumour the less likely it is to spread (Broder 1921). Presence of perineural spread is associated with at least 50% metastatic disease.

PRINCIPLES OF RESECTION

It is clear therefore that in planning the margin of resection the above factors must be borne in mind. Low-grade tumours can be resected with as little as a 5 mm margin beyond visible or palpable tumour, whereas high-grade lesions will require a 10 mm margin at least. In these patients, combination of radiotherapy and surgery should be considered.

The shape of the excisional defect is not a vital issue *provided that the planned margins of resection are maintained*. A triangular defect lends itself more readily to direct closure; W–shaped defects are created in an effort to widen the lateral margins without lengthening the vertical scar and crossing the labiomental line; and rectangular excisions are commonly used as an integral part of many reconstructive procedures, Karapandzic step technique or Freeman's advancement flap.

PRINCIPLES OF RECONSTRUCTION

The principles of lip reconstruction were clearly stated by Sir Harold Gillies in 1920:

'The restoration is designed from within outwards. The lining membrane must be considered first, then the supporting structures, and finally the skin covering.'

To date, these edicts remain unchanged. Our current understanding of the aesthetic units of the lip, the importance of a functioning oral sphincter and, above all, the presence of adequate sensation in the reconstructed lip, has significantly improved our ability to recognise the problems that must be addressed. The use of identical or similar tissues for reconstruction becomes the obvious avenue to follow: *repair like with like*. The importance of correct muscle orientation has been emphasised by Johanson et al (1974) as well as by Karapandzic (1974).

RECONSTRUCTION OF THE VERMILION

Vermilionectomy, the advancement of labial mucosa outwards to replace sun-damaged vermilion, is a common procedure (Emmett 1980). Following this operation, lip function is sometimes significantly disturbed, with complaints of dribbling and paraesthesia being the most frequent. The common factor in all patients is an impairment of sensation in the new vermilion with two-point discrimination values often ranging from 6 to 12 mm (normal values range from 3 to 8 mm, Fogel & Stranc 1984).

To minimise this loss of sensation, it is necessary to elevate the mucosal flap carefully in a plane between submucosa and orbicularis oris with maximal freeing in the midline, gradually reducing the degree of dissection as the flap is mobilised laterally. In instances of unstable vermilion without overt malignant changes, vermilionectomy and direct suture of mucosa to the skin without undermining reduce the likelihood of troublesome sensory disturbances. However, lips thus treated are often narrow (Taylor 1989).

RECONSTRUCTION OF FULL-THICKNESS LOWER LIP DEFECTS

Methods of repair of full–thickness defects fall into three categories based on the amount of the lip that is to be excised:
I.   Defects of up to one-third of the lip
II.   Defects of one-third to one-half of the lip
III. Defects of greater than one-half of the lip

I. Defects of up to one-third of the lip

Up to one-third of the lip can be removed by a simple wedge excision without significant functional or cosmetic defect. This is particularly so in elderly patients, due to the increasing laxity of the tissues. Layered closure is essential to restore the continuity of the orbicularis oris.

II. Defects of one-third to one-half of the lip

Reconstruction of one-third to one-half of the lip can be

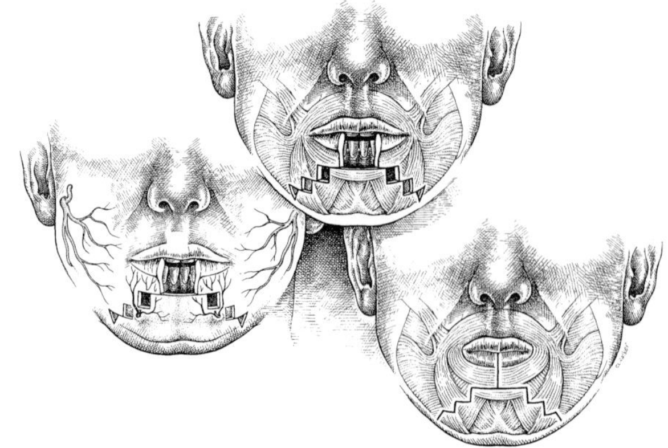

Fig. 2.3   Johanson's lip reconstruction. Note the excellent muscle realignment and preservation of both motor and sensory nerve supply.

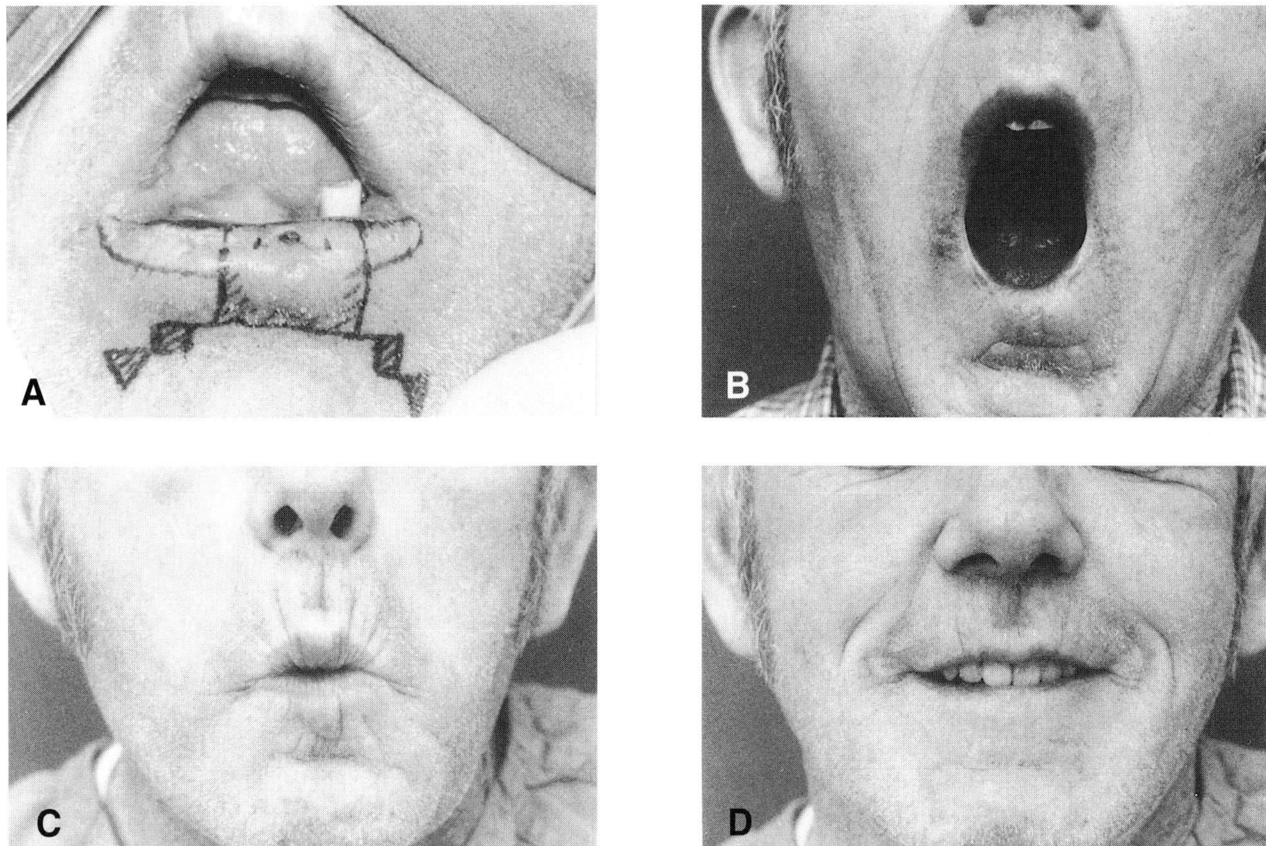

Fig. 2.4 **A** Plan of lip resection and vermilionectomy. **B–D** Function 3 years after surgery. **B** mouth fully open. **C** full contraction of the orbicularis. **D** lips during smile.

achieved using residual lip tissues (lip sharing techniques). Results are satisfactory both aesthetically and functionally.

(a) Johanson's step technique

This method of reconstruction (Fig. 2.3) is applicable to lower lip defects only. The lesion is removed as a rectangle and the repair is carried out with lateral full-thickness advancement flaps from the remaining lower lip (Johanson et al 1974). The migration is facilitated by stepwise excision of skin and subcutaneous tissue. Excision is approximately half the width of the defect until a point is reached where the

tissues will permit advancement without tension.

Larger central defects up to half the lip will require bilateral advancements with full-thickness lip excision of the first rectangle only. Careful layered closure with reconstruction of the orbicularis is essential. The reconstructed lip should be firmly perched on top of the chin. The final scars should generally follow the labiomental line.

This method may be combined with vermilion excision (Fig. 2.4). Results are very gratifying when the defect does not exceed half the lip; following larger resections a degree of microstomia is inevitable. Functional results are good. Studies of lip function 3 years after surgery are shown in

Table 2.1 Lip function 3 years after Johanson's reconstruction

Parameter	Measurement	Mean ± S. D.		
Lower lip height (mm)	25	25	±	5
Intercommissural distance at rest (mm)	65	65	±	5
Soft tissue gape (mm)	53	50	±	11
Elasticity index	48	55	±	12
Oral aperture (cm)	28	32	±	5
Two-point discrimination of the reconstructed lip (mm)★	6	2.5	±	1
Pommeter (g)	450	399	±	152
Disability: none				

★ The two-point discrimination of 6 mm in this patient is the result of vermilionectomy. The usual figure following Johanson's step technique of reconstruction is that expected for the patient's age, which is 2–3 mm.

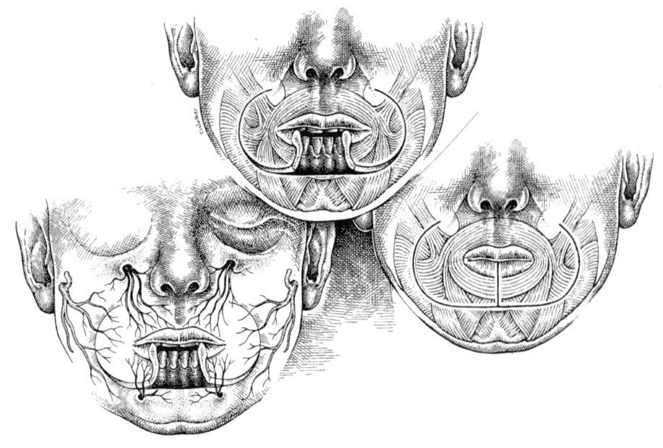

Fig. 2.5 Karapandzic manoeuvre. Note the preservation of the nerve supply to the lip flaps and muscle alignment.

Table 2.1. Simultaneous cervical lymphadenectomy can also be safely carried out.

(b) The Karapandzic lip reconstruction

This manoeuvre (Fig. 2.5) can be used on either the upper or lower lips. It depends on the creation of paired lip flaps based on the branches of the facial artery. The skin incisions parallel the lip margin at a distance equal to the depth of the defect. Careful preoperative marking of the incision, especially in the region of the commissure, will result in the preservation of the original lip height. A careless incision may produce either too high, or too low a lip, an unsightly and unnecessary deformity.

Although the superficial muscles of facial expression are divided, the sensory and motor nerves which run in close proximity to the main arteries are spared. Careful surgery and use of magnification will help to preserve many of these important structures. The mucosal incision parallels that of the skin, but is very much more conservative: rarely more than 2 cm.

All wounds are closed in layers from within outwards, allowing reconstruction of the oral sphincter and reattachment of the extrinsic lip muscles (Fig. 2.6). Best results are achieved in median defects that do not exceed 4 cm.

Larger defects reconstructed by this method will result in microstomia requiring commissurotomy. Functional results are good (Fig. 2.7). Studies of lip function 5 years after surgery are illustrated in Table 2.2. Simultaneous cervical lymphadenectomy is safe.

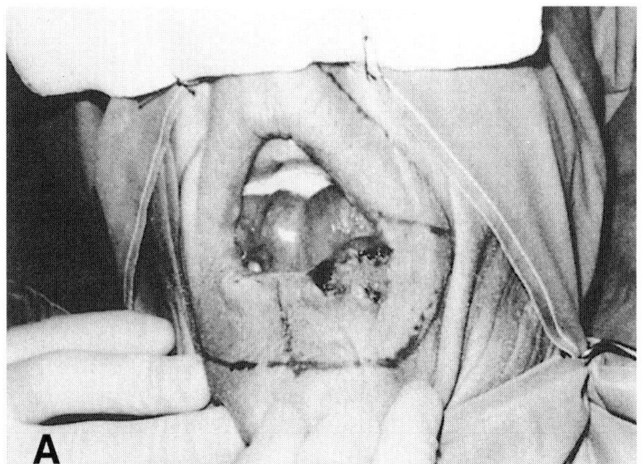
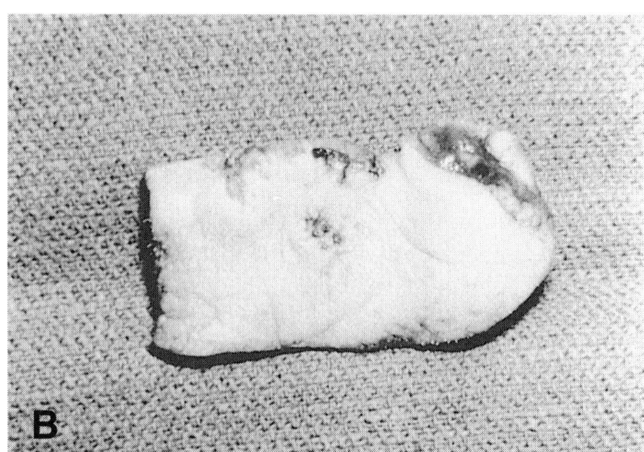
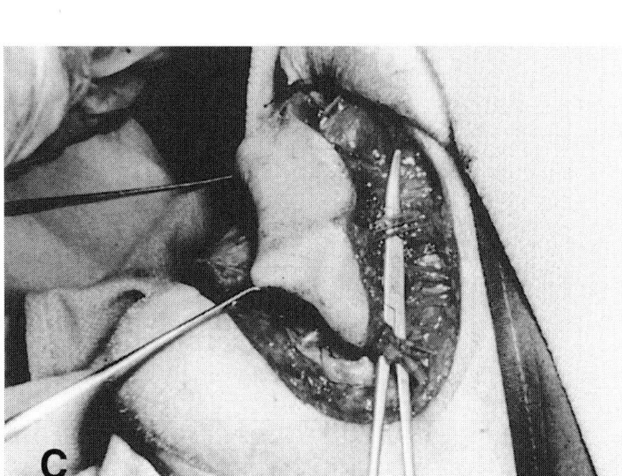
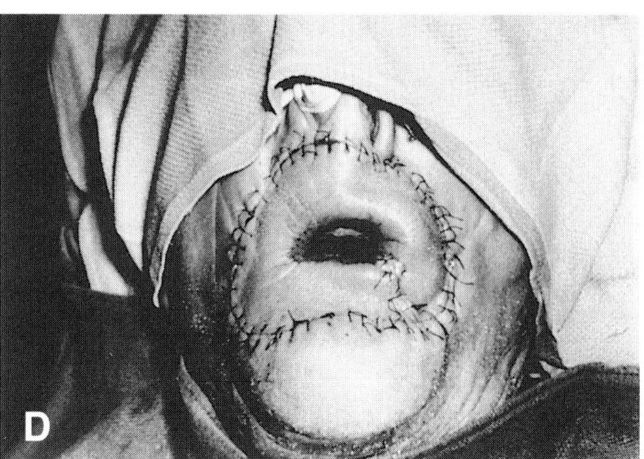

Fig. 2.6 **A** Carcinoma of the lower lip close to the left oral commissure. **B** Resected specimen. **C** Mobilised left upper lip. Note the preservation of the neurovascular pedicles. **D** Wound closure.

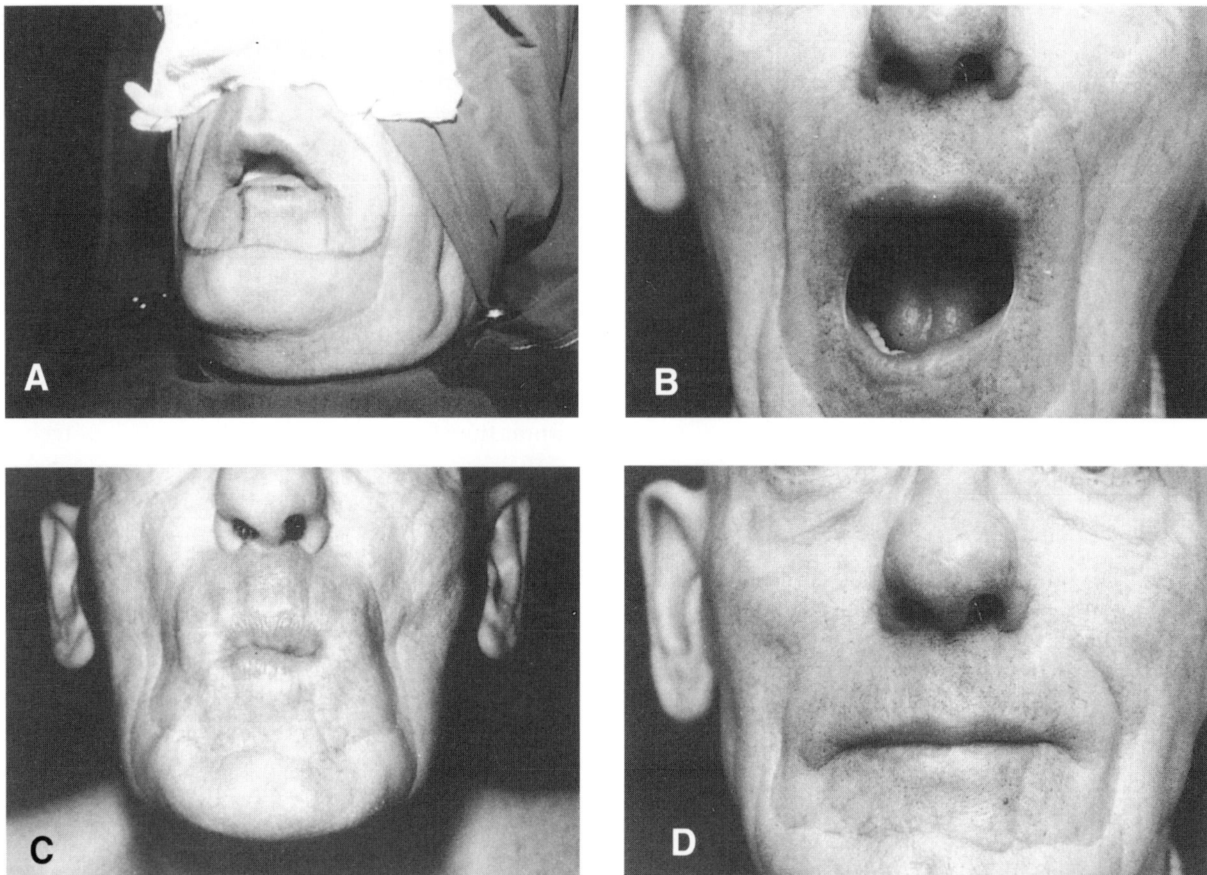

Fig. 2.7 Lip function in a 60-year-old man 5 years after resection of the left half of the lower lip. **A** Plan of surgery. **B** Full mouth opening. Note the slight weakness of the left depressor. **C** Full lip contraction. **D** Smile.

(c) Abbe and Estlander flaps

The transfer of tissues from the intact lip to the other via a narrow pedicle containing the labial artery can be used for defects of either upper or lower lip (Fig. 2.8). The flap is usually half the width of the defect. The Estlander switch is used in defects immediately adjacent to the commissure and the transfer is completed in one stage.

Once the outline of the excision is made, the Abbe flap (which should measure one-half of the width of the defect) is marked on the opposite lip (Fig. 2.9). The flap must be sited to one or other side of the defect, so that the pedicle can be kept close to the centre of the defect.

To raise the flap, a full-thickness vertical incision is made on the side opposite the pedicle. Note the location of the labial artery, as this will help later in preparing the pedicle. The full-thickness incision and definition of the flap should continue until the vermilion in the region of the proposed pedicle is reached.

Careful dissection, without necessarily exposing the labial vessels, facilitates the division of the pedicle, allows immediate matching of the vermilion–skin junction, both at

Table 2.2 Lip function 5 years after Karapandzic manoeuvre in a 65-year-old man

Parameter	Measurement	Mean ± S. D.
Lower lip height (mm)	24	23 ± 5
Intercommissural distance at rest (mm)	65	66 ± 6
Soft tissue gape (mm)	38	44 ± 11
Elasticity index	44	45 ± 12
Oral aperture (cm)	25	27 ± 7.6
Two-point discrimination of the reconstructed lip (mm)	4	3 ± 1
Pommeter (g)	250	290 ± 95
Disability: none		

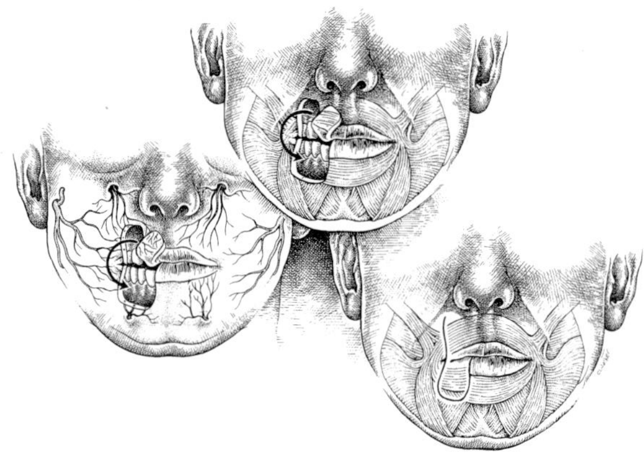

Fig. 2.8   Abbe flap. Note the reasonable muscle realignment.

donor and recipient sites, and adds greatly to the aesthetic quality of the reconstruction.

This form of reconstruction can be used in defects of up to half the lip; using it with larger defects will lead to microstomia. This procedure can be safely undertaken in concert with neck dissection, though this is not a usual practice. Functional results are satisfactory (Fig. 2.10). Studies of lip function 1 year after surgery are shown in Table 2.3.

III. Defects of greater than one-half of the lip

In the majority of patients, there is not enough local tissue to allow satisfactory reconstruction. Adjacent or distant transfers must be used. Regardless of technique, at

Table 2.3   Lower lip function 3 years after Abbe flap

Parameter	Measurement	Mean ± S. D.
Lower lip height (mm)	21	23 ± 5
Intercommissural distance at rest (mm)	60	66 ± 6
Soft tissue gape (mm)	38	44 ± 11
Elasticity index	28	45 ± 12
Oral aperture (cm)	20	27 ± 7.6
Two-point discrimination of the reconstructed lip (mm)	>10	3 ± 1
Pommeter (g)	150	290 ± 95
Disability: occasional drooling		

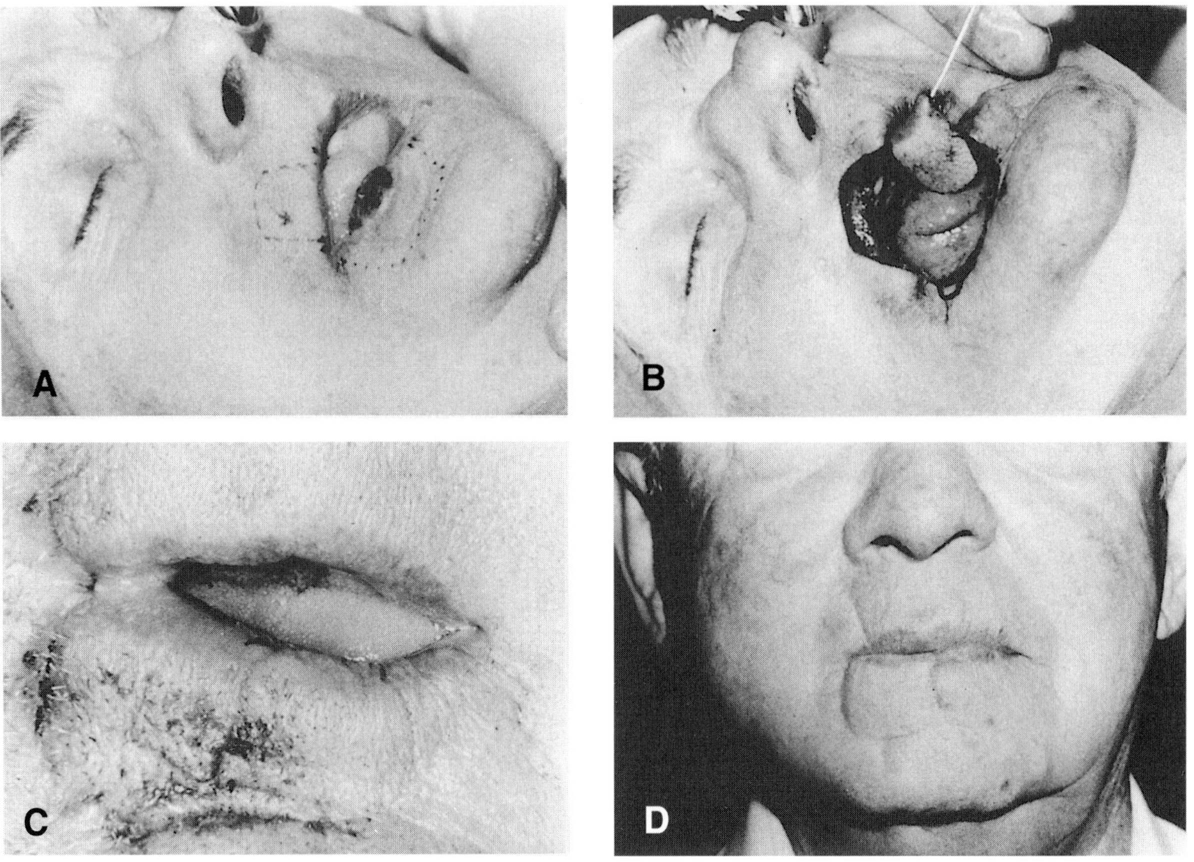

Fig. 2.9   **A** Carcinoma of the lower lip in a 63-year-old-man. **B** The right half of the lip is resected. Note that the Abbe flap is raised well into the vermilion. **C** Appearance of lip just prior to the division of the narrow pedicle. **D** Appearance of lips at rest.

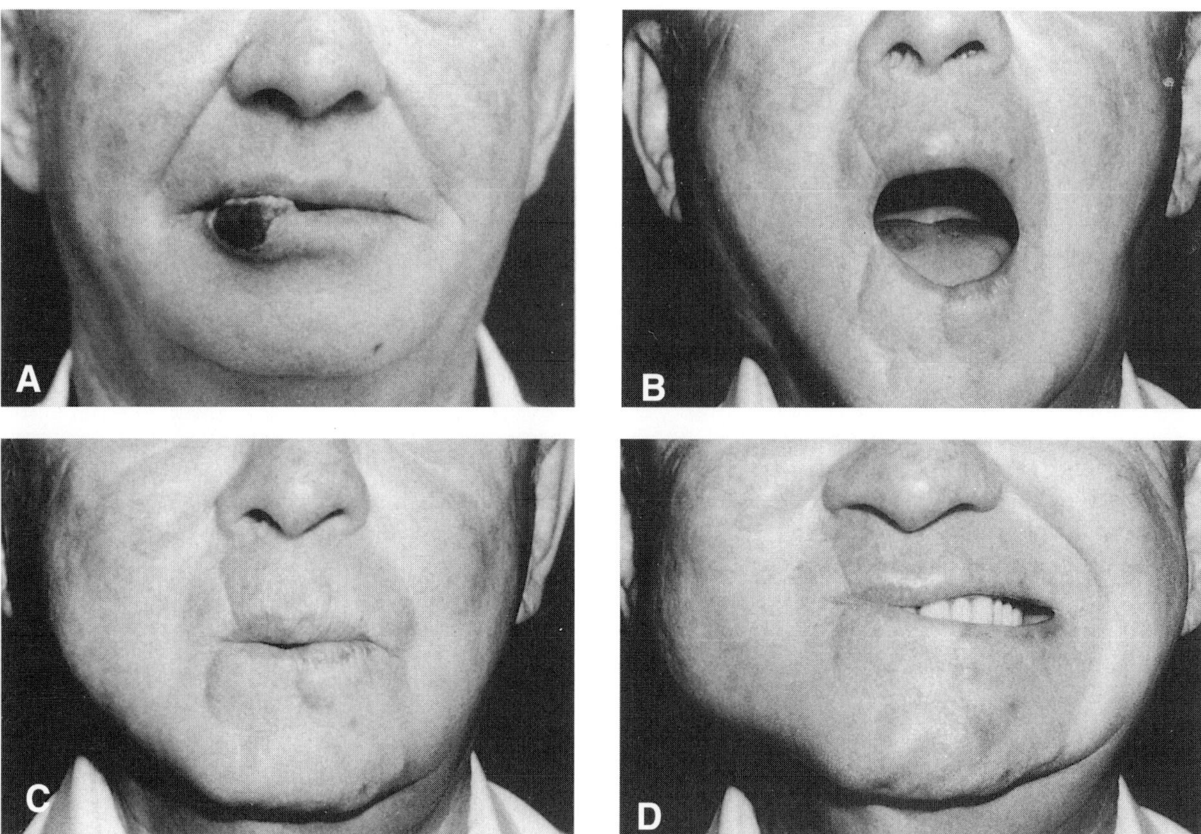

Fig. 2.10 A Preoperative lip at rest. **B** Appearance 3 years after surgery, with full mouth opening. **C** Lips at full contraction. **D** Lips in maximal retraction. Note the incomplete reinnervation of the flap.

our present stage of knowledge, all results are less than optimal.

(a) Reconstruction using cheek tissues

(i) Freeman's modification of Bernard's lip reconstruction. Unlike Bernard's incision which runs horizontally from the commissure and the lower margin of the defect, Freeman's modification (Freeman 1958) allows the direction of the upper incision to remain unchanged,

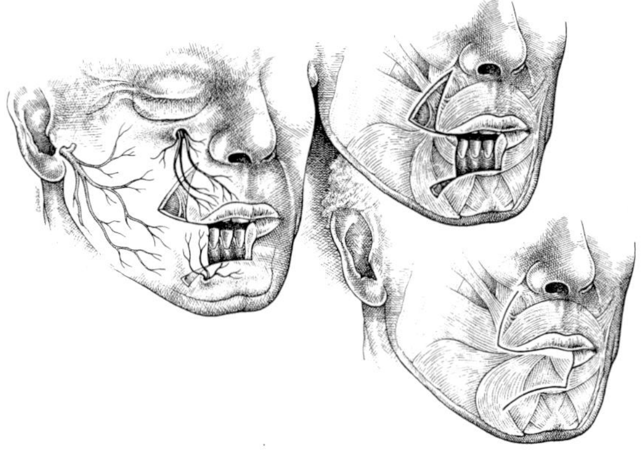

Fig. 2.11 Freeman's cheiloplasty. Note that this method fails to restore the continuity of the orbicularis oris.

while the lower incision follows the mentolabial line (Fig. 2.11). Also, the tissues sacrificed only include skin and fat, instead of the through and through excisions of cheek tissues advocated by Bernard (Fig. 2.12). Extensive undermining of mucosa and skin in the region of the commissure allows identification, isolation and reconstruction of the musculature. The vermilion is reconstructed from the mobilized cheek mucosa.

If the orbicularis ring cannot be reformed, medial translocation of these fibres produces a bizarre appearance during contracture of the sphincter as is seen when this procedure is used for defect exceeding one-half of the lip (Fig. 2.13).

This method, when used bilaterally, is capable of effecting total lower lip reconstruction. When neck dissection is necessary, it is preferable to allow a delay of 2 to 3 weeks before attempting the same. Results of studies of lip function in the patient shown in Figure 2.13 are given in Table 2.4.

(ii) Steeple flap reconstruction of the lip. After marking the extent of the excision, the defect is converted into a rectangle with the short side indicating the height of the resected lip, the long border marking the length of the excised lip (Fig. 2.14). The island flap is marked out by extending the lower line of the excised lip. Vertical sides of the island, equal to the length of the resected lip, are marked.

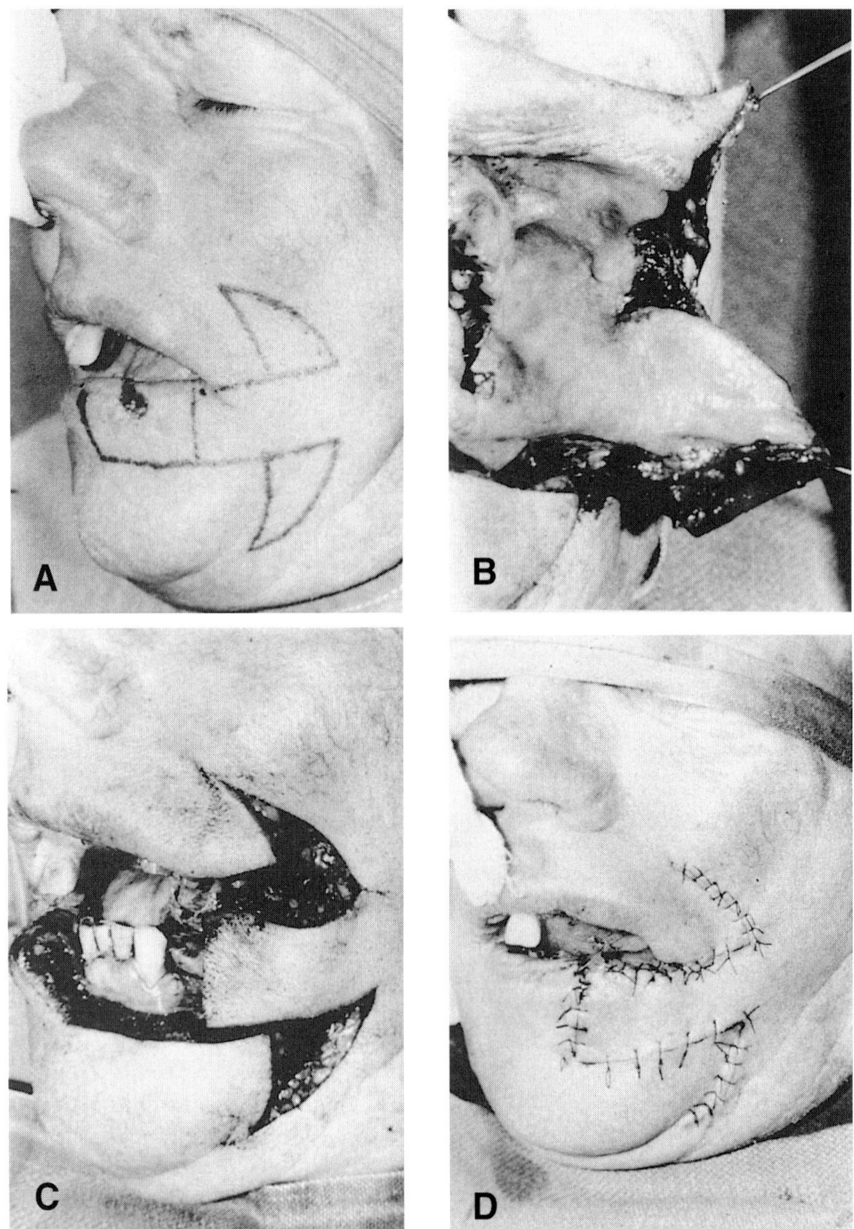

Fig. 2.12 **A** 69-year-old man with carcinoma of the lower lip. **B** The mucosal incision allows for restoration of the vermilion, sparing Stensen's duct. **C** The resected left half of the lower lip. **D** The wound closed.

Table 2.4   Lip function 1 year after surgery in a 69-year-old man presenting with an aggressive squamous cell carcinoma of the lower lip

Parameter	Measurement	Mean ± S. D.
Lower lip height (mm)	30	23 ± 5
Intercommissural distance at rest (mm)	70	66 ± 6
Soft tissue gape (mm)	65	44 ± 11
Elasticity index	23	45 ± 12
Oral aperture (cm)	40	27 ± 7.6
Two-point discrimination of the reconstructed lip (mm)	5	3 ± 1
Pommeter (g)	230	290 ± 95
Disability: occasional drooling		

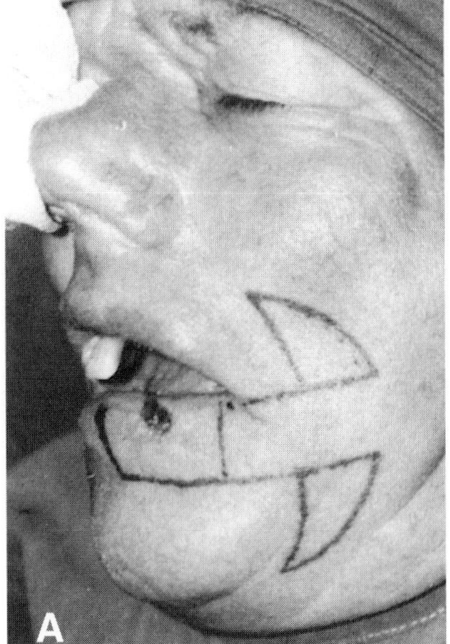

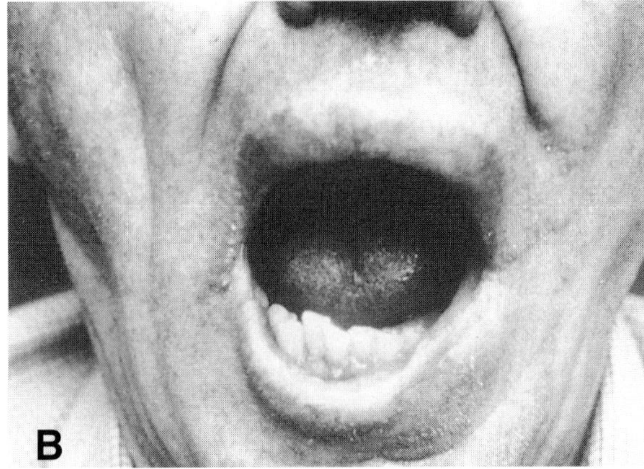

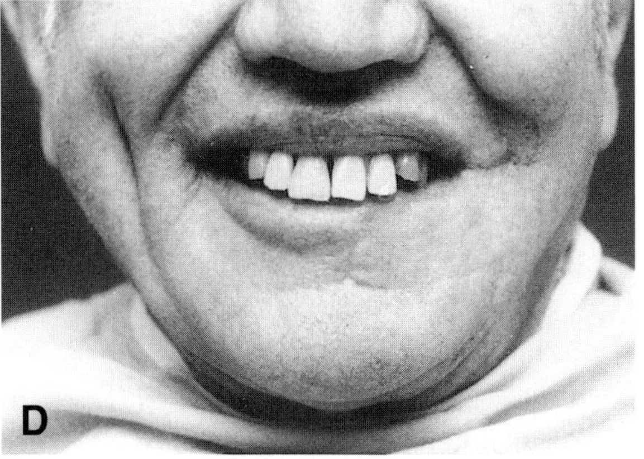

Fig. 2.13 **A** Plan of a surgery. **B** Appearance 1 year after surgery, mouth fully open. **C** Lips in full contraction. Note the bizarre appearance caused by malalignment of the muscle fibres. **D** Lips in lateral retraction.

A skin triangle is marked at the top to allow straight line wound closure. The facial artery and its labial branches are located and marked. A Doppler probe is of considerable help at this stage (Fig. 2.14).

Once the lesion has been excised, the skin and subcuta-

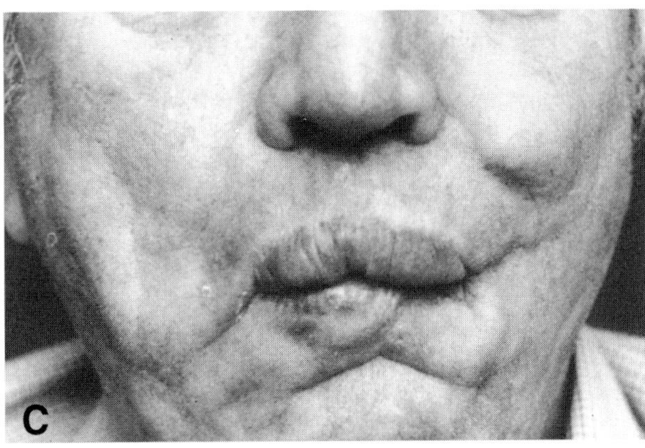

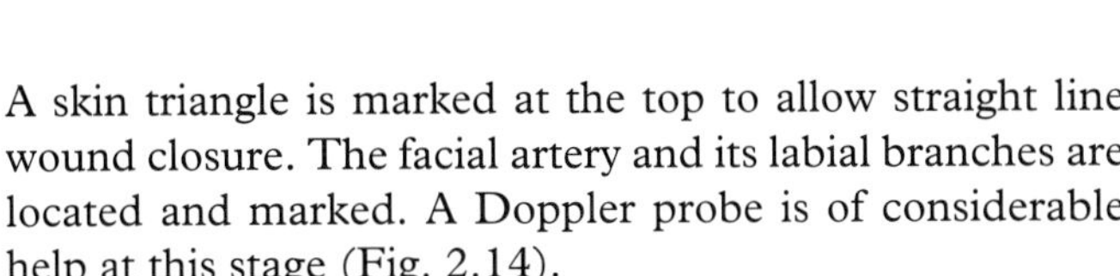

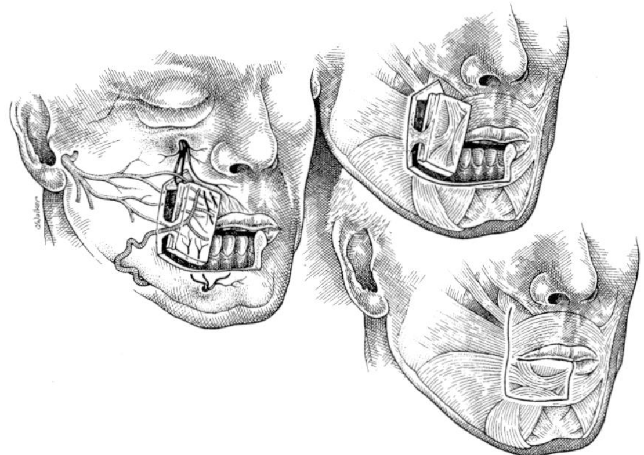

Fig. 2.14 Steeple flap reconstruction of the lower lip. Note the almost total denervation and failure of adequate reconstruction of the orbicularis oris.

neous tissues are incised around the flap and the incision is deepened to full thickness superiorly and inferiorly. The facial artery is identified on the superomedial aspect of the flap and is tied. Tension on the tied vessel helps the precise and safe location of the artery on the lateral side. The obliquely running fibres of the depressor anguli oris also act as a useful marker for the facial vessels, which lie immediately behind and deep to this muscle.

Once the vessel is located, incisions above and below it are deepened to full thickness to within 5 mm of the vessel. Mucosa deep to the artery is divided, allowing transposition of the cheek tissues to their new site. This leads to virtually complete sensory and motor denervation of the tissues, except for those branches of the facial nerve that run in the immediate proximity of the facial artery.

The planning of the mucosal incisions for reconstruction of the vermilion relates directly to the site of the entry of the facial artery into the flap. When the artery enters the flap low, cheek tissues are tumbled into the lip defect with mucosa along the lateral border cut to excess to provide material for the reconstruction of the vermilion (Fig. 2.15).

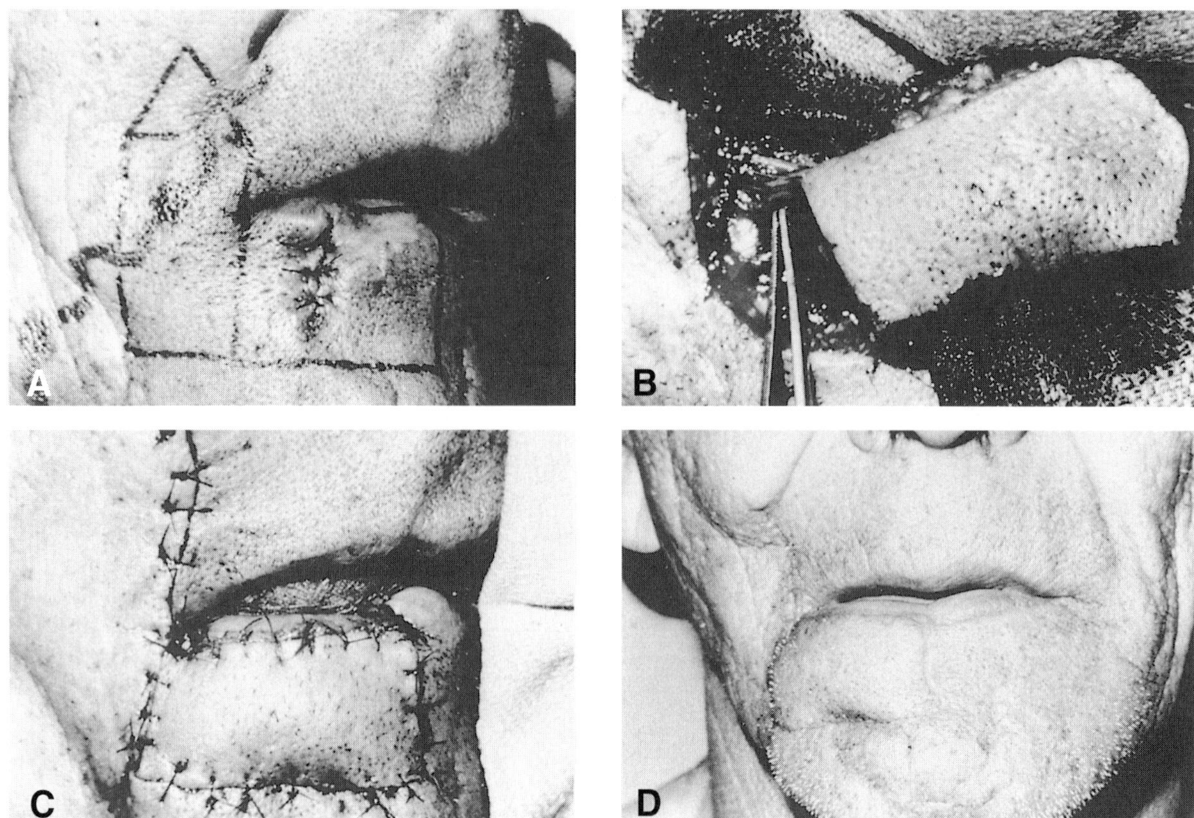

Fig. 2.15 **A** Plan of resection and repair of a biopsy proven squamous cell carcinoma of the lower lip. **B** Island flap used for reconstruction, fully isolated except for its vascular pedicle. **C** Incisions closed. **D** Lips at rest 2 years later.

When the artery enters the flap high, the cheek tissues slide into the cheek defect and the mucosa along the medial border of the island is used for the vermilion reconstruction.

This method can be used only in lower lip defects. Loss of up to three-quarters of the lower lip can be repaired by a single flap, without microstomia or significant denervation of the muscles of the upper lip. Total loss of the lower lip requires the use of bilateral flaps.

Simultaneous lip reconstruction by this method and block dissection of the neck should not be undertaken. Though physical reconstruction of the lip curtain is very adequate with no evidence of microstomia and fair muscle strength, the loss of sensation is a severe drawback, which

Table 2.5 Functional profile 2 years after surgery in a 45-year-old man

Parameter	Measurement	Mean ± S. D.
Lower lip height (mm)	22	25 ± 5
Intercommissural		
distance at rest (mm)	66	65 ± 5
Soft tissue gape (mm)	40	50 ± 11
Elasticity index	30	55 ± 12
Oral aperture (cm)	25	22 ± 5
Two-point discrimination		
of the reconstructed lip (mm)	>10	3 ± 1
Pommeter (g)	170	399 ± 152
Disability: occasional drooling		

patients can only partly compensate for by using their normally innervated tongue. Results of studies of lip function 2 years after surgery are found in Table 2.5. The main disadvantage of the method, apart from significant denervation, is the residual oedema which persists in the reconstructed lip.

(b) Microsurgical reconstruction of the lips

The use of the radial artery flap is indicated only in massive lip defects involving more than three-quarters of the lip. The use of the palmaris tendon helps to maintain the height of the reconstructed lower lip (Fig. 2.16). Anastomosis of the sensory nerve with the mental nerve is always advisable to provide some sensation in the reconstructed lip. Lips reconstructed with forearm skin will, at best, have the same sensory two-point discrimination as the donor site (Lister 1977), which is far less sensitive than a normal lip. Table 2.6 shows functional assessment 3.5 months after surgery.

RECONSTRUCTION OF FULL-THICKNESS UPPER LIP DEFECTS

Tumours of the upper lip occur less frequently than those of the lower lip therefore the problem of reconstruction is

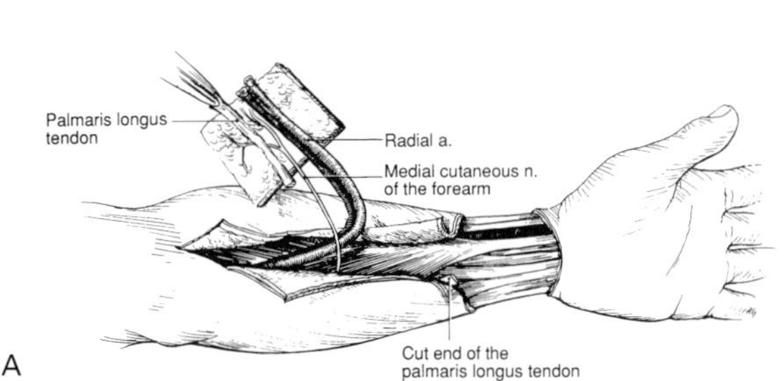
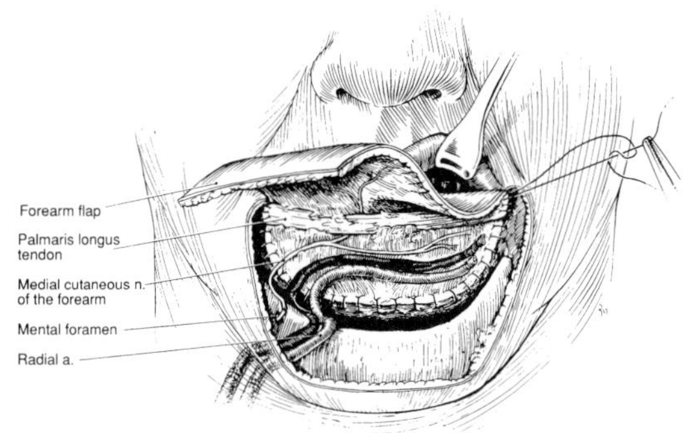

Fig. 2.16 Plan of microsurgical lip reconstruction. **A** Forearm detail. **B** Closure of oral aspect and lateral stabilisation using a palmaris longus sling. Note the neurovascular pedicle. (Reproduced with permission from R C Sadove et al 1991.)

encountered relatively rarely. Excision of up to one-third of the lip length can be closed directly in layers. Karapandzic's manoeuvre or an Abbe type of flap can be used in defects of up to one-half of the lip curtain. Larger defects require tissue to be brought from a distance using either a staged method or direct microsurgical transfer of a radial artery forearm flap (Fig. 2.17).

LIP REHABILITATION

The surgical event of lip reconstruction per se is not the end of the story. Restoration of normal or near normal appearance is an obvious concern during the planning of surgery. However, the method of choice should be that which allows maximum preservation of lip function as well as conserving aesthetic units. Following even the most minor lip resection, the lips need to be rehabilitated in order to restore fine muscle control and to secure the optimal sensitivity.

Muscle control can be substantially improved through the use of appropriate exercises to increase the strength of the orbicularis oris: a patient, who had been involved in a

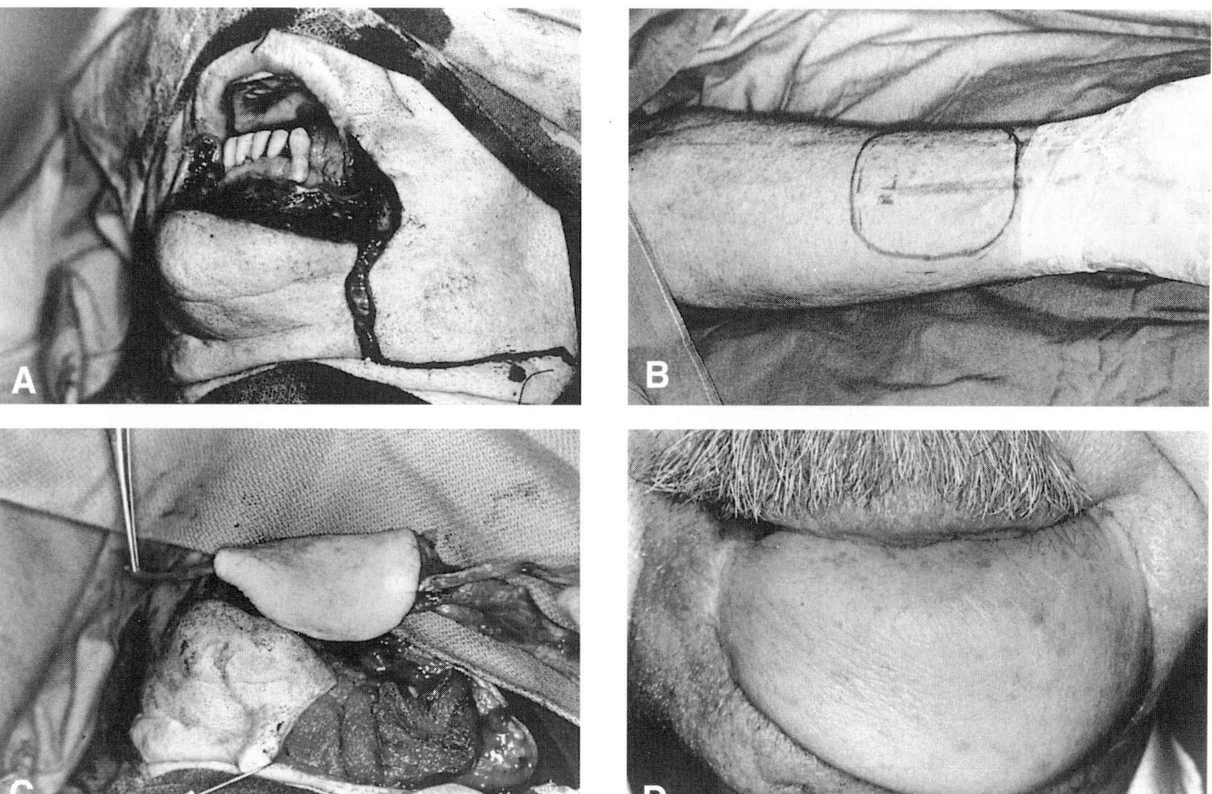

Fig. 2.17 **A** 72-year-old man following subtotal lower lip resection. **B** Outline of radial artery flap. **C** 'Lip' being transferred, held by palmaris longus tendon. **D** New lip at rest 3.5 months after surgery. (Case of M. Zeismann, Department of Plastic Surgery, Health Sciences Centre, Winnipeg, Manitoba, Canada.)

Table 2.6   Early lip function after microsurgical reconstruction*

Parameter	Measurement	Mean ± S. D.
Lower lip height (mm)	10	23 ± 5
Intercommissural		
distance at rest (mm)	85	66 ± 6
Soft tissue gape (mm)	45	44 ± 11
Elasticity index	41	45 ± 12
Oral aperture (cm)	34	27 ± 8
Two-point discrimination		
of the reconstructed lip (mm)	>10	3 ± 1
Pommeter (g)	120	290 ± 95
Disability: moderately		
severe dribbling and some		
difficulty with eating		

*This is an early result: the patient will improve as the swelling resolves and the height of the lip curtain increases, either through the tightening of the palmaris sling or the deepening of the sulcus. Some sensory recovery will take place.

road traffic accident 6 months earlier, was referred to me with vague but persistent complaints of aching and pain in the region of the right corner of the mouth. She had suffered lacerations of the right cheek leading to a partial palsy of the lip muscles. On examination her pommeter reading was 102 g (a normal value for her age would be 390 g). She was given a set of exercises to strengthen the lip muscles, which were performed regularly and enthusiastically. Within 3 months she was symptom-free and had a reading of 350 g.

It is difficult, if not impossible, to improve the sensitivity of a reconstructed lip, again emphasising the need for the selection of the method that best conserves lip sensation. In patients whose lower lip sensation is severely compromised leading to problems with oral continence, use of the sensate tongue unobtrusively resting against the lower lip can minimise the impairment.

Restoration of normal or near normal appearance should be of paramount importance during the planning of the original surgery, when due emphasis should be given to the preservation of the maximum lip function as well as conservation of aesthetic units. Secondary revisionary surgery never gives as good a result.

CONCLUSIONS

Though there are many methods of lower lip reconstruction as has already been indicated, in the author's opinion, based on functional outcome, the following outline is recommended:

- defects of up to one-third of the lip: direct layered closure or if too much tension exists, step technique of Johansen;
- defects of one-third to one-half of the lip: step technique of Johansen or Karapandzic, both are equally good;
- defects greater than one-half of the lip; defects one-half to three-quarters: step technique or Karapandzic can be used, but microstomia is inevitable with the need for secondary commissurotomy;
- subtotal defects of the lip: innervated, suspended radial artery flap or bilateral Steeple flaps are both reasonable options.

REFERENCES

Abbe R 1898 A new plastic operation for the relief of deformity due to double harelip. Medical Records of New York 53: 477

Bernard C 1852 Cancer de la lèvre inférieure: restauration à l'aide de lambeaux quadrilataires–latéreaux. Querison 5: 162–164

Broders A C 1921 Squamous cell epithelioma of the skin. Annals of Surgery 73: 141–160

Burow C A 1855 Beschreibung einer Neuen Transplantation Methode. Nuack, Berlin

Dieffenbach J F 1834 Chirurgische Erfahrungen Series 3 4: 101

Emmett A J J 1980 Operative plastic and reconstructive surgery. Churchill Livingstone, Edinburgh, p 607

Estlander J A 1872 En metod att fran den ena lappen fylla substans-forluster i den andran och i kinder. Norologial Medical Arkive 1V: 1

Fogel M, Stranc M F 1984 Lip function: a study of normal parameters. British Journal of Plastic Surgery 37: 542–549

Freedman A M, Hidalgo D A 1990 Full–thickness cheek and lip reconstruction with a radial forearm free flap. Annals of Plastic Surgery 25: 287–294

Freeman B S 1958 Myoplastic modification of the Bernard cheiloplast. Plastic and Reconstructive Surgery 21: 453–460

Frierson H F, Cooper P H 1986 Prognostic factors in squamous cell carcinoma of the lower lip. Human Pathology 17: 346–354

Gillies H 1920 Plastic Surgery. Frowde Hodder & Stoughton, London, p 8

Gillies H, Millard D R 1957 The principles and art of plastic surgery. Little & Brown, Boston, p 507

Johanson B, Aspeluer E, Breine U, Holmstrom H 1974 Surgical treatment of non–traumatic lower lip lesions with special reference to the step technique. Scandinavian Journal of Reconstructive Surgery 8: 232–240

Karapandzic M 1974 Reconstruction of lip defects by local arterial flaps. British Journal of Plastic Surgery 27: 93–97

Kwa R R, Campana K, Moy R L 1992 Biology of cutaneous squamous cell carcinoma. Journal of the American Academy of Dermatology 26: 1–26

Lister G 1977 The hand: diagnosis and indications. Churchill Livingstone, Edinburgh, p 71

May H 1946 The modified Dieffenbach operation for closure of large defects of the lower lip and chin. Plastic and Reconstructive Surgery 1: 194–200

Penn I 1980 Immunosuppression and skin cancer. Clinics of Plastic Surgery 7: 361–368

Reidiger D, Ehrenfeld M, Cornelius C P 1989 Microsurgical tissue transplantation. Quintessence Publishing, Chicago, p 189

Sadove R C, Edward A L, McGrath P C 1991 Reconstruction of the lower lip and chin with the composite radial forearm–palmaris longus free flap. Plastic and Reconstructive Surgery 88: 209–214

Stranc M F, Fogel M 1984 Lip function: a study of oral competence. British Journal of Plastic Surgery 37: 550–557

Stranc M F, Fogel M, Dische S 1987 Comparison of lip function: surgery vs radiotherapy. British Journal of Plastic Surgery 40: 598–604

Stranc M F, Robertson G A 1983 Steeple flap reconstruction of the lower lip. Annals of Plastic Surgery 10: 4–11

Szymanowski J 1858 Zur plastischen chirurgie. Zeitschrift für praktische Heilkunde 60: 127

Taylor G I 1989 Personal Communication

Von Bruns 1859 Handbuch der praktischen Chirurgie. Laupp & Siebeck, Tubigen, p 778

Section 1

3. The surgical approach to the mandible

Alan D. McGregor

INTRODUCTION

In the surgical treatment of intraoral cancer, the mandible presents the surgeon with two problems. First, it may be involved in the disease, so removal of part of the bone may be necessary on pathological grounds. Second, if not involved by the disease, it remains a considerable obstacle to adequate access to the primary tumour within the oral cavity. A satisfactory approach taking into account and solving both these problems has evolved only relatively recently, due largely to studies investigating the patterns of blood supply and tumour spread to the mandile, and to the coincidental development of modern microsurgical reconstructive techniques.

ANATOMY

The mandible develops in two halves, which meet and fuse in the midline at the symphysis. Each half consists of a horizontal part (the body) and a vertical, muscle-bearing part (the ramus), often termed the horizontal ramus and ascending ramus respectively.

The horizontal ramus of the mandible has two parts. The upper, tooth-bearing part is the alveolar part and is covered with adherent mucoperiosteum. The lower or basal part has no mucosal covering. On the lingual aspect, the mucosa is reflected off the mandible at the mylohyoid line to which the mylohyoid muscle is attached. On the buccal/labial surface, the mucoperiosteum is reflected off the mandible just above the level of the mental foramen to form the lingual sulcus anteriorly and the lower buccal sulcus posterolaterally. The mylohyoid line is an approximate surface marking of the mandibular canal, which runs through the mandible from the mandibular foramen on the buccal aspect of the ascending ramus to the mental foramen on the lingual aspect of the horizontal ramus at the level of the first premolar tooth (Fig. 3.1). The mandibular canal transmits the inferior alveolar artery, a branch of the maxillary artery, and the inferior alveolar nerve, a branch of the mandibular division of the trigeminal nerve. These pass through the bone giving branches to bone and teeth. At the mental foramen, both nerve and artery give off branches which emerge through the foramen to supply the chin and lower lip. These are known as the mental nerve and artery.

Although the inferior alveolar artery is the main nutrient artery to the mandible, it is not the only source of blood supply to the bone. In common with most other bones in the body, the mandible is supplied by *penetrating vessels*, which pass straight through the cortex to supply the medullary cavity and the inner part of the cortex, and *periosteal vessels*, which supply the outer part of the cortex. These two latter sources of blood supply are closely associated with the soft tissues attached to the mandible and can be regarded from the surgical point of view as a single source, which is usually referred to as the periosteal blood supply. There is evidence to suggest that the importance of the inferior alveolar artery diminishes through adult life (Bradley 1972, McGregor & MacDonald 1989b) and that its main role is to supply the teeth and alveolar bone of the mandibular body (Castelli 1963). Consequently the periosteal blood supply becomes increasingly important.

The main arterial source of blood supply to the periosteal surface of the mandible is the facial artery via buccal and submandibular branches (McGregor & MacDonald, in press). The facial artery is divided in the course of cervical lymph node clearance, but it is assumed that the blood supply is maintained by anastomoses within the distribution of the external carotid artery.

The inferior alveolar vein is a small structure and venous drainage is largely via periosteal veins to the anterior and posterior facial veins, with some drainage from the upper ramus to the pterygoid venous plexus (Cohen 1959).

Although periosteum is drained by lymphatics, it appears that bone has no lymphatic drainage (Anderson 1960).

CHANGES IN THE MANDIBLE AFTER DENTAL EXTRACTION

A proportion of patients who develop oral cancer are edentulous. Loss of teeth results in a number of changes in

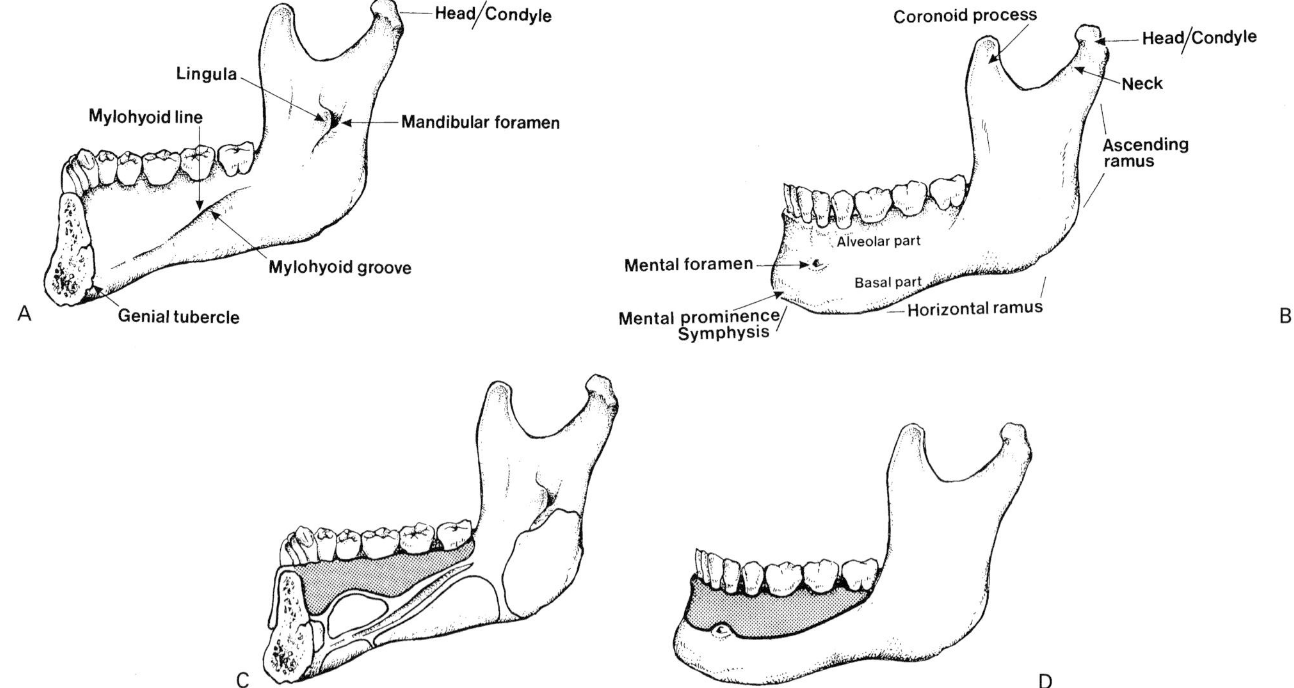

Fig. 3.1 A–D The surgical anatomy of the dentate mandible.

the mandible of considerable importance to the surgeon who is treating their tumour.

Extraction of a tooth is followed by bleeding into the socket, with resultant formation of a blood clot, and healing of the mucosa over socket. The blood clot then organises and, subsequently, ossifies (Schram 1929). Cortical bone forms over the occlusal surface but this never results in a complete layer, possibly due to lack of an osteogenic periosteum. As a result, a variable number of gaps persist in the cortex on the occlusal surface (Nakamoto 1968) with the result that there is no complete bone barrier between the mucosa and the cancellous bone of the medulla (McGregor & MacDonald 1987).

Dental extraction is also followed by progressive resorption of alveolar bone (Atwood 1971), a process which is accelerated slightly in denture wearers (Campbell 1960). The basal segment of the bone is not resorbed to a significant extent, loss of height being confined to the alveolar part of the horizontal ramus. As a result, the occlusal surface becomes progressively closer to the level of the floor of the mouth formed by the mucosa reflected over the mylohyoid muscle and the sublingual and submandibular glands.

In extreme cases, the upper border of the mandible lies virtually flush with the floor of the mouth at the level of the mylohyoid line (Edwards 1954), bringing the genial tubercle, mandibular canal and mental foramen on to the occlusal surface (Fig. 3.2). The effect is to expose the inferior alveolar nerve and artery on the occlusal surface of the mandible with only a covering of mucosa. This is the classic 'pipe–stem' mandible and represents the ultimate degree to which resorption can occur. The height of the genial tubercle and mental foramen above the lower border has been measured at 13–14 mm (Shiller & Wiswell 1954, Edwards 1954) so this figure represents the extreme lower limit of the vertical height of the edentulous body.

Resorption of alveolar bone appears to be less severe in partially dentate mandibles, particularly in those which meet the teeth of the upper jaw in occlusion.

ACCESS TO THE ORAL CAVITY

In a proportion of intraoral tumours, involvement of the mandible is so advanced that a full-thickness segment of bone must be resected. This coincidentally facilitates access to the oral cavity. The majority of patients with oral cancer have no tumour spread to bone. In such cases, there is no indication for bone resection on pathological grounds, so the mandible then functions as rigid obstacle impeding access to the oral cavity. Two approaches have evolved to cope with this problem—the pull-through technique and osteotomy of the body of the mandible with lateral swing of the hemimandible.

THE PULL-THROUGH TECHNIQUE

The pull-through technique (Slaughter 1951) entails incision of the periosteum along the lower border of the body of the mandible, incision of the mucoperiosteum on the lingual aspect of the alveolus and separation of the structures attached to the lingual surface by subperiosteal dissection.

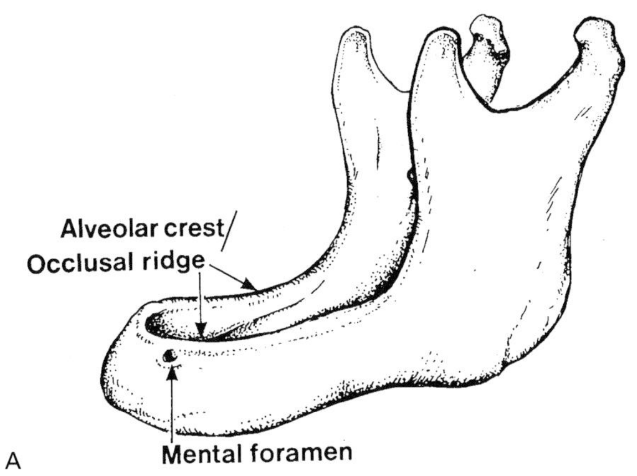

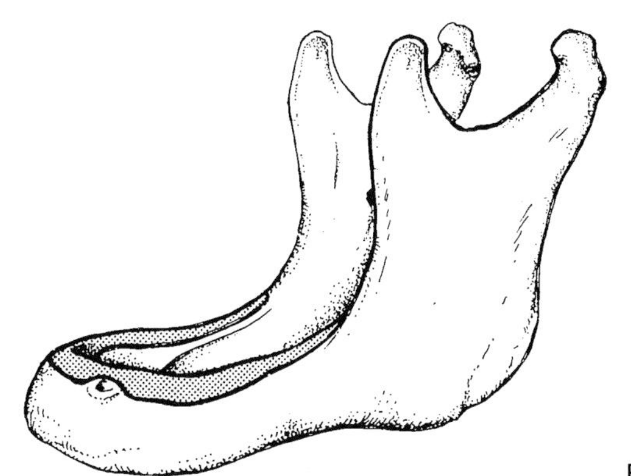

Fig. 3.2 The surgical anatomy of the edentulous mandible.

This frees the lateral attachments of the tongue and floor of mouth, which are then delivered downwards into the neck, in this way providing access to any part of the tongue. The mandible retains its blood supply via the inferior alveolar artery and vessels from the buccal/labial periosteal surface. This method has the advantage of avoiding an incision in the lip and chin, although a submandibular incision is required for exposure. It has the disadvantage of being suitable only for the carcinoma of the tongue which does not involve the mandible. The technique can also be extended around the whole body of the mandible to allow delivery of the entire tongue into the neck. It is possible, in addition, to separate the lingual/buccal attachments over the entire mandibular body and to elevate the chin and lip as a visor flap, thus exposing the whole body. This has the disadvantage that the flap thus raised often fails to adhere and function as before, particularly the mental prominence, so that lip continence and function are often impaired.

MANDIBULAR OSTEOTOMY AND SWING

Osteotomy of the mandible was originally used by Roux in 1836 (Butlin 1985). The bone can be divided at the symphysis or laterally, either anterior to the mental foramen (paramedian osteotomy) or posterior to the mental foramen (lateral osteotomy). Lateral osteotomy has the disadvantage of dividing the inferior alveolar nerve and artery without providing better exposure than paramedian osteotomy (Fig. 3.3).

The paramedian approach (McGregor & MacDonald 1983) is the most useful because, apart from mucosa, the mylohyoid muscle alone need be divided for the lesser mandibular segment to 'swing' outwards. The geniohyoid and genioglossus muscles remain attached to the peri-symphyseal mandible, thus ensuring tongue stability. The soft tissues, particularly on the buccal and labial surface, remain attached to the mandible maintaining the blood supply via periosteal vessels and the inferior alveolar artery. Paramedian osteotomy has the disadvantage of requiring an incision in the lip and chin, but the advantages of providing exposure as far back as the pharynx, applicability to all primary intraoral sites with the exception of the buccal areas and of allowing simultaneous management of the mandible involved by tumour.

Symphyseal osteotomy is the approach of choice on occasions but in most instances it has no particular advantage over paramedian osteotomy which is now the routine approach of choice (Dubner & Spiro 1991).

Use of an osteotomy requires a skin incision over the chin which extends upwards into and splits the lip. The lip-splitting incision can be placed anywhere on the lip but the best position aesthetically is in the midline. The chin can be incised either vertically in the midline (Kremen 1951) or using an incision which curves round the mental prominence (McGregor & MacDonald 1983) (Fig. 3.4). The latter approach gives a better cosmetic result, the vertical incision tending to leave a visually prominent furrow in the mental prominence. It also provides direct access to the mandible just medial to the mental foramen. Fashioning the osteotomy at this point preserves the mental nerve and its distribution to the lip.

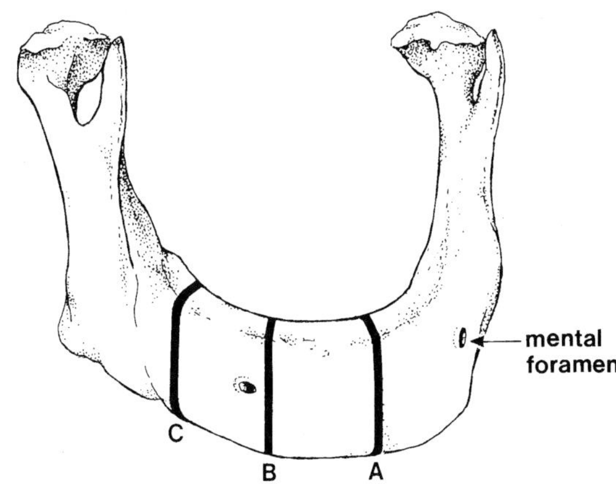

Fig. 3.3 Types of mandibular osteotomy classified according to site. **A** Symphyseal. **B** Paramedian. **C** Lateral.

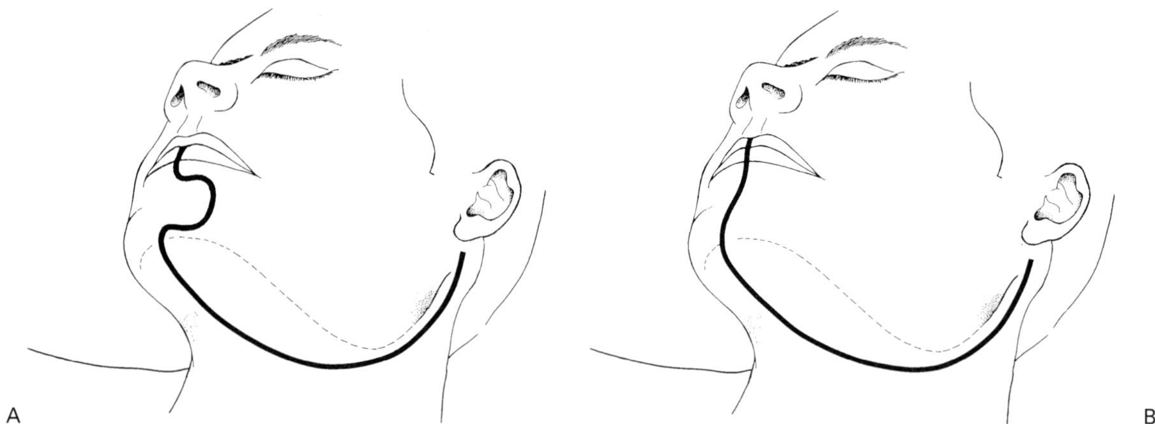

Fig. 3.4 Alternative lip incisions for exposure of the mandibular preparatory to mandible osteotomy. **A** Circummental approach. **B** Midline incision.

Several techniques of fashioning an osteotomy have been described. These can be classified as simple vertical osteotomy, step osteotomy and those incorporating a sagittal split (Fig. 3.5). There is no evidence to suggest that any of these methods has any advantage over the others, and the choice of technique lies with the surgeon.

The osteotomy can be fixed by means of plate and screws or wires (either interosseous wire or interosseous wire and Kirschner wire) (Fig. 3.6). There is to date, no evidence that any of these has any advantage over the others, either in terms of successful union of the osteotomy or complication rate. The choice of technique lies with the operator.

Siting the osteotomy in the edentulous patient in such a way as to avoid injury to the mental nerve can be difficult, though use of the incision around the mental prominence leads to the appropriate part of the body as a rule. In the dentate mandible, the presence of teeth can act as landmarks when correlated with radiological studies, though a dentate mandible does present some technical problems. A step osteotomy carries the risk of exposing the roots of teeth and a sagittal split certainly would. The wisest choice may be vertical division of the bone. The interdental papilla is divided down to the bone, and the mucoperiosteum is incised and mobilised only sufficiently to expose the mandible, which is then divided. The usual site is between the second incisor and canine where the roots diverge (Fig. 3.7), although a better position may have been created by a previous dental extraction. If the mandible is edentulous at the chosen osteotomy site, the mucoperiosteum is incised and stripped by subperiosteal dissection for a few millimetres on either side of the planned osteotomy.

A power-driven oscillating or reciprocating saw is to be preferred to a Gigli saw for fashioning the osteotomy because of its greater accuracy. To avoid unnecessary damage to the bone by heat, the field should be well irrigated and the speed of the saw should be as slow as is compatible with achieving division of the predominantly cortical bone. Unnecessary separation of periosteum from bone is to be avoided in order to promote uncomplicated bone healing.

In most instances, exposure of the mandible is preceded by some form of neck dissection. A submandibular incision will therefore have been employed to obtain access to the submandibular area. When such an incision has not been

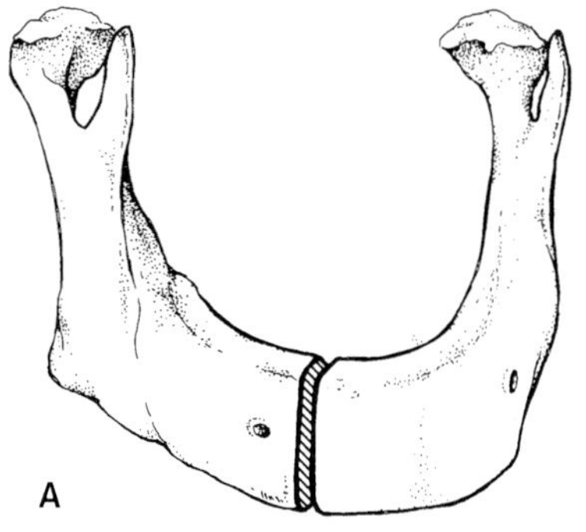
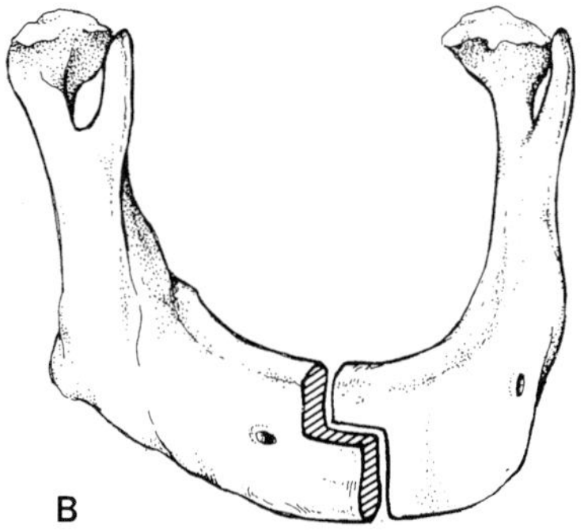
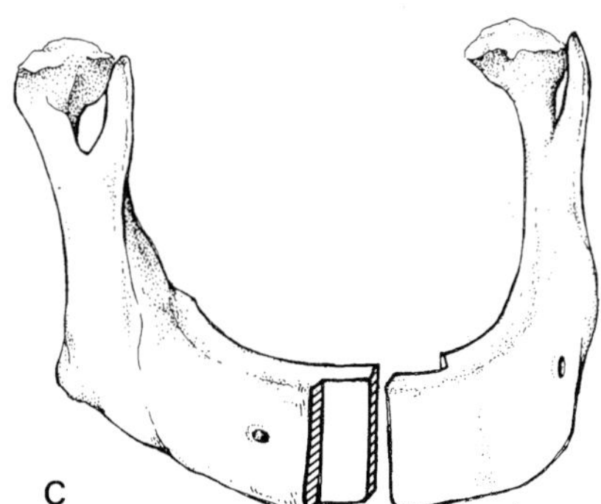

Fig. 3.5 Types of mandibular osteotomy. **A** Vertical osteotomy. **B** Step osteotomy. **C** Osteotomy incorporating a sagittal split. This can be varied as a step osteotomy.

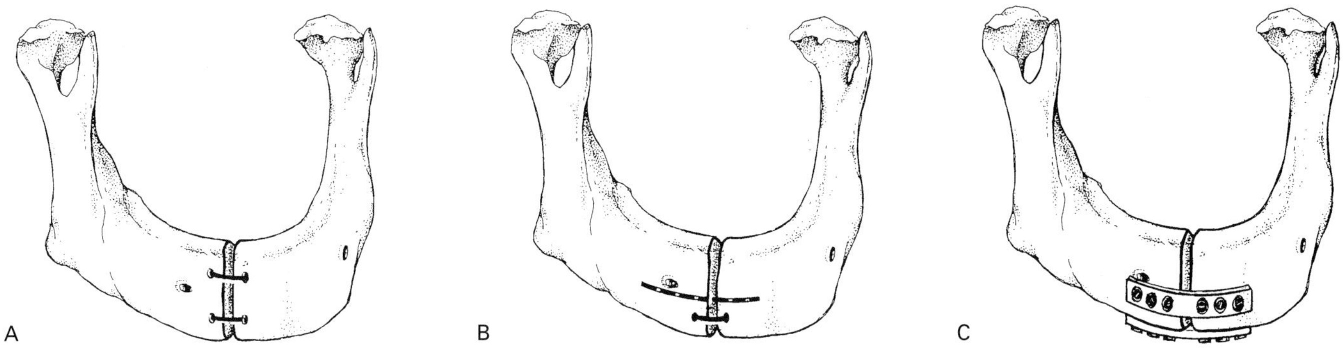

Fig. 3.6 Types of fixation after mandibular osteotomy. **A** Loop wire fixation. **B** Interosseous and Kirschner wire. **C** Plate and screws.

created for this purpose, a submandibular incision will be required to allow either a pull–though or an osteotomy and mandibular swing.

TUMOUR SPREAD TO THE MANDIBLE

Squamous cell carcinoma is the most common tumour arising in the oral cavity and our present knowledge of tumour spread and management relates to it. In the discussion that follows, it will be assumed that squamous cell carcinoma is the tumour involved.

Squamous cell carcinoma can spread from its primary mucosal site to involve all tissues in the head and neck, but the pattern and mechanism of spread varies as follows:

through soft tissues — infiltrative
into bone — infiltrative
along lymphatics — embolic
along nerves — permeative

Infiltrative and permeative spread both occur in continuity from the main primary tumour and this must be taken into account in planning and carrying out surgical removal — involved tissues must be removed en bloc. Embolic spread along lymphatics to lymph nodes (Willis 1967) means that lymph node management can be undertaken independently of the primary tumour.

Much debate in the past has centred around the role of periosteal lymphatics in the management of the mandible in oral cancer and the question is still raised occasionally. The term itself is open to interpretation and it is not clear precisely what is meant. 'Periosteal lymphatics' can relate to two structures. It might apply to those vessels which drain the periosteum of the mandible, or to lymphatics which pass close to or through periosteum but which drain mucosa of the oral cavity, such as described by Polya & von Navratil (1902). There is no evidence to indicate that tumour either spreads to the mandible along lymphatic vessels or that tumour spreads from the mandible to lymph nodes via periosteal lymphatics. Indeed all the evidence is to the contrary. Tumour can spread from primary mucosal sites along lymphatics and, if these vessels have a close

anatomical relationship to the mandible, tumour metastases inevitably pass close to periosteum as they pass to lymph nodes. Because such spread is embolic, the periosteum is not involved and has no potential as a site of recurrence — bone and periosteum need not be excised as part of managing lymphatic spread of squamous cell carcinoma as has been suggested (Kremen 1951). Bone and periosteum need be excised only if directly infiltrated by tumour.

The greatest influences on the pattern of bone invasion are the presence or absence of teeth and whether or not the bone has been previously irradiated.

DENTAL STATUS

Under normal circumstances, periosteum appears to be

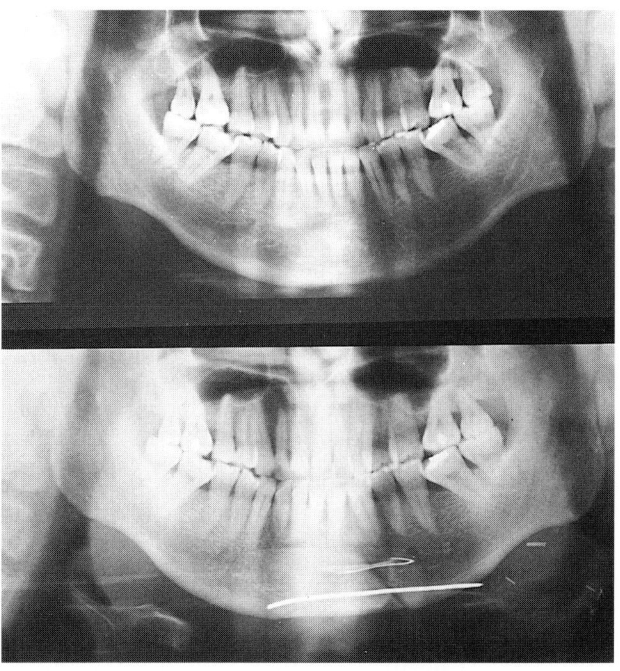

Fig. 3.7 Orthopantogram (OPT) showing site of osteotomy between second incisor and canine.

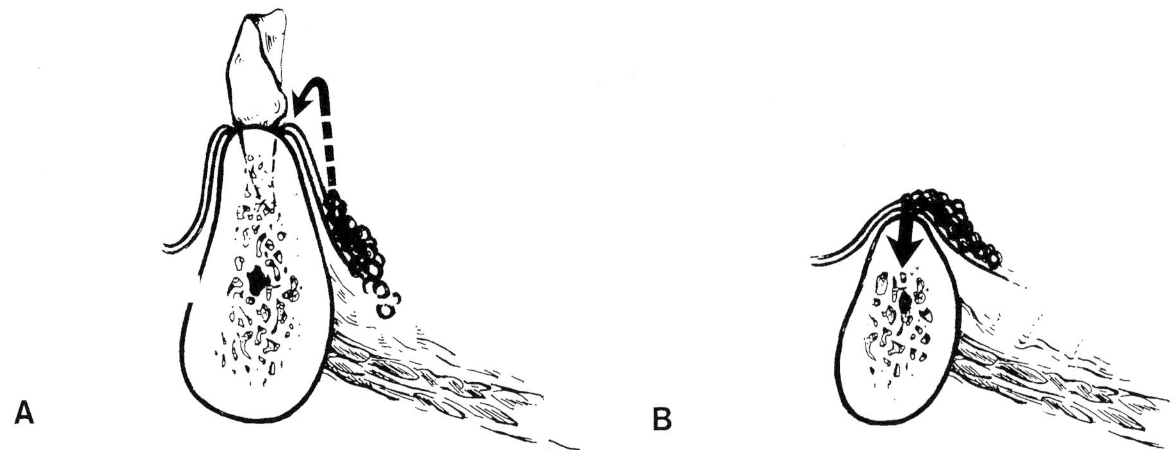

Fig. 3.8 Tumour entry into the occlusal surface of the mandible. **A** Dentate. **B** Edentulous. Tumour invasion of the edentulous mandible is likely to occur at an earlier stage than invasion of the dentate mandible.

very resistant to infiltration by tumour, the formation of periosteal new bone having been observed in response to the presence of squamous cell carcinoma (McGregor & MacDonald 1988b). This reaction has not been observed on the alveolar aspect of the mandible though it has been reported on lingual, labial/buccal and inferior surfaces. Such a lack of response on the occlusal ridge taken in combination with the gaps in the bone on this surface suggests a potential route for tumour spread to the bone through the alveolus.

Loss of vertical mandibular height due to progressive alveolar bone resorption brings the occlusal surface closer to the mucosa of the floor of the mouth. The pattern of tumour spread across this part of the oral cavity has been described as superficial and radial in the early stages rather than deeply invasive (McGregor & MacDonald 1987). This they attributed to resistance to infiltrative tumour growth by the mylohyoid muscle and the submandibular and sublingual salivary glands. The mucosa of an occlusal ridge which is close to the plane of the floor of the mouth will inevitably be involved by tumour spread at an earlier stage than the mucosa on the occlusal surface of a mandible showing less advanced alveolar bone resorption (Fig. 3.8). The amount of alveolar bone, and the vertical height of the body, is always greatest in the dentate mandible. The commonest clinical symptom of tumour spread to the dentate mandible is loosening of teeth, which suggests that the alveolus may also be an important route of tumour spread to the dentate bone.

REACTION IN THE MANDIBLE TO TUMOUR

A number of changes in the mandible have been described in association with the close proximity of squamous cell carcinoma to the mandible. New bone formation is seen on the periosteal and endosteal aspects of the lingual, inferior and buccal/labial surfaces. Tumour invasion is associated with loss of haemopoietic marrow and replacement by fibrous tissue (McGregor & MacDonald 1988b). The underlying mechanism of these processes is unknown.

Such new bone appears to be more resistant to resorption in the presence of tumour than mature cortical bone, but the precise significance of this behaviour and of these reactions is not known.

Changes seen in the mandible after radiotherapy are largely similar to those described in other bones and are not modified by the presence of tumour. The haemopoietic marrow and fat of the medullary cavity are replaced by telangiectatic blood vessels and postradiation fibroblasts in a rather amorphous, oedematous fibrous tissue. Osteoblasts in endosteum and periosteum persist but appear relatively inert. Active new bone deposition in response to tumour has not been reported (McGregor & MacDonald 1988b).

Osteoclastic function appears to be unimpaired by radiation. This is the means by which tumour infiltrates bone—in reality, resorption precedes tumour ingrowth.

TUMOUR SPREAD TO THE MANDIBLE

The desire to limit mandibular resection to what is required on purely pathological grounds has prompted a number of studies on tumour entry to the mandible. Differences have been identified between the patterns of spread to the non-irradiated and to the irradiated mandible, which are of considerable relevance to the surgical management (McGregor & MacDonald 1988a). In both instances, tumour spread to the bone is by direct infiltration, not by metastasis (Marchetta et al 1964, 1971).

The commonest route of entry of squamous cell carcinoma to the non-irradiated mandible is through the occlusal surface (McGregor & MacDonald 1987, McGregor &

MacDonald 1988a). Unequivocal data are available only for the edentulous and partially dentate mandible. In the edentulous bone, the earliest stage of tumour spread is through the gaps in the bone on the alveolar surface. In the partially dentate bone, invasion also occurs most frequently through the edentulous part of the alveolus. The pattern of tumour spread to the fully dentate mandible has not yet been fully clarified, though there is strong histological evidence to suggest that tumour enters tooth sockets along the periodontal membrane (Totsuka et al 1991).

Although the alveolus is the most frequent route of tumour entry to the non-irradiated mandible, other gaps exist in the cortex, as a result of which there is no bone barrier between extraosseous soft tissues and the medullary cavity. The best example of this is the foramina through which nerves and vessels pass into and out of the bone. The best known are the named genial, mental and mandibular foramina, though many others exist (Sutton 1974). Tumour spread does occur though these foramina, but this tends to be at a late stage of tumour spread to the mandible.

Two histological patterns of invasion have been described. Depending on whether tumour infiltration of cortical bone is a prominent feature, these have been termed erosive and infiltrating (Slootweg & Muller 1981). Differentiation between the two patterns is extremely difficult on radiological and clinical grounds (Muller & Slootweg 1990) and, as yet, there is no evidence to suggest that these patterns are of relevance to either management or prognosis. The mechanism accounting for the two patterns also remains to be clarified.

The alveolus is reported as the commonest route of tumour invasion of the mandible after radiotherapy. In contrast to the non-irradiated mandible, squamous cell carcinoma has also been observed to penetrate any other cortical surfaces with which it comes into direct contact in the course of infiltrative spread through soft tissues. This is thought to be due to either alteration of the pattern of soft tissue spread of tumour from a superficial to an infiltrative growth pattern or alteration of the function of the periosteum, in particular in respect to its resistance to tumour invasion (McGregor & MacDonald 1988a). Most probably both play a role. As a result, more than one focus of invasion of the bone is frequently seen after radiotherapy, often on more than one surface of the mandible. Only the alveolus can be seen on clinical examination, other foci of tumour invasion on the lingual, buccal/labial or inferior surfaces are not readily detectable clinically or, if small, radiologically. Tumour invasion may also be present in the absence of tumour entry via the alveolus—it can be impossible to determine whether tumour has penetrated the mandible under such circumstances.

TUMOUR SPREAD WITHIN THE MANDIBLE

The pattern of tumour spread within the mandible appears to differ little whether or not the bone has been irradiated. Two routes have been described—spread in the medulla between cancellous bony trabeculae and spread in relation to the inferior alveolar nerve. Each is important in its own right because the implications for surgical management are different in each case.

Spread of tumour in the medullary cavity of the non-irradiated mandible is associated with loss of haemopoiesis and replacement by fibrous tissue (McGregor & MacDonald 1988b). Though the precise mechanism is unknown, the observation is of importance to the pathologist and to the surgeon—by implication, the presence of haemopoietic marrow at either lateral resection margin after bone excision means that tumour excision is adequate at these points. More importantly, tumour appears not to extend to a significant extent within the medullary cavity deep to an intact cortex in the body of the mandible. Tumour spread in soft tissues and mucosa on the alveolar surface is invariably more extensive than spread within the bone, and consequently, planning of the lateral bone excision margins in the body of the mandible can be based on the extent of mucosal spread of tumour on the alveolus. An exception to this is the spread of tumour from the horizontal ramus of the mandible to the ascending ramus. The ascending ramus is completely enclosed by cortical bone and the surgeon has no convenient guide to the extent of tumour spread into and within this part of the bone.

In the irradiated mandible, the pattern of spread in the medullary cavity differs little from that seen in the non-irradiated mandible. As radiation results in loss of haemopoietic marrow throughout the irradiated field, no difference is to be seen in the medullary cavity beyond the limits of tumour infiltration. Resection cannot be planned solely on the basis of the extent of tumour in alveolar mucosa because of the other possible routes of entry, and account of these must also be taken when considering how much bone to excise. Resection should be based on the limits of tumour spread within the soft tissues in relation to the mandible.

Direct spread of tumour from the horizontal to the ascending ramus is seen, especially when the site of entry is in the molar region of the body, though the extent of spread appears to be more limited than may have been thought previously. In the non-irradiated mandible, tumour spread is usually limited to the anterior part of the ascending ramus, extending posterior to the mandibular canal only infrequently. Following radiotherapy a similar pattern is seen, but separate foci of direct tumour invasion of the ramus from attached soft tissues are also seen frequently (McGregor & MacDonald, in press).

Nerve-related tumour spread is usually referred to as perineural spread, peri- in this context merely meaning 'in relation to'. The term does not refer to the layer of connective tissue covering the nerve called the perineurium. Spread is seen in endoneurium, perineurium and epineurium. It should be emphasised that spread occurs in potential spaces in the connective tissue—these spaces are not lymphatics because none exist in relation to the inferior alveolar nerve (Larson et al 1966). The importance of this pattern of tumour spread lies in the potential for spread along the nerve beyond the bone (Ballantyne et al 1963). Such permeative spread can reach the trigeminal ganglion and may present as recurrent tumour in the infratemporal fossa. By this stage, eradication of disease is impossible.

Perineural tumour spread is also seen in the hypoglossal and lingual nerves, in addition to smaller unnamed nerves. In these sites, however, tumour is rarely seen to extend beyond the main mass of tumour and appears to have little influence on the outcome of treatment. There is no evidence that it has any bearing on the incidence or pattern of tumour recurrence.

The frequency with which tumour spread is seen in relation to the inferior alveolar nerve varies, and appears to be influenced both by the site of tumour entry to the mandible and by previous radiotherapy. An incidence of 25% has been reported following radiation, rising to over 50% with tumour entering the molar region of the non-irradiated mandible (McGregor & MacDonald 1989a). The precise incidence is of less importance than the fact that it occurs frequently.

In contrast to tumour spread within the medullary cavity, which is often associated with radiological changes, clinical or radiological signs of perineural tumour spread are seen only at a late stage in the disease process. Only the pathologist can make an accurate diagnosis—this must be taken into account when planning resection. Although tumour can extend from soft tissues along the mental nerve to the inferior alveolar nerve, this is a rare occurrence, tumour usually entering the nerve by direct spread from the main mass of tumour within the medullary cavity.

SURGICAL MANAGEMENT

Radiotherapy and chemotherapy have no role to play in primary management of tumour which has spread to involve the mandible. If spread is clearly present or is suspected, treatment should be surgical. Although reliable techniques have been developed for mandibular reconstruction, it remains desirable to preserve as much of the original bone as is compatible with adequate removal of the disease, either to avoid the need for, or to minimise the extent of, reconstruction. Primary malignancy of the mandible is rare. Mandibular involvement by tumour is usually the result of local spread to the bone from a primary intraoral squamous cell carcinoma. Limiting bone resection to what is involved by disease preserves optimum function and cosmesis, but this can prove difficult, especially after radiotherapy. When in doubt, the surgeon should always adopt the more radical treatment option open to him.

Objective assessment of tumour spread can be made by radioisotope scanning, MRI scanning and CAT scanning but none of these has proved superior to radiological and clinical assessment (Muller & Slootweg 1990, Shaha 1991) and the decision on how to manage the mandible lies with the surgeon. The need for mandibular resection must be assessed as the first step, followed by the extent and pattern of resection. On occasion the bone may appear relatively uninvolved or, indeed, uninvaded but the extent of tumour spread in soft tissues around the mandible may be such as to preclude the possibility of avoiding an extensive resection. This is seen most commonly in tumour recurrence after radiotherapy. Under such circumstances, radical bone resection must be undertaken. If less radical resection is required, the surgeon has to consider what must be removed, and how to approach the mandible.

In considering what mandibular resection is necessary, the surgeon has three possible options based both on the pattern of tumour spread into and within the mandible, and whether or not it has been irradiated previously. The options are to resect no mandible, to remove only the upper border or to undertake a segmental resection which can be any amount of bone from part of the body to an entire hemimandible (on occasion including part of the contralateral body). The principal consideration at all times is to obtain adequate tumour clearance. On occasion it is best to defer the decision on resection until operative treatment is being undertaken.

THE NON-IRRADIATED MANDIBLE

If tumour within mucosa does not extend as far as the occlusal ridge of the mandible, the bone can be regarded as free of disease. Bone resection is not indicated on pathological grounds under such circumstances.

If the tumour extends on to the alveolus, it is not possible to determine on clinical grounds whether tumour involves the bone. Periosteal involvement by tumour usually results in adhesion of periosteum to underlying bone, as a consequence of which periosteum cannot be separated from the bone (McGregor 1977). Alveolar mucoperiosteum is normally very adherent to the bone and can be separated only with difficulty. Radiological changes are infrequent, even in the presence of early tumour spread. Under such circumstances, it is wiser to assume that there is superficial invasion of the mandible, for which resection of the upper border of the mandible alone ('rim resection') appears to be adequate treatment (Fleming 1987, Barttelbort et al 1987).

Difficulties arise when superficial bone resorption is seen on the occlusal surface of the mandible on X-ray. The treatment choice lies between rim resection and segmental resection. Bone resorption in association with tumour indicates nothing more than destruction of cortical bone. The extent of medullary tumour spread cannot be assessed clinically or radiologically (Muller & Slootweg 1990). While it is accepted that rim resection can be safe in the presence

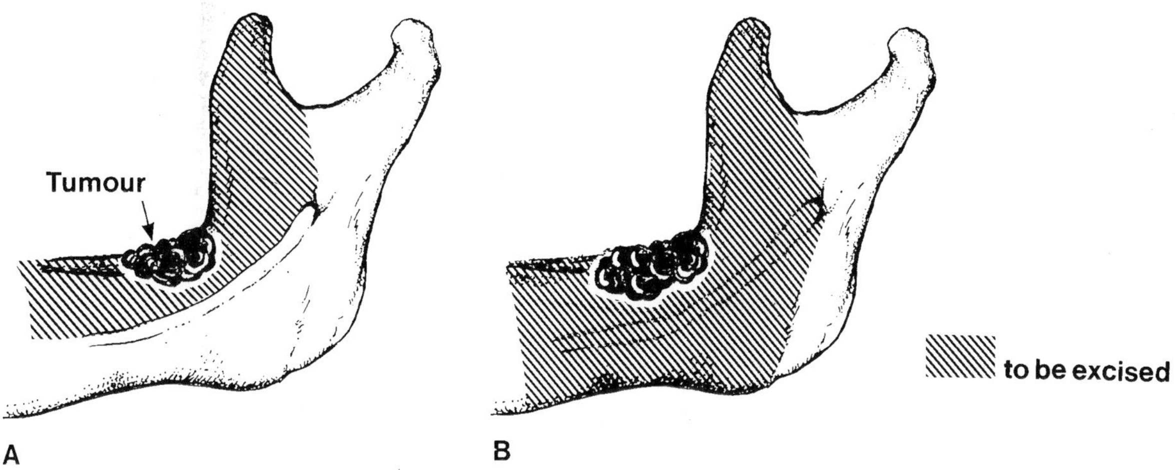

Fig. 3.9 Resection of bone retaining the posterior border of the ascending ramus. **A** Rim resection — reconstruction is unnecessary. **B** Segmental resection — the posterior border of the ascending ramus is preserved facilitating reconstruction of the horizontal ramus.

of early tumour spread (Fleming 1987, Barttelbort et al 1987), the decision as to what type of resection should be undertaken depends largely on the vertical height of the body, assessment of which is based on the position of the alveolus in relation to the mental foramen. The mental foramen is radiologically visible and is the same height (13–14 mm) above the lower border as the genial tubercle on the lingual surface at the symphysis. This also indicates the position of the mandibular canal, which can usually also be seen radiologically, and the inferior alveolar nerve. As the radiological limit of cortical bone resorption comes closer to the mandibular canal, the likelihood of resection of the upper border of the mandible being safe on pathological grounds decreases. It has been proposed that a 1 cm gap on X-ray between the lower extent of bone resorption and the inferior alveolar nerve is the safe limit for rim resection to be undertaken in cases with established bone invasion (Muller & Slootweg 1990). This remains to be proved in clinical practice. In view of the uncertainty, it is wiser for the surgeon in doubt to carry out a segmental resection primarily. If a rim resection is undertaken this must be converted to a segmental resection if the pathologist reports that tumour excision in the bone is incomplete.

Spread of tumour within the medullary cavity from the horizontal to the ascending ramus of the mandible also creates management problems. Pathological studies indicate that the extent of tumour spread in the ascending ramus is frequently less than may have been supposed, often being confined anterior to the mandibular canal (McGregor & MacDonald, in press). As a result it may be safe to retain the posterior border by fashioning a vertical subsigmoid division of the ascending ramus posterior to the mandibular canal, either as part of a segmental resection in combination with removal of part of the horizontal ramus or in combination with a rim resection (Fig. 3.9). Once again, the surgeon

must be prepared to undertake removal of the remaining ramus if the pathologist reports inadequate excision of tumour. This approach has the considerable advantage of both limiting reconstruction to the need to replace the horizontal ramus, which is technically much simpler, and of offering better cosmesis and function by retaining the posterior border and the attached muscles of mastication.

RIM RESECTION

As indicated previously, rim resection is the colloquial surgical term used to denote resection of the alveolus with retention of the basal part of the body. Because of the influence of radiotherapy on the pattern of tumour spread to the mandible, this technique is virtually practicable only in the non-irradiated mandible.

There are two indications for rim resection—surgical convenience and the management of early tumour spread, whether genuine or suspected. The amount of bone and mucosa resected varies depending on the indication.

The alveolar mucoperiosteum is strongly adherent to the occlusal surface of the edentulous mandible, and can be very difficult to separate in the subperiosteal plane from the underlying bone. On occasion tumour or dysplastic change can extend sufficiently close to the alveolus that it becomes necessary to include the alveolar mucosa in the resection to obtain a satisfactory margin of excision. Under these circumstances, when tumour clearly does not involve the mandible, it may be surgically simpler to dissect the mucoperiosteum from the mandible as far as the alveolus and then resect the upper border of the mandible. This simplifies pathological assessment of the resection specimen as alveolar mucosa is easily identified. By resecting the mandible at a slightly lower level than the mucosal incision

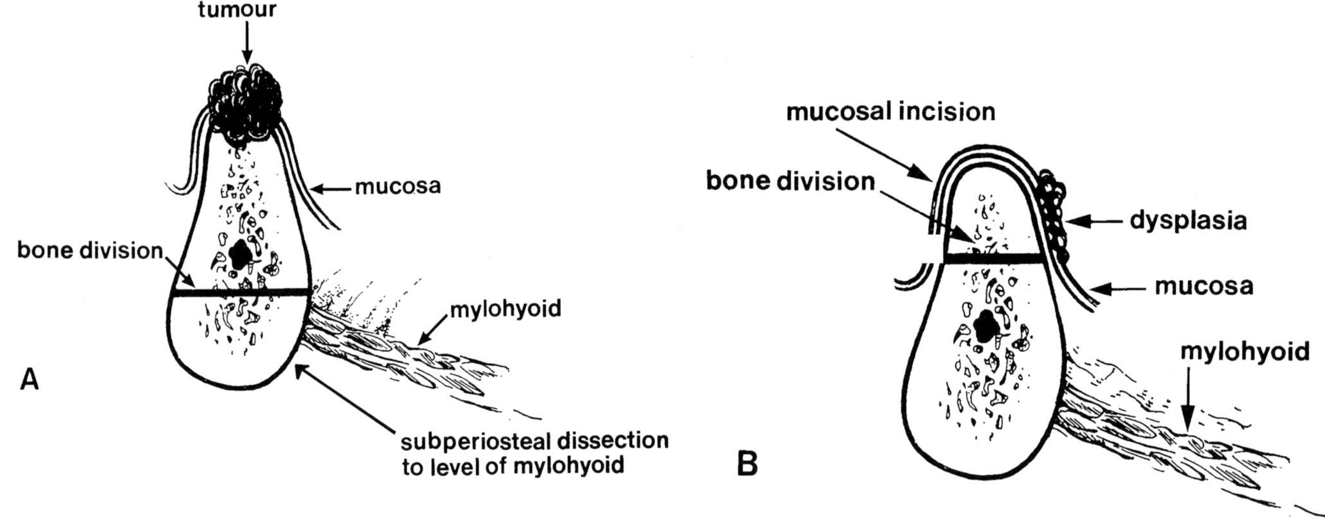

Fig. 3.10 Rim resection. **A** Tumour involving the occlusal surface—resection should include the mandibular canal and contents. **B** Rim resection for 'surgical convenience' to facilitate removal of required mucosa and subsequent repair.

on the non-tumour bearing side, the surgeon simplifies flap repair by giving himself adequate mucosa for subsequent suturing (Fig. 3.10). This is not practicable in the dentate mandible.

In contrast to rim resection for surgical convenience, for which the amount of bone removed is not critical, resection for suspected or genuine early tumour spread must be quite precise. As indicated previously, tumour spread within the mandible can occur in relation to the inferior alveolar nerve or within the medulla between cancellous bony trabeculae. The surgeon must resect sufficient bone to ensure complete removal of the inferior alveolar nerve along with an adequate margin of normal bone. If tumour clearly extends close to the mandibular canal, a rim resection is unlikely to be safe on pathological grounds and segmental resection is indicated.

Rim resection is greatly simplified by mandibular osteotomy. This allows identification of the mandibular foramen on the labial aspect and of the mylohyoid line on the lingual aspect which is the surface marking of the mandibular canal. Because perineural spread can extend beyond the main mass of tumour in the mandible, it is necessary to remove the entire mandibular canal from mental foramen to mandibular foramen. The inferior alveolar nerve should be divided at skull base level to ensure an adequate excision margin, as skip lesions have been described (Larson et al 1966).

It has been suggested that rim resection can be limited to the bone of the horizontal ramus (Barttelbort et al 1987). It has also been suggested that the nerve can be divided more proximally and pulled through the ascending ramus to accommodate this. This is a highly dubious procedure as there is no evidence that all tumour in relation to the nerve will be safely removed without producing seeding of tumour

from the nerve to the bone. If a rim resection is being undertaken on the grounds of early tumour spread, the entire mandibular canal should be removed with overlying alveolus and anterior border of the ramus (Fig. 3.10).

Division of the inferior alveolar nerve renders the lower lip and chin insensate on that side. This rarely represents a major problem for the patient, possibly as a result of some sensory crossover.

THE IRRADIATED MANDIBLE

Rim resection in early invasion of the non-irradiated mandible is practicable because of the predictable pattern of tumour spread to the bone. In contrast, the route of tumour spread to the irradiated mandible is unpredictable, as a result of which there is little prospect for any form of conservative surgery.

The options available are either to resect no bone, if the soft tissue tumour is not in proximity to the bone, or to carry out a full-thickness segmental resection of the mandible. The pattern of tumour infiltration of soft tissues around the mandible is both unpredictable and difficult to assess clinically. As a result, it is usually impossible to determine the degree of bone invasion, consequently resection of bone is best planned to match the soft tissue excision margins.

Osteotomy after radiotherapy may also carry a greater risk of complications for two reasons. First, a higher incidence of non-union is to be expected because of the loss of periosteal and endosteal function. Union may be fibrous rather than bony. Second, the incidence of wound healing problems in the oral cavity with leakage of saliva around the osteotomy site increases the risk of sinus or fistula formation and the risk of radionecrosis.

REFERENCES

Anderson D W 1960 Studies of the lymphatic pathways of bone and bone marrow. Journal of Bone and Joint Surgery 42A: 716

Atwood D A 1971 Reduction of residual ridges: a major oral disease entity. Journal of Prosthetic Dentistry 26: 266

Ballantyne A J, McCarten A B, Ibanez M L 1963 The extension of cancer of the head and neck through peripheral nerves. American Journal of Surgery 106: 651

Barttelbort S W, Bahn S L, Ariyan S 1987 Rim mandibulectomy for cancer of the oral cavity. American Journal of Surgery 154: 423

Bradley J C 1972 Age changes in the vascular supply of the mandible. British Dental Journal 132: 142

Butlin H T 1985 Diseases of the tongue. Cassell and Co Ltd, London, chs 17, 18

Campbell R L 1960 A comparative study of the resorption of the alveolar ridges in denture-wearers and non-denture-wearers. Journal of the American Dental Association 60: 143

Castelli W 1963 Vascular architecture of the human adult mandible. Journal of Dental Research 42: 786

Cohen L 1959 Venous drainage of the mandible. Oral Sugery, Oral Medicine, Oral Pathlology 12: 1447

Dubner S, Spiro R H 1991 Median mandibulotomy: a critical assessment. Head and Neck 13: 389

Edwards L F 1954 The edentulous mandible. Journal of Prosthetic Dentistry 4: 222

Fleming W B 1987 Marginal resection of the mandible in treatment of cancer of the floor of the mouth. Australian and New Zealand Journal of Surgery 57: 521

Kremen A J 1951 Cancer of the tongue—a surgical technique for a primary combined en bloc resection of tongue, floor of mouth and cervical lymphatics. Surgery 30: 227

Larson D L, Rodin A E, Roberts D K, O'Steen W K, Rappeport A S, Lewis S R 1966 Perineural lymphatics: myth or fact. American Journal of Surgery 112: 488

McGregor A D, MacDonald D G 1988a Routes of entry of squamous cell carcinoma to the mandible. Head and Neck Surgery 10: 294

McGregor A D, MacDonald D G 1988b Reactive changes in the mandible in the presence of squamous cell carcinoma. Head and Neck Surgery 10: 378

McGregor A D, MacDonald D G 1989a Patterns of spread of squamous cell carcinoma within the mandible. Head and Neck 11: 457

McGregor A D, MacDonald D G 1989b Age changes in the human inferior alveolar artery—a histological study. British Journal of Oral and Maxillofacial Surgery 27: 371

McGregor A D, MacDonald D G The vascular basis of lateral osteotomy of the mandible. Head and Neck (in press)

McGregor A D, MacDonald D G Patterns of spread of squamous cell carcinoma to the ramus of the mandible. Head and Neck (in press)

McGregor I A 1977 Reconstruction following excision of intraoral and mandibular tumours. In: Converse J H (ed) Reconstructive plastic surgery. W B Saunders, Philadelphia

McGregor I A, MacDonald D G 1983 Mandibular osteotomy in the approach to the oral cavity. Head and Neck Surgery 5: 457

McGregor I A, MacDonald D G 1987 Spread of squamous cell carcinoma to the non-irradiated edentulous mandible—a preliminary report. Head and Neck Surgery 9: 157

Marchetta F C, Sako K, Badillo J 1964 Periosteal lymphatics of the mandible and intraoral carcinoma. American Journal of Surgery 108: 505

Marchetta F C, Sako K, Murphy J B 1971 The periosteum of the mandible and intraoral carcinoma. American Journal of Surgery 122: 711

Muller H, Slootweg P J 1990 Mandibular invasion by oral squamous cell carcinoma. Clinical aspects. Journal of Cranio-Maxillo-Facial Surgery 18: 80

Nakamoto R Y 1968 Bony defects on the residual alveolar ridge. Journal of Prosthetic Dentistry 19: 11

Polya A E, von Navratil D 1902 Untersuchungen uber die Lymphbahnen der Wangenschleimhaut. Deutsche Zeitschrift fur Chirurgie 66: 122

Schram W R 1929 A histological study of repair in the maxillary bones following surgery. Journal of the American Dental Association 16: 1987

Shaha A R 1991 Preoperative evaluation of the mandible in patients with carcinoma of the floor of the mouth. Head and Neck 13: 398

Shiller W R, Wiswell O B 1954 Lingual foramina of the mandible. Anatomical Record 119: 387

Slaughter D P 1951 Discussion after Kremen (1951, above) Surgery 30: 239

Slootweg P J, Muller H 1989 Mandibular invasion by oral squamous cell carcinoma. Journal of Cranio-Maxillo-Facial Surgery 17: 69

Sutton R N 1974 The practical significance of mandibular accessory foramina. Australian Dental Journal 19: 167

Totsuka Y, Usui Y, Tei K, Fukuda H, Shindo M, Lizuka T, Amemiya A 1991 Mandibular involvement by squamous cell carcinoma of the lower alveolus: analysis and comparative study of histologic and radiologic features. Head and Neck 13: 40

Willis R A 1967 Pathology of tumours, 4th edn. Butterworths, London

4. Mandibular reconstruction with osteomyocutaneous flaps

Nilton T. Herter   Paulo R. Godoy   Ricardo G. Kroef

INTRODUCTION AND HISTORICAL REVIEW

The surgical treatment of primary mandibular tumours and tumours of the mouth involving the mandible varies according to the histological type and stage of advancement of the disease. The extent of resection may vary from enucleation to total mandibulectomy. Enucleation, gingivectomy and marginal mandibulectomy do not constitute major difficulties for the surgeon. On the other hand, segmental mandibulectomy, hemimandibulectomy or subtotal mandibulectomy may pose formidable problems particularly if large amounts of skin or soft tissues are removed en bloc.

Immediate mandible reconstruction associated with adequate skin resurfacing and/or reconstruction of intraoral lining and soft tissue replacement may require compound flaps for optimal protection of the bone. A variety of methods are now available including compound local flaps (Snyder et al 1970, Siemssen et al 1978), free bone transfers (Daniel 1977, Ariyan & Finseth 1978, Conley & Gullane 1980) and free osteomyocutaneous flaps (Taylor 1975). The use of vascularised bone transfers appear to be gaining favour among many head and neck surgeons (Cuono & Ariyan 1980). Conley (1972) illustrated several regional compound flaps (bone, muscle, skin) which were available for reconstructive procedures in the head and neck. These included the sternocleidomastoid muscle, the lateral trapezius carrying a segment of the clavicle or scapula and a combination of deltopectoral and pectoralis major flaps attached to a segment of rib.

In Argentina, Demergasso & Piazza (1977, 1979) presented their work on the lateral trapezius myocutaneous flap at the annual meeting of the Argentinian Pathologic Head and Neck Society. Shortly thereafter they described the lateral trapezius osteomyocutaneous flap carrying the spine of the scapula which was used for mandibular reconstruction.

This concept was different from that described by Conley (1972) as the vascular supply to the flap was given by the transverse cervical and suprascapular arteries. Bertotti (1980), Guillamondegui & Larson (1982) and Vila et al (1984) reinforced the use of the lateral trapezius osteomyocutaneous flap in head and neck reconstruction. This flap has been popular in South America and the authors believe that more than 200 patients have undergone mandible reconstruction using this procedure. Hueston & McConchie (1968) first described the pectoralis major myocutaneous flap but it was Ariyan (1979b) who further developed this flap and led to its popularity in head and neck reconstruction. Magee et al (1980) reported that the fifth rib could be carried with the myocutaneous flap for mandibular reconstruction and Cuono & Ariyan (1980) published the first reported case. Viability and active metabolism of the transferred rib was demonstrated by Ariyan (1980b) using tetracycline labelling in the postoperative period. Mendelson (1980) further showed the great versatility and value of the pectoralis myocutaneous flap. Further investigation into the vascular anatomy of the pectoralis muscle and overlying skin and subcutaneous tissue was performed by Freeman et al (1981). Pearlman et al (1983) published 10 cases of mandibular reconstruction using the pectoralis myocutaneous flap carrying a segment of rib attached to the flap. Other authors have developed the pectoralis osteomyocutaneous flap and given additional contributions (Little et al 1983, Azevedo 1987, Bell & Barron 1981, Bhathena & Karavana 1986). The technique was expanded to include a section of pleura attached to the rib so that it could be used for oral lining as a pectoralis major pleural osteomyocutaneous flap (Stromberg 1989). Green et al (1981) reported using the sternum attached to the pectoralis major muscle and Robertson (1986) reported 29 cases of mandibular reconstruction using a similar technique. Analagous to the pectoralis major osteomyocutaneous flap, Azevedo (1987) described the pectoralis minor osteomyocutaneous flap carrying the fifth or sixth rib.

The sternocleidomastoid flap was first described by Owens in 1955 and subsequently by Bakamjian (1963), Littlewood (1967) and Snyder et al (1970). Subsequently, Conley (1972) described a sternocleidomastoid osteomyocutaneous flap which included the medial segment of the clavicle. Siemssen et al (1978) reported the use of a myosseous flap utilising the clavicle attached to the sternocleidomastoid muscle and reported satisfactory results and minimal complications in 18 patients undergoing mandible reconstruction. Subsequently, Ariyan (1979a) described a similar technique but carrying a portion of overlying skin for oral lining. Larson & Goepfert (1982) have pointed out the limitations of the sternocleidomastoid myocutaneous flap in head and neck reconstruction particularly when used in combination with a neck dissection. We have extended the sternocleidomastoid technique for mandible reconstruction and will later describe an original technique which is not yet published. This uses a bilateral 'en bloc' sternocleidomastoid sternoclavicular osteomyocutaneous flap and has been successfully used to reconstruct mandibles in three patients submitted to subtotal mandibulectomy for benign tumours.

PREOPERATIVE PLANNING

By far the majority of patients requiring mandibulectomy present with a large primary or recurrent tumour in the mouth. Often patients have been treated previously by irradiation or surgery and most patients have fungating or excavating tumours infiltrating deeply into the skin of the chin or into the floor of the mouth and tongue. Commonly there is necrosis of the tumour with associated secondary infection. The mandible is infiltrated and shows osteolytic images on radiological studies. Infrequently mandibulectomy may be required for a large osteolytic benign tumour, a compact bone dysplasia, or an osteogenic sarcoma.

In addition to considering the state of the mandible, the site of the malignancy, and histological type will determine the likelihood and presence of cervical lymph node metastases. By far the majority of cases will require some form of neck dissection associated with the resection of the primary tumour.

Cancer resection and reconstructive procedures must be planned together. The surgical ablative procedure for such patients is planned as an enlarged 'commando' operation and often implies a radical neck dissection, mandibulectomy, hemiglossectomy and resection of large amounts of skin and surrounding tissues. While planning the surgery the minimum clearance margin is 2 cm on infiltrated skin and 1 cm on the mucosal surface. The authors recommend the use of multiple frozen sections at the time of surgery.

The operation must be performed 'en bloc' and creates a formidable problem for reconstruction. Large amounts of skin are required for skin resurfacing and oral lining and bone is required for mandibular reconstruction. The bone graft must be tailored and curved to reproduce the arch particularly if the symphysis of the mandible is resected. In the case of hemimandibulectomy an articulation must be created at the temporomandibular joint to enable adequate mandibular function.

Osteomyocutaneous flaps can provide enough skin for both resurfacing the external skin and for replacing intraoral lining in addition to bone for mandibular reconstruction. The soft tissue provides cover and protection for the bone. Among many osteomyocutaneous flaps which can be employed for these purposes the pectoralis major osteomyocutaneous flap is the most versatile but the lateral trapezius and the sternocleidomastoid osteomyocutaneous flaps may have specific and special indications.

Preparation of the patient for major surgery is an important part of preoperative planning. Prior to admission dental care and necessary extraction of infected teeth are performed. Routine tests include cardiovascular and pulmonary function studies, blood chemistry paying particular attention to anaemia, hypoproteinaemia and dehydration. On occasions blood chemistry will identify conditions which require correction prior to surgery and may require hospitalisation for a few days.

The patient is usually admitted to the hospital 24 h prior to surgery. The patient is cross-matched with approximately 2.5 l of available blood. Because of the risk of contamination in such operations, the authors believe that antibiotics should start 24 h before and continue 36 h after the surgical procedure. Carvalho et al (1986) have reported that antiseptic technique using povidone-iodine reduces the incidence of postoperative infections. Becker & Welch (1990) recommend the use of clindamycin 600 mg IV preoperatively and continuation with 900 mg every 8 h for the following 4 days.

The patient is prepared for surgery with the shaving of all hair of the face, mastoid area, neck, shoulder and anterior chest.

Although intranasal intubation is the method of choice patients should be warned as to the likelihood of tracheostomy which may be considered at the beginning or at the end of surgery.

EXCISION TECHNIQUES

Extensive surgical excisions will require en bloc resection of the mandible and cervical lymph nodes using an enlarged commando type of operation. The technique of radical neck dissection in association with mandibulectomy is well known among head and neck surgeons (Crile 1906, Martin 1957, Freund 1967, Elliot 1969, Barbosa 1974). If the skin is not infiltrated by cancer the incision in the neck has a vertical component combined with a transverse line placed in the submandibular triangle beginning at the mastoid process. A split of the lower lip is not mandatory but may provide useful access depending on the extent of excision of the mandible and intraoral lining. If a paddle of skin is to be resected the vertical component starts at the lower line of the circle encompassing the infiltrated skin. Where skin is infiltrated by cancer the platysma muscle is sacrificed and remains attached to the specimen. Bilateral neck dissection may be required, combining a radical neck dissection on one side with supraomohyoid neck dissection on the opposite side.

Table 4.1 Mandible reconstruction using osteomyocutaneous flaps (OMCFs)

Clavicle	—	Sternocleidomastoid OMCF
Scapula	—	Lateral trapezius OMCF
Sternum	—	Pectoralis major OMCF
Rib	—	Pectoralis major OMCF
Lateral rib	—	Pectoralis major OMCF
Rib–pleura	—	Pectoralis major OMCF
Rib	—	Pectoralis minor OMCF

The techniques of neck dissection have been described elsewhere but the importance of considering both excision and reconstruction at the same operation cannot be over-emphasised when considering the lateral trapezius osteo-myocutaneous flap. When this flap is considered for man-dibular reconstruction it is important to isolate and preserve the transverse cervical artery in the posterior cervical trian-gle in the course of performing a neck dissection.

In resection of the mandible it is desirable to save as much chin as possible and also a portion of the ascending ramus bearing the condyle. The mandible should be transected several centimetres beyond any area of attachment of the tumour to the bone. The gum and periosteum are raised from the bone with a periosteal elevator at the point where it is to be divided. The ascending ramus may be disarticulated or transected. Disarticulation is indicated only where tu-mour infiltrates deeply into bone or into the pterygoid fossa. The mandible is transected using an electric saw or Gigli saw and during section of the bone it is essential to stabilise the mandible using suitable Ferguson forceps. After division of the mandible the neck dissection specimen attached to the mandible is displaced outwards and the digastric, mylohyoid and hypoglossal muscles are transected just cephalad to the hyoid bone. The external facial artery is tied and divided so that only the tongue and the floor of the mouth remain attached to the specimen.

Encompassing the tumour may require hemiglossectomy or anterior glossectomy. The lingual and hypoglossal nerves and the lingual artery are divided if necessary. After the last attachment has been completely transected, the entire speci-men of neck dissection, mandible and tongue is removed en bloc. Haemostasis is secured. Routinely the authors soak the operative field with povidone-iodine solution following removal of the surgical specimen.

RECONSTRUCTION TECHNIQUES

A wide variety of osteomyocutaneous flaps (OMCFs) have been used in mandible reconstruction (Table 4.1). Some of these techniques are worthy of further consideration.

THE CLAVICLE–STERNOCLEIDOMASTOID OMCF

The sternocleidomastoid muscle (SCM) has two compo-nents to its inferior insertion. The medial tendinous portion arises from the sternum and the lateral muscular portion from the clavicle. The superior head is inserted into the mastoid process. Innervation of the SCM is from the spinal branch of the spinal accessory nerve and branches from the second and third cervical nerves. The muscle is supplied via a segmental blood supply. The superior pedicle arises from the occipital artery or directly from the external carotid artery and crosses just cephalad to the hypoglossal nerve. The middle artery to the SCM is a branch of the superior thyroid artery and enters the muscle at its anterior border. The inferior pedicle arises from the thyrocervical trunk and penetrates the muscle posteriorly at its clavicular head (Fig. 4.1).

Technique

A paddle of skin over the clavicle is designed together with the cervical incisions required for mandibulectomy and neck dissection. The skin is attached to the underlying muscle and fascia with temporary sutures to prevent shear-ing. The clavicle is freed from the subclavius and pectoralis major muscles and transected laterally and medially with a Gigli saw. The clavicular periosteum is preserved and the clavicle remains attached by the clavicular head of the SCM (Fig. 4.1B). The tendinous head of the SCM should be cut to allow the clavicle to be displaced upwards. Dissection proceeds in a cranial direction and the inferior vascular pedicle to the SCM is ligated. The muscle is freed from its posterior attachment up to the level of C3 which is identified and cut, saving the phrenic nerve. The spinal accessory nerve must also be identified and preserved at the posterior cervical triangle. The middle SCM artery may be identified at the anterior border of the muscle superior to the omohyoid. Often this artery can be preserved to ensure optimal vascularity of the flap.

The flap is elevated and the clavicle bone placed in the mandibular defect (Fig. 4.1C). Siemssen et al (1978) stablised the joints by mortising medially and by plugging distally, reinforcing with wire sutures, but plates can also be used. The length of the clavicle is approximately 8 cm with range of 6–12 cm. Optimal protection for the bone graft is assured by meticulous suturing of the buccal mucosa and the paddle of the skin used for oral lining.

At completion of the operation haemostasis is secured and the neck wounds closed with interrupted simple 000 monofilament nylon sutures with insertion of suction drains in the neck (Fig. 4.1D).

Indications

a. Benign tumours, dysplasia and non-neoplastic condi-tions

b. Primary tumours of the mandible.

Contraindications

a. Metastasis to cervical lymph nodes.

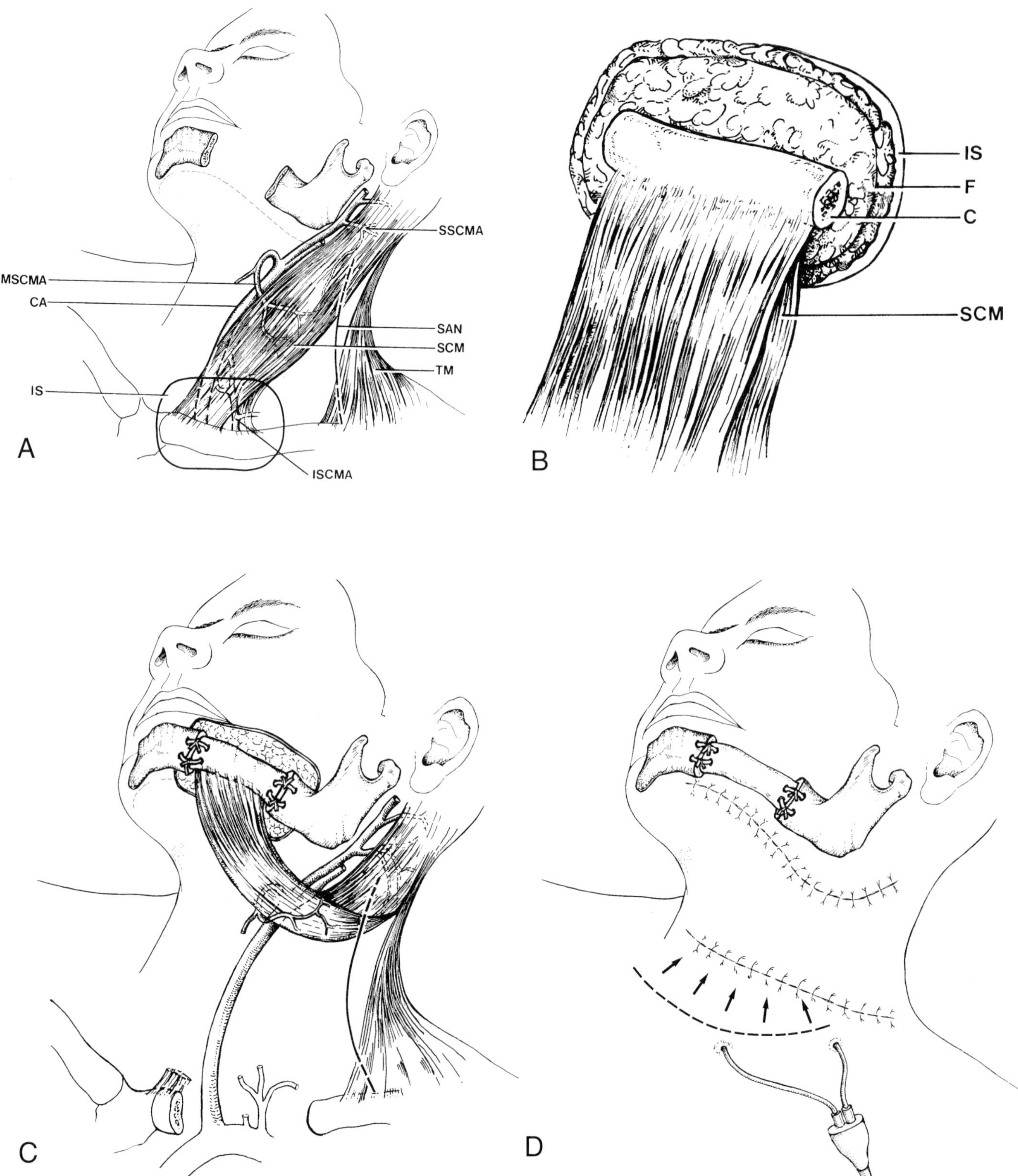

Fig. 4.1 **A** Anatomy of the clavicle-sternocleidomastoid OMCF. Note the three vascular pedicles: the inferior (ISCMA), the middle (MSCMA) and the superior (SSCMA). TM = trapezius muscle; SAN = spinal accessory nerve; SCM = sternocleidomastoid muscle; IS = island of skin, CA = carotid artery. **B** the compound flap includes the sternocleidomastoid (SCM) attached to the clavicle (C), which in turn is attached to the overlying fascia (F) and skin (IS). **C** The flap is transposed preserving the middle and superior vascular pedicles and the spinal accessory nerve. The skin is used to reline the oral cavity and the clavicle fixed to the mandibular stumps. **D** The wounds are closed directly by advancing the skin edges and suction drainage inserted.

Problems and complications

The disadvantages and restrictions of the sternocleidomastoid OMCF are well described by Larson & Goepfert (1982). The arc of the rotation of the flap is limited by the course of the spinal accessory nerve, but a few centimetres can be gained by blunt dissection of the nerve among the muscular fibres. In obese patients and those with a short neck the flap can be very bulky. When an island of skin is taken distal to the clavicle, the deltopectoral flap is destroyed. In such cases, the pectoralis major myocutaneous flap can be used for resurfacing the neck. Although the carotid sheath loses the protection of the SCM, this constitutes no major problem if the pedicle of the flap is superior.

The main problem is the viability of this flap, particularly when it is used for intraoral lining where partial cutaneous loss has been reported as around 50%. In our own experience, of over 15 cases, this complication occurs in approximately 35% of cases. To minimise this problem it is essential to preserve the thin middle sternocleidomastoid artery and to fix the island of skin to the underlying muscle and fascia to prevent shearing.

The most important restriction regarding the use of the sternocleidomastoid myocutaneous flap is its association with neck dissection. Obviously radical neck dissection destroys the flap. However, in patients with N0 or N1 disease with a single submandibular or subdigastric lymph node a modified neck dissection can be performed.

According to Conley & Gullane (1980) the use of the compound flap with bone and muscle has negligible morbidity when the medial head of the clavicle is used. Snyder et al (1970) and Siemssen et al (1978) found that their experience taught them to use the full thickness of the clavicle with the enveloping and intact periosteum. In patients where a partial thickness of the clavicle was used there were problems with fracture, resorption and infection at the donor site as well as at the recipient site. The full thickness of the clavicle is now taken with preservation of the lateral head of the clavicle, which is important from a functional point of view.

THE BILATERAL EN BLOC STERNOCLAVICULAR–STERNOCLEIDOMASTOID OMCF

Anatomy

The anatomy of the SCM has been described above including the classic compound flaps with the medial segment of the clavicle attached to the SCM. Both clavicles join the manubrium of the sternum via the incisura clavicularis and are separated by the incisura jugularis. The manubrium is a well vascularised and thick bone, its blood supply coming via the periosteum. The inferior head of sternocleidomastoid (medial component) inserts into the superior cephalad border of the manubrium. The sternohyoid and sternothyroid muscles insert into the posterior aspect of the bone a few centimetres caudally. The portion of bone between the two clavicles may be transferred together with both medial segments of the clavicles and used for replacing the anterior arch of the mandible. The sternoclavicular joints facilitate the adjustments and insetting of the clavicles and the overlying skin can be used to replace intraoral lining (Fig. 4.2A).

Technique

The patient is positioned in the supine position with a pillow placed underneath the shoulders and a transverse ribbon of skin approximately 4 × 20 cm is outlined over the manubrium and clavicles. This is combined with a midline incision extending from the lower lip to the suprasternal notch (Fig. 4.2A). Using a lower lip midline split, two wide lateral flaps are raised until the posterior border of the SCMs. The platysma is included in these flaps. The mandible and anterior neck are widely exposed enabling mandibulectomy to be performed.

The ribbon of skin is fixed with temporary sutures to the underlying muscle and fascia to avoid avulsion and shearing of the skin during elevation of the flap. This preserves the delicate vascular network between the skin and the muscle. The posterior borders of the SCMs are freed from their posterior attachments paying particular attention to branches of the cervical nerves and the external jugular vein. The inferior sternocleidomastoid arteries are identified and divided as are the connecting veins joining the anterior and the external jugular veins. The superior head of the pectoralis major muscles are detached from the clavicles with electrocautery. The periosteum of the clavicles is preserved at its attachment to the sternocleidomastoid. The clavicles are transected laterally using a Gigli saw and detached from the subclavius muscles. The suprasternal fossa is dissected and the posterior deep surface of the manubrium is exposed. With the clavicles divided they are gently retracted cephalad and freed from any underlying tissue. An avenue is created between the two costoclavicular angles and a Gigli saw is passed behind the manubrium (Fig. 4.2B). The saw is angled downwards and the upper manubrium is transected transversely.

A thick bone graft from the manubrium approximately 3 cm in width can be taken together with the two articulated arms of the clavicles. Both SCMs are dissected upwards until the middle sternocleidomastoid arteries are identified. These arteries arise from the superior thyroid arteries and penetrate each muscle at its anterior border. These vascular pedicles must be preserved. Posteriorly the SCMs are released up to the level of the emergence of the spinal accessory nerves. The compound en bloc flap is now ready for transfer and contains the manubrium and two medioclavicular segments together with overlying skin. The bone is inset between the mandibular stumps and fixation is achieved using plates and plugging. The sternoclavicular joints are opened and the disc and cartilaginous portions resected.

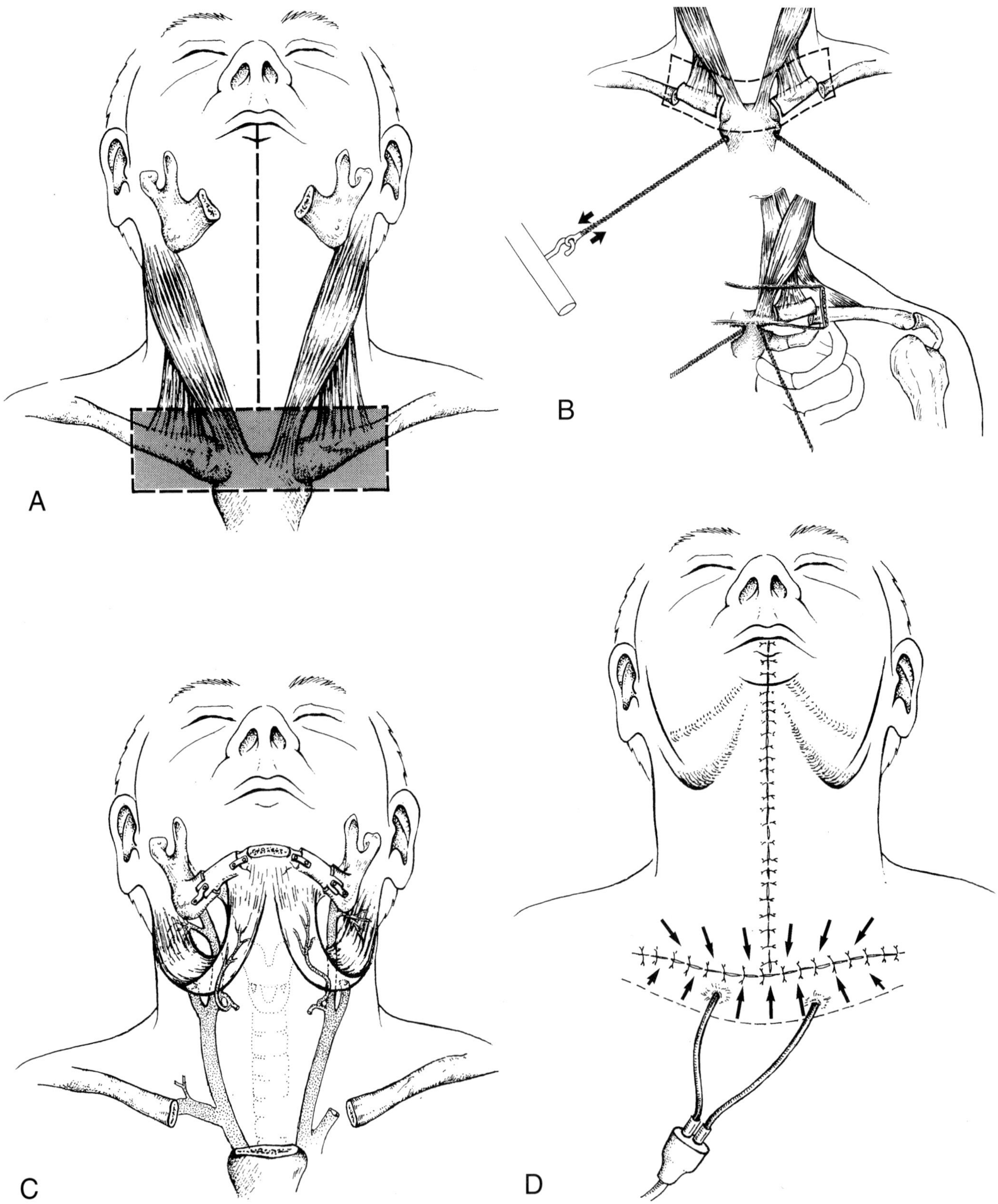

Fig. 4.2 **A** Outline of the bilateral (en bloc) sternoclavicular–sternocleidomastoid OMCF. The flap includes the manubrium and the medial ends of the clavicles together with an overlying horizontal paddle of skin. The verticle lip and chin splitting gives access to the neck and oral cavity. **B** A Gigli saw is used to divide the manubrium. **C** The flap is transposed preserving the superior and middle vascular pedicles of the sternocleidomastoid bilaterally. The cartilaginous portions of the sternoclavicular joints are removed and the bone fixed in position with plates. **D** The wound is closed directly by approximating the skin edges and suction drains are inserted.

Plates are again used for fixation at these joints (Fig. 4.2C). The overlying skin is used to replace intraoral lining and is sutured to the remaining buccal mucosa. Finally the infrahyoid musculature is reattached to the reconstructed mandible by placing some sutures between the remaining infrahyoid muscles and the manubrium.

Following complete haemostasis suction drains are inserted into the neck wounds which are closed with interrupted simple 000 monofilament nylon sutures. The donor area is closed directly by advancing the surrounding skin (Fig. 4.2D).

Indications

Angle-to-angle mandibulectomy particularly in bone tumours or non-neoplastic conditions (Fig. 4.3).

Contraindications

a. Metastasis to cervical lymph nodes.
b. Where a large island of skin is required for external cover.

Problems and complications

As a rule the problems with this compound flap are the same as those described previously for the unilateral flap. However, the use of the cephalad border of the manubrium to replace the anterior mandible requires only a few centimetres of the medial head of the clavicle, minimising the problems with clavicle resection. The upper part of the manubrium has no special function and can be transferred to the head without sequelae. The sternoclavicular joints facilitate shaping the mandible to the required curvature without the necessity to fracture. A good result can be achieved and the ribbon of skin transferred for oral lining appears to be more reliable than that taken with a single ipsilateral muscle. The donor site is closed directly by advancing the surrounding skin.

THE SCAPULA–LATERAL TRAPEZIUS OMCF

Anatomy

The trapezius is flat, triangular muscle, extending over the posterior part of the neck and shoulders. Its lateral head arises from the lateral head of the clavicle, the acromion and the spine of the scapula. The fibres run transversely as a fan inserted into the midline between the external occipital protuberance and the spinal process of T12. Innervation of trapezius is provided by the spinal accessory nerve and branches of C3 and C4.

There are three vascular pedicles supplying this muscle. The main one is the suprascapular artery which lies transversely behind the clavicle and originates from the thyrocervical trunk. The second is the superficial transverse cervical artery arising from the same thyrocervical trunk and the third pedicle is the deep transverse cervical artery arising from the subclavian artery and emerging through the brachial plexus. There are two axial arterial branches from the muscles to the skin over the shoulder and a rich vascular network connecting the trapezius and the periosteum of the spine of the scapula which may be carried with the muscle (Fig. 4.4A).

Technique

An island of skin is outlined around the acromioclavicular joint. This island of skin is encompassed in the incisions required for radical neck dissection. The trapezius muscle is detached from the clavicle with electrocautery early in the surgical procedure. Careful dissection in the retroclavicular fat enables the suprascapular artery to be indentified. The posterior belly of omohyoid is identified and transected. The next step is to detach the deltoid muscles from the spine of the scapula. The spine of the scapula is then exposed and the length of bone required is isolated. The acromioclavicular joint is transected with heavy Mayo scissors or Lister shears. The infraspinatus muscle is retracted downwards to expose the inferior surface of the spine, which can then be transected with a reciprocating Stryker saw and detached from the scapula (Fig. 4.4B). The periosteum of the spine must be preserved and the bone graft maintained attached to the trapezius muscle and to the fatty vascular pedicle which includes the suprascapular artery. Digital dissection enables the supraspinatus muscle to be detached from the spine. The trapezius muscle can now be transected using electrocautery in a direction parallel to the previously identified vascular pedicle. The amount of muscle included in the compound flap is determined by the length of spine required for reconstruction. The distal end of the suprascapular artery is ligated and the flap raised from the shoulder and prepared for transfer.

The full vascular pedicle is inspected comprising the deep transverse cervical artery crossing the brachial plexus, the superficial transverse cervical artery and the suprascapular artery. Depending on the length of flap required for reconstruction, the deep or superficial transverse cervical arteries may be ligated. The main arterial supply for the flap is the suprascapular artery whose pedicle must be preserved with all retroclavicular areolar fat.

The suprascapular nerve lies deep in the retroclavicular fossa overlying the subclavius muscle and posterior to the vascular pedicle. This nerve must be preserved as it is essential in maintaining the tone of the supraspinatus muscle and the attachment of the humerus to the scapula. If the spinal accessory nerve is intact following the neck dissection it may be preserved by tailoring the flap, transecting the trapezius muscle just caudal to the penetration of the nerve into the muscle.

After releasing the last muscular attachment the com-

compound flap is transferred to the oral cavity. The island of skin for oral lining is sutured first of all and the bone graft inserted between the remaining mandibular stumps. Prior to wire fixation the bone is tailored for better adjustment. If a hemimandibulectomy had been performed the new ascending ramus is plugged into the temporalis fossa and fixed to the zygomatic arch with a wire suture (Fig. 4.4C).

The island of skin can also be used for external resurfacing using a de-epithelised ribbon between the intraoral and external components.

The donor site must be closed meticulously. The infraspinatus muscle is sutured to the supraspinatus muscle and fixed to the deltoid muscle using non-absorbable sutures (Fig. 4.4D). The deltoid muscle is then inserted into the

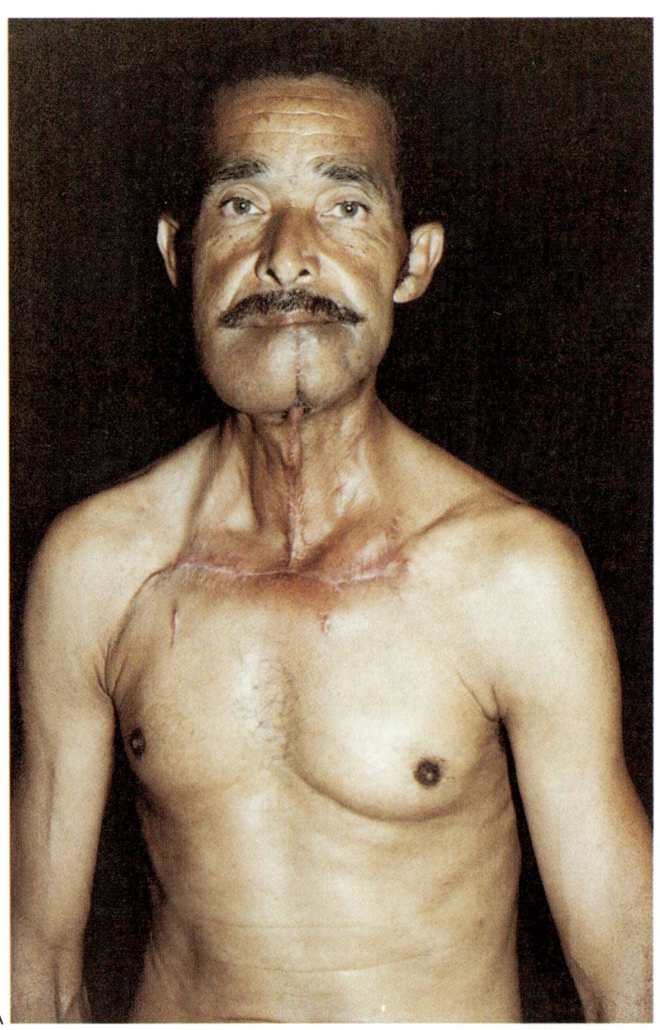

A

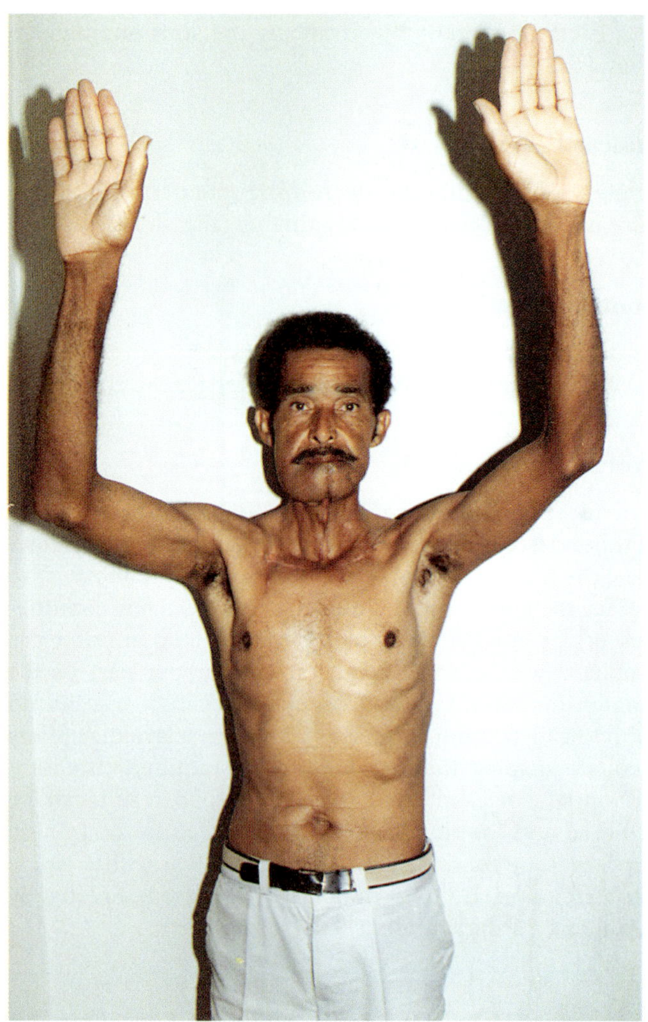

B

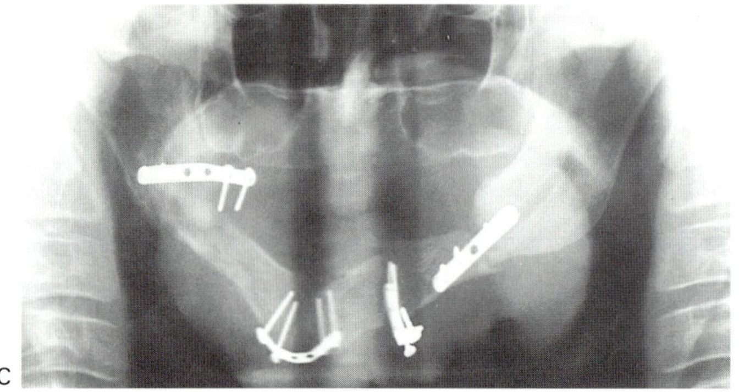

C

Fig. 4.3 **A** Total symphyseal reconstruction using the bilateral en bloc sternoclavicular–sternocleidomastoid. **B** Good shoulder mobility and function is retained despite resection of the medial ends of clavicle and upper portion of manubrium. **C** The bone is fixed in position using plates. Plates are similarly used to obtain the curvature of the mandible following resection of the cartilaginous portions of the sternoclavicular joints.

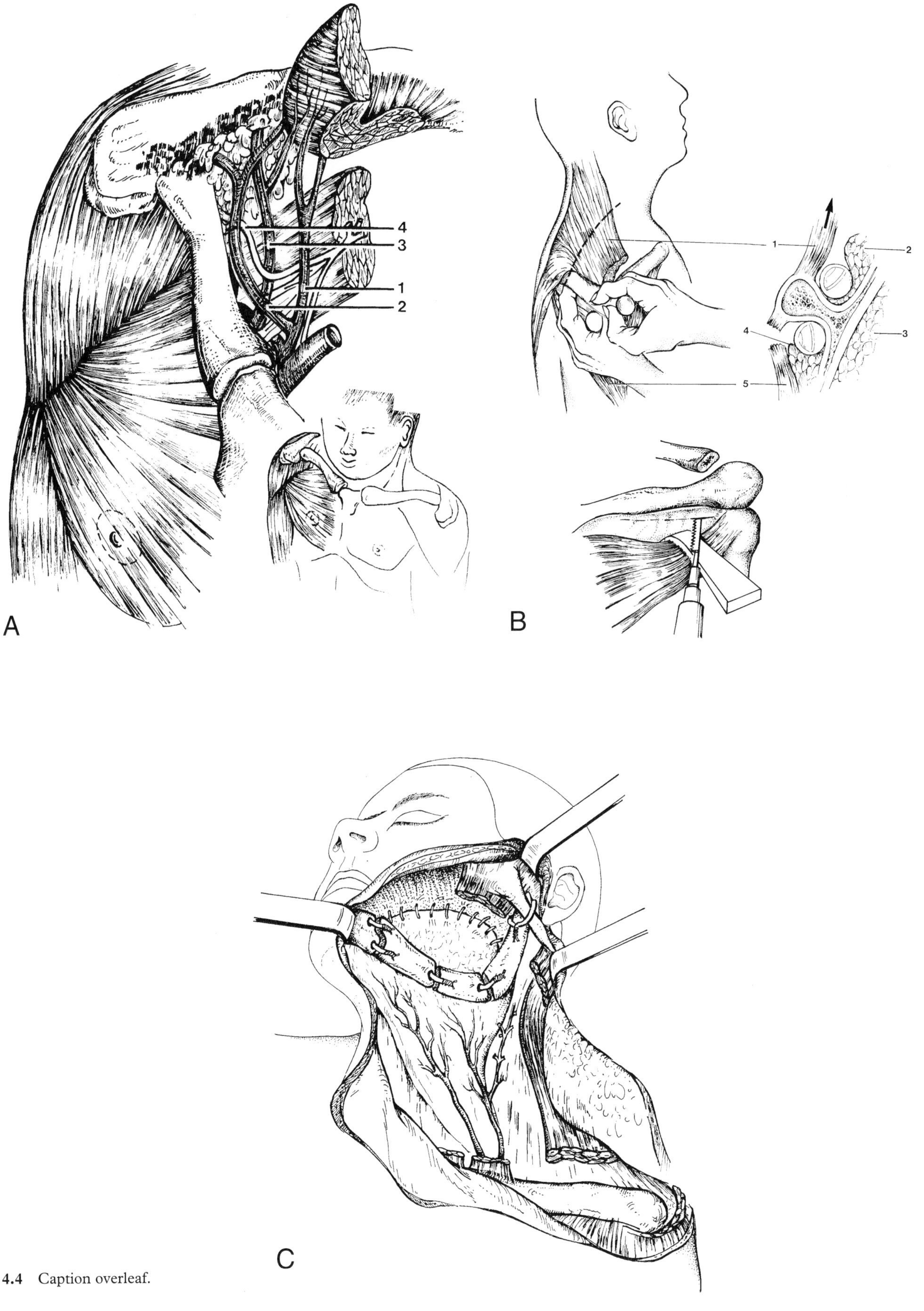

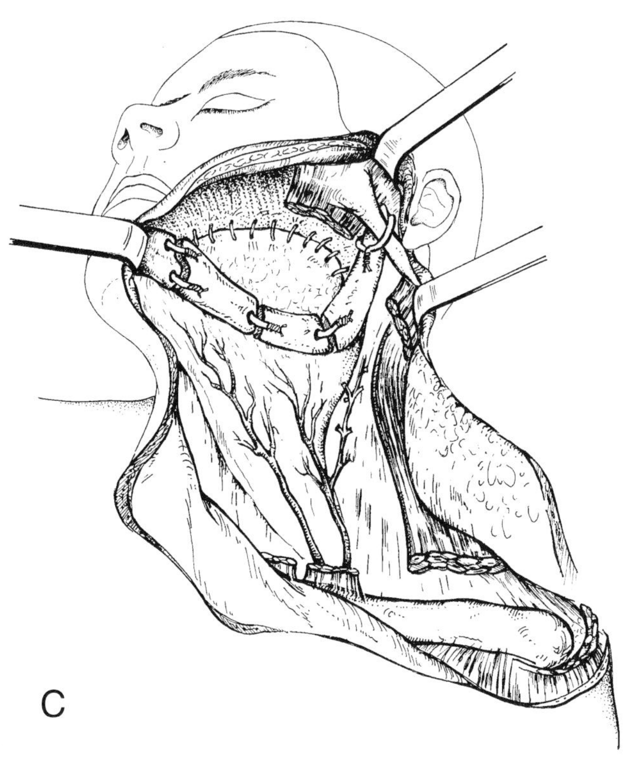

Fig. 4.4 Caption overleaf.

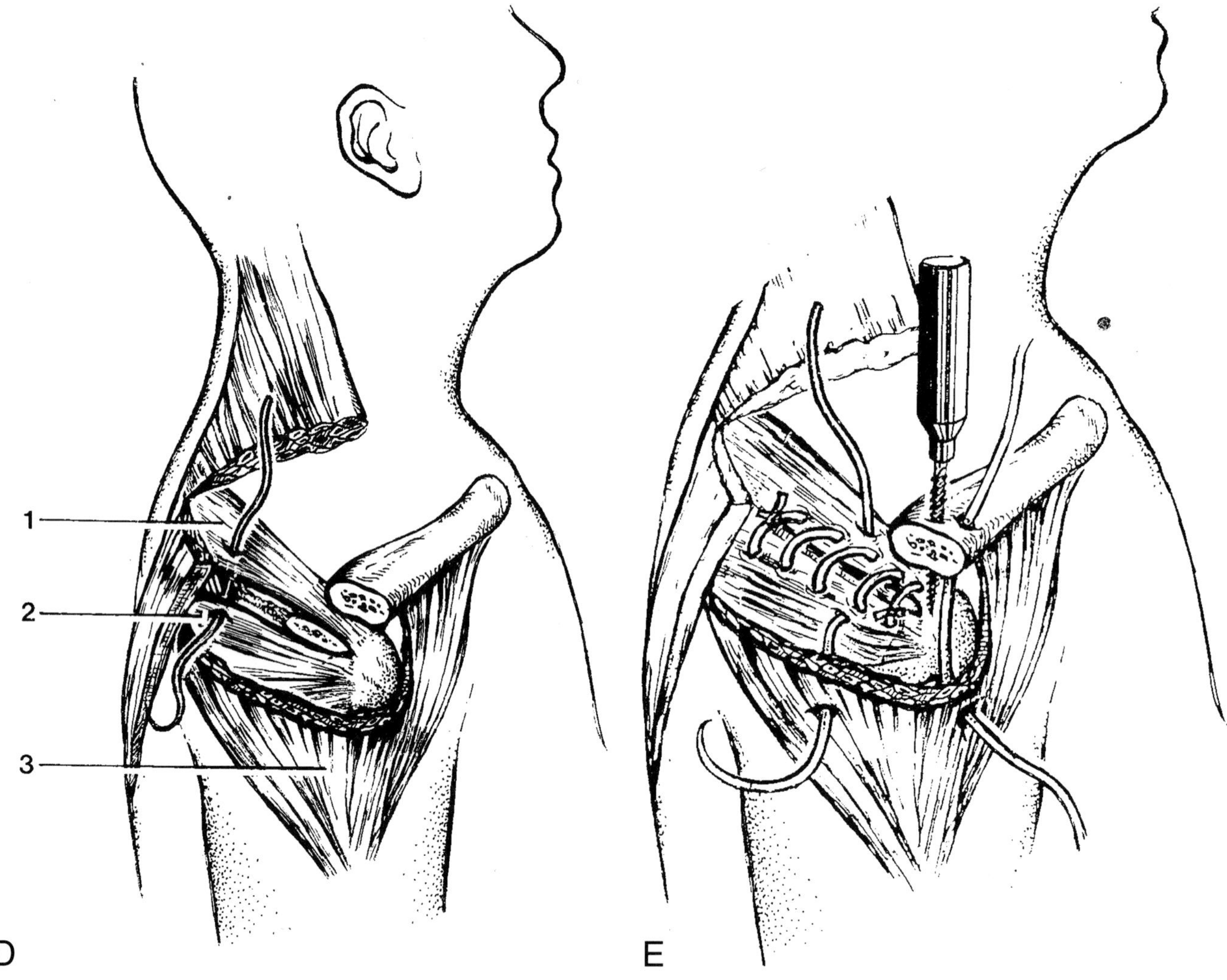

Fig. 4.4   A   Vascular anatomy of the scapula-lateral trapezius OMCF. 1 = the suprascapular artery; 2 = the superficial tansverse cervical artery; 3 = the deep transverse cervical artery emerging through the brachial plexus 4 = the suprascapular nerve. **B** Digital dissection deep to trapezius muscle (1). The spine of the scapula is isolated by gently dissecting off the supraspinatus muscle (2) and the infraspinatus muscle (4). The deltoid muscle (5) is divided from its attachment to the spine. The subscapularis muscle (3) remains intact on the deep inner surface of the scapula. With the spine exposed it can be transected using a reciprocating Stryker saw. **C** The composite flap is transferred. The spine of the scapula has undergone osteotomy to change direction to form the ascending and horizontal ramus. The new ascending ramus is fixed to the zygomatic arch using a wire suture. **D** Meticulous closure of the donor defect is required. The supraspinatus muscle (1) is sutured to the infraspinatus muscle (2) and both are sutured to the deltoid muscle (3). **E** The deltoid is fixed to the clavicle via multiple drill holes in the bone. (Reproduced with permission from Demergasso & Piazza 1979)

clavicle via multiple drill holes in the bone and non-absorbable sutures (Fig. 4.4E). Once haemostasis is secured the neck wounds are closed and suction drains inserted. The donor area can often be closed following mobilisation of the surrounding skin or a skin graft can be used or part of the wound left open to heal by secondary intention.

Indications

a.   Anterior arch of mandible
b.   Lateral ramus of mandible
c.   Anterior arch and lateral ramus (Fig. 4.5)
d.   Hemimandibulectomy
e.   Intraoral lining and external skin resurfacing.

Contraindications

Division and ligation of the suprascapular artery.

Problems and complications

The main advantages of the lateral trapezius OMCF is its rich vascularity and versatility in mandible reconstruction. Only a few centimetres of spine of the scapula may be taken for small bone reconstructions or almost the whole spine for subtotal mandibular reconstruction. The compound flap is ideal for reconstruction of the anterior arch providing at the same time skin for lining and outer resurfacing.

In patients previously submitted to a radical neck

dissection in which the superficial transverse cervical artery has been ligated the remaining suprascapular artery assures satisfactory viability of the flap. In such cases, careful dissection of the retroclavicular areas is required to prevent damage to the suprascapular artery. When the spinal accessory nerve has been cut it is extremely important to preserve the suprascapular nerve to minimise functional disturbances and pain in the shoulder. In such cases, it is perhaps better to choose another method of reconstruction as the potential loss of the 11th nerve is the most significant problem and patients must be commenced on vigorous physiotherapy for shoulder rehabilitation.

The island of skin of the lateral trapezius OMCF may be divided in two to provide skin for oral lining and outer resurfacing. The flap is usually thin enough and there is little excess weight and bulk. Closure of the donor defect is difficult but there is no major problem in secondary intention healing as there are no vital structures in the area. In

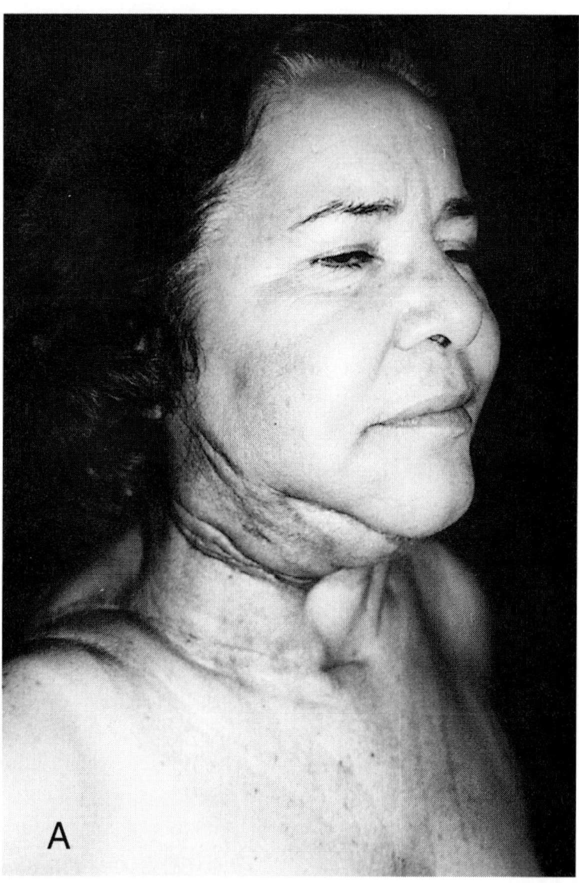

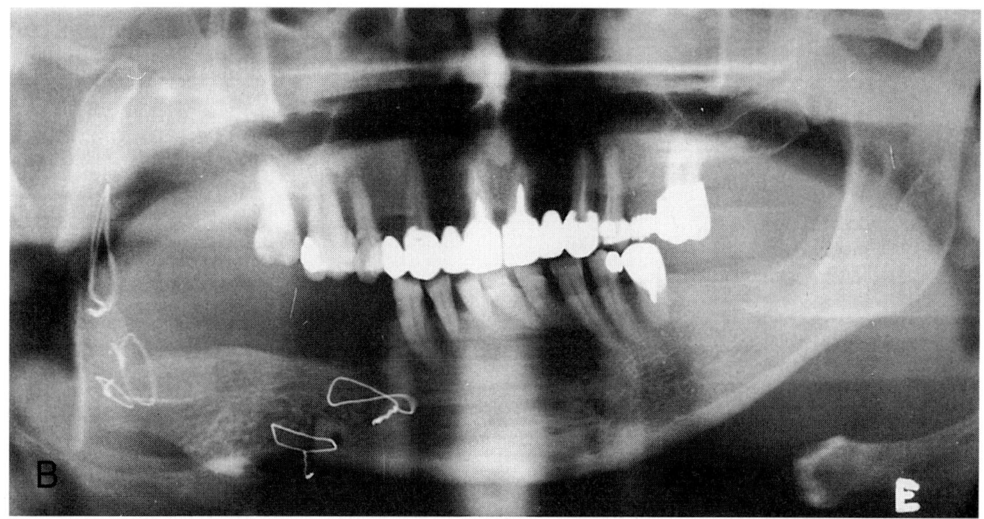

Fig. 4.5
Caption overleaf.

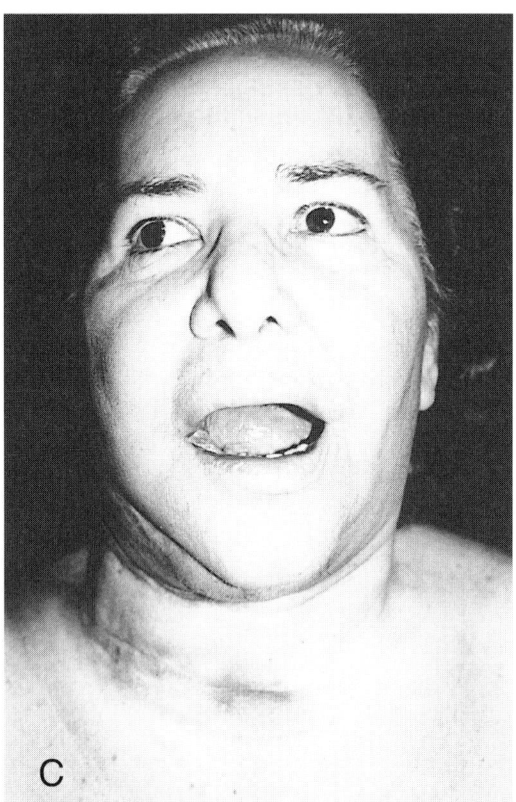
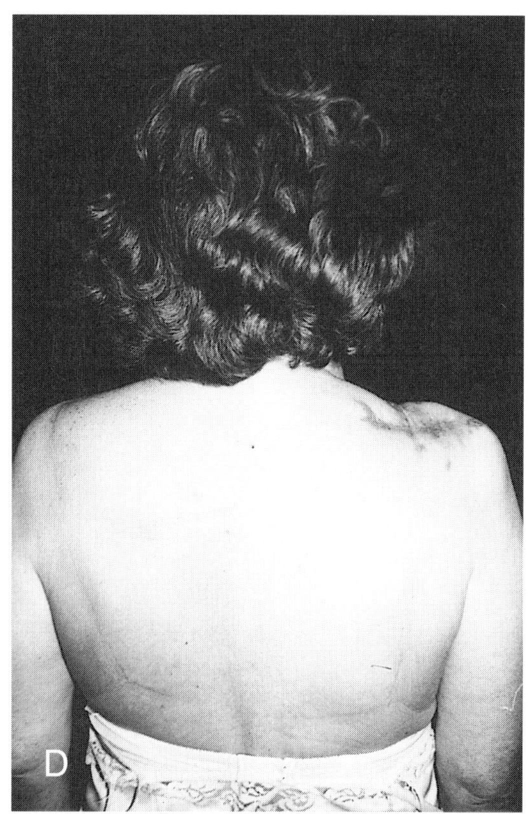

Fig. 4.5 **A** Reconstruction of the right mandible with a scapula–trapezius OMCF. **B** OPT shows the extent of the mandible reconstruction. A formal osteotomy in the scapula is required to shape the reconstructed mandible. **C** Good jaw mobility and mouth opening is achieved. **D** The donor defect has been closed directly.

some cases the defect can be closed using a skin graft.

The most important complication in mandible reconstruction is partial or total loss of the flap. Careful dissection of the suprascapular and transverse cervical arteries is essential. These arteries should be ligated only after they have given their perforating branches to the trapezius muscle. This is on the back where they enter the deep planes of the shoulders. To avoid ischaemia of the bone it is necessary to preserve carefully the periosteum of the spine of the scapula and the vascular network carried by the insertion of the trapezius into the spine. Minor complications have generally been associated with local wound problems such as seroma and localised infection, limited wound dehiscence and partial loss of the skin graft at the donor site. This flap requires careful planning and appropriate positioning of the patient at the beginning of the operation. It is rather laborious and requires an advanced degree of surgical skill.

THE STERNUM–PECTORALIS MAJOR OMCF

Anatomy

The pectoralis major is a triangular muscle comprising three heads. The superior head arises from the medial segment of the clavicle. The medial head arises from the sternum and from the adjacent cartilaginous portions of the second to the sixth ribs. The caudal head arises from the aponeurosis of the external oblique muscle and upper rectus sheath with extensions to the sixth rib. The free border of the muscle inserts inferiorly into the medial head of the sixth rib. The muscle is inserted laterally into the greater tuberosity of the humerus.

Innervation of the pectoralis major muscle is provided by lateral and medial pectoral nerves. The blood supply arises from three sources. The major pedicle is the pectoral branch of the thoracoacromial artery. A second pedicle is the lateral thoracic artery and the third the superior thoracic artery (Fig. 4.6A). These vascular pedicles assure optimal perfusion of the muscle and overlying skin. In addition there is an extensive vascular network connecting muscle and periosteum of the sternum and ribs as reported by Medgyesi (1973) and Ariyan (1980b).

Technique

A vertical paddle of skin measuring approximately 5 x 10 cm centred over the sternum and the chondrosternal joints is outlined. This is combined with two transverse thoracic incisions placed as a reverse deltopectoral flap with the lower incision located just below the inferior border of the pectoralis major muscle. The skin flap of the pectoralis major is raised and the muscle exposed. The paddle of skin is fixed to the underlying muscle and fascia by temporary sutures to avoid avulsion of the skin during elevation of the flap. This manoeuvre maintains the delicate vascular network between muscle and skin (Fig. 4.6A). A longitudinal incision is made on the sternum using a Stryker oscillating saw extending

through the outer table. The length of the sternal bone graft required is taken as low as possible in the sternum to allow a wide arc of rotation up to the mouth without tension. Two transverse cuts are made from the midline to the ipsilateral border of the sternum. The muscle is elevated from the costochondral junctions and using a curved osteotome the compound flap is detached and elevated. Some perforating vessels arising from the internal mammary artery are ligated.

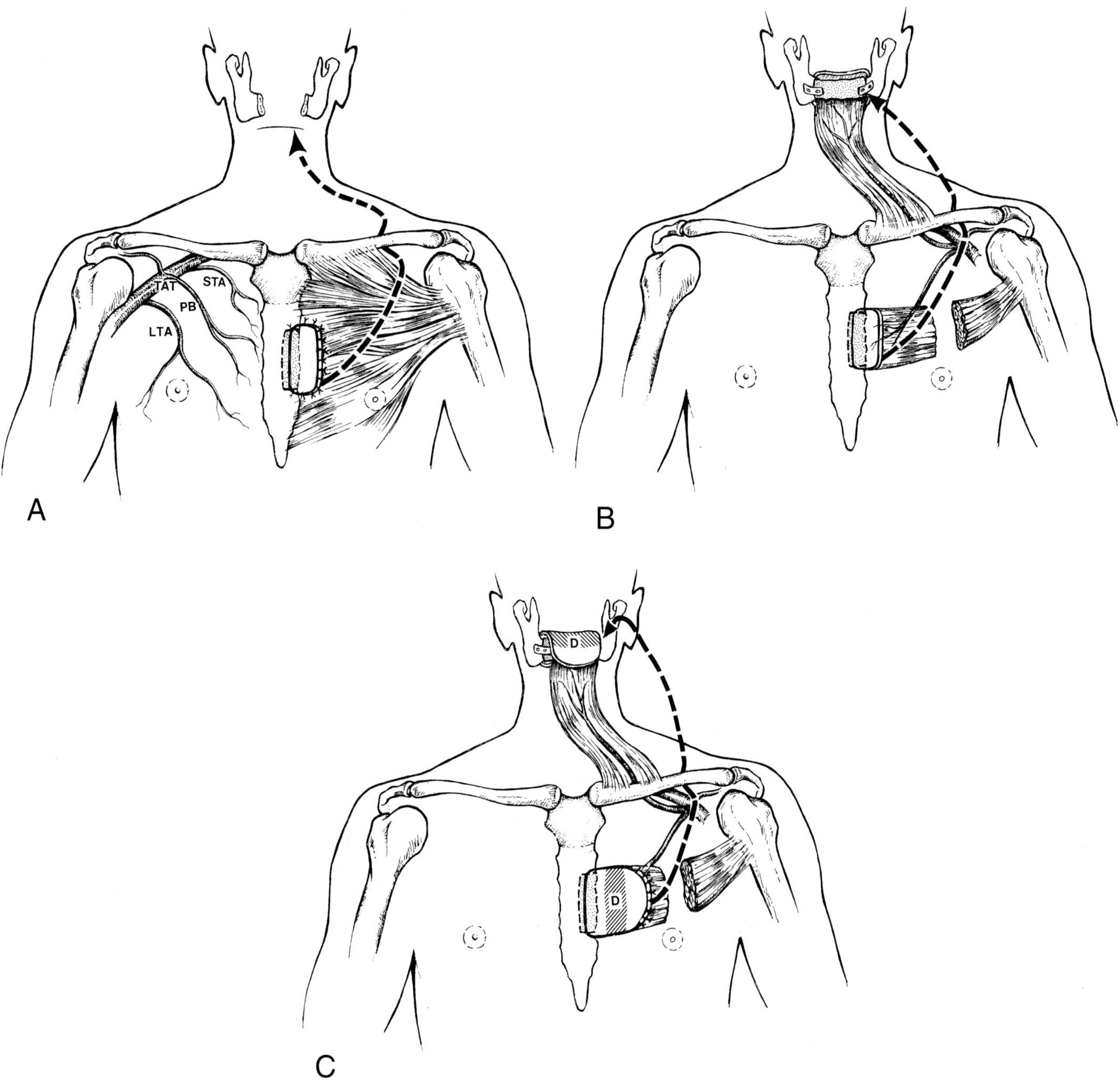

Fig. 4.6 **A** Vascular anatomy of the sternum–pectoralis major OMCF showing the position of the superior thoracic artery (STA), the pectoral branch (PB) from the thoracoacromial trunk (TAT) and the lateral thoracic artery (LTA). **B** The composite flap is transferred into the neck underneath the clavicle. The skin paddle is used for intraoral reconstruction. **C** Using a larger skin paddle, both intraoral lining and external skin cover can be achieved by de-epithelialising the middle area (**D**).

Laterally in the deep fascia of the muscle arising under the clavicle the pectoral branch of the acromiothoracic artery is identified and preserved as it is the main artery to the muscle. The insertion of pectoralis major to the humerus is transected laterally. Wherever possible the lateral thoracic artery is identified and preserved.

The pectoral nerves are divided releasing the muscle from its posterior attachment. Finally, the muscular belly of the pectoralis major is separated from its clavicular head and the flap is mobilised ready for transfer.

The flap is brought into the neck either anterior or posterior to the clavicle. The latter manoeuvre gains a few centimetres more in length. The bone graft is plugged between remaining mandibular stumps and fixed with wire sutures or plates. The bone can be curved to reproduce the contours of the mandible (Fig. 4.6B).

The paddle of skin allows reconstruction of the floor of the mouth. Green et al (1981) recommend folding the distal part of the compound flap on itself to protect the cancellous surface of the sternal bone graft with muscle. The skin paddle can be used to replace intraoral lining (Fig. 4.6C) and where required a second paddle of skin can be used for external skin cover by de-epithelialising a segment between the two islands of skin. After final haemostasis the wounds are closed inserting suction drainage to both neck and chest.

Indications

a. Anterior arch of mandible
b. Lateral ramus of mandible
c. Mandibulectomy angle to angle (bilateral flaps)
d. Oral lining and outer skin cover.

Contraindications

Pectus excavatum.

Problems and complications

The technique depends on the rich vascularisation of the pectoralis major muscle and the firm attachment of this muscle to the sternum. It involves only the medial head of the pectoralis major muscle and the skin can be used for inner lining and outer skin cover. The length of the arc of rotation of this flap is less than that for the pectoralis major–rib OMCF. Transferring this flap, however, by the retro-clavicular route may compensate for this difference. Sometimes the sternum can be exceptionally thin and in one of our cases there was resorption. We have also seen a case where there was a granulomatous reaction at the donor site which required electrocautery.

THE RIB–PECTORALIS MAJOR OMCF

Technique

An appropriate island of skin is outlined on the anterior chest wall overlying the mammary region and situated around or just below the nipple. This island is often centred over the fifth or sixth rib extending 6–8 cm caudally. The skin island is combined with incisions for a deltopectoral approach and the incisions required for mandibulectomy and neck dissection. The island of skin is incised and the pectoralis major muscle is identified. The deltopectoral flap is then raised to expose the pectoralis major muscle completely. It is advisable to fix the skin island to the underlying muscle and fascia with temporary sutures to avoid avulsion and damage of the vascular connections between the muscle and the skin. Lateral and medial to the skin island the pectoralis muscle is transected to expose ribs until the sixth rib is reached (Fig. 4.7A).

The dissection begins distally some 2–8 cm inferior to the sixth rib, incising the aponeurosis of the external oblique abdominis muscle and the rectus sheath, and progressing cranially under these fascia until the sixth rib is reached. The sixth intercostal muscle (internal and external) is detached from the inferior border of the rib, preserving the periosteum which remains attached to the rib. The rib is divided medially at the costosternal junction and as far laterally as necessary depending on the length of bone required. A finger is insinuated behind the rib to detach the pleura carefully from its undersurface. The fifth intercostal muscle is detached from the fifth rib, allowing it to remain attached to the sixth rib. The dissection proceeds upwards under the anterior periosteal fascial layer to the level of the third intercostal space. It is extremely important at this stage to preserve the insertions of pectoralis major muscle to the sixth rib and to the detached periosteum of the fifth and fourth ribs. Insertions of the pectoralis minor into this block of tissue are divided distally freeing the compound flap, which can be elevated allowing identification of the vascular pedicle on the deep surface of the pectoralis major muscle. Superior to the island of skin, the pectoralis major muscle is transected on each side of the pectoral branch of the thoracoacromial trunk. This ribbon of muscle protects the vessels. Lateral to the pectoral branch of the thoracoacromial trunk, the lateral thoracic artery can be identified and divided if necessary. The pectoral nerves are also divided and the flap mobilised ready for transfer. The compound flap comprises skin, pectoralis major muscle, fascia and periosteum from the third intercostal space to 6 cm below the sixth rib, the fifth intercostal muscles and the sixth rib (Fig. 4.7B). Prior to transfer the subclavius muscle is transected and detached from the clavicle. This diminishes the length of transfer from the chest to the face. The compound flap is transferred with a half twist of the pedicle, which is necessary to adjust the curvature of the rib to the mandibular defect. The rib is plugged between the mandibular stumps and fixed with wire sutures or plates. The distal portion of skin is used for inner lining and where necessary using de-epithelialisation a second island can be used for external skin resurfacing. Often a big island of skin

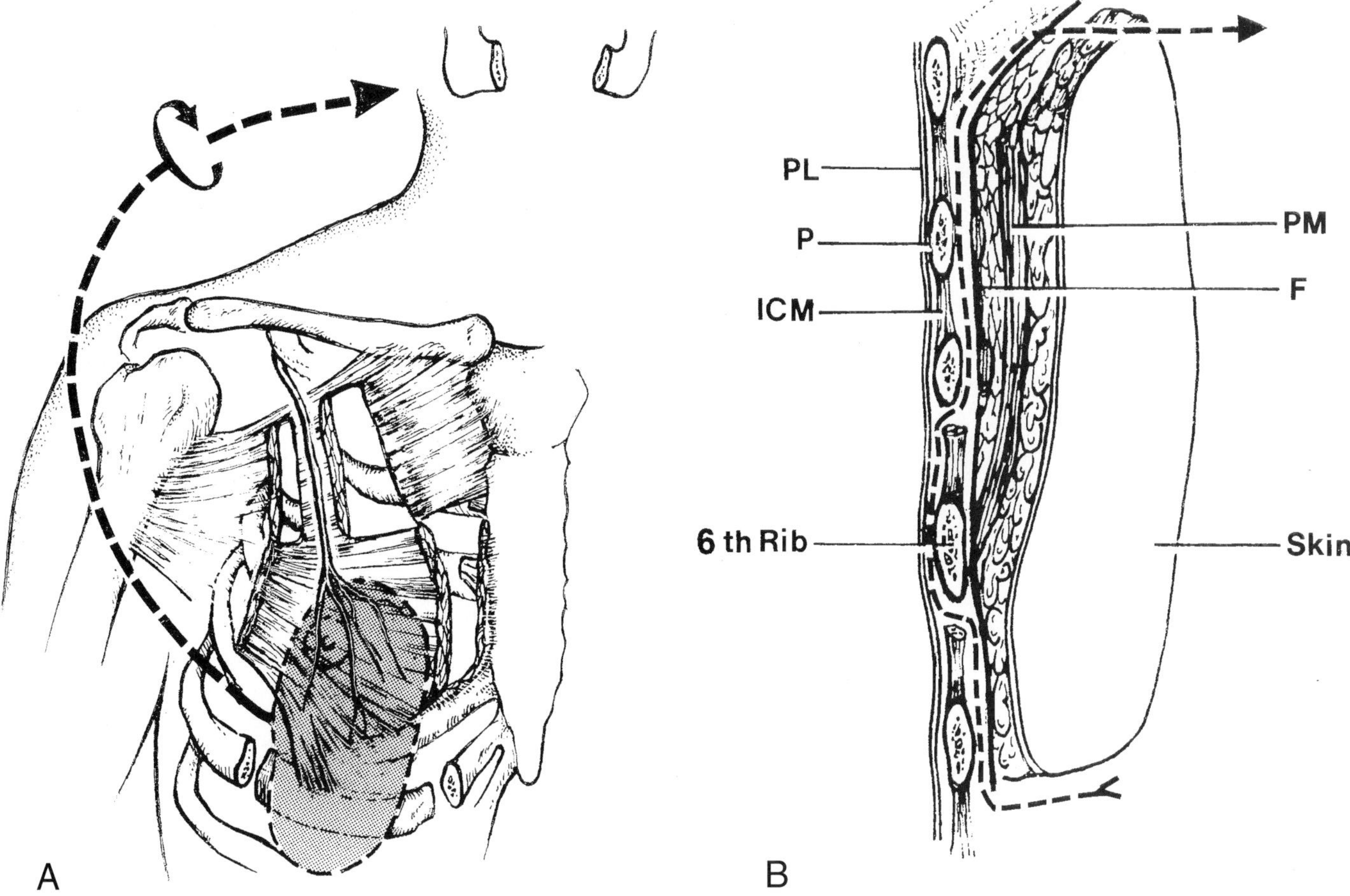

Fig. 4.7 **A** Outline for the rib–pectoralis major OMCF based on the pectoral branch from the thoracoacromial trunk. **B** Plane of dissection for the composite rib flap. The pleura (PL) should be left intact. The composite flap includes skin, pectoralis major (PM), fascia (F), periosteum (P) and the rib with its neighbouring intecostal muscle (ICM).

is used for composite defects requiring intraoral lining and skin in cases where the whole chin, cheek and lower lip are resected.

The donor area is closed by advancing the surrounding skin flaps. For extensive defects the rib can be transected laterally and used to reconstruct the chest defect. The latissimus dorsi and external oblique muscles can also be used to close the defect. Following careful haemostasis the wounds are closed with interrupted 000 monofilament nylon sutures with suction drains inserted into the chest and neck wounds.

Indications

a. Anterior arch of mandible
b. Lateral ramus of mandible
c. Anterior arch and lateral ramus
d. Mandibulectomy angle to angle (Fig. 4.8)
e. Large resections involving chin, cervical skin, lip, cheek, and soft tissues of mouth and mandible (Fig. 4.9)
f. Benign and malignant tumours of the mandible.

Contraindications

a. Systemic disease or poor general medical condition of the patient.

Problems and complications

The pectoralis major OMCF with rib is a difficult flap to elevate. It requires care and attention, particularly in the deep layers to preserve the pleura intact. Where the pleura is breached and the lung collapses then a postoperative chest drain is required. Great care is taken to avoid any shearing forces that will disrupt the delicate vascularity or vascular connections between the muscle, rib and the overlying skin. Where a large amount of tissue is required it may not be possible to close a wound directly. In such instances, there will be an unclosed defect and this should be placed in the area that offers the fewest risks. This essentially means that pleura or lung should not be left exposed. If patients require secondary surgery to close the defect this may result in the delay of subsequent treatment such as radiotherapy.

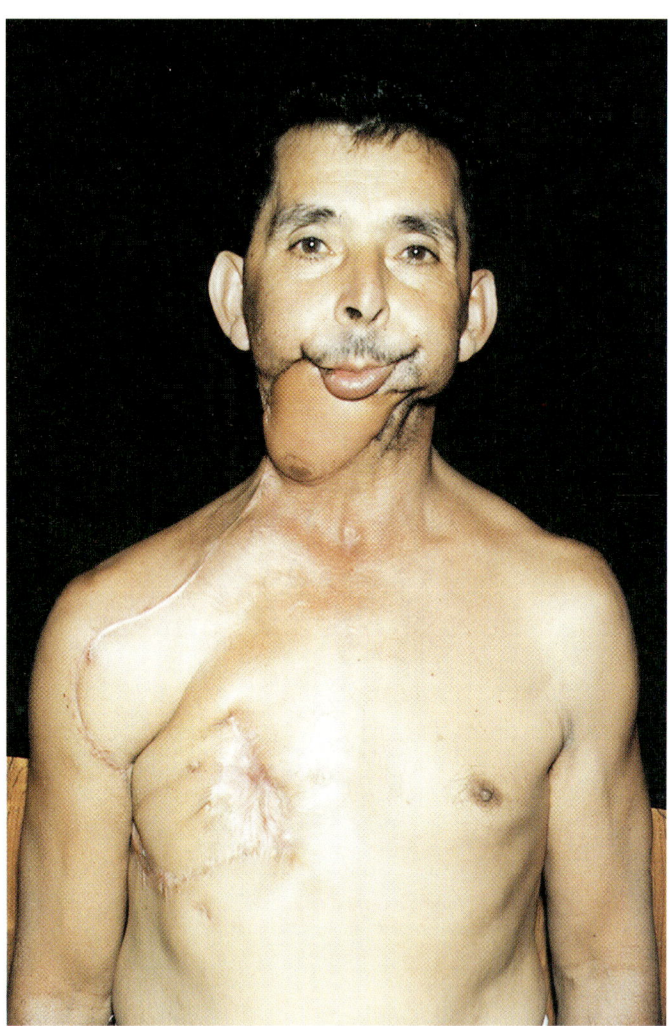
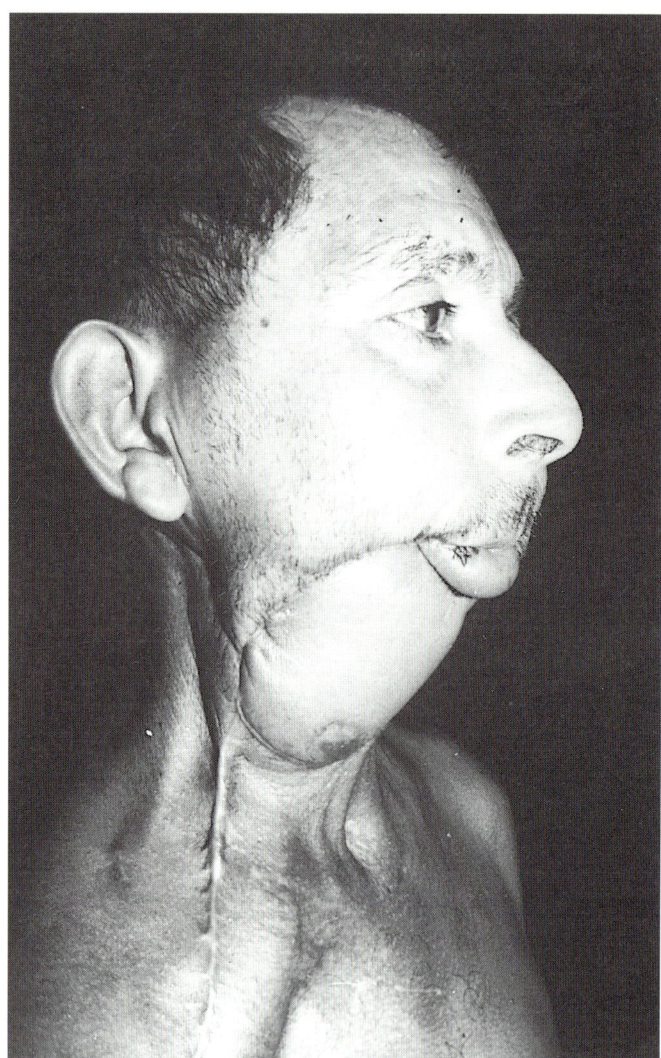

Fig. 4.8 **A & B** Extensive resection of mandible symphysis and right horizontal ramus including oral mucosa and overlying skin. Successful reconstruction has been achieved using a composite rib pectoralis major flap.

The pectoralis major composite flap is quite bulky and the excessive weight of the tissues may result in dehiscence at the recipient site, particularly in patients who have undergone previous irradiation or who have a nutritional defect.

Occasionally the flap may be totally or partially lost, perhaps as a result of poor technique, haematoma, vessel spasm or some other unidentified cause. In patients who have a short thorax and a long neck the rotation of the flap may be difficult and the flap too short and therefore inadequate. Wherever possible the nipple areolar complex should not be taken with the skin island of this flap unless it is absolutely necessary. In such cases, the nipple should be resected at a second stage as soon as possible to avoid asthetic compromise and embarrassment.

THE RIB PLEURA–PECTORALIS MAJOR OMCF

The addition of pleura to the osteomyocutaneous pectoralis

major flap can provide tissue for intraoral lining. The pleura has no bulk. This extension of the technique has proved a valuable addition to the head and neck reconstructive surgeon (Stromberg 1989). In using the compound flap the chest is obviously opened and a chest drain must be inserted postoperatively. It is also vitally important to ensure meticulous wound closure of the donor site.

THE RIB–PECTORALIS MINOR OMCF

Anatomy

The pectoralis minor is a triangular muscle which lies behind the pectoralis major. Its inferior head arises from segments of the third, fourth, fifth and sixth ribs. The muscle is inserted into the coracoid process of the scapula. Innervation of pectoralis minor is by the medial anterior thoracic nerve (medial pectoral nerve). The blood supply is from

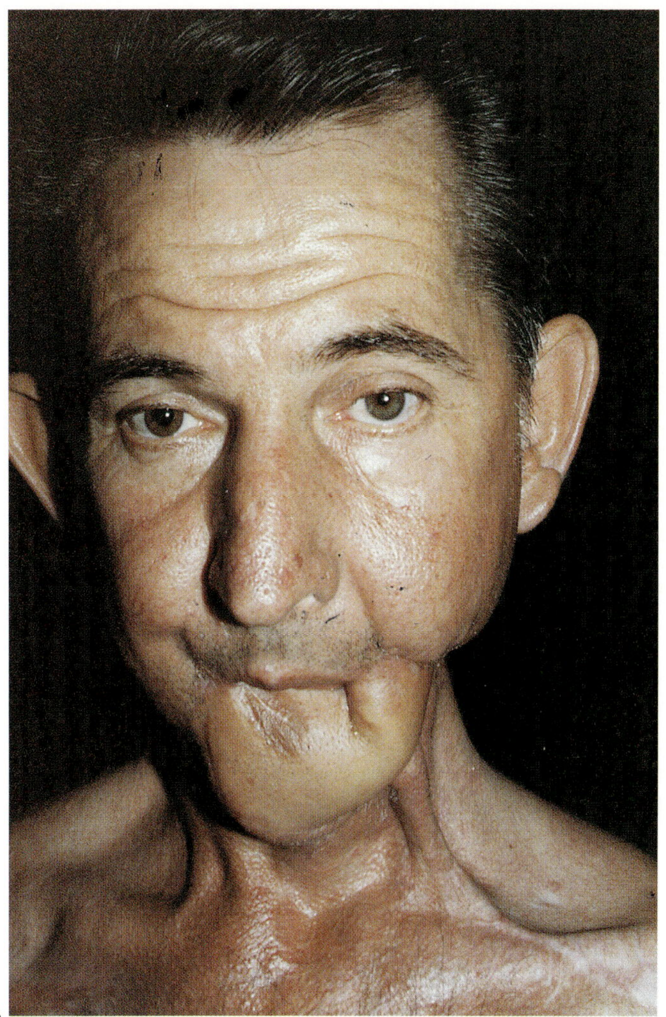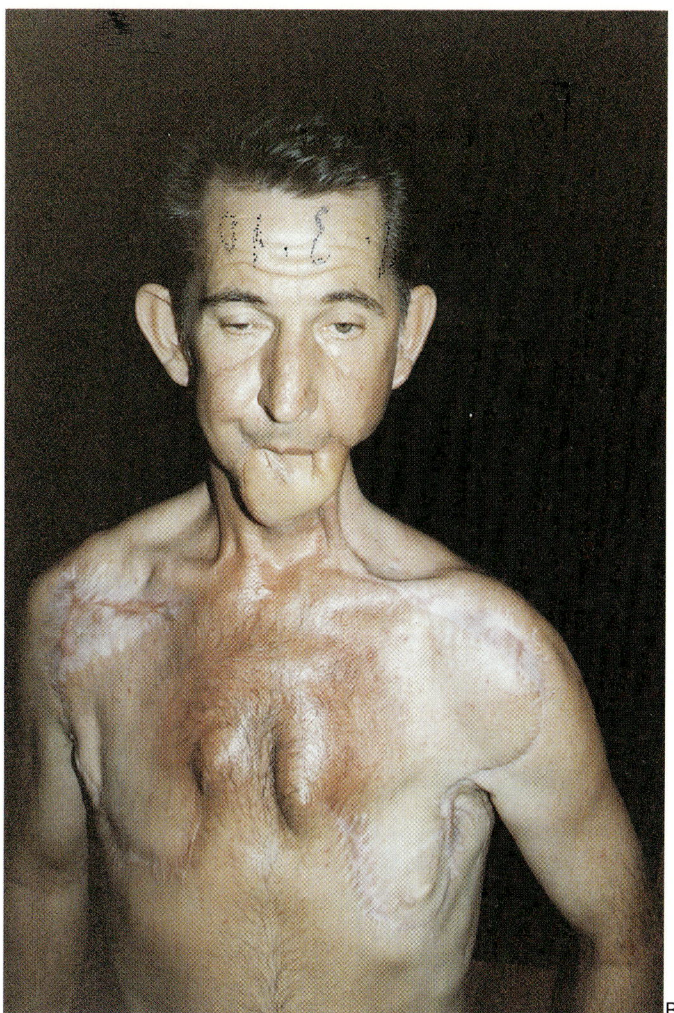

Fig. 4.9 A Reconstruction of the symphysis, floor of mouth and chin using bilateral rib–pectoralis major flaps. **B** All wounds have been closed directly combining the excision with the deltopectoral approach for elevating the composite flap.

small arteries, the pectoralis minor arteries which can arise from the second part of the axillary artery or lateral to the origin of thoracoacromial trunk or from the main thoracoacromial trunk itself. Often the lateral thoracic artery is the main vascular supply for pectoralis minor. Venous drainage accompanies the arterial branches as venae comitantes. There is a rich vascular network connecting these arteries with the third, fourth and fifth intercostal muscles, the fourth, fifth and sixth ribs and fibres of serratus anterior muscle, the inferior head of pectoralis major and the overlying skin (Fig. 4.10).

Technique

A paddle of skin is outlined over the fifth or sixth rib just below and lateral to the nipple areolar complex, in conjunction with an oblique skin incision placed at the anterior axillary line. The pectoralis major is identified and retracted medially and superiorly permitting the acromiothoracic

trunk to be visualised. The inferior head of pectoralis major is transected at the level of the superior limit of the skin paddle and retracted upwards. The pectoralis minor is easily identified. The costocoracoid fascia is opened and the pectoralis minor muscle transected close to the coracoid process. Deep to the muscles the pectoralis minor arteries can be found arising from the axillary artery. The long thoracic and thoracodorsal nerves are identified and preserved as are the thoracodorsal vessels. The areolar fat of the axilla is included in the pedicle of pectoralis minor and not dissected.

The paddle of skin is isolated, including the underlying muscular components, particularly the superior head of external oblique abdominis muscle and anterior digitations of serratus anterior (medial to the long thoracic nerve and the inferior head of pectoralis major). These muscles remain attached to the rib and fascia. The fifth or sixth intercostal muscles are transected medially and detached from the inferior border of the rib. The rib is transected medially and

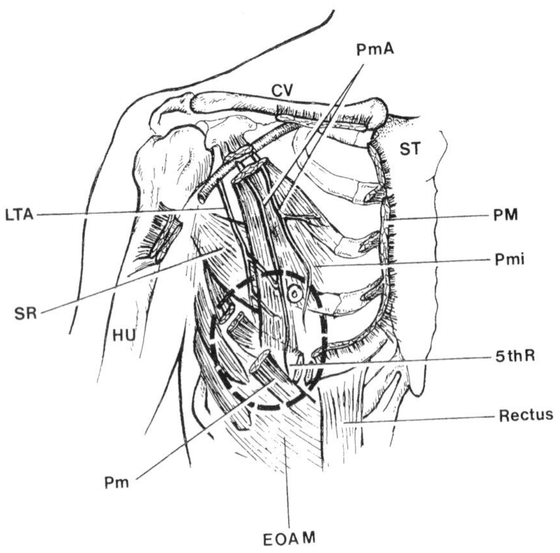

Fig. 4.10 Anatomy of the rib–pectoralis minor OMCF. ST = sternum; PM = pectoralis major; Pm = pectoralis minor; 5thR = fifth rib; Rectus = rectus abdominis; EOAM = external oblique abdominis muscle; SR = serratus; HU = humerus; LTA = lateral thoracic artery; CV = clavicle; PmA = pectoralis minor arteries.

laterally and the pleura is detached carefully upwards until the neighbouring rib. The compound flap includes the rib (fifth or sixth), the adjacent superior intercostal muscle, the fascia and the external periosteum of the two superior adjacent ribs and intercostal muscles (Fig. 4.10). The subclavius muscle is detached from the clavicle in a subperiosteal plane. The flap is raised and passed into the neck posterior to the clavicle after ligating the acromial branch of the acromiothoracic trunk and the cephalic vein. This manoeuvre makes is possible to gain 3 to 4 cm in length of the flap. The compound flap is transferred to the neck and the rib inserted between the mandibular stumps with wire sutures. The paddle of skin is used for outer covering but when it is used for intraoral lining the rib must be rotated 180° to adjust for the curvature of the mandible.

Haemostasis is secured and the operative field and the neck wound closed after suction drainage is inserted. If skin is required for both lining and outer resurfacing, the pectoralis minor flap can be built up together with the pectoralis major myocutaneous flap to provide the necessary skin for the reconstructive procedure.

Indications

a. Anterior or lateral mandible defects
b. Partial mandibulectomy associated with single external cover or intraoral lining.

Contraindications

Large soft tissue defects including skin.

Problems and complications

The rib–pectoralis minor OMCF is a difficult flap to raise and requires considerable surgical expertise and experience. It has a variable vascular pedicle and the arc of rotation is much less than that of the pectoralis major. The muscle insertions into the fourth and fifth ribs, however, are well defined assuring good vascularisation to the bone. There is little bulk and perhaps the best indication for this flap is as a myo-osseus flap. It is certainly not indicated in extensive reconstructions.

It has the advantage of providing less donor site morbidity both in terms of aesthetics and function. It may be combined in larger resections with the pectoralis major to provide sufficient soft tissue bulk.

THE LATERAL RIB–PECTORALIS MAJOR OMCF

Anatomy

The anatomy of the pectoralis major muscle has been described previously. There is, however, a rich vascular network between the thoracic branch of the thoracoacromial trunk (i.e. the pectoral branch) and the lateral thoracic artery. This has been extensively investigated and reported by Freeman et al (1981).

Technique

The best description of the pectoralis major–lateral rib OMCF has been reported by Little et al (1983). Basically the technique of building this compound flap is similar to other techniques involving the rib–pectoralis major muscle. Some differences, however, must be emphasised. The island of skin is placed over the fifth rib laterally just below the nipple areolar complex. The lower head of pectoralis minor muscle is preserved, remaining attached to the fifth rib and surrounding fascia and intercostal muscle. Anterior digitations from serratus anterior (anterior to the long thoracic nerve) and the fascia of external oblique abdominis muscle are included in the block. This caudal extension of the dissection has a variable length from 2–8 cm below the fifth rib. The lower head of pectoralis major muscle with the overlying skin island is included in the block but the island of skin exceeds the inferior limits of the muscle for a few centimetres (Fig. 4.11). Pectoralis minor arteries and the lateral thoracic artery are ligated before they enter the muscle. This ensures a wide and anastomotic network with the thoracic branch (pectoral branch) of the thoracoacromial trunk. This branch is the main vascular supply to this compound flap and the entire pedicle is skeletonised from the upper border of the skin island to its origin from the axillary artery. There is only one essential difference between the pectoralis major lateral–rib OMCF and the pectoralis minor rib OMCF. The rib–pectoralis minor is vascularised by pectoralis minor on the thoracic arteries

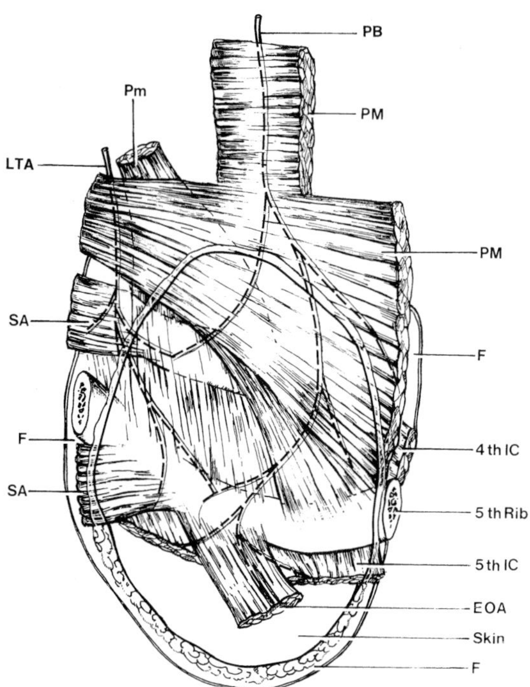

Fig. 4.11 Anatomy of the lateral rib–pectoralis major OMCF. The main vascular pedicle is the pectoral branch arising from the thoracoacromial trunk. PB = pectoralis branch; PM = pectoralis major; F = fat; IC = intercostal muscles; EOA = external oblique abdominis; SA = serratus anterior; LTA = lateral thoracic artery; Pm = pectoralis minor.

whereas the pectoralis major–lateral rib is vascularised by the thoracoacromial trunk. Little et al (1983) have suggested that the flap in truth is a lateral rib–pectoralis major–pectoralis minor OMCF.

Indications

a. Large defects involving the mandible and soft tissues
b. Outer resurfacing and oral lining.

Contraindications

There are no specific contraindications.

Problems and complications

The problems and complications of this flap are similar to those previously described for both the pectoralis major–rib flap and for the pectoralis minor–rib OMCF.

POSTOPERATIVE MANAGEMENT AND COMPLICATIONS

Careful postoperative monitoring is an essential part of any surgical procedure and this must also apply to head and neck surgery. There are, however, other problems particularly related to the head and neck. Haemostasis is an essential part of the operative procedure and by far the majority of head and neck operations require suction drainage in the early postoperative period. Haematomas are not very common but if an abrupt or large haematoma occurs it should be drained immediately as the danger is that it may compress and obstruct the vascular pedicles of the reconstruction. Similarly, ribbons placed around the neck to secure the position of a tracheostomy cannula should be avoided. Such ribbons can have a severe constricting effect particularly with postoperative oedema, which may result in constriction of the vascular pedicle of pedicle flap reconstructions. In the early postoperative period, the tongue is usually fixed and there may be difficulty in controlling saliva. Attention must be focused in preserving the airway and avoiding aspiration.

The flap may partially fail or necrose and such necrosis may be related to infection, or a vascular cause and subsequent ischaemia. Necrosis is usually related to local infection and manifests itself at about the fifth day. There is initial erythematous reaction in the dermis–epidermis and subsequent darkening of the skin leading to necrosis. This is often accompanied by a foetid smell. A common cause is anaerobic bacteria and results in a bubbly appearance at many island sites in the tissues of the flap with subsequent yellow discolouration and necrosis. Vascular compromise as a result of venous thrombosis, arterial obstruction or strangulation of the pedicle will result in necrosis but this is a fairly infrequent cause. The final cause of necrosis is due to inadequate circulating blood supply, most commonly resulting from transoperative or immediate postoperative ischaemia. This may be the result of anaemia, vasoconstrictor drugs or failure to control circulating blood volume, blood pressure and cardiac output.

Chronic infection appearing as osteomyelitis is a problem which can appear much later, despite adequate preoperative and peroperative antibiotic treatment and precautions such as removing diseased teeth and excision of tumour and infected bone. Osteomyelitis of the stumps of the mandible can occur and furthermore there is a risk of infection and loss of part or all of the osseous reconstruction.

Table 4.2 Mandible reconstruction using osteomyocutaneous flaps (OMCFs)

Flap	No. of cases
Lateral trapezius OMCF	20
Rib–pectoralis major	9
Rib–pectoralis minor	3
Lateral rib–pectoralis major	3
Sternum pectoralis major	3
Bilateral sternoclavicular	4
Rib–latissimus dorsi	3
Total	45

Table 4.3 Comparison of the different osteomyocutaneous flaps for mandibular reconstruction

Attribute/OMCF	CSC	SCSC	SLT	RPM	RPm	LRPM	RPPM	SPM
Difficulty in execution	++	++	++++	+++	+++	++	+++	+++
Versatility	+	+	+++	+++	+	++	+++	+++
Blood supply	+	++	++++	+++	++	+++	+++	+++
Sequelae	+	+	+++	+	+	+	+	+
Bulk	+ (+)	+ (+)	+	+++	++	+++	+++	+++
Skin for cover	+	++	+++	++++	++	+++	++++	+++
Oncological limitations	+++	+++	+	0	0	0	0	0
Donor defect	+	+	+++	++	++	++	++	+++
Surgical expertise	++	+	+++	++++	+	++	++	+

CSC = Clavicle–sternocleidomastoid; SCSC = bilateral sternoclavicular–sternocleidomastoid; SLT = scapula–lateral trapezius; RPM = rib–pectoralis major; RPm = rib–pectoralis minor; LRPM = lateral rib–pectoralis major; RPPM = rib–pleura–pectoralis major; SPM = sternum–pectoralis major.

One further problem is bone resorption, particularly in older patients, in patients with nutritional defects, or in cases where there has been a failure to achieve rigid osteosynthesis. Bone resorption does not occur very often to any significant degree and often an intense local fibrosis takes place, preserving the mandibular conformation and integrity.

The head and neck service of Santa Rita Hospital in Porto Alegre has performed approximately 300 myocutaneous flaps for head and neck reconstruction in the past 5 years. Of these, 45 have been OMCFs used for mandible reconstruction (Table 4.2). Surgery was performed with the intent for cure in 82% and for palliation in the remaining 18%. Recurrence within 12 months in this series was 31%. By far the majority of cases were successfully reconstructed but there was evidence of necrosis in 10.7% of the cases.

FUTURE DEVELOPMENTS

The OMCFs have enabled great progress in head and neck surgery in the last decade. They have enabled surgeons to enlarge the concepts of operability and also represent a significant decrease in cost and hospitalisation time. It has never before been possible to resect with oncological and anatomical thoroughness confident with so many reconstructive possibilities, increasing the cure rate of tumours and giving patients a life with dignity. Particularly in mandible reconstruction, the various OMCFs make it possible to reconstruct so that patients will swallow properly, maintain oral competence and control of their saliva and have an acceptable aesthetic appearance.

The wide variety of flaps that can be used is evidence that there is not one sovereign flap. Each technique has its advantages and disadvantages which vary in relation to the security of the vascular supply, the simplicity of execution, the difficulty and complications in closing the donor defect, the possibilities in covering bigger areas of chin skin and mucosa, and the ability to combine with techniques such as radical neck dissection (Table 4.3). Each patient is unique and individual and the precise indication for one patient may not be ideal for another.

The best surgeon will be the one who masters the greatest number of techniques since he will have more scientific substrate and discernment to indicate the best flap for each patient. It is to be hoped that in the future, existing techniques will be improved with increasing clinical experience and that there will be development of newer and better techniques.

REFERENCES

Ariyan S 1979a One-stage reconstruction for defects of the mouth using a sternomastoid myocutaneous flap. Plastic and Reconstructive Surgery 63: 618
Ariyan S 1979b The pectoralis major myocutaneous flap. Plastic and Reconstructive Surgery 63: 73
Ariyan S 1980a The sternocleidomastoid myocutaneous flap. Laryngoscope 90: 676
Ariyan S 1980b The viability of rib grafts transplanted with periosteal blood supply. Plastic and Reconstructive Surgery 65: 140
Ariyan S, Finseth F 1978 The anterior chest approach for obtaining free osteocutaneous rib grafts. Plastic and Reconstructive Surgery 62: 676
Azevedo J F 1987 Pectoralis minor flaps : an experimental study and clinical applications of osteomuscular, osteomyocutaneous and myocutaneous flaps. Head and Neck Surgery 9: 211
Bakamjian V 1963 A technique for primary reconstruction of the palate after radical maxillectomy for cancer. Plastic and Reconstructive Surgery 31:103
Barbosa J F 1974 Surgical treatment of head and neck tumours, 1st edn, Grune, New York
Becker G D, Welch W D 1990 Quantitative bacteriology of intraoperative wound tussues in contaminated surgery. Head and Neck Surgery 12(14): 293
Bell M S G, Barron P T 1981 The rib-pectoralis major osteomyocutaneous flap. Annals of Plastic Surgery 6: 347
Bertotti J A 1980 Trapezius musculocutaneous island flap in repair of

major head and neck cancer. Plastic and Reconstructive Surgery 65: 16

Bhathena H, Karavana N M 1986 One-stage total mandibular reconstruction with rib, pectoralis major osteomyocutaneous flap. Head and Neck Surgery 8: 311

Carvalho M B, Kanda J L, Kowalski L P et al 1986 Povidone–iodine in head and neck surgery. Revista Brasileira de Cirurgia de Cabeça e Pescoço 10 (1,2,3,): 42–46

Conley J 1972 Use of composite flaps containing bone for major repair in head and neck. Plastic and Reconstuctive Surgery 49: 522

Conley J, Gullane J P 1980 The sternocleidomastoid muscle flap. Head and Neck Surgery 2: 308

Crile G H 1906 Excision of cancer of head and neck, with special reference to the plan of dissection based on 132 operations. Journal of the American Medical Association 47: 1790

Cuono B C, Ariyan S 1980 Immediate reconstruction of a composite mandibular defect with a regional osteomyocutaneous flap. Plastic and Reconstructive Surgery 65: 477–483

Daniel R K 1977 Free rib transfer by microvascular anastomoses. Plastic and Recontructive Surgery 59: 737

Demergasso F, Piazza M 1977 Colgajo cutaneo aislado a pediculo muscular en cirugia reconstructiva por cancer de cabeza y cuello. Tecnica original. Revista Argentina de Cirurgia 32: 27

Demergasso F, Piazza M 1979 The trapezius flap in reconstruction surgery for head and neck. An original technique. American Journal of Surgery 138: 533–536

Elliott R A 1969 Technique of radical neck dissection. In: Gaisford J C (ed.) Symposium on cancer of head and neck. Mosby St Louis, p 39

Freeman J L, Walker E P, Wilson J S P et al 1981 The vascular anatomy of the pectoralis major myocutaneous flap. British Journal of Plastic Surgery 34(1): 3–10

Freund H R 1967 Principles of head and neck surgery, 1st edn. Appleton, New York

Green M F, Gibson J R, Bryson J R et al 1981 A one-stage correction of mandibular defects using a split sternum pectoralis major myocutaneous transfer. British Journal of Plastic Surgery 34: 11–16

Guillamondegui O M, Larson D L 1982 The lateral trapezius musculocutaneous flap: its use in head and neck reconstruction. Plastic and Reconstructive Surgery 67: 143–150

Hueston J T, McConchie I H 1968 A compound pectoral flap. Australian and New Zealand Journal of Surgery 38: 61–63

Larson D L, Goepfert H 1982 Limitations of the sternocleidomastoid musculocutaneous flap in head and neck cancer reconstruction. Plastic and Reconstructive Surgery 70: 328–335

Little J W, McCulloch D T, Lyons J P 1983 The lateral pectoral composite flap in one-stage reconstruction of irradiated mandible. Plastic and Reconstructive Surgery 71: 326–335

Littlewood M 1967 Compound skin and sternomastoid flaps for repair in extensive carcinoma of head and neck. British Journal of Plastic Surgery 20: 403

Magee W P, Gilbert D A, McInnis W D 1980 Extended muscle and musculocutaneous flaps. Clinics in Plastic Surgery 7(1): 57

Martin H E 1957 Surgery of head and neck tumors. Harper, New York

Medgyesi S 1973 Observations on pedicle bone grafts in goats. Scandinavian Journal of Plastic and Reconstructive Surgery 15: 369–374

Mendelson B C 1980 The pectoralis major island flap: an important new flap for head and neck reconstruction. British Journal of Plastic Surgery 33: 318

Owens N 1955 Compound neck pedicle designed for repair of massive facial defects. Plastic and Recontructive Surgery 15: 369–374

Pearlman N W, Albin R E, O'Donnell R S 1983 Mandibular reconstruction in irradiated patient utilizing myosseouscutaneous flaps. American Journal of Surgery 146: 474–477

Robertson G A 1986 The role of sternum in osteomyocutaneous reconstruction of major mandibular defects. American Journal of Surgery 152: 367–370

Siemssen S O, Kirkby M D, O Connor T P F et al 1978 Immediate reconstruction of a resected segment of the lower jaw, using a compound flap of clavicle and sternomastoid muscle. Plastic and Reconstructive Surgery 61: 724

Snyder C C, Bateman J M, Davis C W et al 1970 Mandibulo-facial restoration with osteocutaneous flaps. Plastic and Reconstructive Surgery 45: 14

Stromberg V B 1989 The pleural osteomuscular flap in oropharyngeal reconstruction. Laryngoscope 99: 339–341

Taylor G I 1975 The free vascularized bone graft: a clinical extension of microvascular techniques. Plastic and Reconstructive Surgery 55: 533

Vila C N, Salazar J Z, Dezotti D M et al 1984 Reconstruction experience with myocutaneous and osteomyocutaneous skin flaps in oncological surgery of the head and neck. Journal of Maxillary and Facial Surgery 12: 107–113

5. Mandibular reconstruction with vascularised bone

David S. Soutar

INTRODUCTION AND HISTORICAL REVIEW

Autogenous bone has been used in mandibular reconstruction for over 100 years and the development of such conventional bone grafts will be dealt with subsequently (Chapter 6). The history of vascularised bone transfer is much more recent and takes its origin from the development of microvascular surgery and free tissue transfer. The first free flap using microvascular techniques was, in fact, for intraoral reconstruction and was presented by Kaplan at a meeting in 1971 and subsequently reported in the literature (Kaplan et al 1973). Since that time there has been a virtual explosion in microvascular reconstructive techniques so that now a wide variety of differing tissues can be successfully transplanted and revitalised by anastomosing their blood supply.

Traditionally the rib had been used extensively as a conventional non-vascularised bone graft and it is perhaps not surprising that the rib was one of the first bones to be extensively investigated for its vascular properties. This resulted in the rib being the first vascularised free bone transfer described for mandibular reconstruction (Daniel 1977). Further donor sites for bone transfer paralleled the development of skin flaps. The groin flap which had been the first skin flap used in free tissue transfer led to the development of a composite flap including a segment of bone (Taylor & Watson 1978). Further investigation into the blood supply of the iliac crest as a donor site for bone (Taylor et al 1979a, 1979b) led to the description of the deep circumflex iliac artery groin flap, which subsequently became a popular method of mandible reconstruction.

Several other donor sites which had been initially described as skin flaps were subsequently shown to be useful in composite tissue transfer including vascularised bone. These included the dorsalis pedis flap including metatarsal (Rosen et al 1979, McLeod & Robinson 1982); the scapular flap (Teot et al 1981, Swartz et al 1986), the radial forearm flap (Soutar et al 1983, Soutar & Widdowson 1986), the ulnar forearm flap (Lovie et al 1984) and the lateral arm flap (Katsaros et al 1984).

One further very important donor site for vascularised bone proved to be the fibula. This was initially described as a free bone transfer suitable for replacement of long bones (Taylor et al 1975). Subsequently Chen & Yan (1983) showed that the overlying skin could be taken with the fibula and this opened up the way for the use of this bone in composite resections involving the mandible (Hidalgo 1989).

There are now a wide variety of donor sites for vascularised bone suitable for transfer and revitalisation using microvascular surgical techniques, (Webster & Soutar 1986). It is inevitable that such complicated surgical techniques should be compared with the simpler conventional bone grafting techniques. Vascularised bone, however, offers the reconstructive surgeon significant advantages over non-vascularised autogenous bone grafts.

THE FATE OF TRANSPLANTED AUTOGENOUS BONE

Conventional autogenous bone grafts depend for their survival on the condition of the recipient bed, which should be free from tissue damage or infection (Adekeye 1978, Kudo & Fujioka 1978). Furthermore, the success of autogenous bone grafts is dependent on the transplantation of live surface cells to produce osteogenesis and these cells can be adversely affected by the recipient environment (Manchester 1972, Ham & Gordon 1952, Gray & Elves 1981). To increase the surface area of live surface cells in the transplantation, there has been a tendency towards using cancellous bone chips rather than corticocancellous blocks of bone for mandibular reconstruction. It has been suggested that the cancellous surface of any bone grafts should be placed against the best vascularised recipient bed to aid revascularisation (Thomson & Casson 1970).

There has been considerable debate as to whether early or delayed revascularisation is advantageous but current opinion tends to favour early revascularisation with incorporation of the bone graft into its anatomical site (Burwell 1965). Cancellous bone is thought to be superior to cortical bone in this respect and calvarial bone grafts have increased in popularity because of their early revascularisation (Zins &

Whitaker 1983). A further problem with conventional bone grafting techniques has been the tendency to resorb with the passage of time. Calvarial bone has been shown to maintain its bone mass more effectively than endochondral bone presumably due to its early revascularisation. Furthermore, there is evidence to suggest that where periosteum is preserved there is a tendency for bone grafts to resorb less quickly (Peer 1955, Knize 1974).

The transfer of autogenous bone which can be revascularised by microvascular surgical techniques offers significant advantages by maintaining its own blood supply and vascularity. Such grafts maintain their original mass and also appear to maintain their intrinsic bone growth unabated (Ostrup & Tam 1975, Cutting & McCarthy 1983, La Trenta et al 1987). Such vascularised bone transfers are not dependent on their surroundings unlike other conventional bone grafts which rely on the vascularity of the recipient area (Puckett et al 1979, Moore et al 1984). Furthermore such microvascular free bone transfers show a more rapid rate of healing and subsequent strength and tolerance to stress than conventional autograft bone (Puckett et al 1979, Haw et al 1978, Berggren et al 1982). The normal bony architecture can be maintained with the survival of the original osteogenic cells (Moore et al 1984).

The advantages of vascularised bone in unfavourable recipient sites is now well documented (Ostrup & Fredrickson 1975, Daniel 1978, Taylor 1983, Weiland et al 1984, Rosen et al 1985, Wood 1986).

The majority of cases requiring mandible reconstruction present the head and neck surgeon with an unfavourable recipient bed either at the time of excision with contamination from the oral cavity or subsequently because of prior irradiation or scarring as a result of previous surgery. All these factors contribute significantly to failure of conventional bone grafts (Conley 1972, Adekeye 1978, Conley 1953, Kudo & Fujioka 1978, Millard et al 1970, Kruger 1982). To increase the survival of conventional bone grafts these authors have suggested improving the neighbouring soft tissue with the import of flaps or to delay reconstruction so that an extraoral approach avoiding contamination from the oral cavity can be performed at a later date.

Unfortunately much of the comparison between vascularised and non-vascularised autogenous bone grafts for mandible reconstruction have been made from published reports of a wide variety of mandibular defects resulting from trauma, chronic infection, congenital deformity and benign and malignant tumours. In benign conditions, a wide variety of reconstructive methods can be used employing multiple stages as required. On the other hand, when the mandible is involved with a malignant process, most commonly direct spread from the oral cavity, the prognosis is very poor (Langdon et al 1977, Wald & Calcaterra 1983, Platz et al 1985, Soderholm et al 1991). This probably relates to the fact that segmental excision of the mandible is required only in advanced disease (T3 T4). Radical surgical excision and postoperative radiotherapy offer these patients the best possible chance of 'cure'. There is therefore some urgency for the head and neck surgeon to reconstruct the defect and so minimise disfigurement and morbidity.

SURGICAL MANAGEMENT

Patients requiring mandibular resection for malignancy are at significant risk with regard to both mortality and morbidity (Robins et al 1975, Flynn 1977). Futhermore, as stated above, the cure rates and survival rates for such patients are poor with involvement of the mandible indicative of advanced disease. A careful preoperative evaluation is therefore an essential prerequisite and a multidisciplinary approach is essential. The author works as part of a head and neck team which includes the expertise of radiotherapy and oncology, oral and maxillofacial surgery, otolaryngology, plastic surgery and associated medical specialties of speech therapy, dietetics and nurse counselling. Each member of the team has an important role to play. From a clinical point of view, clinical assessment and TNM staging of disease is of vital importance. Pain, particularly that radiating to the ear or into the temple region, and abnormalities of sensation of the lower lip should be regarded as poor prognostic signs. Trismus is also generally associated with advanced disease involving the mandible.

Because of the difficulty of examining such patients the author favours the use of an examination under anaesthetic to clinically stage disease. Preoperative X-rays are mandatory and these should include an orthopantogram and where necessary lateral and occlusal views. Advice of the oral maxillofacial surgeon should be sought with regard to dentition and where mandible resection is planned, the advisability of retaining any remaining teeth should be clarified. The author has also found technetium-99M bone scans to be of some value (Ahuja et al 1990). CT scans and MRI scans are not used routinely in intraoral investigation but can be of value in assessing erosion of the mandible from external structures, notably the parotid and advanced cervical lymph node metastasis.

Identifying the amount of mandible to be resected as part of the oncological procedure is only part of the surgical problem. The surgeon has to consider the functional and cosmetic morbidity that such surgery will inflict on the patient. In choosing a method of reconstruction, the surgeon should have clear aims as to what he hopes to achieve in the way of functional stability, cosmetic appearance and subsequent denture rehabilitation. The advent of osseointegrated implants (see Chapter 22) may very well influence the choice of bony reconstruction.

Conscious of the poor prognosis of patients with advanced intraoral cancer, our head and neck team has advocated a policy of radical surgery with immediate reconstruction followed by postoperative radiotherapy (Robertson et al 1986). This radical treatment has necessitated a change in policy towards immediate reconstruction using vascularised bone grafts which have the ability to withstand postoperative radiation (Soutar & Widdowson 1986, Jewer et al 1989, Boyd et al 1990). Conventional bone grafting techniques were no longer applicable as they would not survive early radical postoperative radiation (Branemark et al 1975, Weinstein 1968). One further concern was that by adopting this radical approach there would be an increase in the incidence of osteoradionecrosis. A recent review of 188 patients with advanced intraoral tumours who underwent combined modality treatment showed osteoradionecrosis in 6.7%, with no demonstrable increase in those patients undergoing immediate reconstruction of the mandible (Ahmad et al 1992).

Each patient has to be assessed on an individual basis because of the risks associated with this type of surgery. In the final analysis, a decision is made whether the patient is fit to undergo surgery. If this is the case, then the author believes that there should be no compromise and the patient should have the best possible surgery with regard to both excision and reconstruction. There is no excuse for undertaking a compromise operation to shorten the length of anaesthetic and operating time. This only results in incomplete excision and unsatisfactory reconstruction. If the patient is unfit to undergo major surgery then alternative methods of treatment should be sought in the form of chemotherapy and/or radiotherapy.

EXCISION

By far the commonest reason for resecting the mandible is as a result of direct invasion from an intraoral carcinoma. Despite all our preoperative investigations, it is frequently very difficult to determine the exact extent of the bony resection except in cases which show gross evidence of neoplastic infiltration of the mandible. It is the intraoral part of the mandible that causes most problems as this is the site of the primary tumour and also the method by which squamous cell carcinoma invades the mandible through the occlusal surface (see Chapter 3). It should also be remembered that any tumour requiring excision of the bone is by nature an advanced lesion and in the author's practice a neck dissection is routinely performed whether the neck is clinically positive or clinically negative. Access to the mandible therefore can be achieved via the neck and it is therefore tempting to consider excision using a pull through technique. The problem with this approach is that the most important border of the mandible, i.e. the occlusal surface is not clearly identified and resection is performed in a blind manner. For lateral and posterior intraoral lesions, the author prefers to use a mandibular swing approach using a lip split and lateral mandibulotomy to gain access to the oral cavity (McGregor 1986). This gives excellent exposure of the oral cavity for precise and accurate excision of the intraoral tumour and the important occlusal surface of the

mandible. It should be remembered that despite all our preoperative investigations there remain cases in which there is doubt as to whether the mandible is truly involved with tumour and the options of upper border resection, rim resection or segmental resection have been addressed previously (Chapter 3).

It is currently the author's practice that where there is radiological evidence of invasion of bone then a segmental bone resection is performed. In cases where there is doubt as to whether the bone is involved or not, either in preoperative investigation or at the time of surgery, then a rim resection of the mandible is performed and in large tumours (T3, T4) this would include clearance of the inferior dental canal and the inferior alveolar nerve. If subsequent histology should show gross invasion of bone or an unusual histological pattern of disease then a second operation with a more radical removal of the bone should be performed.

Good access to the oral cavity not only facilitates tumour excision but also reconstruction, particularly by ensuring a watertight intraoral wound closure.

In anteriorly situated tumours in the floor of mouth and symphyseal region, satisfactory exposure of the oral cavity can be achieved without the necessity to perform a lip or chin split, although lip split can facilitate exposure when a rim resection of the symphysis is being performed. If a segmental excision of this mandibular symphysis is to be carried out then the majority of cases, in the author's experience, show gross disease in preoperative evaluation. It is easiest to approach the mandible via the neck where osteotomies can be performed laterally at the extent of resection of the mandible. Once the osteotomies are complete, the specimen can be delivered readily into the neck.

RECONSTRUCTION

Jewer et al (1989) have described a method for classifying mandibular defects. This classification divides the mandible into a central segment (C), which includes the lower canines, a lateral segment (L), which does not include the condyle, and a lateral segment (H), which does include the condyle. This HCL system of classifying mandibular defects although useful does not supply the surgeon with sufficient information to plan his reconstruction. The major problem using vascularised free bone is that the majority of donor bones are straight and require formal osteotomies to conform to the natural curvatures of the mandible. The iliac crest is the one exception as the curve of the ilium can be used to great effect in hemimandible reconstruction. In considering reconstruction of the bone therefore it is important for the surgeon to realise how many osteotomies will be required to alter the shape of the bone and obtain a satisfactory mandibular contour. Furthermore in the author's practice, the majority of patients has proved to be edentulous and this has given rise to difficulties in determining the limits of the central segment.

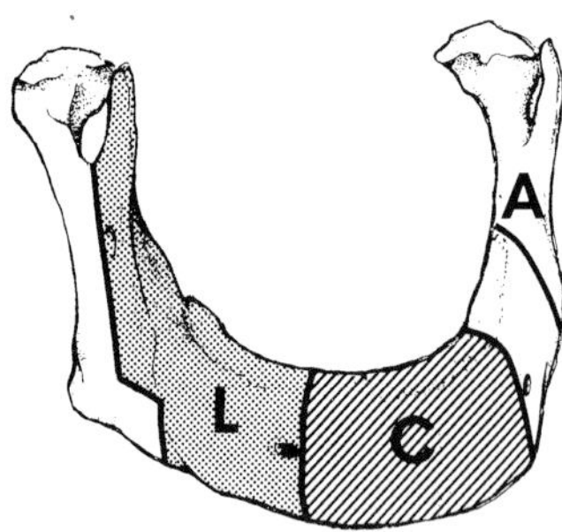

Fig. 5.1 Classification of defects in the mandible. (For key, see text.)

The author has modified the original classification of Jewer et al (1989) as follows: C = central segment extending from mental foramen to mental foramen and divided in the midline into left (Cl) and right (Cr); L = the lateral segment of the mandible from the mental foramen to the lingula preserving the condyle and posterior ascending ramus; A = the ascending ramus of the mandible (Fig. 5.1). Using this system, a standard right hemimandibulectomy = ALCr and implies two changes in direction that the bony reconstruction will have to accommodate. A pure lateral defect (L) could be reconstructed using a straight bone whereas LCl denotes reconstruction of the left mandible requiring an osteotomy to maintain chin prominence. The shape of the bony defect and the number of osteotomies that might be required to recreate that shape is a major influence on the choice of donor bone. Equally important, however, is the necessity to provide soft tissue cover either to reconstruct the external skin or to replace intraoral lining.

Careful planning of the flap is essential to avoid problems in insetting the flap and performing the microvascular anastomosis. In such situations being both the excisional surgeon as well as the reconstructive surgeon has particular benefits. Routinely the author uses two teams of surgeons, one performing the excision of the tumour and the isolation of vessels in the neck while the other simultaneously commences elevation of the flap. The two teams are interchangeable at significant points in the operative procedure. The soft tissue defect can usually be mapped out early in the surgical procedure to allow commencement of elevation of the flap and isolation of its vascular pedicle. Contouring of the bone, however, has to await resection of the mandible. Once the specimen has been resected a template is made of the resected portion of mandible using a long champey-type plate which is bent to the contours of the lower inferior border of the excised mandible (Fig. 5.2). This plate is resterilised and used at the donor site to shape and contour the bone. All osteotomy work is performed at the donor site while the bone maintains its vascularity on its pedicle. The plate is used only as a template and is not used to bridge the defect in the mandible. Only once all the osteotomy work is perfomed and the shape of the mandible is complete, together with its soft tissue flap, is the flap ready to be transferred. In this way devascularisation of the bone is kept to a minimum.

Despite the wide variety of donor sites for vascularised bone, the author has found four bones consistently useful

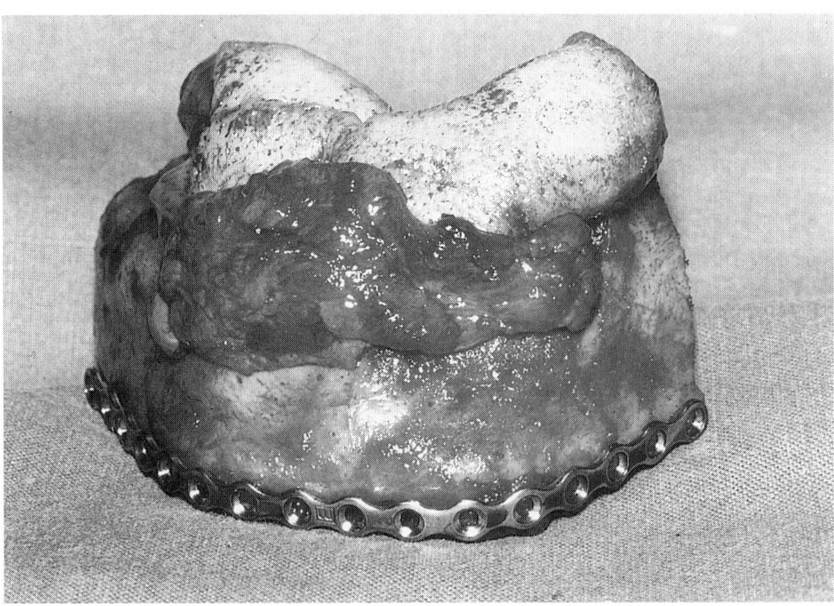

Fig. 5.2 A metal plate is shaped to the outer border of the excised specimen to act as a template for reconstruction.

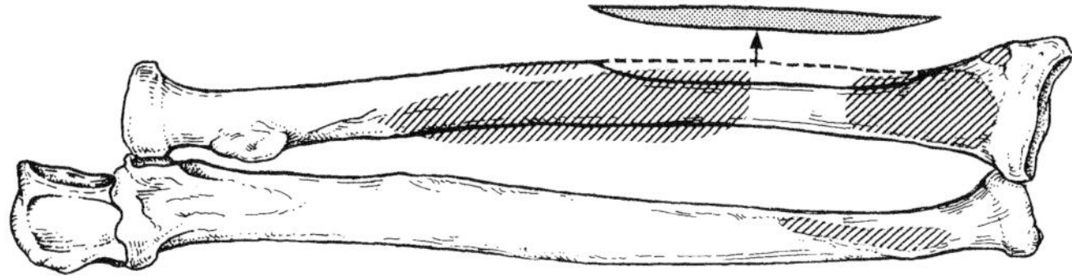

Fig. 5.3 A boat-shaped segment of radius can be removed from its lateral border.

and reliable. These are the radius, the iliac crest, the scapula and the fibula.

Radius

The radius receives a periosteal blood supply from the radial artery via perforators which pass in the lateral intermuscular septum and small vessels which pass through the flexor pollicus longus to supply the bone. The available segment of bone lies between the insertion of pronator teres proximally and brachioradialis distally (Fig. 5.3). This gives an available length of approximately 12 cm in the adult. No more than one-third of the cross-section of the radius should be removed to avoid weakening the bone and risking subsequent fracture (Bardsley et al 1990). Preoperatively an Allen test must be performed to ensure that the hand will maintain its viability following division of the radial artery. Similarly a preoperative X-ray to assess the thickness of the radius and exclude any pathology in the bone such as previous fracture is mandatory. Since the original description of the composite osteocutaneous flap used for mandible reconstruction (Soutar et al 1983, Soutar & Widdowson 1986), there have been several modifications (Soutar & Ray 1992). To avoid weakening the radius, wedge or boat-shaped osteotomies should be perfomed and right-angled cuts avoided. The bone is cortical and is therefore very strong and there is no need to take more than 25–30% of the circumference of the radius. The technique is most commonly used as a composite flap incorporating a skin paddle for soft tissue reconstruction. Although it is possible to preserve a superficial vein for venous drainage, the author prefers to rely on the venae commitantes for venous drainage and close the defect in the

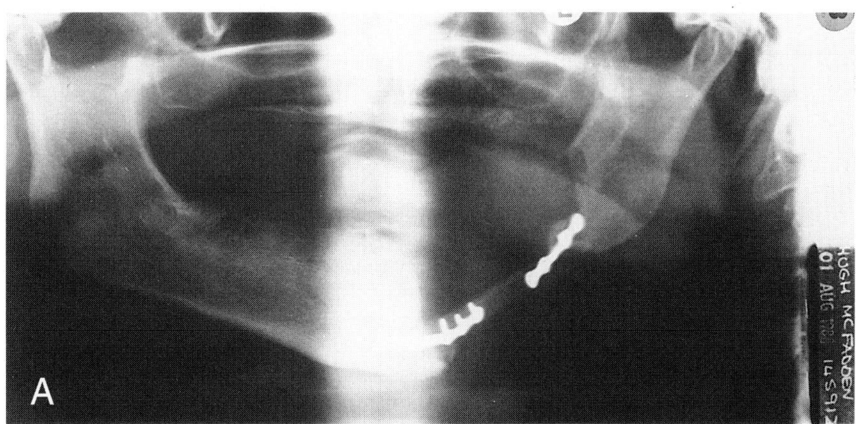

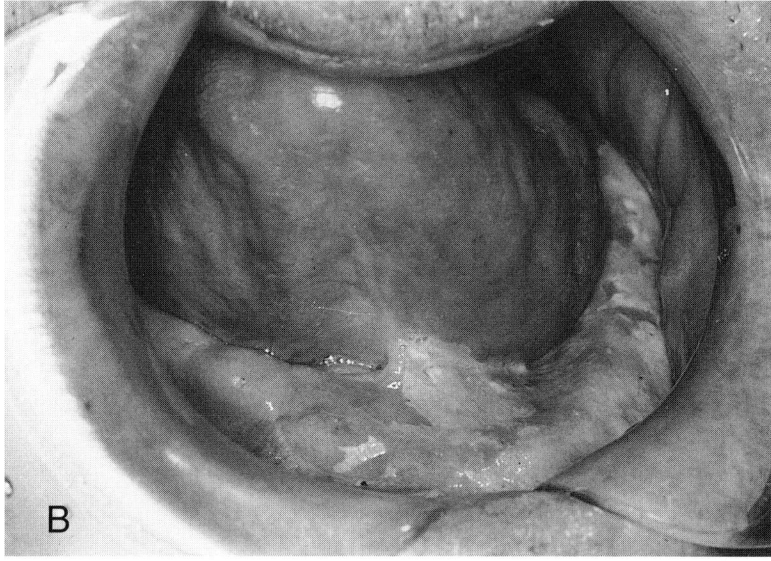

Fig. 5.4 Caption overleaf.

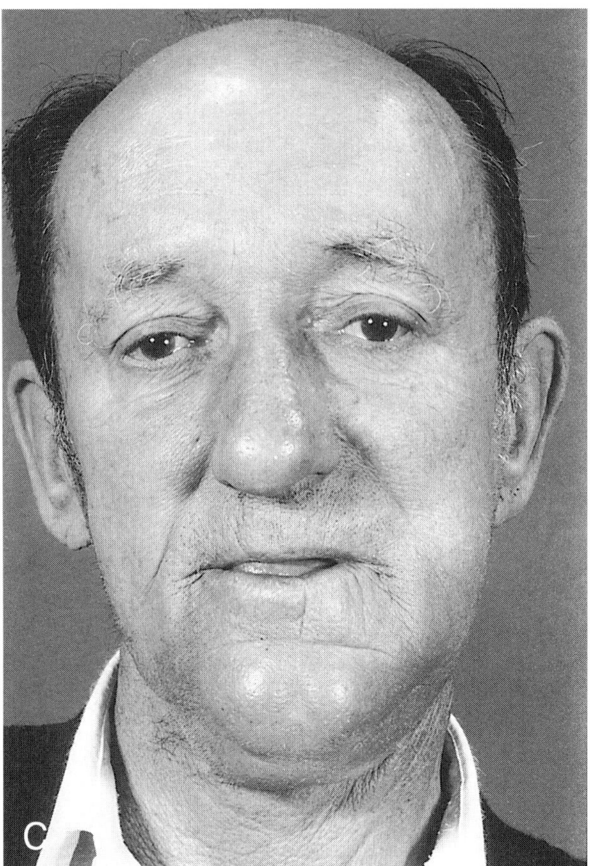

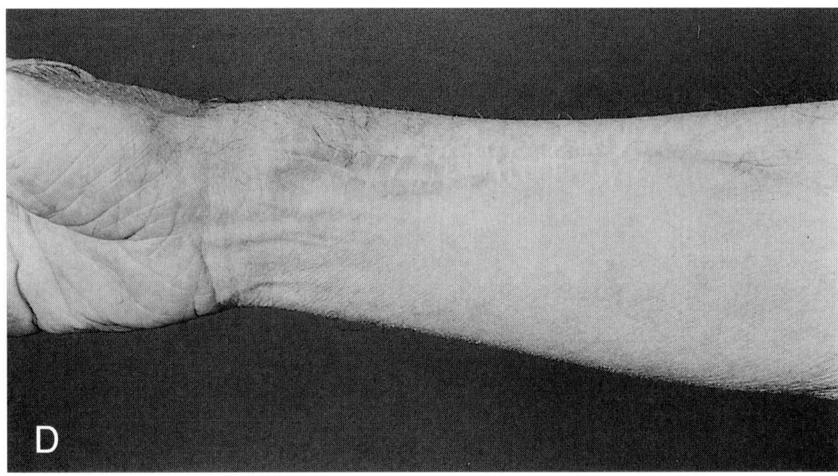

Fig. 5.4 **A** The lateral segment of mandible (L) has been replaced with a thin strip of radius. **B** The forearm skin conforms well to the contours of the oral cavity overlying the reconstructed lower alveolus. **C** The appearance at 6 months. The patient has undergone postoperative radical radiotherapy. **D** The donor defect has been closed directly with an acceptable cosmetic result.

arm directly. This has resulted in much improved cosmetic results at the donor defect (Elliot et al 1988).

The technique is best suited to composite defects of mandible and oral mucosa and the free radial forearm flap is now an established method of intraoral reconstruction (Soutar & McGregor 1986, Swanson et al 1990, Boyd et al 1990). As a composite osteocutaneous flap, it is most useful for dealing with lateral (L) defects of the mandible (Fig. 5.4). The technique is also useful with a single osteotomy for LC defects (Fig. 5.5). A closing wedge osteotomy is performed in the inner surface of the radius preserving the lateral periosteal border with the intermuscular septum and

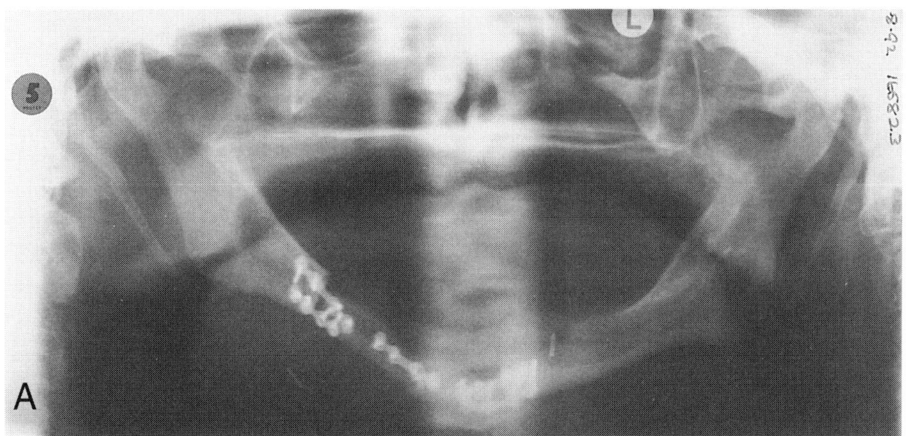

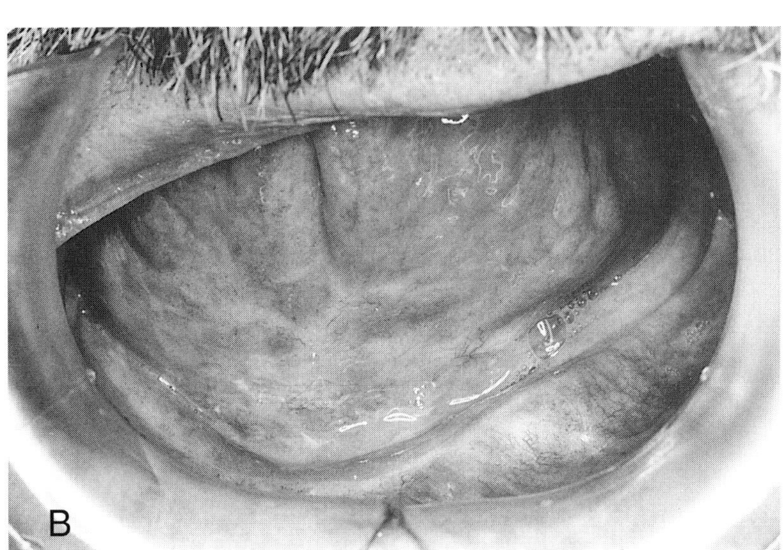

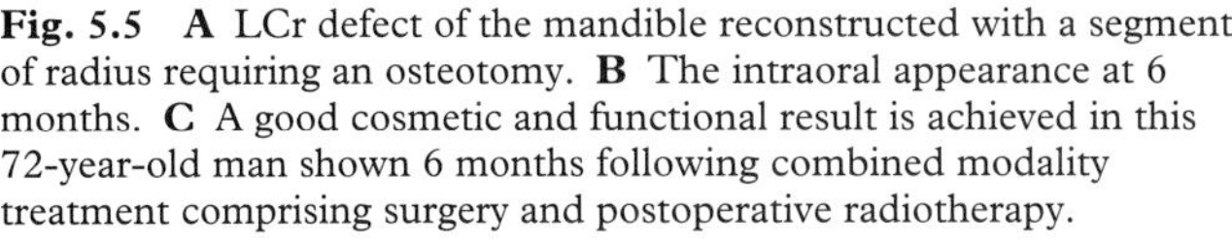

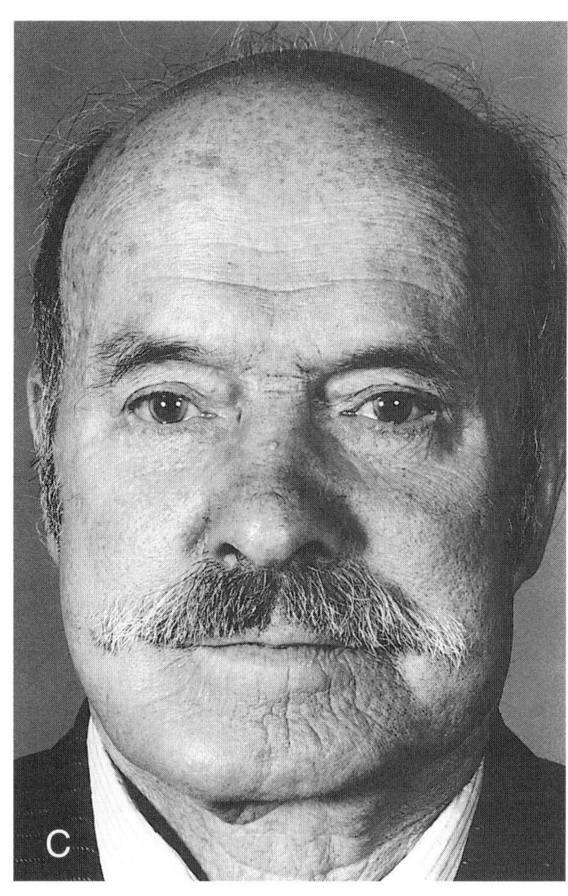

Fig. 5.5 **A** LCr defect of the mandible reconstructed with a segment of radius requiring an osteotomy. **B** The intraoral appearance at 6 months. **C** A good cosmetic and functional result is achieved in this 72-year-old man shown 6 months following combined modality treatment comprising surgery and postoperative radiotherapy.

vascular supply intact. The cortical nature of the bone is ideally suited to small plate and cortical screw fixation. The rigid fixation that can be achieved in these lateral defects gives immediate mandible stability while maintaining continuity. The soft pliable skin of the forearm ideally replaces the intraoral mucosal defect abutting on to the tongue but allowing tongue mobility. The technique is only useful, however, for small-volume defects and there is sometimes a slight flattening of the face on the side of the reconstruction. The early return of oral function and competence, however, more than adequately compensates for this deficiency.

The reliable and predictable vascular anatomy of the radial forearm flap has undoubtedly contributed to its popularity. A long vascular pedicle with good-sized vessels are available to simplify the microvascular anastomosis and

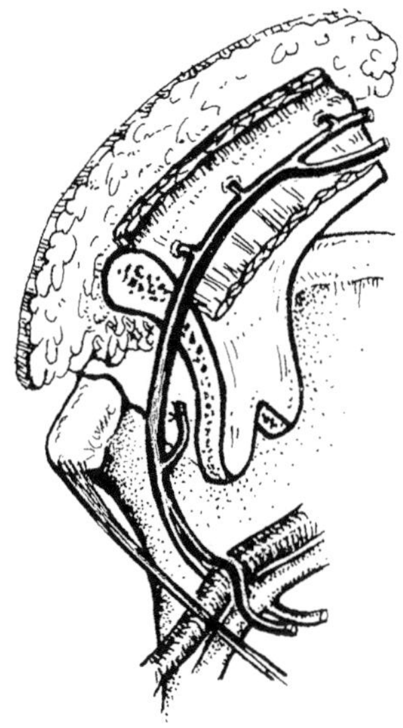

Fig. 5.6 The anatomy of the deep circumflex iliac artery flap.

this technique, in the author's hands, has proved to be one of the most reliable in intraoral reconstruction (Soutar & Ray 1992). Surgery can be performed simultaneously at both donor and recipient sites without the necessity to alter the position of the patient on the operating table. There is also some manoeuvrability in the skin paddle which does not necessarily have to be raised in the same axis as the bone. The bone although rigid is not ideally suited to receive osseointegrated implants because of its small volume but successful cases have been reported (Martin et al 1992).

Iliac crest

Where the radial forearm flap offers an almost ideal soft tissue replacement with its thin pliable skin but less than ideal bone, the reverse is true of the composite iliac crest flap based on the deep circumflex iliac artery (DCIA) (Fig. 5.6). The DCIA arises from the lateral margin of the external iliac artery at the same level as the inferior epigastric artery. It passes laterally towards the anterior superior iliac spine. Just medial to this point it gives off an ascending branch to the abdominal musculature and continues in the curve on the inner plate of the ilium approximately 2 cm below the margin of the iliac crest. It provides perforating branches direct to the inner plate of the iliac bone and provides one of the best vascularised bone donor sites that is available (Taylor et al 1979a, 1979b, Taylor 1982, Bitter et al 1983, David et al 1988, Jewer et al 1989). The overlying skin has a more precarious blood supply and it has been suggested that the composite osteocutaneous flap may require additional anastomosis of the superficial circumflex iliac system to maintain skin viability (Salibian et al 1989).

The bone is ideally suited to hemimandible reconstruction because of the natural curve of the iliac crest. The outer portion of the crest usually forms the lower border of the mandible and it can be designed so that the vascular pedicle enters either at the angle for ipsilateral anastomosis or at the symphysis for contralateral anastomosis. Careful design can allow a hemimandible to be constructed from the iliac crest preserving the anterior superior iliac spine (Fig. 5.7). This significantly improves the donor defect and is particularly important in maintaining the belt line.

As the blood supply enters the inner aspect of the iliac bone it is possible to cut this bone with the same degree of accuracy as for a non-vascularised graft. In this way, precise anatomical reconstruction can be achieved (Fig. 5.8).

The composite flap including the overlying skin is more difficult to use. The skin lies on the outer border of the iliac bone and is therefore best suited to reconstructing the external skin. When used to reconstruct intraoral lining, it has to be rotated over the bone into the intraoral defect. With the already precarious blood supply this perhaps partly explains why this skin has not proved very reliable in intraoral reconstruction (Jewer et al 1989). The skin and subcutaneous tissue together with the muscle cuff overlying the bone are sometimes too bulky to allow sufficient movement of the skin paddle over the bone and frequently provide too much bulk for intraoral reconstruction. Salibian et al (1985) have reported using this bulk to good effect in symphyseal resections with total or subtotal glossectomy. The skin flap bulk can be contoured to simulate the shape of the tongue without displacing the base of the tongue.

An alternative to taking skin as a composite flap with the DCIA is to use the internal oblique muscle which is vascularised by the ascending branch (Ramasastry et al 1984). The muscle can be left either to re-epithelialise or can be skin grafted.

The strength of the DCIA flap is in the quality of vascularised bone and the author prefers to use this technique in cases requiring bone only reconstruction or bone and cheek reconstruction. Difficulties of rotating the skin flap into the oral cavity and the bulk of the soft tissue restrict its use for composite defects involving oral lining. The curve of the iliac crest can be altered by performing osteotomies on its lateral outer cortex. Of necessity these have to be open wedge osteotomies maintaining the inner border with its vascular pedicle intact. Such open osteotomies may require a wedge-shaped portion of iliac crest to be inserted to help maintain the position and angle of the osteotomy.

The bone of the iliac crest is predominantly cancellous with a very thin cortex and is therefore not so rigidly fixed with plate and cortical screws as the more cortical bones and it is sometimes advisable to use simple interosseous wires particularly at osteotomy sites.

The DCIA flap offers a consistently reliable blood supply to the bone but less reliable to the overlying skin. A long

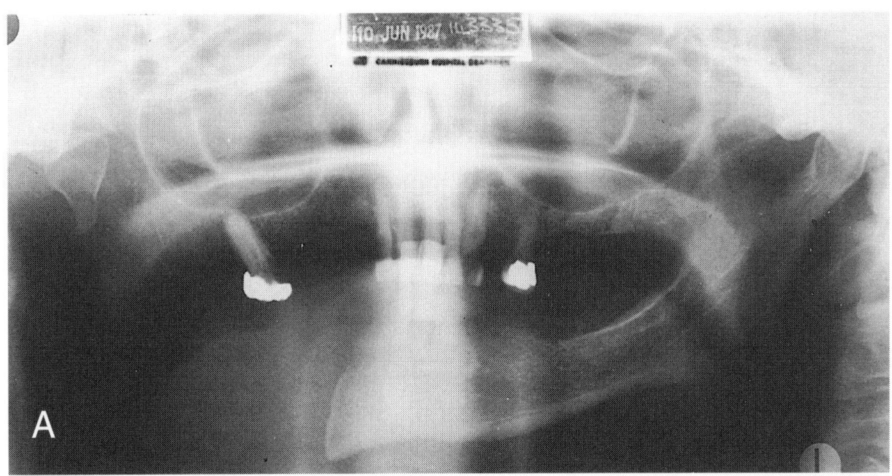

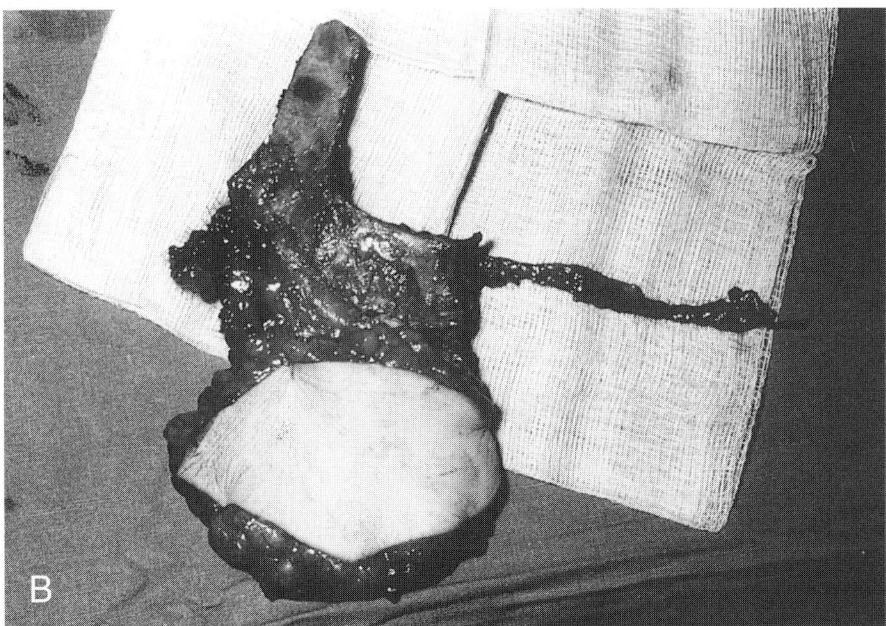

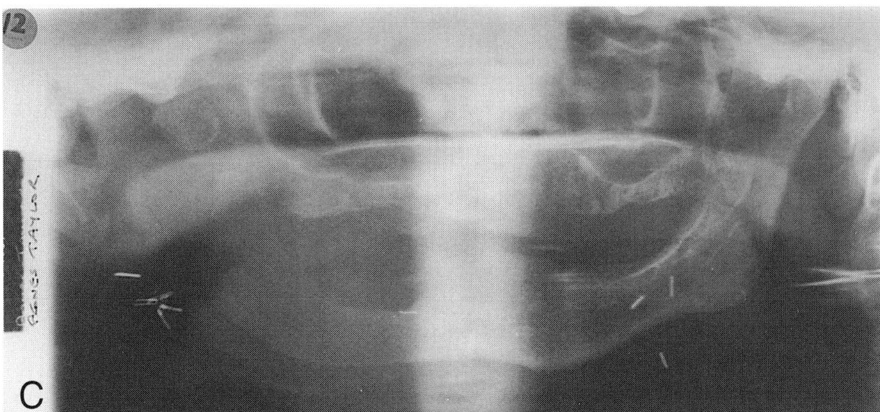

Fig. 5.7 A Mandibular defect resulting from excision of an intraoral tumour and hemimandibulectomy with reconstruction using a pectoralis major myocutaneous flap. **B** A DCIA composite flap has been raised showing the vascular pedicle, the shape of the bone and an overlying paddle of skin and soft tissue. **C** The apperance of the reconstructed mandible is shown at 4 years. **D–G** overleaf: The preoperative appearance (**D** and **E**) contrasts with the postoperative appearance 4 years following surgery (**F** and **G**).

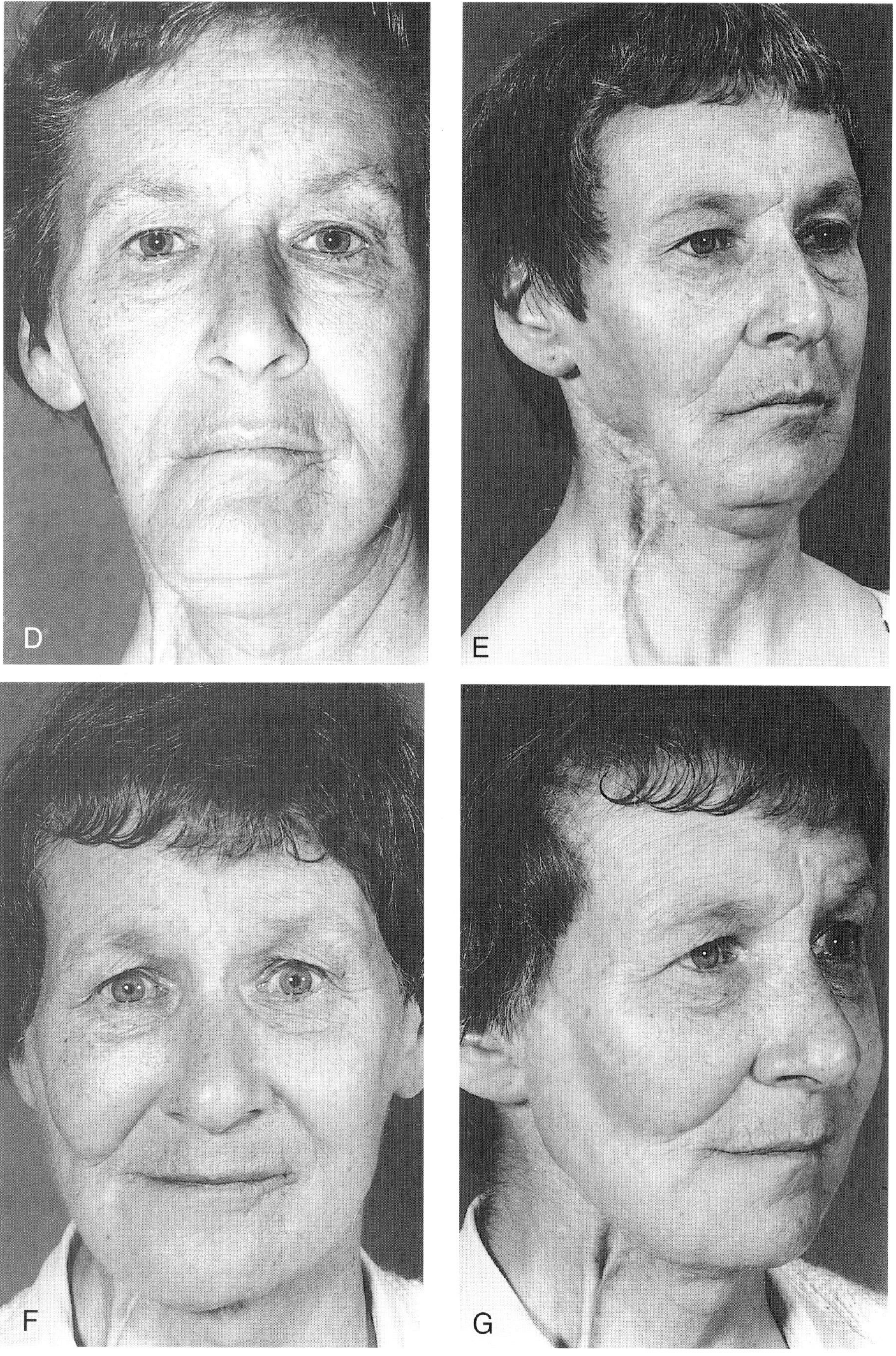

Fig. 5.7

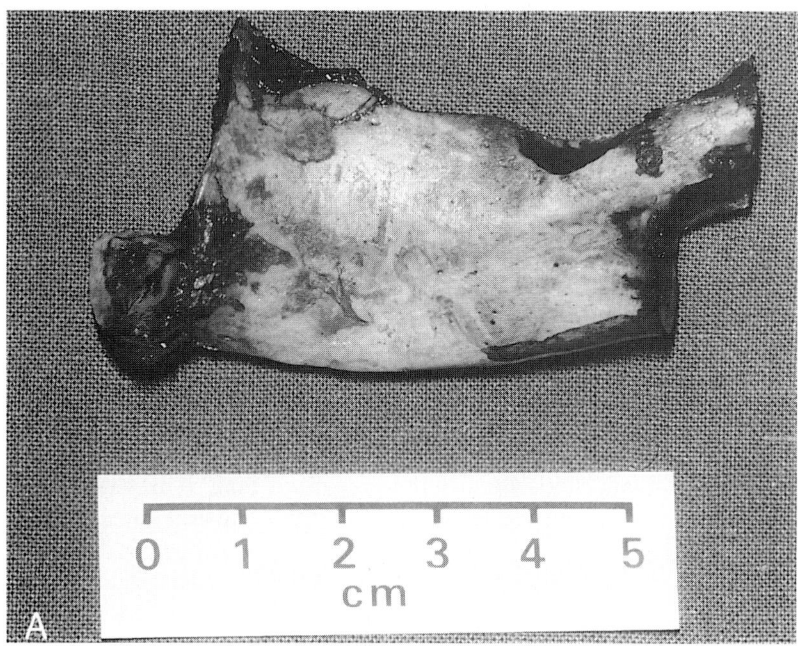

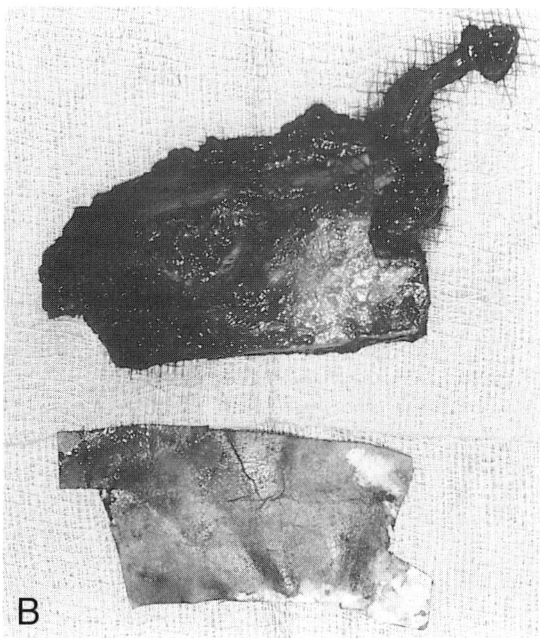

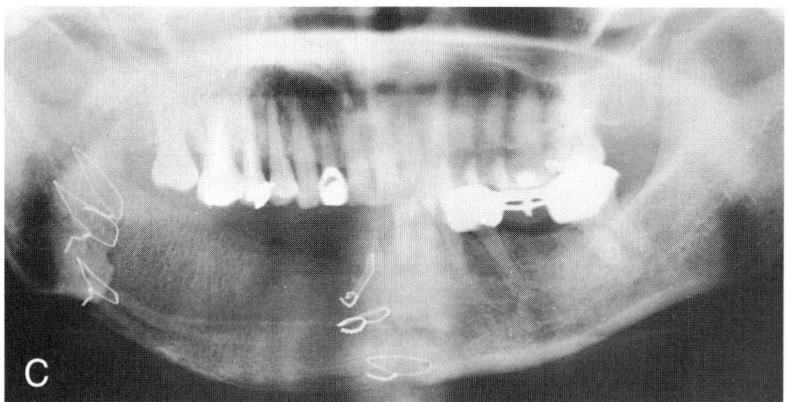

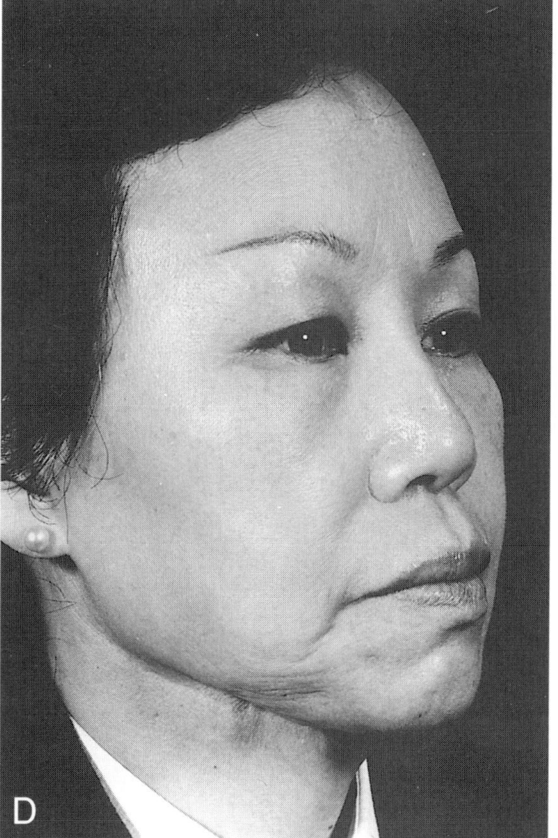

Fig. 5.8 A Resection of a segment of mandible for osteoradionecrosis. **B** Using a template, a precise match for the bone can be raised together with its vascular pedicle. **C** The mandible has been reconstructed and the X-ray appearance at 2 years is shown. **D** The patient has good function and cosmetic appearance. The scars of the skin are the result of abscess formation at the time of an acute episode of osteoradionecrosis.

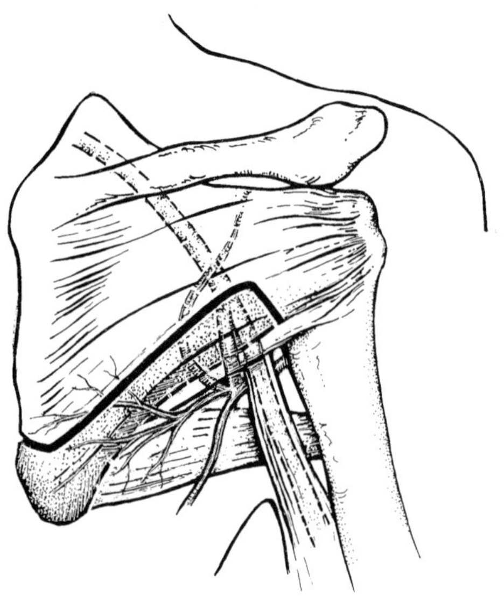

Fig. 5.9 The anatomy of the scapula osteocutaneous flap.

vascular pedicle in excess of 8 cm can be dissected to simplify microvascular anastomosis. Simultaneous operating can be performed at both donor and recipient sites without the necessity to move the position of the patient on the operating table.

The iliac crest vascularised on the DCIA can provide a large volume of very well vascularised bone suitable for mandible reconstruction and subsequent osseointegration of implants (see Chapter 22).

Scapula

The lateral border of the scapula can be raised as an extension of the scapular flap based on the subscapular artery (Swartz et al 1986, Baker 1989). A bone segment approximately 12–14 cm in length and 3 cm in width can be raised from the lateral border of the scapula (Fig. 5.9). The skin of the scapular flap can be raised either as a horizontal transverse scapular flap or as a more vertical parascapular flap and has proved to be very reliable. This is one of the strengths of the scapular flap as a composite osteocutaneous flap. The skin is not only reliable but can be placed at a distance from the bone allowing a high degree of manoeuvrability with regard to bone and soft tissue reconstruction (Fig. 5.10). The bone is good quality corticocancellous bone but is relatively thin. It is straight and therefore requires an osteotomy to change direction. Because of its cortical component it is readily fixed by small plates and cortical screws allowing immediate rigid fixation. The skin of the back is rather thick to provide a good intraoral lining and sometimes the cutaneous flap can be quite bulky. This can, however, be used to good effect in reconstruction of symphyseal defects where the bulk of the skin flap can be used in a similar fashion to that described by Salibian et al (1985) for the DCIA flap. The author has found the scapular osteocutaneous flap most useful for limited symphyseal resections. The 3-cm lateral border of scapula adequately compensates for mandibular height, which is useful in maintaining the chin and lip position. The bone, however, is somewhat thin to accommodate osseointegrated implants should this be required at a later date.

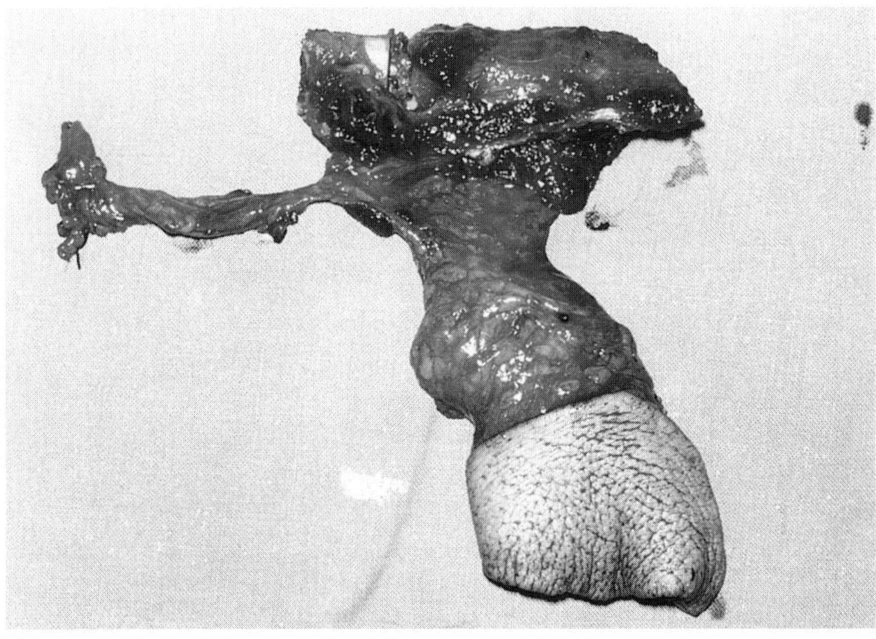

Fig. 5.10 The skin paddle and bone raised on the same vascular pedicle. Careful planning can allow for significant manoeuvrability of both skin and bone.

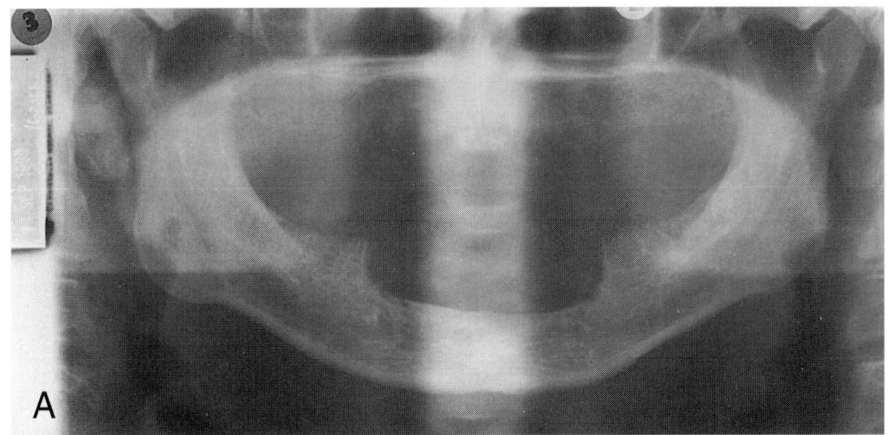

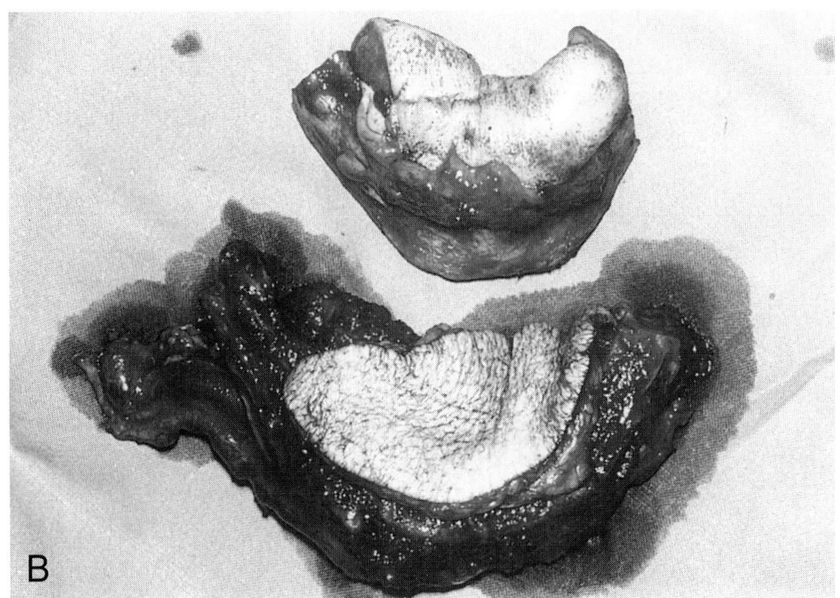

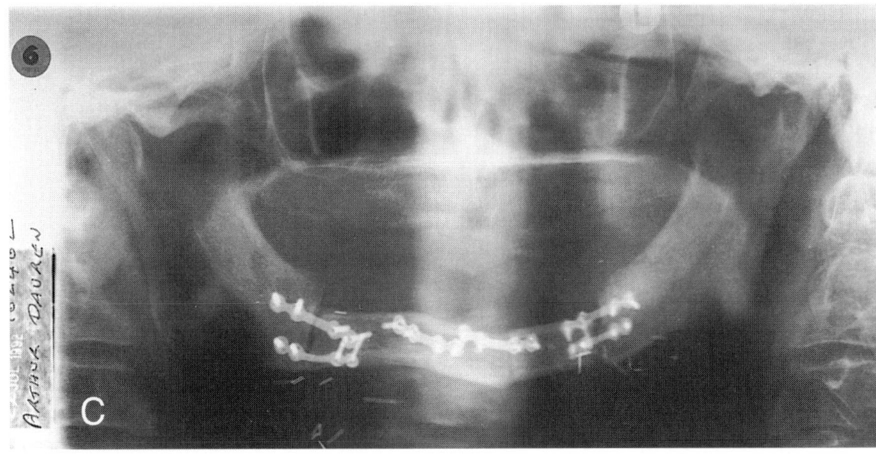

Fig. 5.11
Caption overleaf

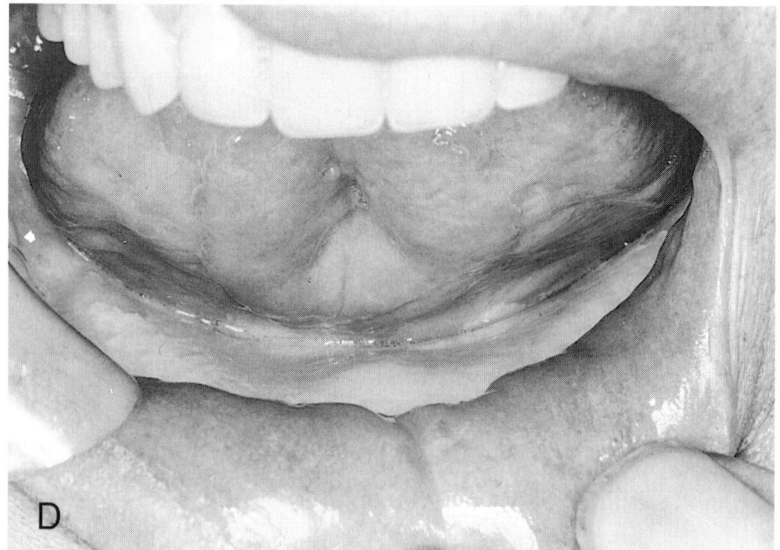

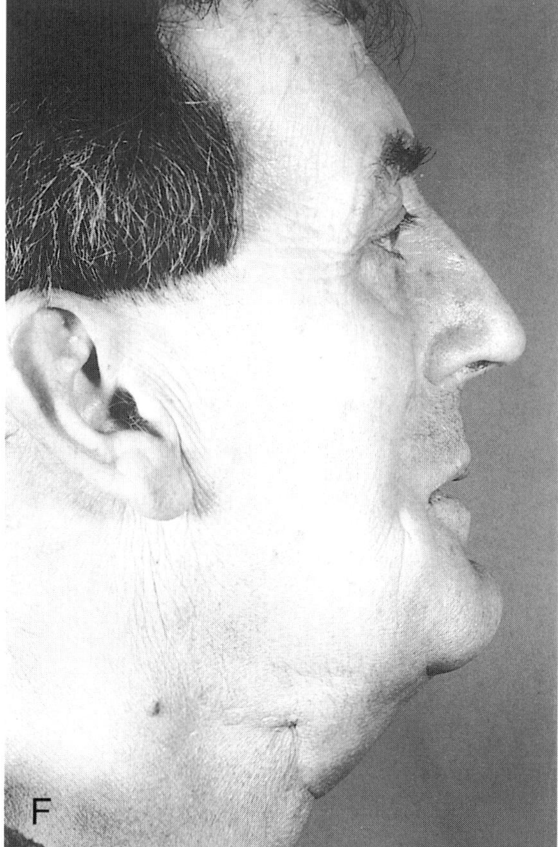

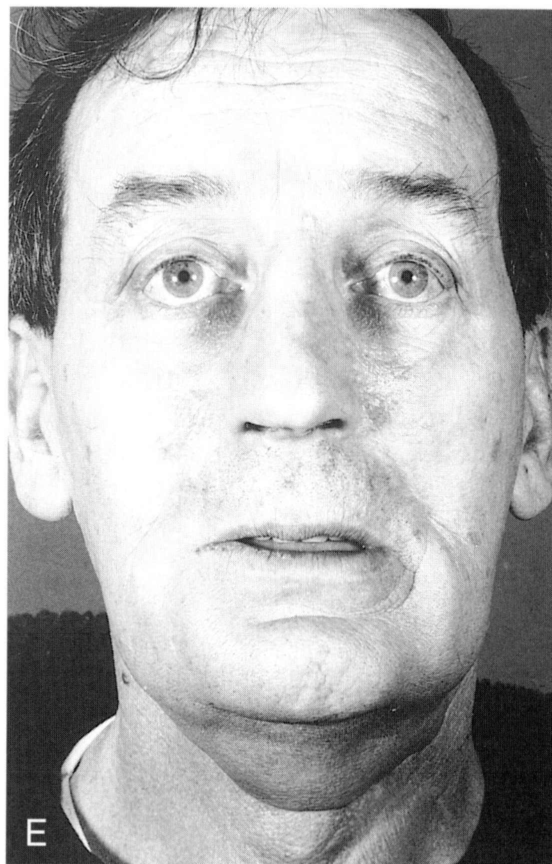

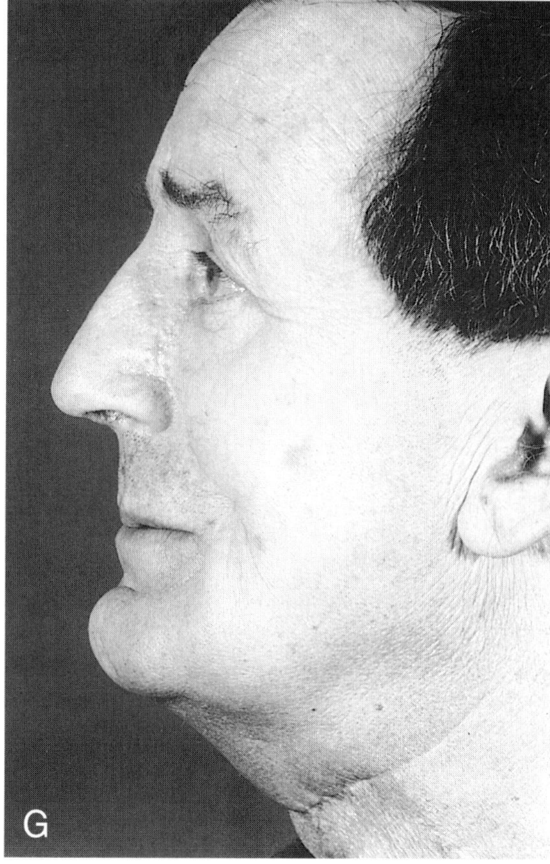

Fig. 5.11 A This patient had undergone excision of the floor of mouth including a rim resection of the mandible as shown and reconstruction using nasolabial flaps. Histology showed the presence of tumour within the mandible. **B** A more radical excision was performed and the fibula osteocutaneous flap contoured to the shape of the defect. **C** The orthopantogram shows the extent of the fibula reconstruction. **D** The skin adequately reconstructs the floor of the mouth. **E, F, G,** A satisfactory reconstruction of the chin has been achieved and the patient remains disease-free 3 years postoperatively.

Both the skin and the bone of this flap, however, are reliably vascularised. A long vascular pedicle can be raised with good-sized vessels simplifying the microsurgical aspects of reconstruction. Despite careful positioning of the patient on the operating table, it is often very difficult to operate at both the donor and the recipient sites simultaneously because of the lack of space available. Care should be taken when raising this flap in conjunction with a radical neck dissection as the resultant shoulder dysfunction can be significantly disabling.

Fibula

The fibula has only recently become a popular method of mandible reconstruction. It was initially described as a vascularised bone transfer (Taylor et al 1975) and subsequently as a composite flap including the overlying peroneal skin (Chen & Yan 1983). It was the introduction of this composite flap that was to prove the stimulus for its use in mandible reconstruction (Hidalgo 1989, Fleming et al 1990). The fibula is supplied by a nutrient branch from the peroneal artery and by segmental periosteal branches of the same artery. It is likely that in the age group of the population requiring mandible reconstruction that the periosteal blood supply is the more important. The island of skin is centred over the fibula in the same axis and allows very little manoeuvrability between the bone and the skin. The skin, however, in most individuals is relatively thin and pliable.

The fibula has proved a very reliable source of vascularised bone and similarly the overlying skin has a reliable vascular pattern. The author prefers the approach described by Gilbert (1979) rather than the originally described by Taylor et al (1975). This lateral approach gives excellent access for both bone only and for composite fibula flaps. The fibula offers the longest length of bone that is available. It is an extremely strong bone with a high cortical component. It is most suited for extensive symphyseal resections where a large length of bone is required. One of the difficulties of working with the fibula, however, is in carrying out the osteotomies because of the dense cortical nature of the bone. Where possible the author prefers to make closing wedge osteotomies preserving as much periosteum as possible intact and safeguarding the vascular pedicle. With experience a wide variety of osteotomies can be performed in the fibula, maintaining its vascular pattern and improving the contour of this bone (Hidalgo 1991, Serra et al 1991). As the skin flap lies along the axis of the bone, it is ideally suited to replace the floor of the mouth in symphyseal reconstruction (Fig. 5.11). Where more bulk is required a section of soleus muscle can also be included with the flap (Baudet et al 1992). The fibula provides a very acceptable donor site (Goodacre et al 1990), but care should be taken to preserve sufficient fibula both proximally and distally to preserve

knee and ankle stability. Proximally care must also be taken to preserve and protect the common peroneal nerve.

The major disadvantage of the fibula is that it has a relatively short vascular pedicle, although this can be lengthened by stripping some of the periosteum and siting the bone graft more distally. In the very elderly, care must be taken to ensure that division of the peroneal arterial supply will not affect the viability of the lower limb or foot.

The cortical nature of this long bone gives it tremendous strength and enables absolute rigid fixation with plates and screws. It is also suitable for subsequent osseointegrated implants and is really in class of its own for extended symphyseal reconstruction.

CONCLUSIONS

Vascularised bone offers significant advantages to the head and neck surgeon over conventional or traditional methods of bone grafting. To all intents and purposes, contamination of the local field when the oral cavity is breached or scarring and contracture associated with radiotherapy, previous trauma, surgery or infection can be ignored as the technique offers the possibility of introducing both vascularised bone and well vascularised soft tissue at the same time. Immediate reconstruction of major defects involving the mandible is therefore now possible with success rates much superior to those achieved in the same situation by conventional techniques. Such surgery, although complicated, has not proved to have any increase in mortality. With immediate reconstruction the morbidity for patients with a very poor prognosis is significantly reduced. Microvascular surgery has opened up new horizons in head and neck reconstruction such that defects which were previously unimaginable can now satisfactorily be reconstructed. This may require more complicated techniques involving one or more free flaps (Fig. 5.12).

Unfortunately there is no ideal solution for mandible reconstruction. Many of the vascularised bones require significant effort to recreate the correct contour and shape of the mandible by performing specialised and somewhat difficult osteotomies while at the same time maintaining vascularity and viability. Inclusion of skin as a composite flap is not always ideal for either intraoral reconstruction or reconstruction of the external cheek or chin. Despite these drawbacks, microvascular bone transfer has permitted surgeons to be more aggressive in their excision and to complement this with combined modality treatment. The rapid rate of wound healing in particular has enabled early postoperative radiotherapy to be performed within a matter of weeks of surgery. It is to be hoped that by adopting a more aggressive approach that the survival of this poor prognostic group of patients will be improved or at least the morbidity associated with treatment will be diminished.

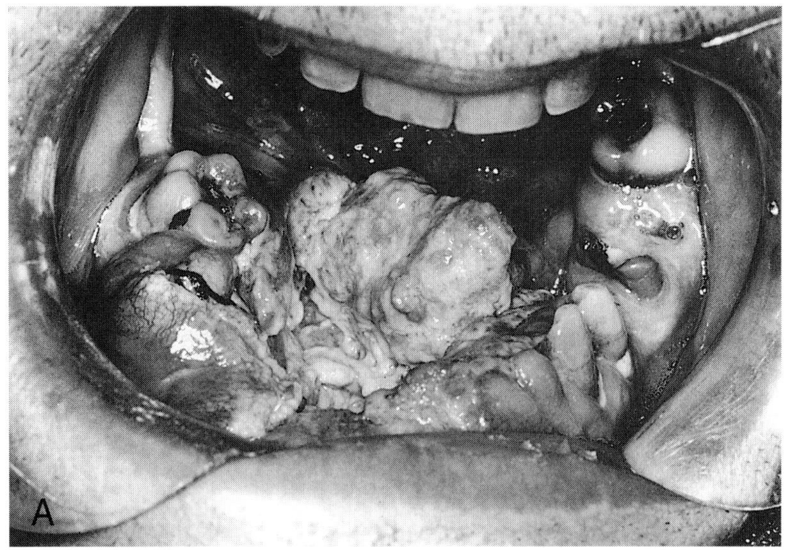

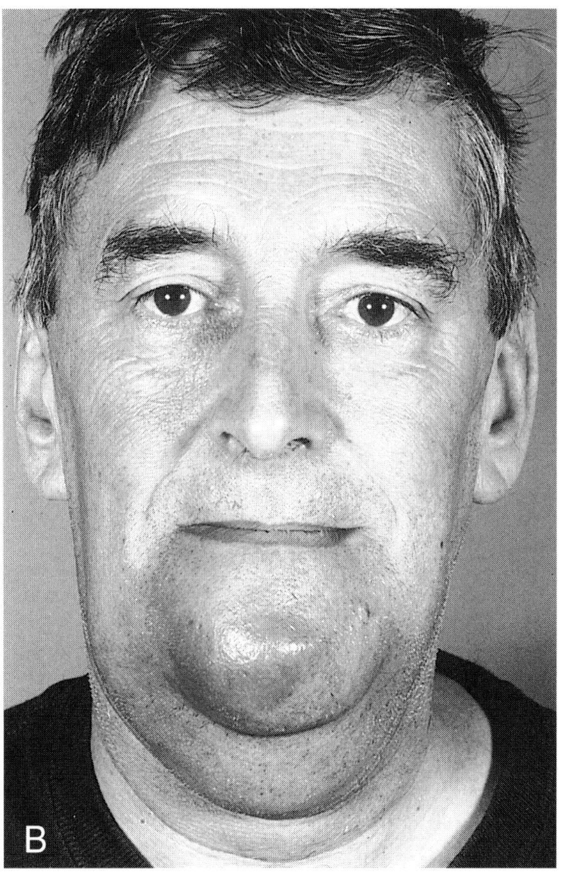

Fig. 5.12 Caption on page 76

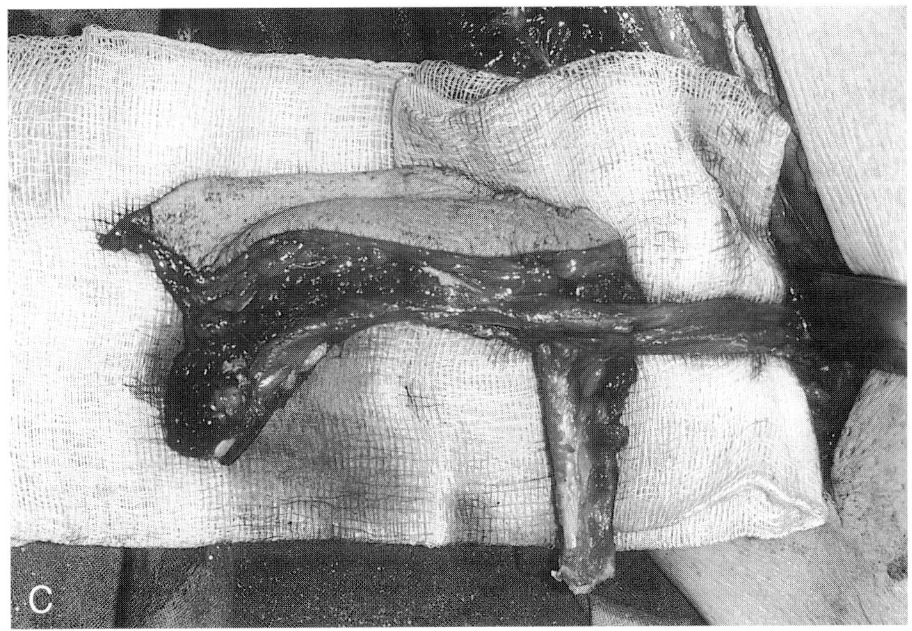

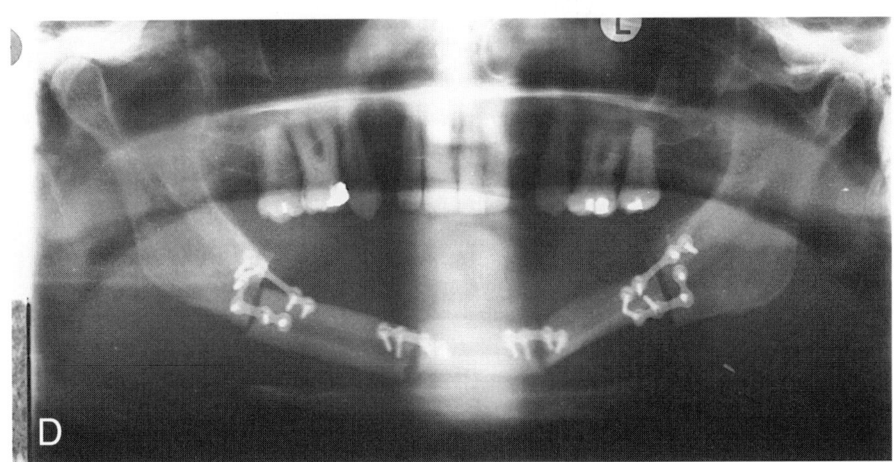

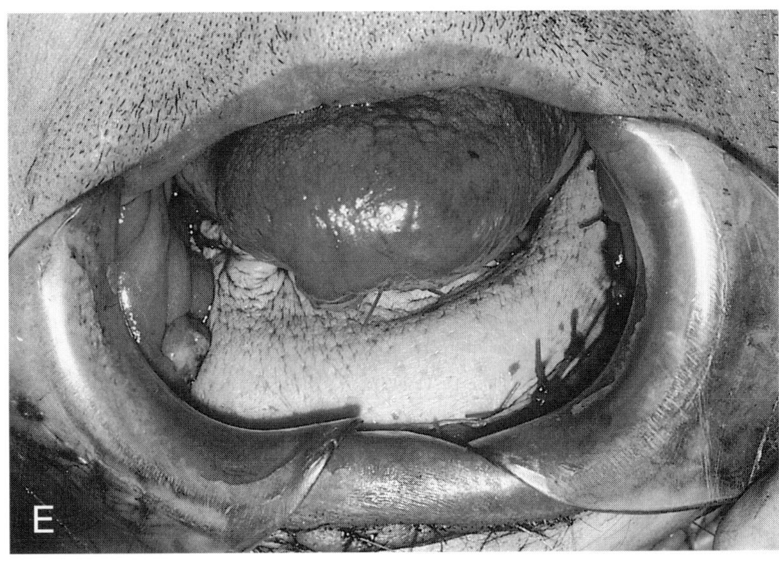

Fig. 5.12 Caption on page 76

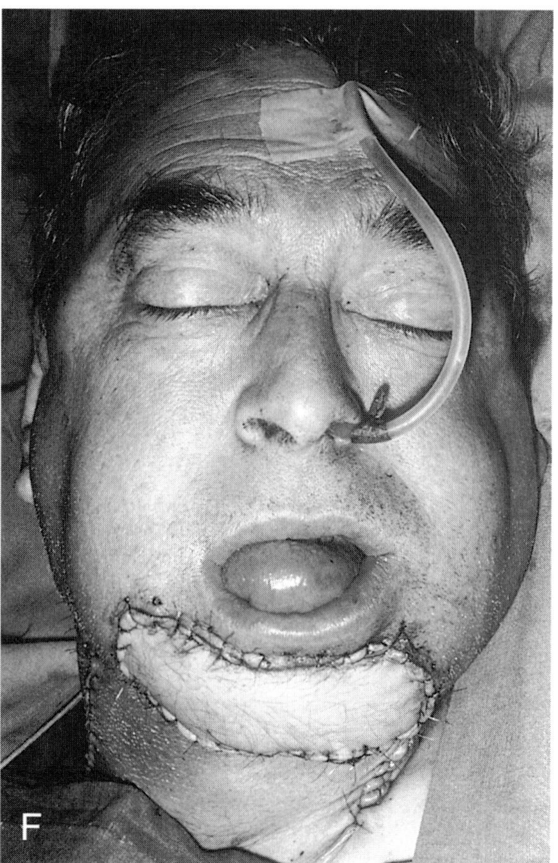

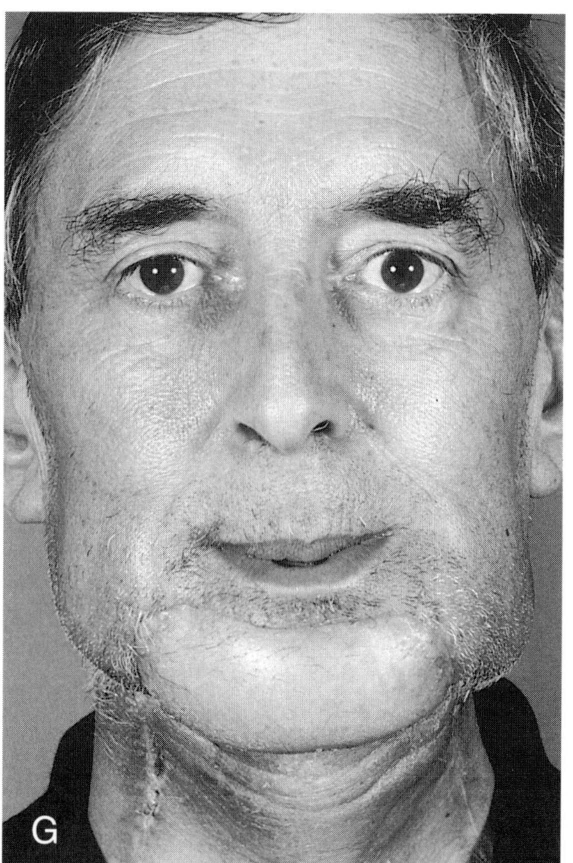

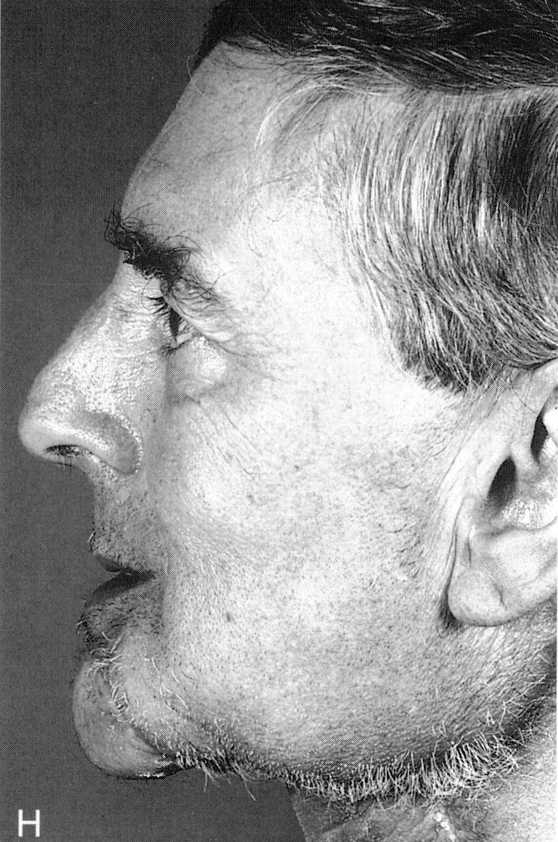

Fig. 5.12 A & B An extensive squamous cell carcinoma of the floor of mouth involving the symphysis of the mandbile and the chin. Excision involved the symphysis of the mandible, floor of mouth and skin of the chin. **C** A fibula osteocutaneous flap is prepared and contoured on the leg. **D** The orthopantogram shows the extent of the reconstruction of the bone. **E** The peroneal skin was used to replace the floor of the mouth. **F** A radial forearm flap was used as a separate free flap to reconstruct the external chin. **G & H** The appearance 3 weeks postoperatively. Even at this early stage there is a satisfactory cosmetic and functional result and the patient is ready to commence radio-therapy.

REFERENCES

Adekeye E O 1978 Reconstruction of mandibular defects by autogenous bone grafts: a review of 37 cases. Journal of Oral Surgery 36: 125

Ahmad M S S, Rao G S S, Robertson A G, Soutar D S 1992 The incidence and management of osteoradionecrosis following combined modality treatment for intraoral cancer. Unpublished data.

Ahuja R B, Soutar D S, Moule B et al 1990 Comparative study of technetium-99M bone scans and orthopantomography in determining mandible invasion in intraoral squamous cell carcinoma. Head and Neck 12: 237

Baker S R 1989 Scapular flaps. In: Baker S (ed) Microsurgical reconstrucion of the head and neck. Churchill Livingstone, New York

Bardsley A F, Soutar D S, Elliot D et al 1990 Reducing morbidity in the radial forearm flap donor site. Plastic and Reconstructive Surgery 86: 287

Baudet J, Martin D, Persichetti P 1993 Bone defects in the lower limb. In: Soutar D S (ed) Microvascular surgery and free tissue transfer. Edward Arnold, London

Berggren A, Weiland A J, Dorfman H 1982 Free vascularised bone grafts: factors affecting their survival and ability to heal to recipient bone defects. Plastic and Reconstructive Surgery 69: 19

Bitter K, Schlesinger S, Westerman U 1983 The iliac bone or osteocutaneous transplant pedicled to the deep circumflex iliac artery. Journal of Maxillofacial Surgery 11: 241

Boyd J B, Rosen I B, Freeman J et al 1990 The iliac crest and the radial forearm flap in vascularised oral mandibular reconstruction. American Journal of Surgery 159: 301

Branemark P I, Lindström J, Hallen O et al 1975 Reconstruction of the defective mandible. Scandinavian Journal of Plastic and Reconstructive Surgery 9: 116

Burwell R G 1965 Osteogenesis in cancellous bone grafts considered in terms of cellular changes, basic mechanisms and the perspective of growth-control and its possible aberrations. Clinical Orthopaedics 40: 35

Chen Z W, Yan W 1983 The study and clinical application of the osteocutaneous flap of fibula. Microsurgery 1: 4

Conley J J 1953 A technique of immediate bone grafting in the treatment of benign and malignant tumours of the mandible and a review of 17 consecutive cases. Cancer 6: 568

Conley J 1972 Use of composite flaps containing bone for major repairs in the head and neck. Plastic and Reconstructive Surgery 49: 522

Cutting C B, McCarthy J G 1983 Comparison of residual osseous mass between vascularised and non-vascularised onlay bone transfers. Plastic and Reconstructive Surgery 72: 672

Daniel R K 1977 Free rib transfer with microvascular anastomoses. Plastic and Reconstructive Surgey 59: 737

Daniel R K 1978 Mandibular reconstruction with free tissue transfers. Annals of Plastic Surgery 1: 346

David D J, Tan E, Katsaros J et al 1988 Mandibular reconstruction with vascularised iliac crest: a ten year experience. Plastic and Reconstructive Surgery 82: 792

Elliot D, Bardsley A F, Batchelor A G et al 1988 Direct closure of the radial forearm flap donor defect. British Journal of Plastic Surgery 41: 358

Fleming A F S, Brough M D, Evans N D et al 1990 Mandibular reconstruction using a vascularised fibula. British Journal of Plastic Surgery 43: 403

Flynn N B 1977 Morbidity and mortality of mandibular resection for malignant disease. American Journal of Surgery 134: 510

Gilbert A 1979 Vascularised transfer of the fibula shaft. International Journal of Microsurgery 1: 100

Goodacre T E E, Walker C J, Jawad A S et al 1990 Donor site morbidity following osteocutaneous free fibula transfer. British Journal of Plastic Surgery 43: 410

Gray J C, Elves M W 1981 Osteogenesis in bone grafts after short term storage and topical antibiotic treatment. Journal of Bone and Joint Surgery 63B: 441

Ham A, Gordon S 1952 The origin of bone that forms in association with cancellous chips transplanted into muscle. British Journal of Plastic Surgery 5: 154

Haw C S, O'Brien B, Kurata T 1978 The microsurgical revascularisation of resected segments of tibia in the dog. Journal of Bone and Joint Surgery 60B: 226

Hidalgo D A 1989 Fibula free flap: a new method of mandibular reconstruction. Plastic and Reconstructive Surgery 84: 71

Hidalgo D A 1991 Aesthetic improvements in free flap mandible reconstruction. Plastic and Reconstructive Surgery 88: 574

Jewer D D, Boyd J B, Manktelow R T et al 1989 Orofacial and mandibular reconstruction with the iliac crest free flap: a review of 60 cases and a new method of classification. Plastic and Reconstructive Surgery 84: 391

Kaplan E L, Buncke H J, Muray D E 1973 Distant transfer of cutaneous island flaps in humans by microvascular anastomoses. Plastic and Recostructive Surgery 52: 301

Katsaros J, Schusterman M, Beppu M et al 1984 The lateral arm flap: anatomy and clinical applications. Annals of Plastic Surgery 12: 489

Knize D M 1974 The influence of periosteum and calcitonin on onlay bone graft survival. Plastic and Reconstructive Surgery 53: 190

Kruger E 1982 Reconstruction of bone and soft tissue in extensive facial defects. Journal of Oral and Maxillofacial surgery 40: 714

Kudo K, Fujioka Y 1978 Review of bone grafting for reconstruction of discontinuity defects in the mandible. Journal of Oral Surgery 36: 791

Langdon J D, Harvey P W, Rapidis A D et al 1977 Oral cancer: the behaviour and response to treatment of 194 cases. Journal of Maxillofacial Surgery 5: 221

La Trenta G S, McCarthy J G, Cutting C B 1987 The growth of vascularised onlay bone transfers. Annals of Plastic Surgery 18: 511

Lovie M J, Duncan G M, Glasson D W 1984 The ulnar artery forearm free flap. British Journal of Plastic Surgery 37: 486

Manchester W M 1972 Some technical improvements in the reconstruction of the mandible and temporomandibular joint. Plastic and Reconstructive Surgery 50: 249

Martin I C, Cawood J I, Vaughan E D, Barnard N 1992 Enclosseous implants in the irradiated composite radial forearm free flap. Journal of Oral Maxillofacial Surgery 21: 266

McGregor I A 1986 The surgical approach to the mouth. In: McGregor I A, McGregor F M (eds) Cancer of the face and mouth. Churchill Livingstone, Edinburgh

McLeod A M, Robinson D W 1982 Reconstruction of defects involving the mandible and floor of mouth by free osteocutaneous flaps derived from the foot. British Journal of Plastic Surgery 35: 239

Millard D R, Garst W P, Campbell R C et al 1970 Composite lower jaw reconstruction. Plastic and Reconstructive Surgery 46: 22

Moore J B, Mazur J M, Zehr D et al 1984 A biochemical comparison of vascularised and conventional autogenous bone grafts. Plastic and Reconstructive Surgery 73: 382

Ostrup L T, Fredrickson J M 1975 Reconstruction of mandibular defects after radiation using a free living bone graft transferred by microvascular anastomosis: an experimental study. Plastic and Reconstructive Surgery 55: 563

Ostrup L T, Tam C S 1975 Bone formation in a free living bone graft transferred by microvascular anastomoses. Scandinavian Journal of Plastic Surgery 9: 101

Peer L A 1955 Transplantation of tissue. Williams & Wilkins, Baltimore

Platz H, Fries R, Hudec M 1985 Retrospective DOSAK study on carcinomas of the oral cavity: results and consequences. Journal of Maxillofacial Surgery 13: 147

Puckett L L, Hurvitz J S, Metzler M H et al 1979 Bone formation by revascularised periosteal bone grafts compared with traditional grafts. Plastic and Reconstructive Surgery 64: 361

Ramasastry S S, Tucker J B, Swartz W M, Hurwitz D J 1984 The internal oblique muscle flap: an anatomic and clinical study. Plastic and Reconstructive Surgery 73: 721

Robertson A G, McGregor I A, Soutar D S et al 1986 Postoperative radiotherapy in the management of advanced intraoral cancers. Clinical Radiology 37: 173

Robins R E, Budden M K, MacDougall J A 1975 Analysis of mortality and morbidity in 100 composite resections for oral carcinoma. American Journal of Surgery 130: 178

Rosen I B, Bell M S, Barron P et al 1979 Use of microvascular flaps including free osteocutaneous flaps in reconstruction after composite resection for radiation-recurrent oral cancer. Americal Journal of Surgery 138: 544

Rosen I B, Manktelow R Y, Zuker R M et al 1985 Application of microvascular free osteocutaneous flaps in the mangement of postradiation recurrent oral cancer. American Journal of Surgery 150: 474

Salibian A H, Rappaport I, Allison G 1985 Functional oromandibular reconstruction with the microvascular composite groin flap. Plastic and Reconstructive Surgery 76: 819

Salibian A H, Allison G, Rappaport I et al 1989 Functional microvascular reconstruction after total and subtotal glossectomy. In: Karcher H (ed) Functional surgery of the head neck. Druck Verlagsgesellschaft

Serra J M, Paloma V, Masa F et al 1991 The vascularised fibula graft in mandibular reconstruction. Journal of Oral and Maxillofacial Surgery 49: 244

Soderholm A L, Lindquist C, Sankila R et al 1991 Evaluation of various treatments for carcinoma of the mandibular region. British Journal of Oral and Maxillofacial Surgery 29: 223

Soutar D S, Scheker L R, Tanner N S B et al 1983 The radial forearm flap: a versatile method for intraoral reconstruction. British Journal of Plastic Surgery 36: 1

Soutar D S, Widdowson P W 1986 Immediate reconstruction of the mandible using a vascularised segment of radius. Head and Neck Surgery 8: 232

Soutar D S, McGregor I A 1986 The radial forearm flap in intraoral reconstruction: the experience of 60 consecutive cases. Plastic and Reconstructive Surgery 78: 1

Soutar D S, Ray A K 1992 The radial forearm flap in head and neck reconstruction In: Jackson I T, Sommerlad B C (eds) Recent advances in plastic Surgery—4. Churchill Livingstone, Edinburgh

Swanson E, Boyd J B, Manktelow R T 1990 The radial forearm flap: reconstructive applications and donor site complications in 35 consecutive cases. Plastic and Reconstructive Surgery 85: 258

Swartz W M, Banis J C, Newton E D et al 1986 The osteocutaneous scapular flap for mandibular and maxillary reconstruction. Plastic and Reconstructive Surgery 77: 530

Taylor G I, Miller G T H, Ham F J 1975 The free vascularised bone graft: a clinical extension of microvascular tehniques. Plastic and Reconstructive Surgery 55: 533

Taylor G I, Watson N 1978 One stage repair of compound leg defects with free revascularised flaps of groin skin and iliac bone. Plastic and Reconstructive Surgery 61: 494

Taylor G I, Townsend P, Corlett R 1979a Superiority of the deep circumflex iliac vessels as the supply for free groin flaps: experimental work. Plastic and Reconstructive Surgery 64: 595

Taylor G I, Townsend P, Corlett R 1979b Superiority of the deep circumflex iliac vessels as the supply for free groin flaps: clinical work. Plastic and Reconstructive Surgery 64: 745

Taylor G I 1982 Reconstruction of the mandible with free composite iliac bone grafts. Annals of Plastic Surgery 9: 361

Taylor G I 1983 The current status of free vascularised bone grafts. Clinics in Plastic Surgery 10: 185

Teot I, Bosse J P, Moufarrege R et al 1981 The scapular crest pedicled bone graft. International Journal of Micorsurgery 3: 257

Thomson M, Casson J A 1970 Experimental onlay bone grafts to the jaws. Plastic and Reconstructive Surgery 46: 341

Wald R M, Calcaterra T C 1983 Lower alveolar carcinoma: segmental versus marginal resection. Archives of Otolaryngology 109: 578

Webster M H C, Soutar D S 1986 Practical guide to free tissue transfer. Butterworth, London

Weiland A J, Phillips T W, Randolph M A 1984 Bone grafts: a radiologic, histologic and biomechanical model comparing autografts, allografts and free vascularised bone grafts. Plastic and Reconstructive Surgery 74: 368

Weinstein I R 1968 Bone grafting after mandible resection. Journal of Oral Surgery 26: 17

Wood M B 1986 Free vascularised bone transfers for nonunions, segmental gaps and following tumour resection. Orthopaedics 9: 810

Zins J E, Whitaker L A 1983 Membranous versus endochondral bone: implications for craniofacial reconstruction. Plastic and Reconstructive Surgery 72: 778

6. Mandibular reconstruction with conventional bone graft

Rammohan Tiwari

HISTORICAL REVIEW

The use of autogenous bone for reconstruction of the mandible is one of the oldest methods in use. According to Hamblen (1978) the use of bone graft was first described by McEwan in 1880. One of the earliest reports was by Bardenheur in 1892 with the use of rib and tibial grafts. He also published a case of mandibular reconstruction with an osteocutaneous forehead flap. Six decades passed before the significance of his technique was realised. In 1900 Skyhoff employed free grafts for mandibular reconstruction. It was not until World War II that the value of autogenous bone grafts for mandibular reconstruction was recognized and became popular. Blocker and Stout (1947) reported experience on 1010 bone grafts taken from various donor sites including tibia, rib and iliac crest by various workers, for the purpose of mandibular reconstruction. Although this experience was entirely on traumatic cases, it is nevertheless one of the largest series reported. They reported an overall success rate of over 90% Their report brought to the forefront the reliability of the iliac crest for this purpose.

In the sixties, the use of the rib for mandibular reconstruction was popular and frequently reported in the literature (Ketchum et al 1974, McCullough & Fredrickson 1972) for this purpose. The superior osteogenic potential of cancellous bone and its paucity in a rib graft however, limited its use. In recent years Piggot & Logan (1983) and Wersall et al (1984) have reported extensively on the successful use of rib grafts for mandibular reconstruction. Sanders & Cox (1976) and Sanders (1982) reported its use in augmentation rib grafting of the mandible.

Since the iliac crest offers a much greater potential as a source of cancellous bone, and the ilium can easily provide compact as well as cancellous bone equivalent to a half of the mandible, this became the favourite site for autogenous bone grafts for the purpose of mandibular reconstruction (Lindemann 1916). Its use has been extensively reported in the literature either as compact, cancellous or particulate bone by Adamo & Szal (1979), Boyne & Zarem (1976), Millard et al (1971) and Manchester (1965). Lindström's

report on the use of preformed autologous bone graft for mandibular reconstruction was a significant step (Lindström et al 1981).

BONE GRAFT SURVIVAL

The fate of autogenous bone grafts is a subject that has attracted the attention of research workers as well as clinicians for several centuries. According to Chase & Herndon (1955) the first scientific report on the subject of osteogenesis was of Duhamel in 1742. They also refer to the significant contribution of Axhausen on the role of the periosteum in osteogenesis (Axhausen 1909). He put forward the concept that after a massive transfer of autogenous bone the transplanted bone dies but that most of the periosteum survives and is a source of lively osteogenesis. These observations have stood the test of time. In normal circumstances the periosteum does not seem to have any osteogenic function, but in the presence of a stimulus such as a fracture or surgical trauma the potentialities of the periosteum to form osteoblasts is revived. In recent years Mowlem observed that the bone should be regarded not as a tissue, but as an organ consisting of two parts. One part is cellular, active and living, while the other part is inorganic, passive and inanimate (Mowlem 1963). Mowlem stressed the value of a vascular environment and the presence of the necessary stimulus for the graft to survive and to modulate itself to the required form in a particular part of the body. In recent years calvarial bone flaps for cranifacial reconstruction have been used in the belief that cranial bones, being of membranous origin similar to those of the facial skeleton, are more rapidly vascularized than bone of endochondral origin (Kusiak et al 1981). However, this view has been challenged, and Cohen et al (1989) in a controlled study concluded that the success of bone grafting depends on the use of meticulous surgical technique, simultaneous closure of coexisting fistulae, use of cancellous bone particles only and coverage of grafts with well vascularized flaps. The source of bone grafts does not seem primarily to influence the success of the outcome. According to Burwell, the outcome of autologous free bone graft is known to depend upon factors such as graft cell survival, the revascularization rate and the osteogenic potential at the host site (Burwell 1969). The survival of compact bone graft is dependent on an intact blood supply, and the few cells buried in its dense calcified matrix cannot survive free transplantation. After a few days an autologous graft is effectively dead. Nevertheless, it provides an osteogenic stimulus to the bed in which it is placed, causing osteogenic cells of the host to proliferate. Herein lies the importance of a well vascularized bed for the graft. Many investigators believe that the periosteum contains osteoblasts and should therefore be carefully preserved both at the recipient site as well as over the graft. Cancellous bone contains more cells and although many of these cells will not survive grafting some will remain viable by diffusion of nutrients from the tissue fluids. These surface cells have the ability to proliferate and differentiate into osteoblasts. Vessels grow in from the periosteum and the medulla, and the new bone is laid down on the surface. The graft is first anchored by this activity at its peripheries and then gradually invaded by revascularization of the old Haversian system to remove dead bone by osteoclastic activity and replace it with new living bone formed by osteoblastic cells.

EXCISIONAL TECHNIQUES

The last two decades have seen much progress in the field of mandibular reconstruction. Primary reconstruction with microvascular free bone or composite grafts has now become a first choice and is practised extensively. Other techniques, such as allografts and the use of metal plates in combination with myocutaneous flaps, have also been used extensively (Gullane 1991). In a cancer operation, the mandible may have to be sacrificed at one of the following sites: the ascending ramus, the horizontal ramus and the arch. Loss of even a part of the mandibular continuity affects the functional abilities of the patient with regard to speech, swallowing and competence of the oral commisure as well as aesthetic appearance to a varying degree. This disability is least with the loss of the ascending ramus, moderate when the horizontal ramus is involved and severe when the arch of the lower jaw is sacrificed. Several decades ago Byers

(1954) stressed the need for conservation of the mandibular bone. He proposed segmental resection, but opposed disarticulation. A marginal resection whenever oncologically safe is preferable to segmental resection. Sacrifice of bone of the mandible may be either for a primary tumour of the mandible or because of secondary involvement of the bone with cancer. The tumour may be too close to the mandible or may be growing along the inferior dental canal. These are invariably large tumours not uncommon in somewhat older patients with an edentate atrophic mandible. Radiotherapy following surgery often forms an integral part of the treatment. Unless a free vascularized composite flap or a metal plate can be used, reconstruction with simple autogenous grafts is preferably deferred until well after the radiation reaction has come to rest. Some clinicians take the view that if the patient is unsuitable for a free vascularized graft, he/she should be treated as a palliative problem. These patients often have nutritional and medical problems. This consideration along with the already mentioned availability of modern methods of primary reconstruction account for the fewer non-vascularized simple bone grafts used over the last decade. It is important therefore to individualize the reconstructive management of every case to acheive optimum results. The increased risk of graft failure in radiated patients has led to the use of hyperbaric oxygen (Marx & Ames 1982). They reported a 91.6% success rate for grafts using 30 hours of preoperative and 15 hours of postoperative hyperbaric oxygen with 100% oxygen administered at 2.4 times absolute atmospheric pressure for 1.5 hours at each treatment for 30 sittings.

PRIMARY VERSUS SECONDARY RECONSTRUCTION

Primary reconstruction is the method of choice while using an autogenous bone graft. It has the advantage that the vascularity of the recipient bed is not compromised and there is little scar tissue formation. Apart from this, the bone fragments are healthy, reasonably vascularized, and can easily be aligned in the desired position. On the other hand, primary reconstruction adds to the length of the procedure. The important consideration, however, is the fact that the

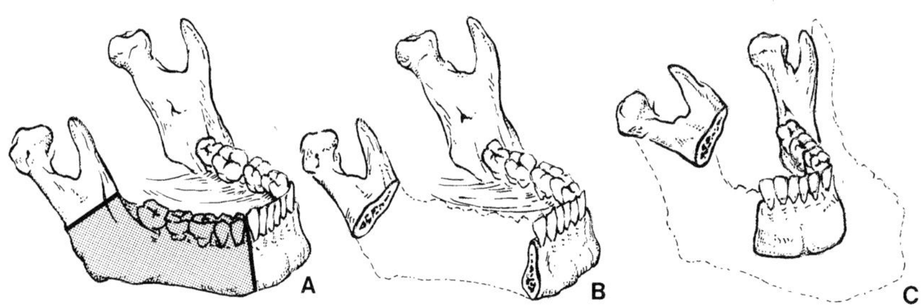

Fig. 6.1 Changes after segmental mandibular resection. The remaining mandibular segments deviate towards the defect, because of the unopposed pull of the remaining muscles of mastication and scar contracture.

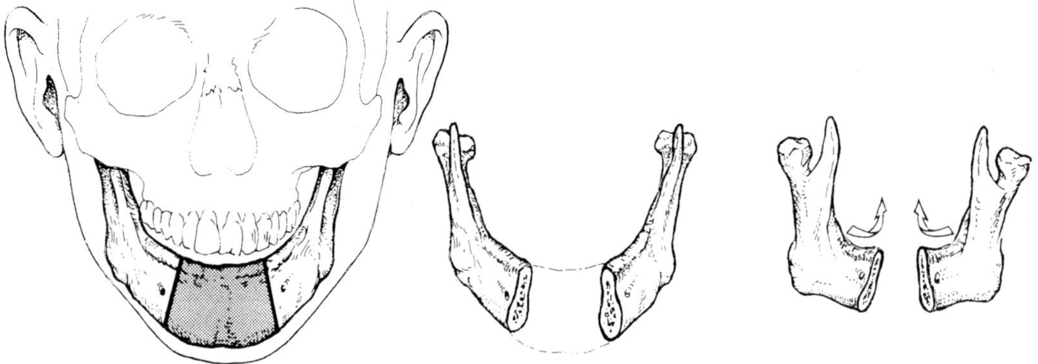

Fig. 6.2 Changes following resection of the anterior arch. Both segments are pulled medially and upwards by contraction of the pterygoid muscles.

recipient bed is contaminated. The advantage of secondary reconstruction is that a temporary delay will ensure that the graft will be placed in a non-contaminated area. The patient's general condition and nutritional status by this time would have been improved. Radiation impedes the growth of osteocytes, retards bone healing and can lead to loss of the graft. Therefore, when the patient has to be radiated, secondary reconstruction is preferred. Following lateral segmental resection, the remaining segment deviates towards the defect because of scar contracture and the unopposed pull of the remaining muscles of mastication (Fig. 6.1). It must be said, however, that patients occasionally like to postpone this second reconstruction procedure simply because they are unable to muster the necessary

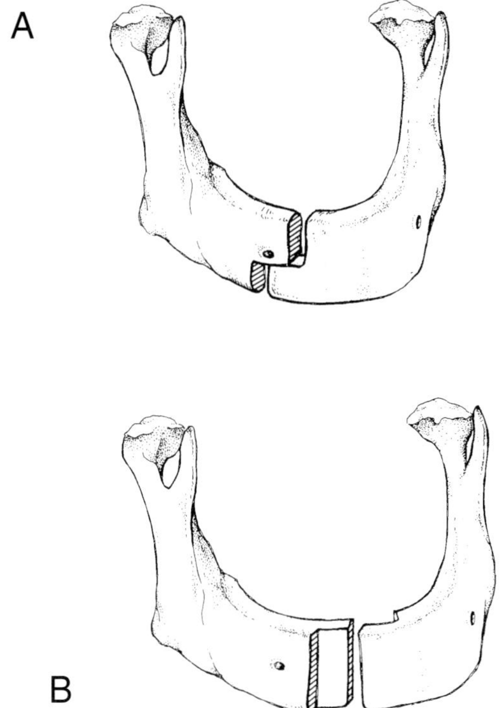

Fig. 6.3 **(A, B)** Planning cuts at the time of excision.

self-confidence, having undergone major surgery and radiotherapy. Technically, secondary reconstruction can occasionally pose problems, especially if the remaining ascending ramus is small and retracted anterosuperiorly. It is the ultimate prognosis with regard to the tumour that outweighs all other considerations. If the prognosis is poor, one can afford to delay the reconstruction until such time that the chance of recurrence is remote. On the other hand, where the prognosis is favourable an early reconstruction is advisable. Defects of anterior arch need to be treated as a priority. Following resection of the anterior arch, both segments are pulled upwards and medially by the pterygoids (Fig. 6.2). Anterior mandibulectomy can precipitate the development of sleep apnoea (Panje & Holmes 1984). Primary mandibular reconstruction is considered after segmental resection for benign or locally malignant tumours of odontogenic origin by some (Cohen & Schultz 1985). There is very little soft tissue loss in these resections. A water-tight closure of the oral mucosa is an essential prerequisite. Iliac crest is the favourite donor site, although rib is preferred by some because of its capability for bone regeneration, especially if some periosteum is preserved at the donor site.

THE PROCEDURE

Before actually excising the tumour a careful study of the radiological findings and CT scans along with the clinical findings with regard to the primary tumour must be undertaken. Within reasonable limits it is safer to err to the side of slightly larger excision than otherwise. Keeping in mind the nature of reconstruction, the cuts are made. In a broad horizontal ramus, for instance, it is wise to make a 'stepwise' cut so that the graft can be made to fit and rest on it (Fig. 6.3A). Alternatively, a deep sulcus can be created to engage the graft which can be appropriately shaped (Fig. 6.3B). In reconstruction of a half of the mandible, the size of the graft can be mapped out with the help of a 1-to-1 CT scan and carved out of the ilium (Fig. 6.4).

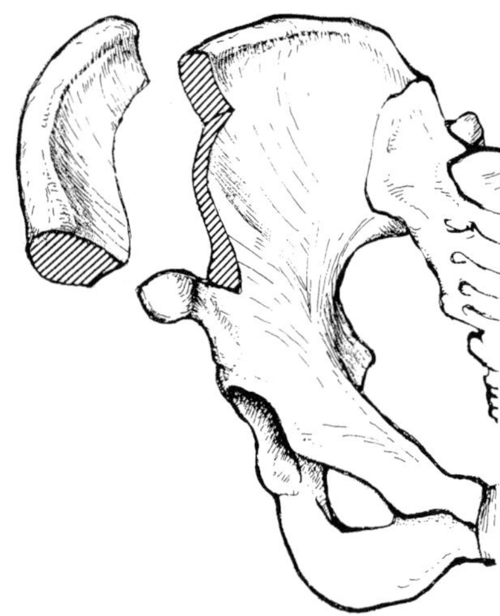

Fig. 6.4 The ilial bone graft.

The configuration of the ilium permits the design of a hemimandible on it with the anterosuperior iliac spine as the angle of the mandible (Fig. 6.5). The cranial end can be shaped to resemble a condyle. Fibrous union and formation of a pseudocapsule usually allows a good range of movement. When the reconstruction involves the anterior arch, every effort should be made to create the form of the chin. The graft may need to be bent. This can be achieved by keeping the outer periosteum intact and making wedge cuts into the inner surface of the cancellous bone (Millard et al 1971) (Fig. 6.6). When a rib is used for reconstruction, the designed curvature either for the ramus or the arch can be obtained by making multiple sections through the posterior cortex. The rib graft is then 'skewed' with a bent Kirschner wire to obtain the desired shape (Piggot & Logan 1983). Irrespective of what kind of bone graft is harvested, its length must preferably be about 2 cm more than that of the defect so as to compensate for the loss of bone during the process

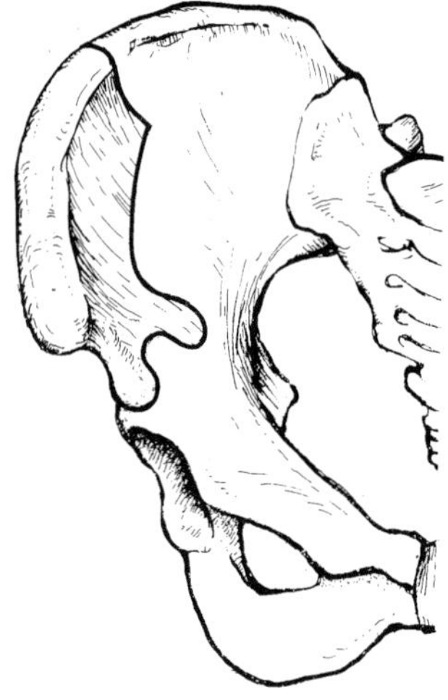

Fig. 6.5 Planning a hemimandible bone graft from the ilium.

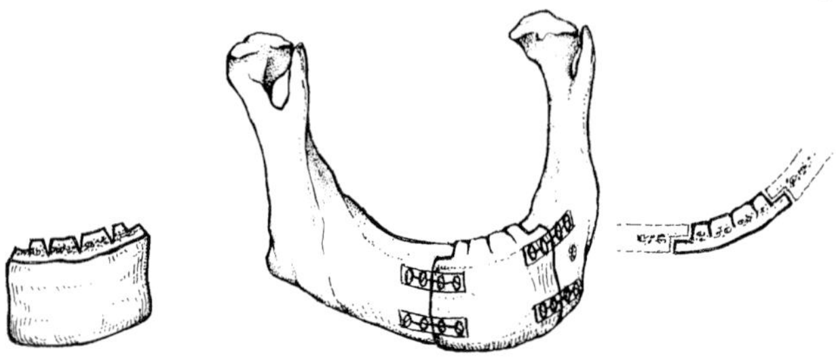

Fig. 6.6 Modelling and fixation of the graft for anterior arch.

of modelling the graft to the shape of the defect. When a secondary reconstruction is planned it is vital that the alignment of the remaining mandibular segments are maintained after primary surgery. In a dentate patient this can be achieved by intermaxillary fixation using cast vitallium splints. In an edentulous patient monobloc acrylic appliances are constructed by the prosthodontist. A temporary tracheotomy is advisable after intermaxillary fixation. When an insufficient length of the horizontal ramus is left on one side for the appliance to be placed, fixation is not necessary, provided the pterygoid and the temporalis muscles have been severed from the stump. External biphasic splints are used by some in edentulous patients.

Exposure of the mandibular stumps for secondary reconstruction is performed through the pre-existing suprahyoid scar. Care is needed in the dissection. The carotid vessels may be exposed as most of these patients have had an en bloc neck dissection. If the internal jugular vein had been preserved, it is vulnerable. The vascular pedicle of the myocutaneous flap needs to be preserved if blood supply to the recipient bed is to be optimally safeguarded. Injury to the oral mucosa should be avoided at all costs, and, should this occur it is better to postpone further surgery until the fistula has healed. Some surgeons prefer to harvest the graft only after the recipient bed has been prepared. The graft is excised out of the ilium with an electric saw to obtain accurate sharp cuts. Cancellous bone obtained in addition to the graft, as well as the graft, is stored in gauze soaked in the patient's own blood. Perfect bony contact is essential. The mandibular stumps are burred away until bleeding is encountered. Mention has been made of appropriate shaping of the graft and the stumps to achieve maximum contact. Cancellous bone revascularizes more quickly than cortical bone. Additional chips of cancellous bone at the site of contact help to restore vascularization and provide stability, and the dead space is obliterated. The bony ends must be well immobilized. Champey plates with three screws on either side are adequate, although some surgeons prefer a complete A0 plating (Fig. 6.7). Other alternatives, such as Gunning splints secured with circumzygomatic and circummandibular wires, are used. External fixation, such as More's biphasic splint, is preferred by some. The advantage of this latter technique is that intraoral splinting is avoided. The procedure is carried out under antibiotic

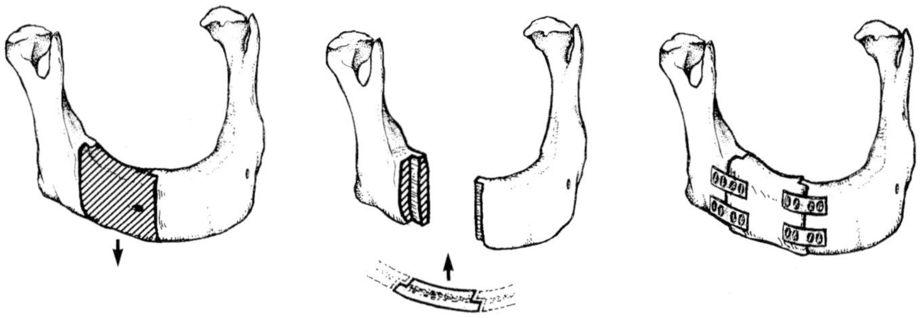

Fig. 6.7 Modelling, excision and fixation of bone graft, horizontal ramus.

cover. It is advisable to plan this surgery as the very first operation of the day so that minimum bacterial contamination is likely. Adequate drainage with vacuum drains is provided and kept in place until no further exudate is being produced. A high protein fluid diet providing adequate calories is prescribed.

Tracheotomy is kept until the intermaxillary fixation is removed. It may be plugged and used only when needed—for instance, for pulmonary toilet. In the absence of an intermaxillary fixation the patient is decannulated at about 10 days after surgery.

Once the wound has healed satisfactorily, and there is evidence of bony union clinically and radiologically, usually after a period of 3–6 months, the patient is seen along with maxillofacial colleagues with a view to a vestibuloplasty in order to create a buccogingival sulcus and a suitable bed for a dental prosthesis. The scar tissue adjacent to the transplant is superficially removed and a split skin graft is laid. This is, by itself, a short procedure and requires a minimal hospital stay.

PROBLEMS AND COMPLICATIONS

When the procedure is carried out on a properly selected patient in the manner described above few complications are encountered. Most patients complain of pain in the region of the donor site, on the hip or the rib-cage. Because of the presence of a large muscle mass both around the hip and the thorax, haematoma of the donor site is sometimes encountered. This is best avoided, for it can lead to secondary infection and delayed recovery. Meticulous haemostasis of the muscles and the bone with adequate and efficient

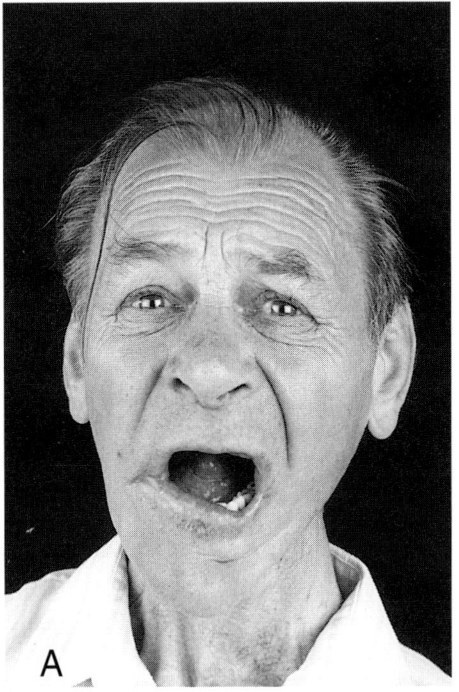
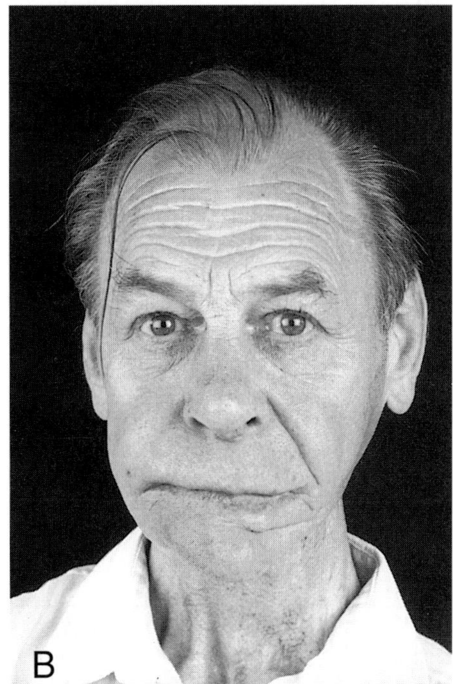

Fig. 6.8 (A, B) Clinical photograph of a patient 5 years after excision and postoperative radiation for T4NO squamous-cell carcinoma of the floor of the mouth. Secondary reconstruction of the mandibular segment with subsequent prosthodontic rehabilitation.

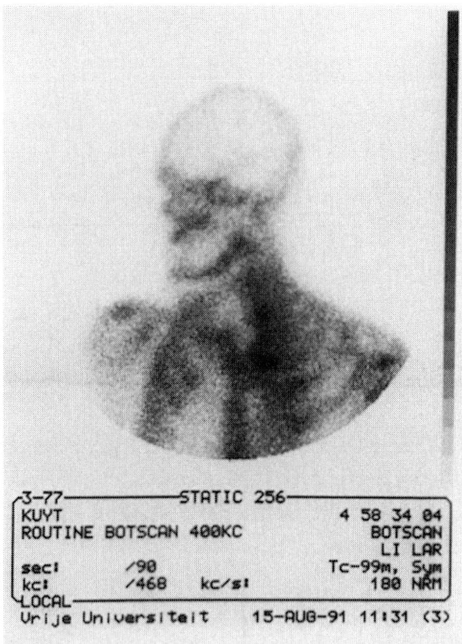

Fig. 6.9 Scintigraphy of the same patient as in Figure 6.8 showing uptake of 99m Tc some months postoperatively.

drainage is essential. Early removal of vacuum drains may lead to seroma formation. Although the use of bone wax is not advised in the literature, the author has used it regularly for haemostasis for several years without any complications.

Injury to the vessels of the neck and the flaps should be avoided during preparation of the donor site. It is important to find the right planes, which may not be easy because of the fibrosis. Injury to the branches of the facial nerve while preparing the recipient area and the stumps can be avoided by keeping in mind the course of the nerves and being in the right plane. Indiscriminate use of diathermy and the hot knife should be avoided. The skin flap in these radiated, often elderly, patients is thin and it is better to avoid retraction with heavy and sharp retractors. Avoidance of all communication with the oral cavity has already been referred to and is vital for the success of the procedure.

Early ambulation is encouraged. The management of general complications, such as pulmonary embolism and others, is beyond the scope of this discussion and is the same as that after any major surgical procedure. As a preventive measure, patients receive 5000 units of heparin subcutaneously for 10 days or until they are well mobilized.

EVALUATION

An accurate assessment of results is difficult in the absence of a protocol. The criteria for success vary from the mere 'take' of the transplant to the fitting of a dental prosthesis,

its use and the patient's ability to bite on it. There is no doubt that a successful 'take' of a bone transplant improves a patient's appearance, self-confidence and body image. His or her ability to wear a dental prosthesis not only has cosmetic value, but also improves speech and social acceptance (Fig. 6.8).

Radiography and scintigraphy have been the standard methods of evaluation after bone transplantation. The use of scintigraphy for obtaining evidence of successful uptake of the graft has, however, been questioned by some. Berggren and his colleagues demonstrated that conventional bone grafts had positive scintiscans 11 days to 3 weeks postoperatively (Berggren et al 1982). These observations were also reported earlier by Bos (1979).

Technetium-99m scanning and tetracycline labelling are considered 'reliable' methods of evaluation (Fig. 6.9). In conventional bone grafting, long-term results show that a varying proportion of grafts are partially or totally nonfunctional and may have to be removed. The results reported vary from 15–40%.

In a personal series of 18 autogenous bone transplants from the iliac crest, the author encountered 16% long-term failures with a follow up of 3 to 9 years. Of the patients, 54% were able to wear a dental prosthesis and were satisfied with their cosmetic and functional results (Tiwari et al 1993). Some 30% of the patients—in spite of a good functional transplant—could not be evaluated satisfactorily from the point of view of reconstruction because of tumour recurrence or other disease-associated problems, a fact that must remain in our thoughts whenever considering reconstruction in patients who have had cancer.

In the management of oral cancer the clinician has to weigh up the benefits and drawbacks of primary versus secondary reconstruction. Primary reconstruction has the advantage that it reduces the number of operations; it is the most convincing evidence possible for the patient of the surgeon's expectation of a cure; in the event of failure it gives the longest and best palliation; it reduces the total cost; it keeps the patient physically and socially acceptable within his/her social circle; and it maintains the features and functions unlikely to be regained by late reconstruction. Against this, the drawbacks of an immediate reconstruction are that it may cover recurrence of tumour; it may make repeated reconstruction necessary later; it may pre-empt the best repair method prior to cure; it may make the initial operation too long; and it may open up new tissue planes with possible seeding of tumour.

Postoperative radiotherapy is the single most important factor against primary conventional reconstruction. The final decision rests on the dexterity and experience of the treating surgeon, the stage of the disease process and the condition of the individual patient.

REFERENCES

Adamo A K, Szal R L 1979 Timing results and complications of reconstructive surgery. Journal of Oral Surgery 37: 755–763

Axhausen G 1909 Die histologischen und klinischen Gesetze der freien Osteoplastik auf Grund von Thierversuchen. Archief fur Klinische Chirurgie 88: 23–145

Bardenheur F 1892 Verhandlung der Deutsch Gesellschaft Zentralbibliothek. Chirurgie 21: 68

Berggren A, Weiland A J, Ostrup L T 1982 Bone scintigraphy in evaluting the viability of composite bone grafts revascularized by microvascular anatomoses, conventional autogenous bone grafts, and free non-revascularized periosteal grafts. Journal of Bone and Joint Surgery 64: 799–809

Blocker T C, Stout R A 1949 Mandibular reconstruction, World War II. Plastic and Reconstructive Surgery 4: 153

Bos K E 1979 Bone scintigraphy of experimental composite bone grafts revascularized by microvascular anastomoses. Plastic and Reconstructive Surgery 64: 353–360

Boyne P S, Zarem H 1976 Osseous reconstruction of the resected mandible. American Journal of Surgery 132: 49

Burwell R G 1969 The fate of bone grafts. In: Apeley A G (ed) Recent advances in orthopaedics. Churchill Livingstone, London, p 115

Byers L T 1954 Surgical management of mandible invaded by oral cancer. Surgery Gynaecology and Obstetrics 98: 564–570

Chase S W, Herndon C H 1955 The fate of autogenous and homogenous bone grafts. Journal of Bone and Joint Surgery 37A: 809–841

Cohen M, Schultz R C 1985 Mandibular reconstruction. Clinics in Plastic Surgery 12: 411–422

Cohen M, Figueroa A A, Aduss H 1989 The role of gingival periosteal flaps in the repair of alveolar clefts. Plastic and Reconstructive Surgery 83: 812–819

Cohen M, Figueroa A A, Harviza Y, Schafer M E, Aduss H 1991 Iliac versus cranial bone for secondary grafting of residual alveolar clefts. Plastic and Reconstructive Surgery 87: 423–427

Duhamel H L 1742 Sur le development et la crue des os des animaux. Mémoire de l'Academie Royale des Sciences Paris 55: 354–370

Gullane P 1991 Primary mandibular reconstruction: analysis of 64 cases and evaluation of interface radiation dosimetry on bridging plates. Laryngoscope 101: suppl 54

Hamblen D L 1978 Bone. In: Ledingham I M, Mackay C (eds) Jamieson and Kay's, Textbook of surgical physiology. Churchill Livingstone, Edinburgh, pp 194–209

Ketchum L D, Masters F W, Robinson D W 1974 Mandibular reconstruction using a composite island rib flap. Plastic and Reconstructive Surgery 53: 471–476

Kusiak J F, Zins J E, Ring E, Whitaker L 1981 Early vascularization of membranous bone grafts. Surgical Forum 32: 567–568

Lindemann A 1916 Bruhn's Ergebnisse aus dem Dusseldorfer Lazarett. Wiesbaden, Kieferschuss Verletzungen p 213

Lindström J, Branemark P L, Albrektsson T 1981 Mandibular reconstruction using the preformed autologous bone graft. Scandinavian Journal of Plastic and Reconstructive Surgery 15: 29–38

McCullough D W, Fredrickson J M 1972 Neovascularized rib grafts to reconstruct mandibular defects. Surgical Forum 23: 492–494

Manchester W M 1965 Immediate reconstruction of the mandible and temporomandibular joint. British Journal of Plastic Surgery 18: 291

Marx R E, Ames J R 1982 The use of hyperbaric oxygen in bony reconstruction of the irradiated and tissue deficient patient. Journal of Oral and Maxillofacial Surgery 40: 412–420

Millard R D, Deane M, Ganst W P 1971 Bending an iliac bone graft for anterior mandibular arch repair. Plastic and Reconstructive Surgery 48: 600

Millard R D, Maisels D O, Batstone J H 1967 Immediate repair of radical resection of the anterior arch of the lower jaw. Plastic and Reconstructive Surgery 39: 153

Mowlem R 1963 Bone grafting. British Journal of Plastic Surgery 16: 293–304

Panje W R, Holmes D K 1984 Mandibulectomy without reconstruction can cause sleep apnoea. Laryngoscope 94: 1591–1594

Piggot T A, Logan A M 1983 Mandibular reconstruction with simple bonegraft. British Journal of Plastic Surgery 36: 9

Sanders B 1982 Augmentation rib grafting to the inferior border of the mandible. Head and Neck Surgery 4: 324–329

Sanders B, Cox R 1976 Inferior border rib grafting for augmentation of the atrophic edentulous mandible. Journal of Oral Surgery 34: 897–900

Skyhoff W 1900 Zur Frage der Knocken-plastik am Unterkiefer. Zentralbibliothek Chirurgie 35: 881

Tiwari R M, van der Waal I, Snow G B 1993 Reconstruction of the mandible with simple bone graft. An evaluation. European Archives of Otolaryngology (in press)

Wersall J, Bergstedt H, Korlof B, Lind M G 1984 Split rib graft for reconstruction of the mandible. Otolaryngology—Head and Neck Surgery 92: 270–276

7. **Mandibular reconstruction, bone transplants and implants**

Robert E. Marx

INTRODUCTION

In no portion of the body is lost tissue more grieved, and its reconstruction more desired, than it is in the face and jaws. In particular, the mandible is so much a part of the functions involved in eating, speech and swallowing that a person is truly crippled without it. Those who have lost a significant portion of their mandible due to tumour or trauma are often forced to endure gastrostomy feedings to maintain basic nutritional requirement or to use commercial prepared liquid diets at best. Although loss of the mandible is also associated with a significant cosmetic deformity, our lengthy experience has been that the patient's focused and often times desperate concern is not so much one of appearance but one of regaining a semblance of their eating ability. Their focused goal is almost always to be able to wear a denture prosthesis and to be able to chew once again. The surgeon must, therefore, develop a treatment plan that will predictably lead to that goal. That is, to not only reconstruct the mandible but to do it in such a way as to make it able to support a denture prosthesis, align it to the arch form of the maxillae, and ensure that it lasts. In short, the surgeon must combine the scientific knowledge of reconstructive surgery with the technical artistry to achieve it and then prepare the reconstructed jaw using a knowledge of dental prostheses to truly rehabilitate the patient.

BIOLOGY OF BONE TRANSPLANTATION

Mandibular reconstruction is mostly required for malignant-tumour-related defects, benign-tumour-related defects, traumatic avulsive defects, and osteoradionecrosis-related defects. Each length and location of mandibular continuity defect, and each varied condition of the soft tissue, requires a special consideration and a specific approach. Therefore, each continuity reconstruction must be individualized for each patient's defect. However, the basic biological principles of reconstructive surgery are universal. These may be built upon and used to satisfy each individual patient's need.

Bony reconstruction of the mandible requires the transplantation of viable bone from a donor site to that of the mandible. Today's state of the art requires the transplantation of autogenous bone as the primary bone graft material, although allogeneic bone is very useful and recommended as a crib for housing autogenous bone. Allogeneic bone by itself is not sufficient to restore a mandible due to its fate of incorporation then slow resorption as a compatible and sterile but non-viable bone. Bone substitutes such as hydroxyapatite blocks or particles or metallic plates are also unsuitable for definitive mandibular reconstruction. Hydroxyapatite is not bone and lacks the integrity, elasticity and ability to remodel. It is therefore not a consideration in mandibular continuity reconstruction because it is not bone. Bone substitutes cannot support a prosthesis and do not remodel. Metal bridging plates will restore continuity but they are also not bone. They cannot support a prosthesis and do not remodel. They may be useful for an intermediate time to gain stability for 6 months to 2 years before plate loosening, but long-term functional use is not commonly experienced.

The autogenous grafting approaches in use today distil down to three types: corticocancellous blocks, particulate cancellous bone, and free vascularized bone. The most predictable and most truly functional for the patient has been particulate cancellous bone placed in a crib usually of allogeneic bone. The biological and practical failings of the other two can be understood from a bone healing and bone morphology perspective.

Corticocancellous blocks contain mostly mature osteocytes and little marrow mesenchymal cells or true osteoblasts. Osteocytes do not survive free non-vascular transplantation due to the disruption of their delicate canalicular blood supply (Gray & Elves 1979). The only cells capable of forming new bone are the endosteal osteoblasts (Littoral cells of Burwell) and the marrow mesenchymal cells of which there are too few in number (Burwell 1986). The fate of the graft is thus osteocyte death by delayed revascularization and resorption of the cortical bone and trabecular bone mineral matrix. Thus, for mandibular continuity defects

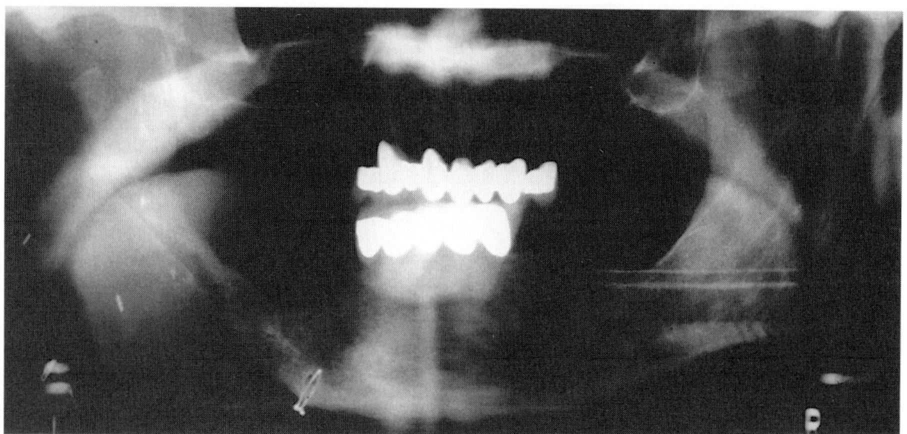

Fig. 7.1 Block cortical cancellous graft with fracutre because of minimal transplantation of osteocompetent cells.

such a graft begins as an initially pleasing radiographic result but, with time, it resorbs with little new bone replacement – either rendering the graft too small for proper function or developing a pathological fracture (Fig. 7.1). Because these grafts transplant too few osteocompetent cells, the obligatory resorption replacement cycle universal to all bone is lacking in the replacement phase. The longer the defect and the more compromised the tissue bed by scar or radiation the more the graft will show evidence resorption.

Microvascular free bone transfers are able to transplant viable osteocytes and periosteum so that the graft will undergo a resorption replacement cycle with all of its own endosteum periosteum, and osteocytes. Such grafts will require new bone formation only at each graft–host interface, as in normal fracture healing. Thus, microvascular free bone transfers are the theoretical ideal in bone grafting. Sadly though, all microvascular bone transfers are either too straight, too small or possess the wrong shape and curvature to be useful for mandibular reconstruction. Such grafts literally transplant a bone which is unusable to the patient and cannot support a prosthesis due to size, arch discrepancies, and arch curvature (Fig. 7.2). They are also mainly tubular bones with less trabecular bone volume and therefore do not osseo-integrate implants well. Microvascular grafts also have the highest degree of donor site morbidity of any graft harvest.

We thus employ a grafting system which produces a usable graft of sufficient size, in the correct arch form, and one that does not impart disability on the patient from its donor harvest (Fig. 7.3). That graft system uses autogenous particulate bone and cancellous marrow (PBCM) within a crib framework. The preferred crib framework is one of allogeneic bone (Burwell 1964, Marx et al 1981).

Autogenous PBCM transplants a high population of marrow endosteal osteoblasts and marrow mesenchymal cells (osteocompetent cells) which will form a new bone ossicle over 4 to 8 weeks. This cellular bone generated from living cells transplanted from usually the posterior ilium is

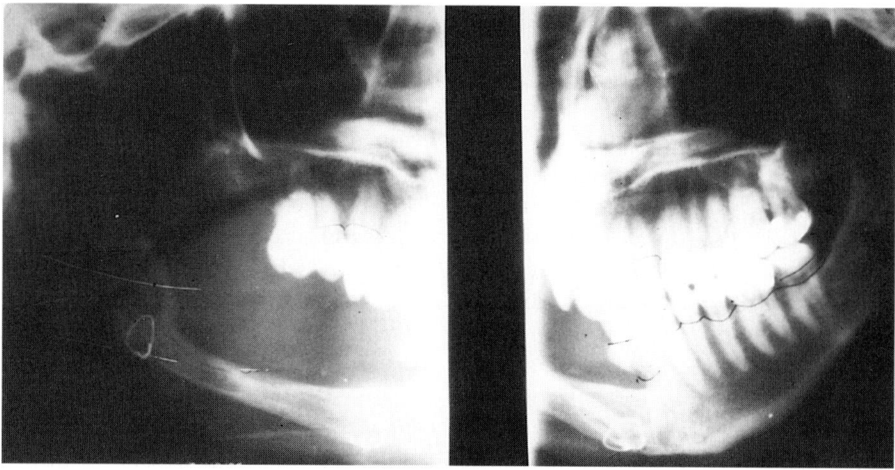

Fig. 7.2 Free microvascular bone graft volumetrically too small and too straight to serve as a functional mandibular reconstruction.

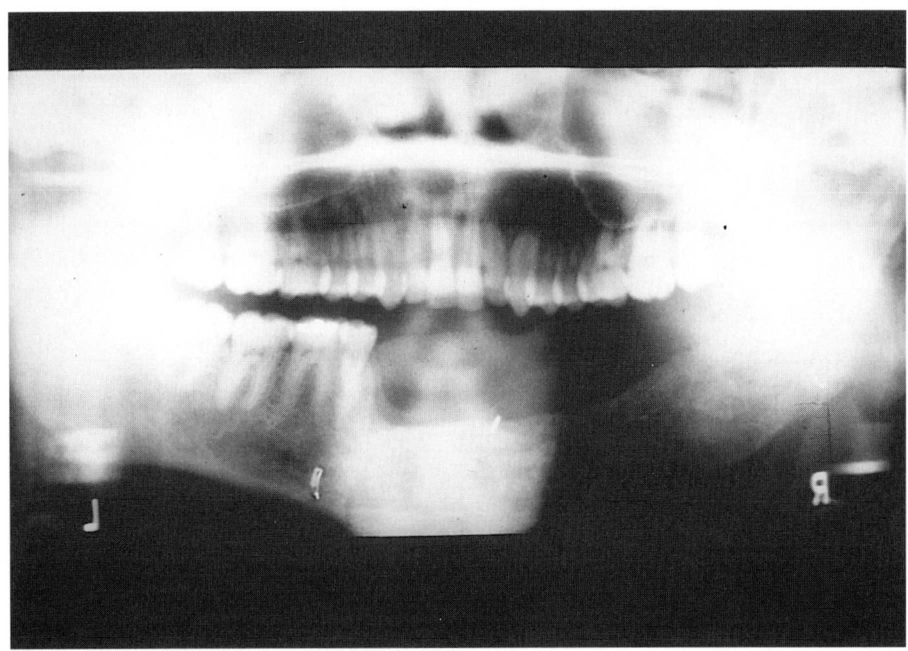

Fig. 7.3 PBCM graft with an allogeneic bone crib with osseous content and morphology supportive of mandibular form and function.

called phase I bone (Axhausen 1956). Phase I bone is derived from the donor bone, it is quantitatively the largest amount the graft will produce, and its amount of bone development is directly proportional to the concentration (cellular density) of the transplanted osteocompetent cells (Friedensten et al 1966). Phase I bone will obligatorily also undergo a resorption–replacement cycle. It will be replaced by a more lamellar and mature bone called phase II bone (Gray et al 1982). Phase II bone forms upon resorption of the phase I bone when osteoclasts trigger the release of osteogenin which stimulates the graft and host mesenchymal cells to form new bone. Such phase II bone is largely formed by the ingrowth of host cells and will develop the endosteum and periosteum which will ensure the longevity of the graft. Phase II bone is thus derived from host cells, it resorbs and replaces phase I bone with a more dense and lamellar bone, and it will determine the longevity of the graft (Gray et al 1982).

Understanding the longevity of graft healing points out the great importance of transplanting cellular marrow elements rather than cortex, condensing the graft material to increase the cellular transplantation, keeping cells viable, and grafting into a vascular and cellular tissue bed that can support the metabolic needs of the graft and at the same time possess the cellular elements which can form a periosteum and endosteum about and within the graft. Practically speaking, this has most often translated into harvesting of bone from the posterior ilium which has the greatest reservoir of cellular bone and the least morbidity of harvest; condensing the graft material in a simple syringe; compacting the graft material into an allogeneic crib with hand-held

instruments; and improving the recipient tissue bed with hyperbaric oxygen if it has been radiated and myocutaneous flaps if it is deficient and very scarred.

The value of allogeneic bone as crib framework for this type of a graft is that is can be fashioned into an ideal mandibular arch form and morphology. Allogeneic bone is also preferred because it does not become encapsulated by a dense scar as do all alloplastic cribs; instead, it becomes incorporated by vascular ingrowth and later resorbed (Marx et al 1981). Such cribs will therefore promote graft periosteal development and later pre-prosthetic surgeries.

PREPARATION OF THE TISSUE BED

Preparation of the tissue in this sense refers to biological preparation more than surgical preparation. The tissue bed that a graft is to be placed into is actually more important than the technique of the bone graft placement. Clearly, the biology of bone transplantation has taught us that the ideal tissue bed needs to be vascular and cellular. It also needs to be infection- and contamination-free. Therefore, attention must first be directed to the soft tissue into which the bone graft will be placed.

Infected or contaminated tissue

Microorganisms residual in the tissue bed or leaking into a potential graft site from an oral communication pose a significant risk to the bone graft. Such microorganisms will lyse bone-forming cells and thrombose vessels leading to either an overtly necrotic graft or one which

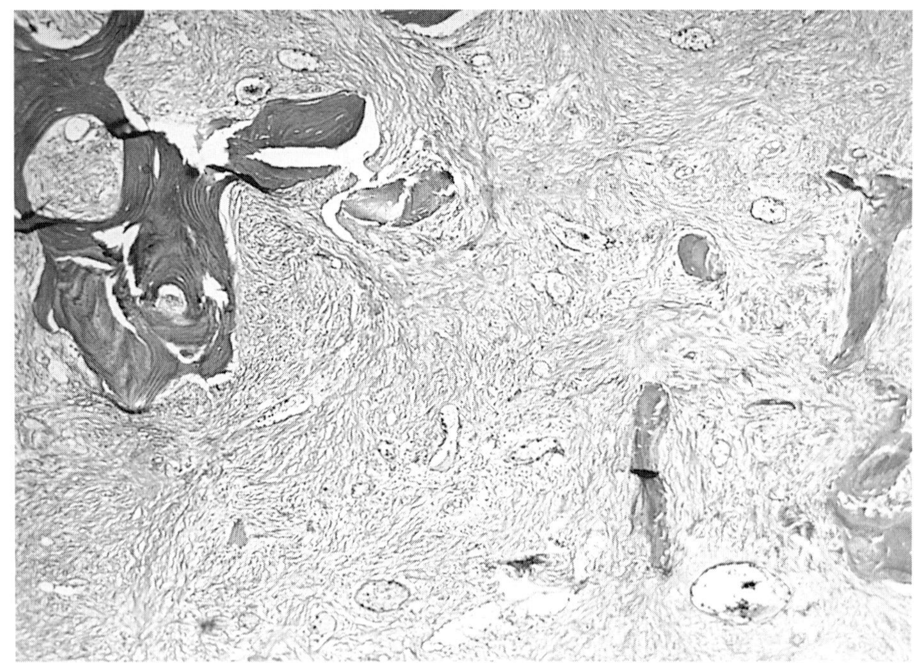

Fig. 7.4   Hypovascular–hypocellular–hypoxic tissue of a radiated tissue bed.

consolidates too little bone to be useful.

Contaminated graft beds require surgical debridement and a full course of culture-specific antibiotics before a graft can be safely placed. Although no specific timetables are known for the duration of antibiotics and the time lapse before a graft can be placed, a useful guideline remains at least 2 weeks of culture-specific antibiotics past the time of clinical healing and a tissue bed maturity of at least 3 months past the time of clinical healing.

Radiated tissue

Grafting into tissue beds which have been radiated is associated with higher incidence of complication such as

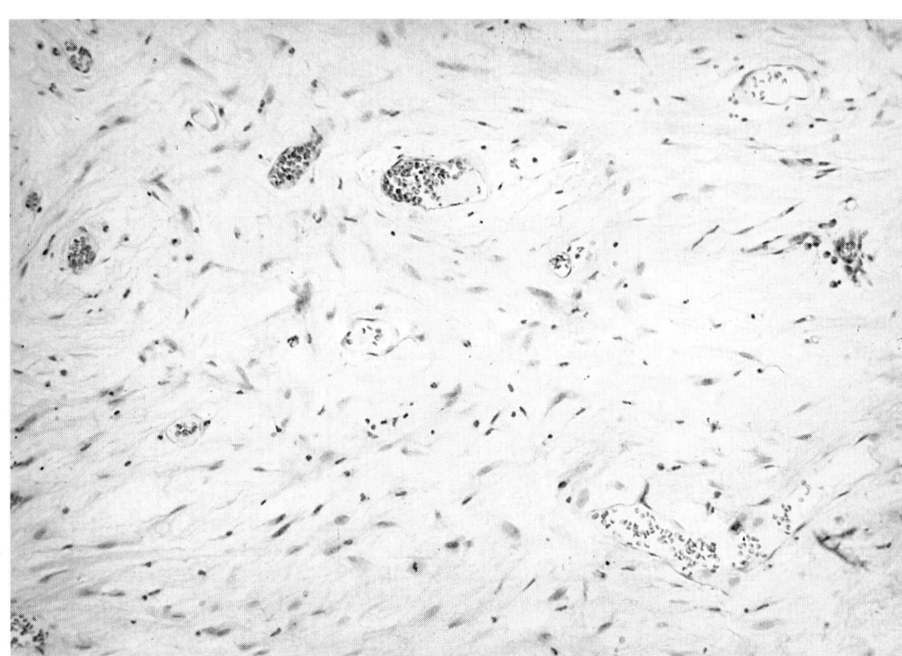

Fig. 7.5   Tissue of Figure 7.7 after hyperbaric-oxygen-induced angiogenesis and fibroplasia.

Table 7.1A Hemimandibular reconstruction in patients who have undergone radiation (≥ 6400 cGy)

	Number of Patients	Complication rate	Met the six criteria for a successful bone graft
Without hyperbaric oxygen	52	11 (22%)	34 (65%)
With hyperbaric oxygen	52	5 (9%)	48 (92%)

Table 7.1B Criteria for successful bone graft

1. Continuity
2. Alveolar bone height
3. Arch form
4. Osseous bulk
5. Maintenance of bone (18 months min)
6. Facial form

infection, dehiscence, and delayed wound healing. This higher incidence of complications arises from the tissue damage effects of radiotherapy creating what has been identified as a hypovascular–hypocellular–hypoxic tissue (Marx & Johnson 1987) (Fig. 7.4). This type of tissue cannot revascularize a particulate graft or heal into a microvascular graft. The hypovascular–hypocellular–hypoxic tissue also can develop an ingrowth of cells to form a phase II endosteum or a phase II periosteum. Therefore, grafts placed into unimproved radiated tissue beds are often observed to undergo delayed resorption, in addition to being more vulnerable to infection and dehiscence.

Radiated tissue is best improved with a presurgical course of hyperbaric oxygen. Hyperbaric oxygen has been shown to cause the development of capillaries within radiated tissue (angiogenesis) and to produce a fibroplasia to reverse, to some degree, the hypovascular–hypocellular–hypoxic tissue of radiation damage (Marx & Johnson 1988) (Fig. 7.5). A specific protocol of 20 sessions presurgical followed by 10 sessions postsurgical has been shown to improve the radiated tissue vascular density from the usual level of 30% of non-radiated tissue to 75% or 80% of non-radiated tissue. This protocol has also been shown to retain the vascular density improvement long term (at least 4 years through follow-up measurements), allowing grafting to take place at times long after the hyperbaric oxygen exposures. A hyperbaric oxygen protocol treats patients at 2.4 ATA (atmosphere of absolute pressure) for 90 oxygen minutes of 100% oxygen, 5 or 6 days per week.

This use of hyperbaric oxygen is indicated in any elective surgery in radiated tissue to promote normal wound healing and lessen the probability of wound infection and dehiscence. It is particularly indicated in bone grafting because its induced angiogenesis promotes bone cell survival and bone development and its fibroplasia supports periosteal and endosteal development which will maintain the graft over the long term. A documentation of the efficacy of hyperbaric oxygen in bone grafting radiated patients is seen in Table 7.1A. This study involved 104 radiated patients undergoing hemimandibular reconstruction with the same surgeons using the same technique. Fifty-two patients underwent the aforementioned hyperbaric oxygen protocol and 52 others did not, in a randomized prospective fashion. As Table 7.1A shows, the group treated with hyperbaric oxygen had a complication rate of 9% , as compared to 22% for the group not treated with hyperbaric oxygen, and a success rate of 92% as compared to 65% for the latter group.

The tissue-deficient bed

While hyperbaric oxygen is able to improve qualitatively a tissue bed, it cannot quantitatively improve it. A tissue bed of 1.5 cm thickness between oral mucosa and skin is needed for bone graft placement. Tissue contractions or scarring from previous surgery, radiation or trauma often need to be replaced or added to so that a sufficient tissue volume for bone graft placement can be achieved. It is not uncommon to see grafts fail due to oral perforation or skin dehiscence because a graft was forced into a tissue bed volumetrically too small to receive it. In such cases, myocutaneous flaps are most useful. The pectoralis major myocutaneous flap, in particular, is the most predictable and has the least donor site morbidity (Ariyan 1979). In particular, a flap design described by Marx and Smith makes this flap the most predictable flap of all and one with a greater perfusion pressure than the original design by Ariyan (Marx & Smith 1990). The design as described preserves all three vessels to the pectoralis major muscle, the thoracoacromial (50% of its blood supply), the lateral thoracic (40% of its blood supply) and the superior thoracic (10% of its blood supply). The preservation of the muscles entire blood flow system, as compared to only 50% as described by most other techniques, allows the surgery to individualize skin paddle designs, use large skin paddles, take skin paddles somewhat off the muscle, and split the skin paddles etc., all with great predictability (Figs 7.6 and 7.7).

As a secondary choice, a trapezius myocutaneous flap is also useful but the operator must be cautious in the cancer patient who has undergone radical neck surgery. In such patients, the transverse cervical artery is often harvested as part of the tumour extirpation. Since the transverse cervical artery is the axial vessel for the trapezius flap, the surgeon assesses its patency in such patients by Doppler assessment or angiography.

The value in myocutaneous flaps related to bone graft placement is that they are able to provide either skin

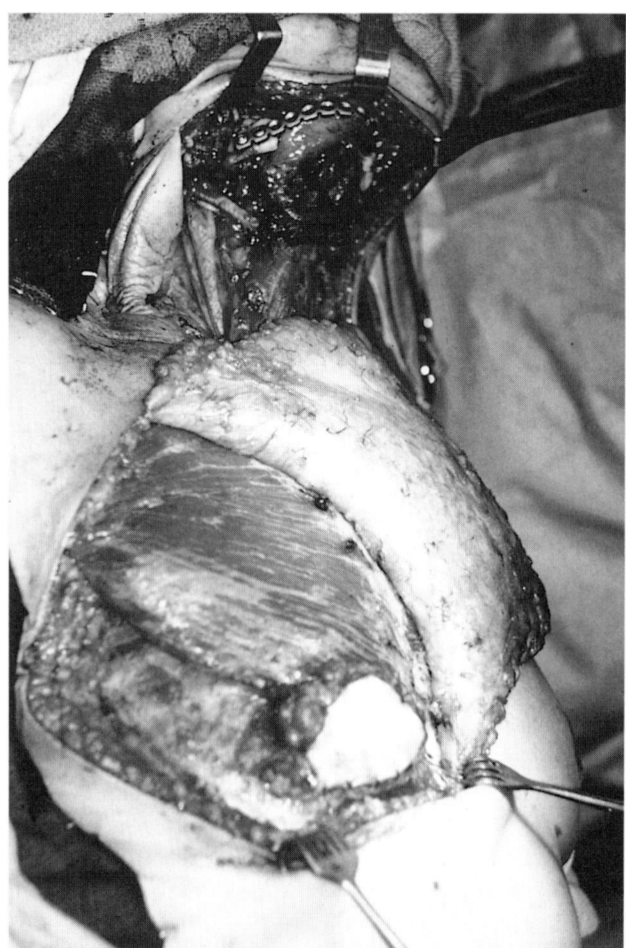

Fig. 7.6 Two-thirds of the skin paddle of a pectoralis major myocutaneous flap may be off the muscle if all three vessels to the muscle are preserved.

cover or oral lining, or both, and a vascular muscle bulk into a deficient area. Once placed they are usually allowed to heal for 3 months before surgically re-entering the area for bone graft placement. By that time, and usually sooner (6 weeks), the flap has developed its secondary blood supply via anastomosis of vessels from the recipient area so that the main pedicle can be transected or the flap dissected into without jeopardizing tissue viability. The flap's vascularity and cellularity, like angiogenesis and fibroplasia of hyperbaric oxygen, will support bone cell survival and bone formation. The added tissue bulk will support facial contour and reduce dehiscence potential as the added lining or cover will allow for a more tension free closure.

In select cases, a soft-tissue microvascular free transfer may be the flap of choice to improve a tissue bed prior to grafting. Although microvascular bone transfers do not serve jaw reconstruction well at all due to size, contour and bone density deficiencies, microvascular soft-tissue transfers can fulfil the soft-tissue needs. A microvascular soft-tissue transfer is chosen over a myocutaneous flap when previous flap use or previous surgery precludes the harvest of a myocutaneous flap. Such is seen in patients who have chest-wall pacemakers, breast implants, or the previous harvest of such flaps. A microvascular soft-tissue flap is also a more preferred flap in cases where lining or cover is required but there is little or no need for tissue bulk. In such cases a radial forearm transfer is an excellent choice.

BONE GRAFTING THE MANDIBLE

The three most common and most difficult mandibular reconstructions are the hemimandibular defect with a condylar proximal segment, the hemimandibular defect without a condylar proximal segment, and the anterior mandibular arch defect. For each of these defects a specific surgical dissection is required, a specific type of crib needs to be fashioned, and a specific type of fixation employed. Since each of these defects—and, for the most part, most tumour- and trauma-related defects—is greater than 5 cm in length, donor bone harvest is best accomplished from the posterior ilium.

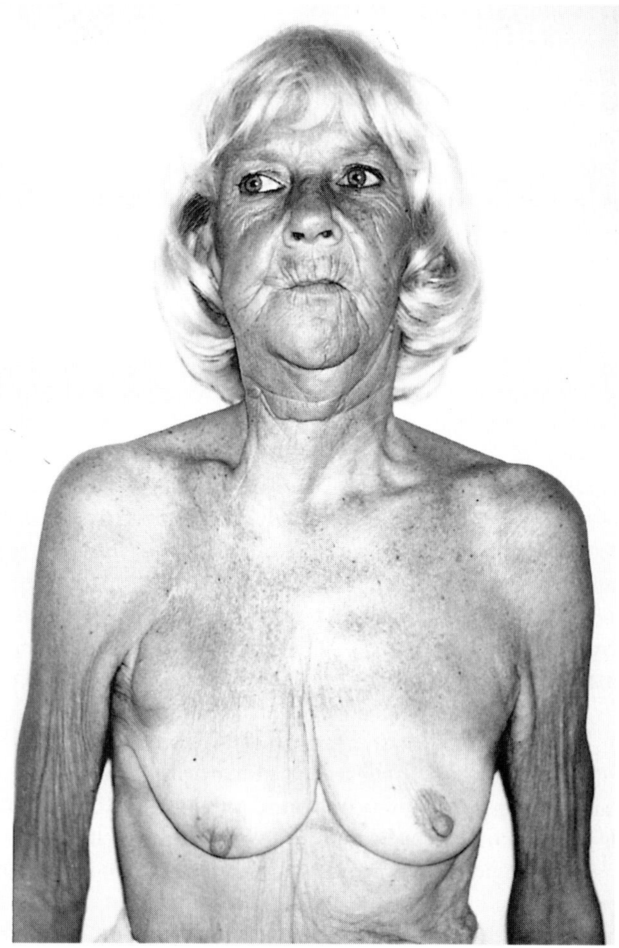

Fig. 7.7 Patient after anterior mandibular resection and a pectoralis major myocutaneous flap. Breast distortion has been avoided and excellent chin reconstruction achieved.

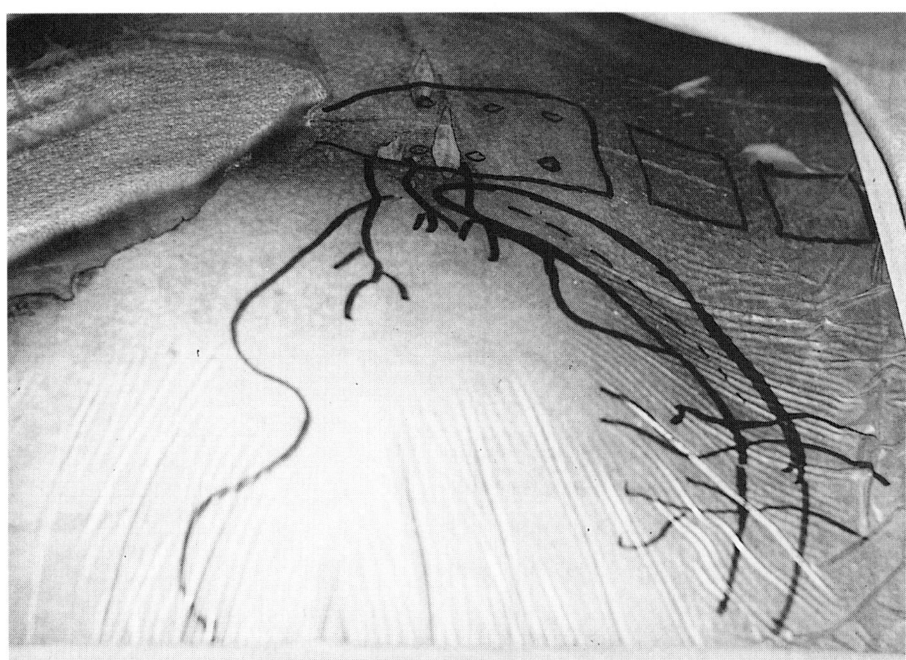

Fig. 7.8   Incisional placement for harvesting bone from the posterior ilium. Note that the middle of the incision is over the insertion of the gluteus maximus and is between the cluneal nerve trunks.

BONE HARVEST FROM THE POSTERIOR ILIUM

The posterior ilium has the advantage of possessing twice as much cancellous bone as the anterior ilium in each individual (Marx & Morales 1988). It also allows for harvest of bone with reduced blood loss by virtue of patient positioning as well as earlier and more complete ambulation due to the absence of gait-specific muscle reflection (Wolfe & Kawamoto 1978, Marx & Morales 1988). The patient is placed in a prone position on the operating table with the arms stretched outward on arm supports. Axillary rolls are placed in each axilla, and a transverse roll is placed under the anterior thigh. With these supports and with the table reverse flexed at 210° the posterior ilium–buttocks area is elevated. This elevation reduces the venous pressure in the posterior ilium and, therefore, the blood loss throughout the surgical harvest.

The incisional approach is a curvilinear incision of about 10 cm following the curvature of the palpable ilium contour. The centre of the incision should be located over the most palpable convex bony contour. This definitive bony elevation is the triangular-shaped insertion of the gluteus maximus (Fig. 7.8). The incision should end inferiorly 3 cm lateral to, and parallel to, the midline. The dissection proceeds through skin and subcutaneous tissue to the external lip of the posterior iliac crest with no major vessels or nerves in the path. There are peripheral sensory nerve branches of the superior cluneal nerves (L1, L2, L3) which pierce the lumbodorsal fascia (also called the thoracodorsal fascia) from above, and middle cluneal nerves (S1, S2, S3) which

arise out of the sacrum and course medio-laterally but these are small terminal sensory branches which have not shown a tendency to develop hyperaesthesia or neuroma formation (Fig. 7.8).

The incision to bone is accomplished at the insertional juncture of the gluteus maximus from below and the lumbodorsal fascia from above. The gluteus maximus tendon is firm and tenacious, and it requires reflection by sharp dissection. The remaining reflection of the lateral cortical plate can be accomplished by periosteal reflection of the posterior extent of the gluteus medius. A 5 cm x 5 cm lateral cortical osteotomy is accomplished with a saline-cooled saw blade, and the cortical–cancellous block is removed with a curved osteotome. The harvested block of bone is temporarily stored in either room-temperature saline or tissue culture medium. It will be particulated in a bone mill and added to the cancellous bone just prior to placement. With the 5 x 5 cm cortical plate removed, sufficient cancellous bone and marrow is gouged and curetted from the ilium (Fig. 7.9). The quantity of harvested bone can be estimated by counting the 5 cm x 5 cm cortical–cancellous block as 25 cc of particulated uncompressed bone and measuring the remainder harvested from the posterior ilium in a graduated cylinder in an uncompressed, loosely placed manner. It has been correlated that 8–10 cc of loosely uncompressed harvested bone is required to reconstruct fully each 1 cm length of mandibular continuity defect.

Once the appropriate amount of bone has been harvested, the sharp bony edges are smoothed, haemostasis is

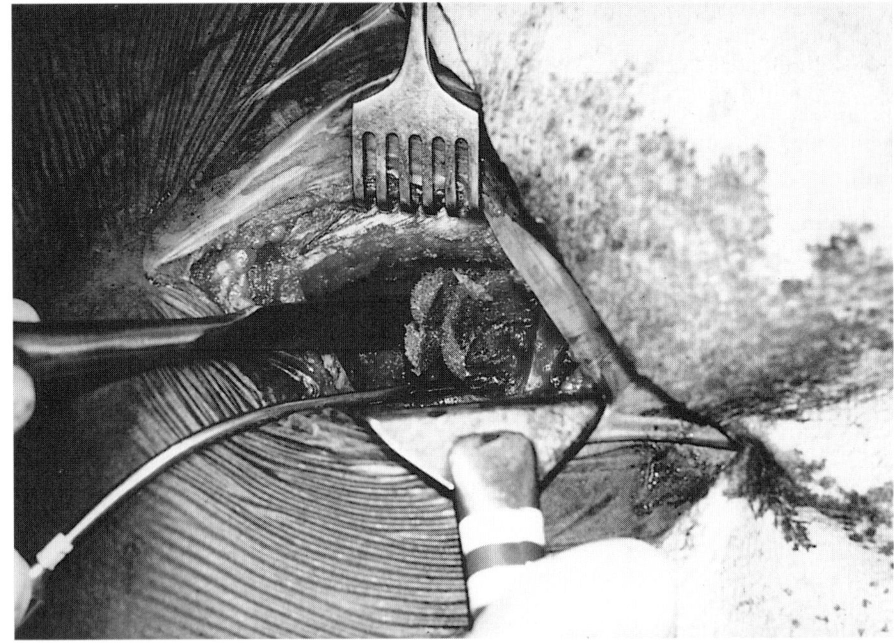

Fig. 7.9 Cancellous bone is removed with a bone gouge by a walking motion through the spongy-textured bone.

gained by a small amount of bone wax and microfibrillar collagen, a drain is placed and layered closure accomplished. It is important to place the drain under low suction only because a high negative pressure will actually promote continued marrow bleeding. It is also recommended that a pressure-dressing be placed as this will further assist haemostasis.

HEMIMANDIBULAR DEFECT WITH PROXIMAL CONDYLAR SEGMENT

The incision design for this surgery should ideally be placed in a skin fold or previous incision 3 cm below the inferior border of the mandible. It should parallel the intended inferior border of the graft and extend about 3 cm beyond each bone edge. The incision extends through the skin layers, the platysma, and the superficial layer of the deep cervical fascia. The facial vein becomes a key anatomical landmark. This vessel is ligated and transected so that the dissection is turned superiorly in a plane deep to this vessel and superficial to the anterior belly of the digastric muscle, the submandibular gland, and the stylohyoid muscle. In patients who have previously undergone neck dissections for cancer, the platysma is atrophied and the fascia and submandibular gland are gone. In those patients, dissection is through scar tissue until either the intermediate tendon or one of the bellies of the digastric muscle is identified.

Periosteum is incised and reflected for at least 3 cm at each bone edge and over the alveolar height. The tissue bed is bluntly dissected between each bone edge to develop a full volume for the graft. Scar often requires excision and the periosteum release to gain a complete development of the graft bed. As a guide in dissection to help avoid an oral perforation, the surgeon can palpate the maxillary teeth or the patient's inserted maxillary denture through the tissue to gain an appreciation of the tissue's thickness. The surgeon can also place a gloved hand in the mouth, or a surgical assistant can place a gloved hand in the mouth to guide the dissection. This must, however, be followed by the complete change of gown and gloves to avoid contamination of the wound.

During dissection of this graft area other members of the operating team prepare the crib. This defect can be reconstructed using either two different orientations of split allogeneic rib or a hemi-ilium form. Both rib cribs require splitting the rib longitudinally after reconstitution in saline. The split ribs will, therefore, yield an outer and an inner cortical strip of which the adherent cancellous bone is removed with a rotary burr. If the proximal host bone segment includes the entire ramus to the angle of the mandible, the allogeneic rib strips are placed to recapitulate the buccal and lingual cortices respectively (Fig. 7.10). If the proximal segments include only the condylar neck or posterior ramus, the allogeneic rib strips are placed at the inferior border and superior alveolar crest (Fig. 7.11). Each rib strip is bent to create the angle contour of the mandible before it is wired into place. In each placement orientation, the lingual edge of the crib is sutured to the deep tissues via burr holes placed into the allogeneic crib. In each orientation the allogeneic rib strips act as a matrix band to allow a more dense cellular compaction of the PBCM bone graft. The orientation difference allows for a more ideal arch curvature

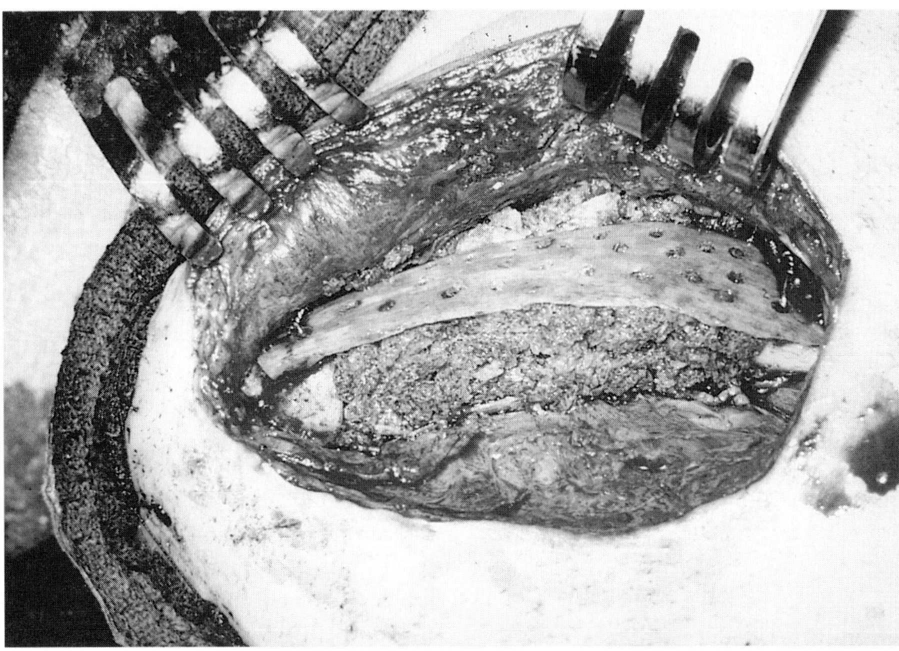

Fig. 7.10 Split allogeneic rib segments in the buccolingual orientation as a crib for an autogenous PBCM graft.

and morphology. It is best for the buccal–lingual orientation to follow the arch curvature around the canine area to the symphysis. The superior–inferior orientation is best used to create the angle–ramus curvature.

In each orientation the PBCM graft material is further particulated by rongeurs or by a bone mill device and loaded into 3 cc and 5 cc syringes. The PBCM graft is thus compacted in the syringes, the tips are cut off, and the graft material is injected between the allogeneic rib strips and then further condensed with hand instruments.

Allogeneic hemi-ilium forms can also be used in this type of defect. The anatomical similarity of the ipsilateral an-

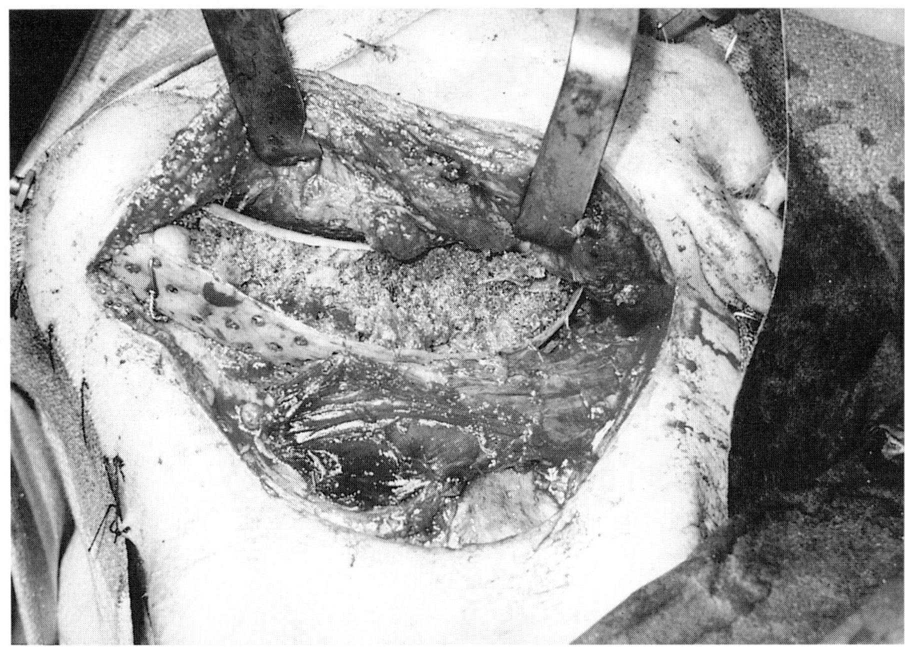

Fig. 7.11 Split allogeneic rib segments in the inferior/superior orientration as a crib for an autogenous PBCM graft.

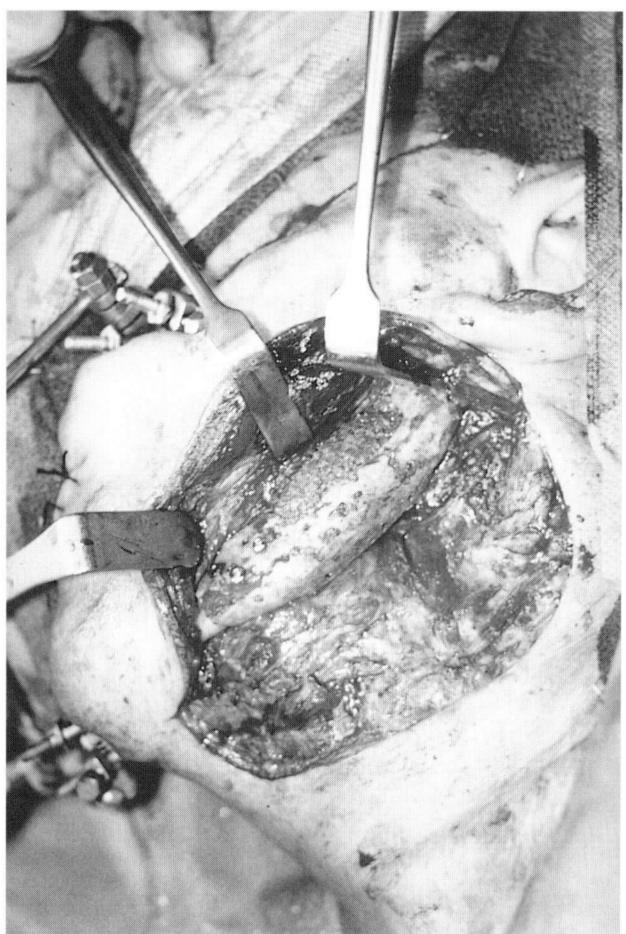

Fig. 7.12 The allogeneic hemi-ilium crib will recapitulate the morphology of the hemimandible. Here the tubercle of the ilium is positioned to create an angle contour.

terior ilium and the contralateral posterior ilium to the hemimandible was first reported by Manchester. Today, this principle is used to develop hemimandible-like cribs from an anterior allogeneic ilium. These cribs are available from most tissue banks today. The crib is hollowed out by rotary burs and fashioned to overlap on the buccal surface of the host bone. The flanges of the crib are cut down to about 1 cm—especially the lingual flange because the majority of revascularization comes from the lingual. The tubercle of the allogeneic anterior ilium is placed where the angle should be located, and the crib is lag-screwed to the host bone. In a similar fashion to the rib segments, the syringe-loaded PBCM is then injected into the crib and further condensed with hand instruments (Fig. 7.12).

Closure is obtained in layers. The most important layer is the first layer, the periosteal layer. The lateral cover flap is brought over the graft and closed to the deep tissue at the inferior border. This envelopes the graft in a vascular tissue envelope. The remaining layers of platysma, dermis, and skin surface are approximated. It is recommended that a drain be placed superficial to the periosteal layer closure and

deep to the platysma layer closure. In order to gain a tension-free closure, most necks require undermining deep to the platysma. The drain is thus placed at the most inferior extent of the undermined neck and exited in the posterior triangle.

Fixation is either by maxillomandibular fixation or via external skeletal pins. With either type of fixation, it is maintained for 6 weeks.

HEMIMANDIBULAR DEFECT INCLUSIVE OF CONDYLE

The incision design and dissection planes for this surgery are similar to the previous defect of a hemimandibular nature with a full proximal segment. In this case, it is sometimes advantageous to also use a pre-auricular incision to guide placement of the graft into the temporal fossa. This dissection is added because of the need to prepare the tissue bed to the temporal fossa. This is accomplished by developing a plane deep to the masseter and superficial to the internal pterygoid muscles. The dissection is best accomplished in a blunt fashion because branches of the pterygoid venous plexus will prolapse into the defect and may create difficult to control bleeding. Branches of the facial nerve will also prolapse into the temporal fossa which will predispose to a frontal nerve paresis.

In this defect, we have found three crib approaches to give consistently excellent functional and cosmetic results. The first approach is to use an allogeneic hemimandible as a crib.

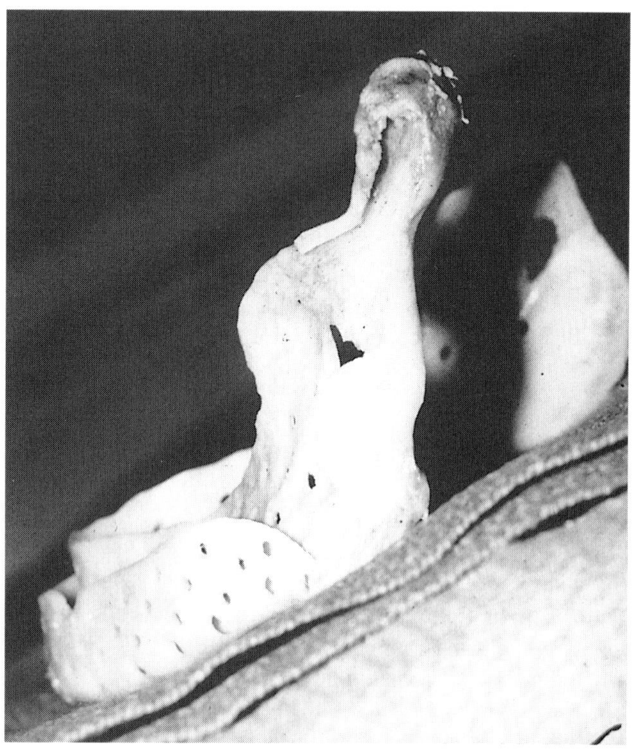

Fig. 7.13 A mandible crib seen here is hollowed at the ramus and condyle to reconstruct the hemimandible inclusive of the condyle.

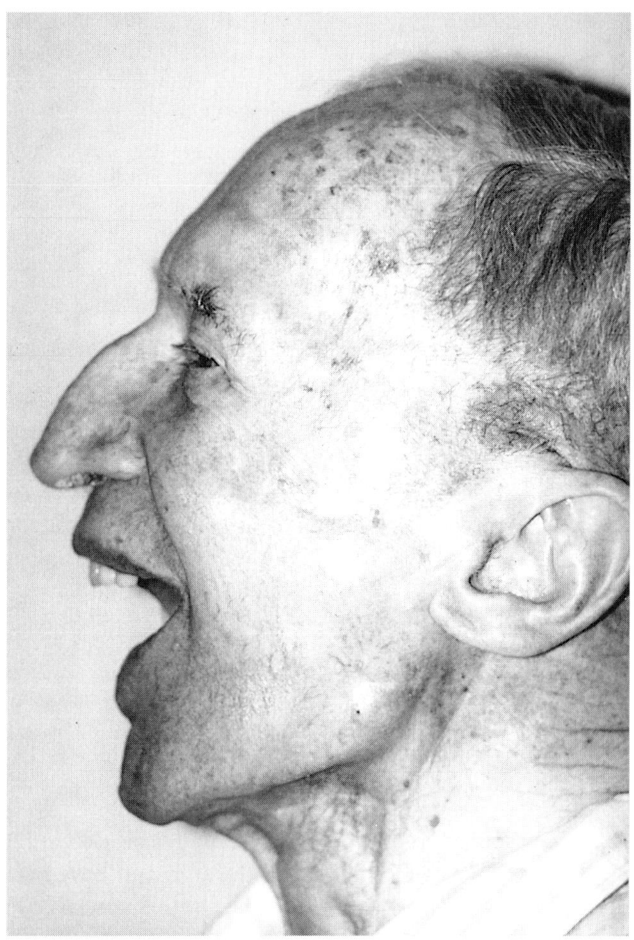

Fig. 7.14 A hemi-ilium crib will create an excellent angle contour and support a full opening as seen here on a 6-year follow-up.

In a similar fashion to other allogeneic bone cribs the specimen is hollowed out after reconstruction and fashioned so as to overlap the buccal cortex of the distal host bone segment. The ramus is hollowed out by removing the lateral cortex but leaves the inferior border and lateral cortical edge of the posterior ramus (Fig. 7.13). The condylar neck is hollowed out by removing the lateral cortex (Fig. 7.13). The condyle is hollowed by removing both the medial and lateral poles and removing the cancellous bone within using a round burr.

Once completely prepared, the crib is lag-screwed to the host bone and cantilevered so that the condyle rests in the fossa. The soft-tissue dissection should leave a small thickness of tissue at the roof of the temporal fossa so that the graft does not articulate directly against bone. The autogenous PBCM graft can then be injected into the crib and further condensed with hand instruments.

An alternative approach is to use the same type of allogeneic hemi-ilium form as was described for the previous defect. This specimen can be obtained with a greater ramus length so that it will extend into the temporal fossa. It then can be hollowed out completely, lag-screwed to the host

bone at the distal segment and filled with autogenous PBCM graft material. With this crib and the hemimandible crib, several trial fits and adjustment are made to adapt the crib to the host bone and gain a good fit into the temporal fossa (Fig. 7.14).

Another approach involves using an adult costochondral graft. An autogenous rib harvest is also used here to create a stable articulation into the temporal fossa. The rib is harvested with 2–3 mm of cartilage, but a full length 12–14 cm of bone. The rib is then scored at its inner cortex and both edges to allow bending. The rib is then fixed to the inferior border of the distal host bone segment and bent to create an angle form. The length is adjusted so that the costochondral end lies in the temporal fossa in a medial-lateral direction. The costochondral rib thus serves as an articulation graft and as a crib. The autogenous PBCM graft is then condensed on top of the costochondral graft to reconstruct the complete alveolar height and ramus width (Figs 7.15 and 7.16).

The closure, fixation and drainage for all three of these approaches is the same as described for the hemimandibular defect with a proximal segment.

ANTERIOR MANDIBULAR ARCH DEFECT

The incision design to approach a continuity defect of the anterior mandibular arch is ideally in a skin fold approximately 3 cm below the intended inferior border and extends 3 cm beyond each proximal host bone edge. In defects which extend posterior to the angle and ramus area, a midline upward vertical extension will offer increased access to develop the graft bed. The dissection proceeds through the various skin layers, the platysma and the superficial layer of the deep cervical fascia. It is well to remember that the platysma is thin and even discontinuous in the midline. The key anatomic landmark is the anterior belly of the digastric on each side. The plane of dissection continues superiorly on these muscles' surfaces and upon the surface of the submandibular gland more posteriorly to the proximal bone ends. Each bone end is exposed for at least 3 cm from the bone edge via a periosteal incision at the inferior border and reflection to the height of the alveolus.

In the midline the dissection needs to dissect a tissue pocket for the graft in the chin. This is accomplished so that the soft-tissue chin will drape around the graft rather than come to rest above it. This is accomplished with a blunt-nose scissors using both blunt and sharp dissection. It is also recommended that the dissection be guided so as to prevent oral perforation by placing a gloved hand in the mouth. Of course, once completed, the operating surgeon or the assistant who guided the surgery from the mouth must change gloves and gown.

If the continuity defect extends only from the mental foramen on one side to the mental foramen on the other side, an allogeneic split rib crib with the buccal–lingual orientation

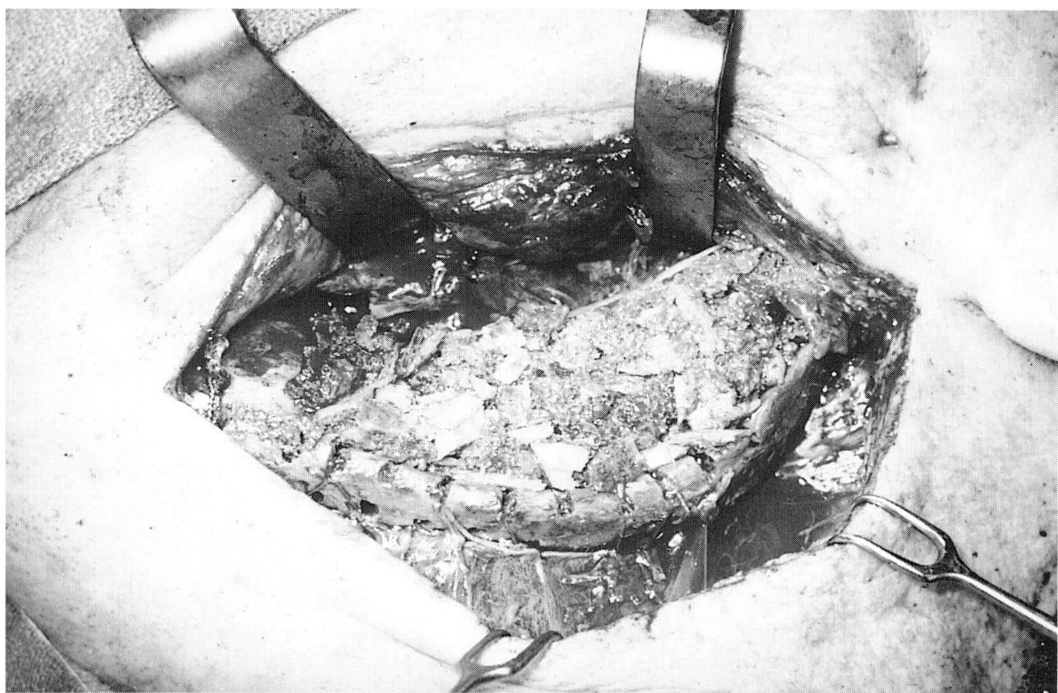

Fig. 7.15 The costochondral graft seen here replaced the inferior border and the articulation; it also acts as a crib for a PBCM graft.

will achieve an excellent arch form and chin contour. If the defect extends posterior to the mental foramen on each side, split rib segments tend to become downwardly displaced due to the greater length. In these cases an allogeneic mandible becomes the best crib (Fig. 7.17).

In the case where split rib segments would be used, each rib cortex is bent to achieve the desired curvature and chin projection. The rib segments are fixed with a single vertical mattress wire on each end placed through two burr holes placed about 1 cm apart vertically. The autogenous PBCM graft is injected between the rib segments and condensed further with hand instruments.

In the case where the allogeneic mandible would be used, the mandible is reconstituted in saline and then hollowed

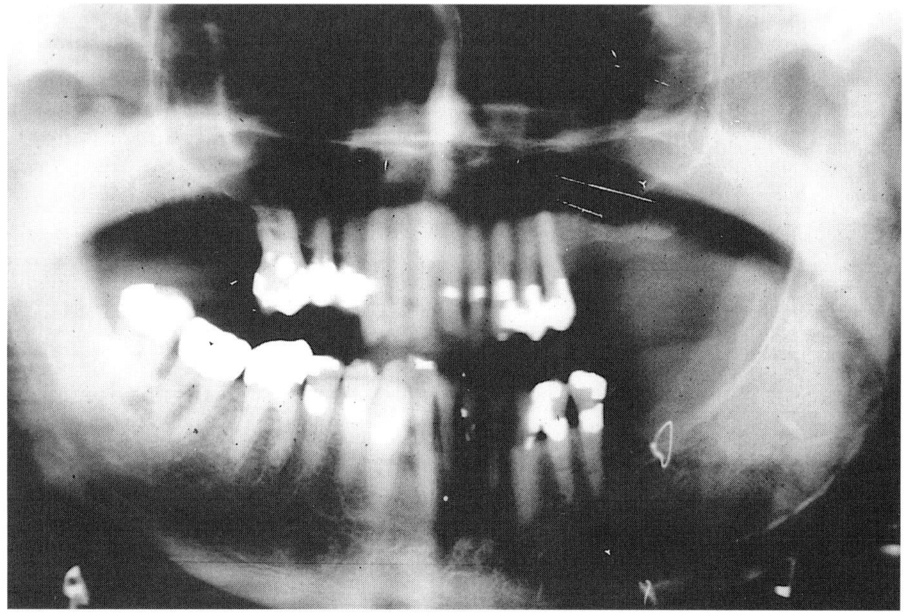

Fig. 7.16 A 5-year follow-up shows a full reconstruction to the fossa.

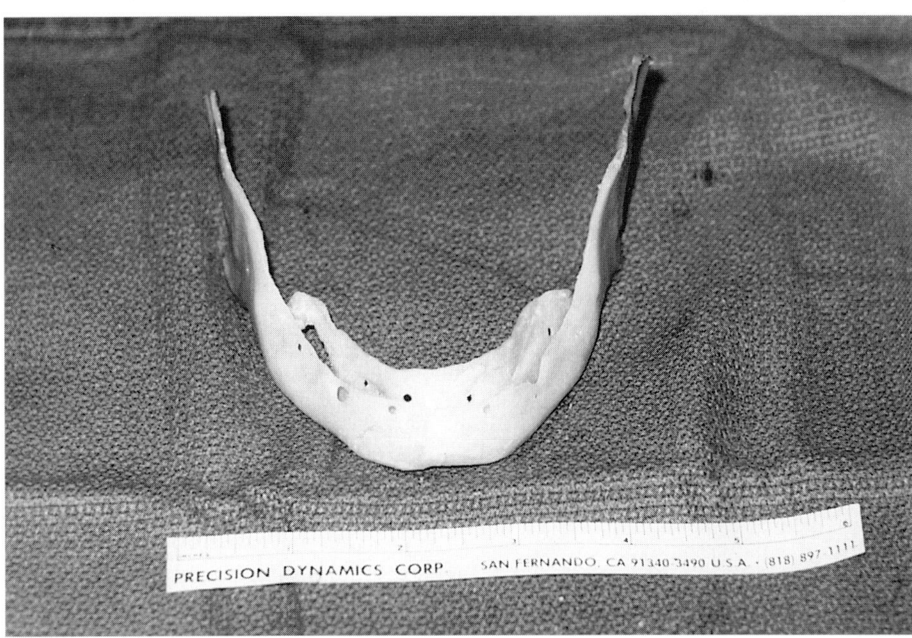

Fig. 7.17 An allogeneic mandible is used for longer span anterior mandibular arch defects.

out with rotary burrs. Since mandibles possess a greater thickness, and have a thicker cortex than ribs or ilium forms, they will take longer to prepare (about 1 hour). The mandible should be hollowed and thinned so that light can pass through it if held up to the light. The lingual flange is reduced to a height of only 0.5 cm and the buccal flange between 1.0 and 1.5 cm. In this manner the buccal flange will achieve the desired mandibular curvature and contour and the more open lingual for blood supply. The allogeneic mandible is fashioned so that it will overlap the buccal surface of the host bone in the body or ramus area. It is lag-screwed to the host mandible. Burr holes should be placed through the inferior border of the allogeneic mandible. In this way the lingual tissues can be sutured directly to the crib,

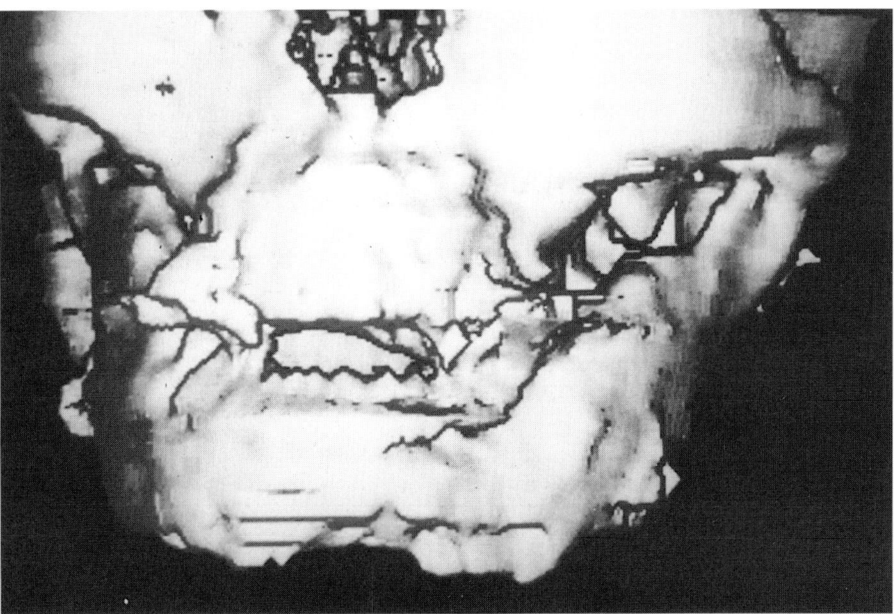

Fig. 7.18 A three-dimensional CT scan of a mandibular graft shows consolidation as well as the morphology in greater detail.

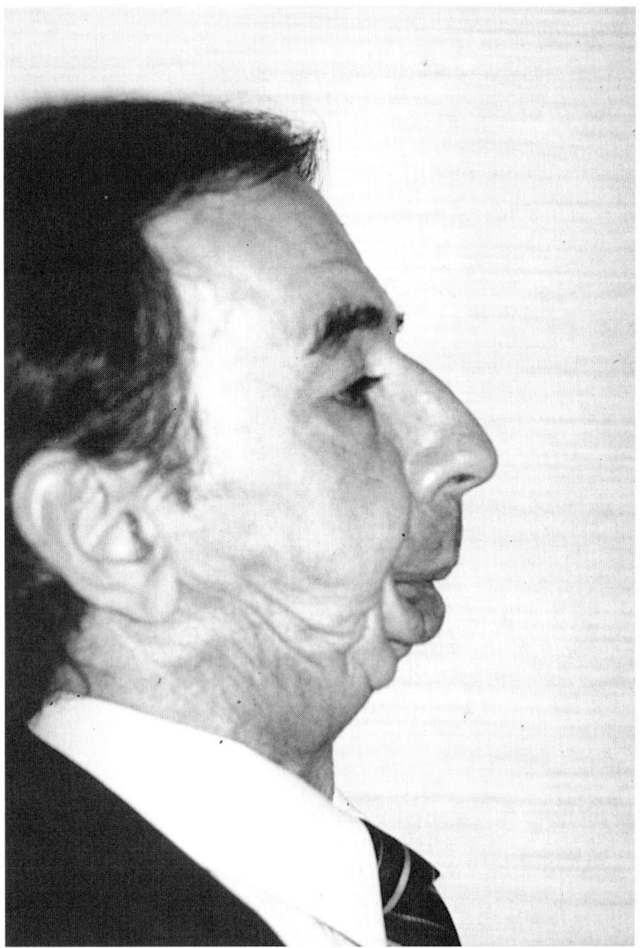

Fig. 7.19 Patient with loss of chin projection prior to mandibular reconstruction.

eliminating dead space and bringing the vascular tissue bed in closer approximation to the graft.

Once the allogeneic mandible crib is fixed in its place, the autogenous PBCM graft is injected into the crib and further condensed with hand instruments (Fig. 7.17) The closure is no different from any of the previous grafts discussed except that special attention needs to be directed to the chin area. The chin needs to be brought over the graft and its deepest layer sutured to the inferior border of the allogeneic crib. If the chin space has been fully prepared, this will place the soft-tissue chin in the correct position (Figs 7.18–7.20). The remaining closure is in the layers of the platysma, dermis and skin. A drain is placed in the neck inferior and parallel to the incision design in the area of the neck which has been undermined to permit a tension-free closure.

Fixation in some cases of anterior mandibular arch continuity defects is not necessary and is impossible to accomplish. In the defects which are edentulous, or extend posterior to the angle region, no fixation other than the crib is required. This is because the suprahyoid musculature is not active and does not re-attach until the bone graft has consolidated somewhat and would, therefore, be able to

resist displacement. In addition, in such cases maxillo-mandibular fixation is impossible, and external skeletal pins would not immobilize the graft–host interface. Therefore, patients are kept on limited jaw movements postoperatively and soft diets for 6 weeks.

In cases where the defect is limited to the anterior area and residual molar teeth exist, maxillomandibular fixation via this dentition is very much required. Posterior teeth must be immobilized because patients will persistently occlude and grind on these teeth due to their relatively greater proprioception compared to adjacent areas, thereby causing deflection of the proximal segments and separating them from the graft.

PRE-PROSTHETIC PROCEDURES TO REHABILI-TATE PATIENTS FUNCTIONALLY

The timing of pre-prosthetic surgery to prepare patients for a prosthesis is based upon revascularization of the graft and consolidation maturity of the bone ossicle. Today, patients go on to either conventional prostheses (non-implant-sup-ported) or implant-supported prostheses. The conventional prostheses usually require a vestibuloplasty procedure which releases scar tissue and creates ridge height and a rounded vestibular depth. Revascularization of PBCM bone grafts begins as early as the third or fourth postoperative day. Prior

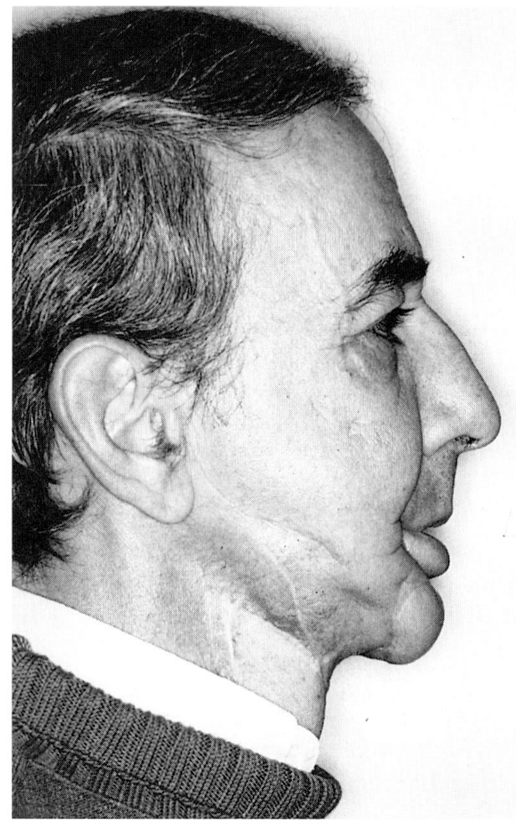

Fig. 7.20 Patient with reconsturcted mandible showing full chin projection and lip competence.

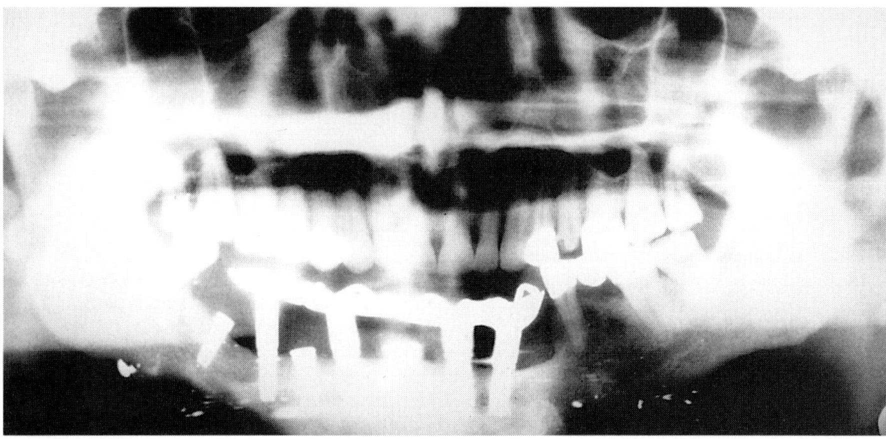

Fig. 7.21 Implants can be placed into bone-graft-consolidated bone as well as they can into non-grafted bone.

to this time, and even during the first week of revascularization, the graft exists to some degree on a plasmatic circulation by diffusion alone. By 3 months the revascularization is not only complete but stable and able to withstand the insults of surgery and the demands of wound healing. Therefore, vestibuloplasty procedures may be accomplished at 3 months or any time after. Bone consolidation continues for various lengths of time. By 6 weeks the ossicle is sufficiently consolidated to release fixation and begin meeting the demands of function. At 6 weeks, phase II bone is actively replacing and remodeling phase I bone. This activity begins to slow down at 3 months, and, although a remodeling continues throughout the graft life as it does in all bones, it is minimal and at a steady state by 6 months. Six months of graft maturity is the current time-frame used for implant placement. Certainly the biology of bone regeneration suggests that implants can be placed at earlier times, and perhaps immediately, but this is as yet not thoroughly tested and researched. A 6 month maturity time has shown consistent clinical results and osseointegration rates equal to non-grafted mandibles.

Vestibuloplasty procedures are accomplished around a bone graft in the same fashion and with the same skin, dermis, or mucosal considerations and splint considerations as exist for vestibuloplasties around the non-grafted mandible. However, the extent and the degree of vestibuloplasty must be modified because of the blood supply characteristics of the grafted mandible. A grafted mandible – as well as a non-grafted mandible which has been radiated – does not have a useful inferior alveolar blood supply. The blood supply in these two situations is almost solely from the attached muscle and periosteum. In particular, the lingual periosteum is the most abundant blood supply. Therefore, it is much preferred that vestibuloplasties be carried out on the buccal rather than the lingual. Too aggressive a dissection on both the buccal and lingual side will eventuate into an avascular necrosis of the graft. The usual vestibuloplasty creates an extensive buccal vestibule and releases the commonly found lip retraction. Split thickness skin grafts are most often used under a splint, although dermis and oral mucosa can also be used. The splint is allowed to remain for 8 days fixed by circummandibular wires or sutures and is then converted to a removable splint to retain the vestibular depth until the prosthodontist can begin the prosthetic phase. The prosthetic phase can begin biologically at 4 weeks after the vestibuloplasty as, by that time, the graft has developed a blood supply from the tissue base and is firmly attached.

The technique of placement of osseo-integrated fixtures is also altered by the blood supply characteristics. Because the blood supply to the grafted mandible is from the buccal and lingual attached periosteum with little cross-over at the crest of the ridge, a mid-crestal incision is preferred and a minimal periosteal reflection is advised (Fig. 7.21). The bone-grafted bone is more dense than a non-grafted mandible and will therefore require additional time to place each drill hole. The operator must remain patient and use sharp burrs and high-torque hand pieces so as not to heat-damage the bone. It is advisable to counter-sink each final drill hole so that the implant has a low profile once seated. The remaining aspects of implant placement, osseo-integration time of 6 months, uncovering, and loading, are the same as for placement into non-grafted mandibles. Our experience with osseo-integrated fixtures into bone-graft

Table 7.2A Implants placed into bone-graft bone loaded ≥ 1 year

Total implants	117
Osseo-integrated	107 (91.5%)
Failed to osseo-integrate	10 (8.5%)

Table 7.2B Implants placed into ungrafted mandibles loaded ≥ 1 year

Total implants	246
Osseo-integrated	235 (92.2%)
Failed to osseo-integrate	11 (7.8%)

continuity defects, as compared to non-grafted mandibles, is shown in Tables 7.2A and 7.2B. Both situations yielded an overall osseo-integration rate of 92% after one year of loading. In other words, bone-graft bone with only slight

modifications in approach can undergo the same pre-prosthetic procedures as a natural mandible, and the patient can be afforded complete rehabilitation based on a stable long-term outcome.

REFERENCES

Ariyan S 1979 The pectoralis major myocutaneous flap: a versatile flap for reconstruction in the head and neck. Plastic and Reconstructive Surgery 63: 73–79

Axhausen W 1956 The osteogenic phases of regeneration of bone: a historical and experimental study. Journal of Bone and Joint Surgery 38A: 593–601

Burwell R G 1964 Studies in the transplantation of bone. The fresh composite homograft-autograft of cancellous bone. Journal of Bone and Joint Surgery 46B: 110–154

Burwell R G 1986 The scientific basis of bone homotransplatation. In: The scientific basis of medicine annual reviews. Oxford University Press. New York, p 147

Friedenstein A J, Piatetsky-Shapiro I I, Petrakova K V 1966 Osteogenesis in transplants of bone marrow cells. Journal of Embryology and Experimental Morphology 16: 381–386

Gray J C, Elves M W 1979 Early osteogenesis in compact bone isografts: a quantitative study of contributions of the different graft cells. Calcified Tissue International 29: 225–237

Gray J C, Elves M W 1982 Donor cells' contribution to osteogenesis in experimental cancellous bone grafts. Clinical Orthopedics 163: 261–271

Marx R E, Johnson R P 1987 Studies in the radiobiology of osteoradionecrosis and their clinical significance. Oral Surgery 64: 379–390

Marx R E, Johnson R P 1988 Problem wounds in oral and maxillofacial surgery: the role of hyperbaric oxygen. In: Davis J C, Hunt T K (eds) Problem wounds: the role of oxygen. Elsevier, New York, pp 65–123

Marx R E, Kline S N 1983 Principles and techniques of bony reconstruction in cancer patients. In: Murphy G P (ed) International advances in surgical oncology. A. H. Liss, New York, pp 167–228

Marx R E, Morales M J 1988 Morbidity from bone harvest in major jaw reconstruction: a randomized trial comparing the lateral anterior and posterior approaches to the ilium. Journal of Oral and Maxillofacial Surgery 48: 196–203

Marx R E, Smith B R 1990 An improved technique for the development of the pectoralis major myocutaneous flap. Journal of Oral and Maxillofacial Surgery 48: 1168–1180

Marx R E, Kline S N, Johnson R P et al 1981 The use of freeze dried allogeneic bone in oral and maxillofacial surgery. Journal of Oral Surgery 39: 264–274

Wolfe S A, Kawamoto H K 1978 Taking the iliac bone graft. Journal of Bone and Joint Surgery 60A: 411–414

8. Prosthodontics

Patricia M. Finlay

INTRODUCTION

Maxillofacial prosthetics is the art and science of anatomical, functional or cosmetic reconstruction by means of non-living substitutes of those regions in the maxilla, mandible and face that are missing or defective because of surgical intervention, trauma, pathology, developmental or congenital malformations (Chalian et al 1972).

The prosthodontist has an important role in the management of patients with head and neck cancer and should be an integral part of the team of health care professionals providing their treatment. The prosthodontist should be involved in the initial treatment planning if a satisfactory functional and aesthetic result is to be achieved. Immediate splints for use at operation can be provided, or impressions can be taken in theatre for future use. Even if a prosthesis is not to be worn by a patient in the immediate postoperative phase, the prosthodontist can assess the condition of natural teeth pre-operatively and advise on the need for removal of those which are carious or peridontally involved and unrestorable. If the patient is to proceed to radiotherapy, removal of diseased teeth becomes especially important, and oral hygiene instruction must be given to the patient and appropriate prophylaxis arranged.

The success of prosthesis depends on the patient's acceptance and willingness to learn, and there is therefore a large psychological element involved. It is of great benefit to both patient and prosthodontist that they meet before surgery so that the patient has prior knowledge of the proposed treatment and of its prolonged nature. If a good relationship is formed at this stage the chances of a prosthodontic success may be increased.

PRE-OPERATIVE ASSESSMENT AND PLANNING

Ideally, prosthodontic treatment of head and neck cancer patients should begin pre-operatively. At the initial assessment in the head and neck clinic the prosthodontist will have the opportunity of discussing with the surgeon the potential site and size of the defect and what structures are likely to remain after the disease is eradicated. The likelihood of the patient's progression to radiotherapy can be discussed with the radiotherapist at this stage. It is important to note what structures would be included in the field of radiotherapy. Perhaps the most important factor when considering the retention of a prosthesis is the presence and condition of remaining natural teeth. The patient's own teeth should be carefully assessed at this stage. The presence of dental pathology, such as caries or periodontal disease, is evaluated. Natural teeth should be preserved wherever possible as they can be utilized to provide retention using metal clasps. Those teeth which cannot be saved should be earmarked for removal at the time of surgery, and the surgeon should be informed. A treatment plan for the teeth which are to remain is formulated. Impressions of both arches are taken and diagnostic casts made. The likely resection margins can be drawn on the diagnostic casts by the surgeon. Surgical splints, if required, can be fabricated from this model and the casts can be utilized in later stages of prosthesis construction. The pre-operative assessment also allows the prosthodontist to meet the patient and explain the procedures which will be involved in constructing their prosthesis. This is especially important to the patient with a tumour in the maxilla as the resulting defect is such a devastating one functionally and aesthetically and the patient can be much encouraged by the knowledge that their prosthesis or obturator will restore function and aesthetics to near normality.

The effects of radiotherapy on the oral tissues

Many patients undergoing treatment for oral malignancy will receive radiotherapy. It is well recognized that irradiated tissues within the oral cavity undergo changes. Epithelium can show thinning or atrophy, and the underlying connective tissue can become fibrosed and less vascular. Bone marrow may also become avascular with progressive fibrous or fatty degeneration. The number of active osteoblasts and osteoclasts is reduced. There is often decreased salivary flow and increased viscosity of saliva due to degeneration of the salivary glands. These changes lead to difficulties in the construction and wearing of dentures. Minimal denture trauma can lead to soft-tissue ulceration with delayed healing, and bone exposure may lead to osteoradionecrosis. There has been much discussion in the past concerning the timing of placement of dentures in irradiated patients. Historically, many prosthodontists and radiotherapists felt that it was necessary to wait for up to 2 to 3 years prior to placement of dentures. Beumer et al (1976), in a study of 88 patients, reported three osteoradionecroses of the mandible attributable to dentures. These all healed within 6 months without incident. There were five soft-tissue necroses secondary to dentures which again healed without complication. They concluded that the risk of developing osteoradionecrosis or soft-tissue necrosis was small and that the risk appears to be least in those patient who were edentulous and experienced denture wearers prior to radiation therapy. Osteoradionecrosis is more likely if patients have teeth in the field or radiation and if pre- or postradiation extractions are performed. The most important factor to consider when deciding on the provision of dentures for irradiated patients should be the condition of the oral mucosa. The mucosa should be healthy prior to commencement of the construction of the prosthesis. The effects of radiation on the oral mucosa usually appear during the first two or three weeks of therapy. Mucositis, a painful inflammation of the oral mucosa, can occur. Candidal infections are common. Patients complain of xerostomia due to decreased salivary production. There is also an increase in the viscosity and pH of the saliva causing a reduction of its normal cleansing and buffering effects. This, coupled with poor oral hygiene due to oral discomfort and a high carbohydrate soft diet can lead to rampant dental caries. Osteoradionecrosis is more commonly found in the mandible due its poorer blood supply.

DENTAL MANAGEMENT OF PATIENTS UNDERGOING HEAD AND NECK SURGERY

At the pre-operative assessment, unrestorable or questionable teeth will have been earmarked for removal at the time of surgery. However, there is a limit to the amount of extensive restorative work that can be done prior to surgery since the surgery will, of necessity, be performed soon after the initial assessment. The patient should be made comfortable and gross dental disease should be eradicated at this stage. Definitive restorations can be carried out at the end of the patient's treatment. Patients who are going for radiotherapy must be entered into an oral hygiene programme. The patient should be seen by a dental hygienist and have a thorough prophylaxis. The patients are instructed on strict oral hygiene procedures. This will include efficient home cleaning, regular review by the hygienist and the use of topical fluoride. This latter is useful in making the teeth more resistant to decay. Fluoride can be applied by the hygienist or at home by the patients in gel form in special carriers. These measures should reduce the possibility of radiation caries and the necessity for subsequent extraction. It is generally accepted that any questionable teeth should be removed before radiotherapy. If, however, any extractions become necessary after radiotherapy they should be done as atraumatically as possible and as long after radiotherapy as practicable and certainly under antibiotic cover. Alveolectomies and alveoplasties must be performed as the bone modelling capacity is reduced after radiotherapy and healing is delayed. If alveolectomy is not performed the risk of bone necrosis increases. This can be a most uncomfortable period for the patient and will certainly delay the provision of a prosthesis. Root canal therapy must be considered as an alternative to extraction. The periodontal condition must also be closely monitored. If the natural teeth are to be used to support the prosthesis, periodontally involved or mobile teeth may be unsuitable for use as abutments. It may be necessary to splint the teeth in order to reduce mobility. It should, however, be remembered that extensive periodontal surgery is not practical in irradiated patients, and any doubtful teeth should be removed.

PROSTHETIC MANAGEMENT

The prosthodontic treatment required and its timing is dependent on the site of the tumour and the treatment modality employed by the surgeon and radiotherapist. It is convenient to divide the prosthodontic treatment as it relates to tumours in the maxilla, mandible and those resulting in facial defects.

MAXILLA

Surgical treatment of tumours in the maxilla may result in defects of the hard or soft palate, or a combination of the two. Defects in the hard palate are easier to deal with prosthodontically than those in the soft palate alone.

Maxillectomy

Hemimaxillectomy resection is particularly devastating for patients. Following the resection, a defect is created which removes the separation between oral and nasal cavities and allows the passage of air and fluids from one to the other. This grossly impairs speech, mastication and deglutition. Speech is hypernasal at best and, at worst, totally unintelligible. Patients have great difficulty in communicating with their carers, friends and relatives. Patients are unable to drink liquids without the imbibed fluid being emitted down the nose, and food of certain consistencies will also be lost this way. The loss of the teeth, alveolus and maxillary bone

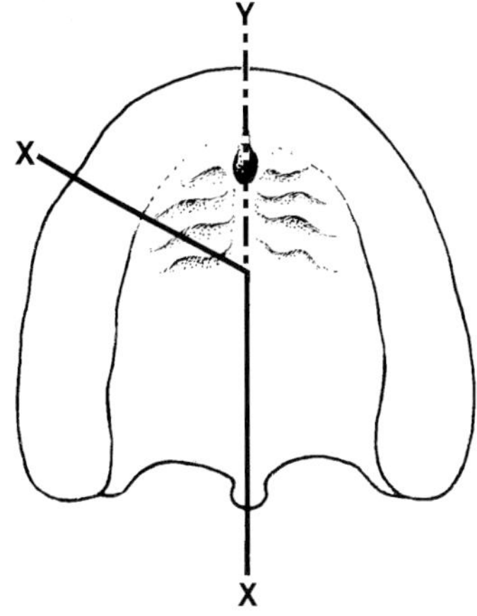

Fig. 8.1 Bony cut (X–X) in this position preserves premaxilla. A prosthesis is much more stable than if a bony cut is made (X–Y).

results in collapse of the soft tissues of the cheek into the defect, resulting in a poor appearance. This coupled with the inability to carry out normal physiological functions, may lead to considerable psychological morbidity. It is therefore imperative that speech, swallowing and mastication be re-instated. This can be accomplished by placement of an obturator prosthesis which re-establishes the separation between the oral and nasal cavities. It is convenient to divide the prosthodontic treatment into three stages:

1. the surgical splint
2. intermediate prosthesis
3. definitive prosthesis produced when healing is complete.

SURGICAL CONSIDERATIONS

The main objective of cancer surgery must be the total removal of the disease, but of major importance also is postoperative rehabilitation. Careful consideration prior to and at the time of surgery can greatly enhance the effective function and appearance of the definitive prosthesis. Many structures useful for the retention of the prosthesis will unfortunately be removed with the disease specimen. However, forethought, and an understanding of the factors which aid retention of the prosthesis, can greatly increase its success. Of paramount importance is the retention of natural teeth. Some teeth will be removed with the tumour, and any unrestorable teeth will also be removed at surgery, but the emphasis here must be placed on preservation of natural teeth wherever possible.

As much hard palate as commensurate with tumour control should be preserved (Fig. 8.1). If possible, the premaxillary segment should be retained. The position of the tumour will determine this but it has been reported

that the majority of tumours are found in the posterior superior antrum, making possible preservation of premaxilla (Shaefer et al 1963). This is important because:

1. The resulting defect is smaller, and thus the prosthesis is smaller and lighter.
2. There is an increased area to support the prosthesis.
3. The maxillary canine is preserved in the dentate patient. This tooth is useful as the crown shape allows for clasp placement and the long root resists torquing forces created by the prosthesis.
4. Support from the ipsilateral side will resist vertical displacement of the prosthesis.

The longevity of the teeth adjacent to the defect can be enhanced by correct placement of the incision and bone cuts (Fig. 8.2). If the cut is placed in the interdental space, the bony support for this tooth on the intact side is compromised. This tooth will become mobile due to further bone resorption and will be lost. If, however, the last tooth on the specimen is extracted prior to making the bony cut, and the bony cut placed through the socket preserving the maximum amount of interdental bone, this will increase the chances of survival of remaining teeth and reduce the risk of inadvertent damage to their roots.

If tumour clearance will allow, the mucosal and bony incisions should not coincide. The mucosal incision should be made 5–6 mm lateral to the planned bony cut (Fig. 8.3). The mucoperiosteum should then be carefully resected to expose the palatal bone. The bone cuts are then made and the maxillary specimen removed. The mucoperiosteum should then be replaced over the cut edge of the defect. Palatal mucosa is better able to resist the pressure of a prosthesis than is the respiratory epithelium which would form if this area was allowed to granulate (Brown 1970). Ulceration and pain in this area under a prosthesis is a common occurrence when this procedure is not followed.

The amount of soft palate remaining after the resection

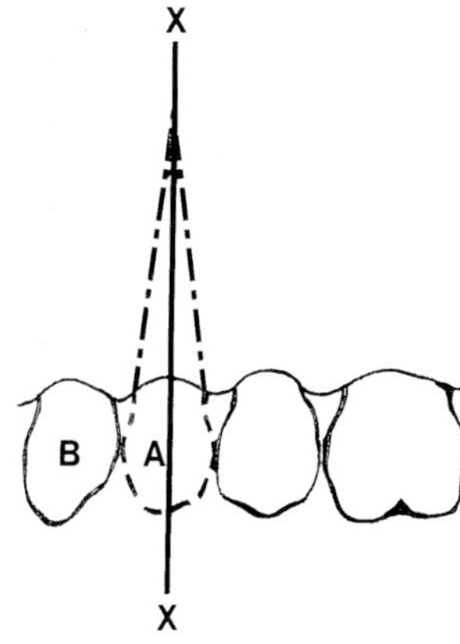

Fig. 8.2 The tooth (A) is removed and the bony cut (X) made through the extraction socket to preserve bone distal to remaining teeth (B).

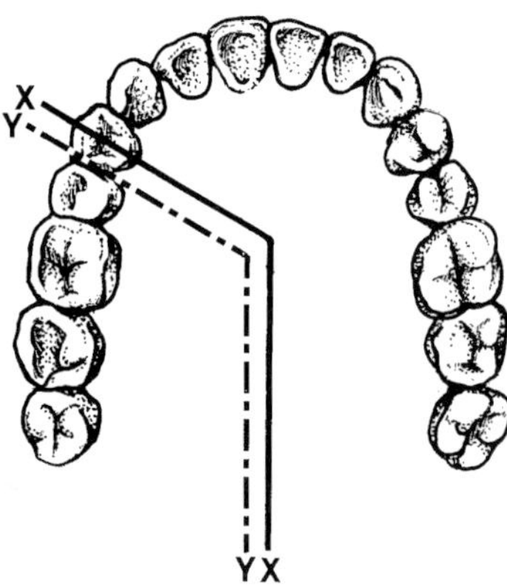

Fig. 8.3   Mucosal incision (Y–Y) 5 mm lateral to bony cut (X–X). Mucosa is then folded over the cut edge of the bone.

is also important. It has been stated that if more than one half of the soft palate requires removal then the entire soft palate should be resected in the dentate patient. If less than 50% of the soft palate remains then it fails to create an adequate seal of the prosthesis and interferes with the correct placement of the obturator into the pharyngeal wall posteriorly and laterally (Harrison 1979, Jacobs & Marunick 1988). If the soft palate is completely removed, an adequate obturator prosthesis can be constructed and will result in better function. In the edentulous patient, however, any remaining soft palate should be preserved as it will provide posterior retention for the prosthesis. If the resection specimen extends posteriorly it may be necessary to remove the coronoid process,

otherwise this will infringe on the obturator on mouth opening and cause inferior displacement of the prosthesis.

Nasal remnants should be removed as respiratory epithelium will not support the prosthesis. Remaining turbinates should be removed to allow the prosthesis to engage areas otherwise not accessible and increase retention and comfort of the prosthesis. The larger cavity is also easier to clean.

After the resection of the maxilla, a split thickness skin graft is placed on the lateral wall of the defect. This creates a scar band on the inner aspect of the cheek which provides lateral retention as the obturator can be made to engage the undercut superior to the band. The skin-grafted area is also better able to resist the pressure from the prosthesis. There is an additional advantage also as the skin graft helps to prevent extra oral contracture, thus resulting in a superior cosmetic result.

Surgical splint

The surgical splint is placed at the time of surgery. Immediate restoration of the maxillary defect with an obturator offers a number of distinct advantages:

1.   The obturator can carry the skin graft used to line the cavity or can carry some other form of surgical packing if desired.
2.   It re-establishes separation between the oral and nasal cavities, thus allowing the patient the functions of speech, deglutition and limited mastication in the postoperative period.

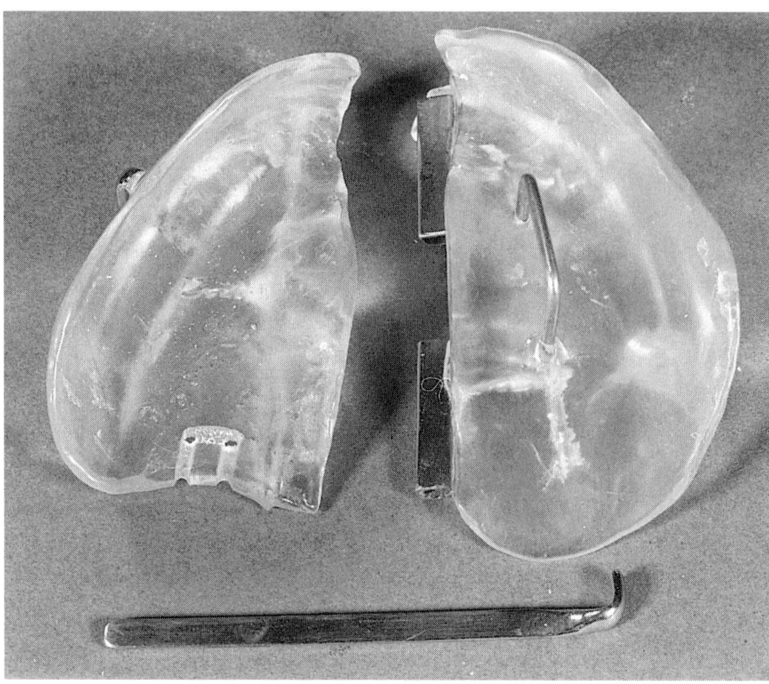

Fig. 8.4   Two-part surgical splint connected with pin and tube. Note goalpost for retention of obturator.

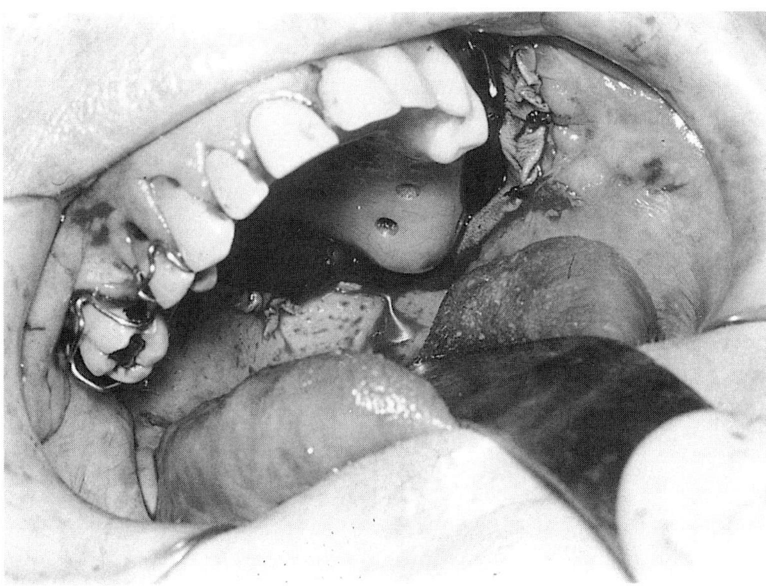

Fig. 8.5 Surgical splint carrying anterior teeth. A split thickness skin graft is sutured to the edges of the defect which is obturated with gutta percha.

3. The obturator stabilizes the defect and reduces the amount of contracture.
4. It minimizes trauma to the defect.
5. The patient's appearance is also improved, and it may enhance the patient's emotional and psychological well-being in this difficult postoperative period.

The design of the surgical splint should be simple and it should be easily and quickly produced. Depending on the surgical schedule there may be limited time for preparation of a splint and thus simplicity and speed is of the essence. The material from which it is made should be easily adjusted and non-irritant to the tissues. The surgical splint is often made of methylmethacrylate, and the obturator portion constructed in theatre from a mouldable quick-setting material such as gutta percha, silicones or tissue conditioners. The splint can be constructed in one or two parts. The two-part splint is useful for larger maxillary defects. It comprises one fixed and one removable section (Fig. 8.4). The two parts are joined using a pin and tube device. The fixed section is wired to the contralateral side using transpalatal wires. This has the major advantage of allowing access to the defect without removing its means of retention. This system allows for ease of inspection of the surgical site by the surgeon and will allow cleaning of the cavity. Impressions of the defect can be taken for an intermediate splint prior to final removal of the surgical splint.

The one-part surgical splint is retained using clasps on the remaining teeth or circumzygomatic or transpalatal wires. The appropriate cleats and hooks are fixed to the surgical splint in the laboratory. Once the defect has been prepared the obturator portion is constructed using either a surgical packing of the surgeon's choice or a resilient temporary denture liner or a material such as gutta percha. The gutta percha is softened in hot water and moulded to the defect. It is then cooled and the skin graft placed over it. Thus, a close adaptation of the skin graft to the defect walls can be achieved (Fig. 8.5). This will reduce the possibility of haematoma formation and enhance the chances of good graft take. The gutta percha is sealed to the surgical splint and wired in place. This procedure can be followed for dentate or edentulous patients. If a silicone material is used the components are mixed and applied to the defect until setting has occurred. Any trimming is then carried out and the surgical splint wired in place. The postoperative period is made more comfortable for the patient by such a technique as he is unaware of the large defect in his mouth, and eating and speech will be easier. The surgical splint is left in place for 3 to 4 weeks until the skin graft has healed. The patient is usually taken back to theatre at this stage for removal of the splint and inspection of the defect. If a two-part splint has been used, the removable part is removed and the cavity inspected and cleaned. Impressions of the defect are taken at this stage and an intermediate prosthesis constructed.

Intermediate prosthesis

An intermediate prosthesis is frequently used after the surgical splint has been removed. Following the initial phase postoperatively, there will be a stage of healing during which the defect will undergo certain dimensional changes for a variable period of up to 6 months. This prosthesis should allow the patient to function but at the same time be constructed in such a way that it can be easily modified during this healing phase. The patients may also progress to radiotherapy, and this prosthesis can be worn whilst undergoing this treatment. It is of prime importance that an obturator be provided to prevent rapid contraction of tissues around the defect. If the defect collapses the eventual prosthesis may be non-functional and of poor cosmetic appearance. It also greatly increases the morale of the patient during the period of radiotherapy if they are able to function normally. In the partially dentate patient, this prosthesis is retained by the natural teeth, but in the edentulous patient the defect is used more extensively for retention and stability. The obturator can be hollowed to decrease its weight. The intermediate prosthesis would normally carry anterior teeth to improve the patient's appearance. However, posterior teeth are generally left off the prosthesis or left out of occlusion to minimize any traumatizing effect from the occlusion on the healing defect.

Definitive prosthesis

The definitive prosthesis is made once healing is complete. This would normally be between 3 and 6 months post–operatively. If the patient has undergone radiotherapy this may delay the provision of the definitive prosthesis. Other factors would be the patient's ability to handle the obturator and his previous denture experience. Those patients who are already comfortable with partial or complete dentures may find it easier to cope with one that carries an obturator.

The edentulous patient

The design of the obturator for the edentulous patient is crucial as hydrostatic forces cannot be relied upon for retention as in normal complete dental prostheses. These

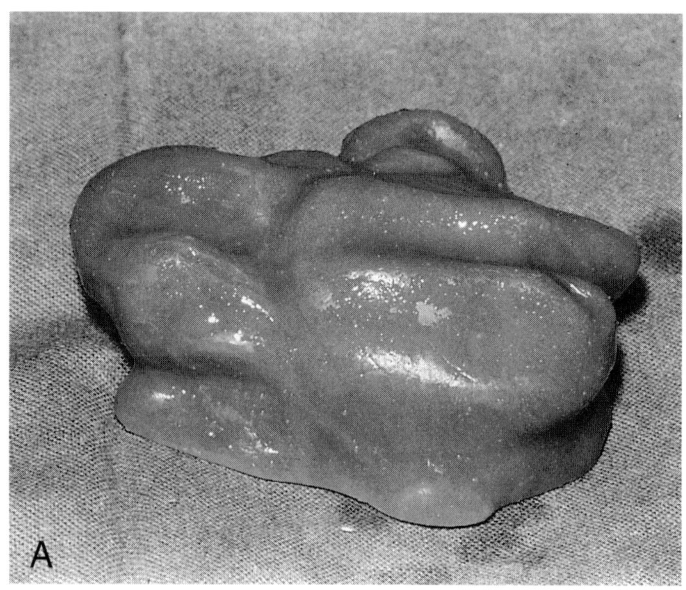

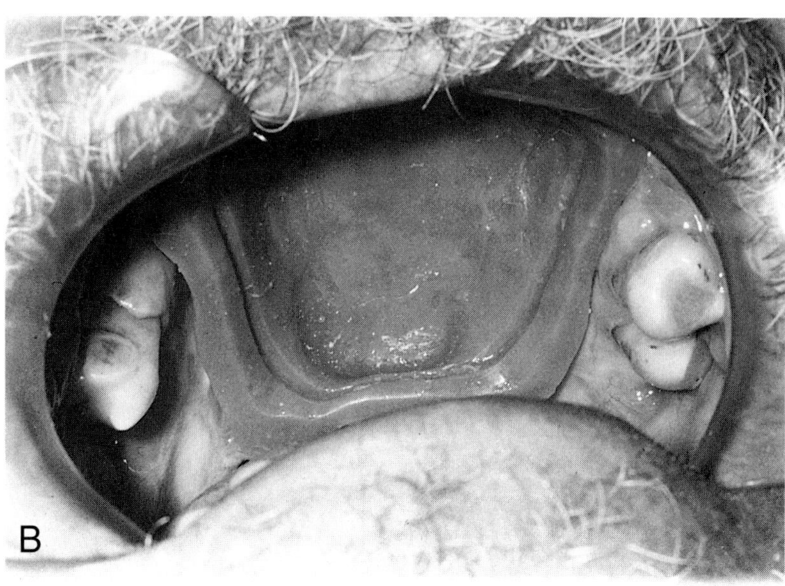

Fig. 8.6

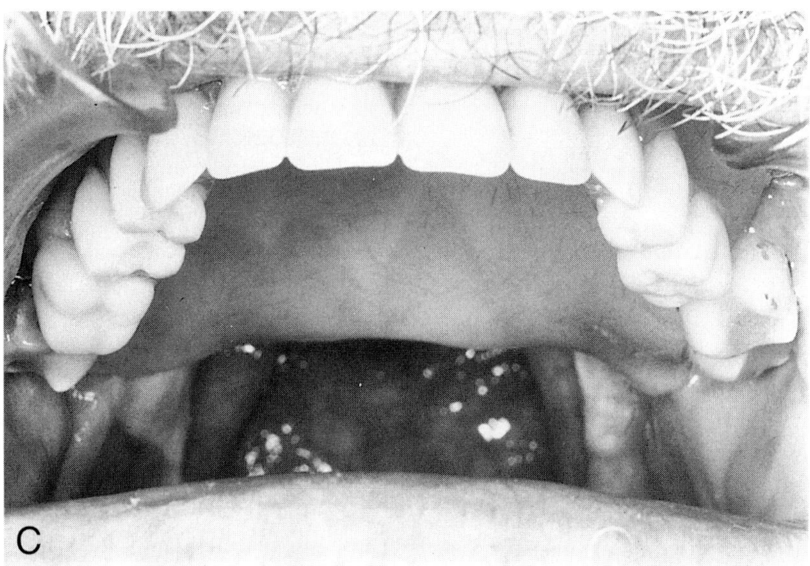

Fig. 8.6 A. Silicone shell to obturate maxillectomy defect. **B.** Silicone shell in situ. **C.** Complete upper denture is in situ. A soft-palate extension requires to be added.

are eliminated by the communication into the nose. The defect itself must be utilized to provide support, retention and stability (Desjardins 1978). The obturator should contact structures within the defect if possible. These include the hard palatal shelf, the soft palate, the lateral wall of the defect and the lateral scar band and the anterior nasal aperture. Stability can also be gained by providing a balanced occlusion. Heat-cured denture bases are extremely useful for recording jaw relationships in this situation. The obturator portion of the prosthesis should also build out the facial contours to improve aesthetics. It should be contoured to achieve a good seal to minimize the entry of liquids into the nasal cavity. The prosthesis should therefore be extended below the lateral scar band and over the soft palate, if present, in order to produce this seal. The obturator should also include a nasal airway which will alow drainage posteriorly and nasal respiration.

Following surgery and radiotherapy, many patients have trismus. If the patient is unable to open the mouth fully, a large obturator fixed to an upper denture cannot be inserted. In these cases, a two-part obturator is a useful alternative. The obturator portion is constructed from a flexible material such as Molloplast B (Regneri & Co, Karlsruhe, Germany) (Fig. 8.6 A and B). The denture portion which carries the teeth is fixed to it by means of a positive connection at the base of the obturator (Fig. 8.6C). The obturator can be compressed and it resumes its normal shape once inside the defect. A nasal airway can easily be incorporated. The denture portion, made from methyl-methacrylate is then fixed into position with ease. The flexible obturator engages undercuts within the defect which could not be utilized by a rigid obturator, thus providing retention and stability. The obturator is hollow, which

decreases the weight and improves vocal resonance. The residual alveolar ridge will provide support, and it is essential that maximum coverage of the ridge is obtained. Support will also be obtained within the defect from structures including the orbital floor, the nasal floor, the nasal septum, the pterygoid plate and the infratemporal fossa. Adequate extension of the prosthesis will provide resistance to rotational movements. A well fitting lower denture is also of benefit to the edentulous patient wearing an obturator, and flat plane occlusion can minimize lateral forces which develop during mastication. The weight of the prosthesis can be additionally decreased by using plastic as opposed to porcelain teeth.

Partially dentate patient

The most effective support and retention can be gained from the remaining natural teeth; the importance of preserving the teeth has already been stressed. Periodontally involved teeth can be splinted to distribute the load over a wide area. The distribution of clasps, connectors and rests can encourage the functional load to be directed down the long axis of the teeth. The amount of retention will depend upon the number and condition of remaining teeth but it is generally accepted that as many retainers as possible should be used to provide maximum stress distribution. The communication into the nasal cavity will again affect the border seal, which is of paramount importance in a normal denture. Undercuts within the defect can again be used to minimize rotational forces.

It is most important to maintain follow-up on a regular basis for these patients. All irradiated patients should be recalled periodically to check the condition of the oral mucosa and fit and comfort of the prosthesis. Oral hygiene should be monitored and the importance of good oral hygiene reinforced.

Soft-palate defects

Defects of the soft palate alone are less common and are more difficult to treat prosthodontically than are those of the hard palate. Surgical splints are not normally placed in conjunction with resection of soft palate tumours. If the soft palate and musculature are removed in part or in total the normal velopharyngeal mechanism is disrupted and closure will not occur causing a communication into the nasal cavity. This leads to hypernasality of speech and nasal regurgitation of fluids. Obturators can be provided to close the oral and nasal cavities during speech and swallowing. Soft palatal defects have been classified into the following categories (Aramany & Myers 1978):

1. Total resection of the soft palate retaining part of the hard palate
2. Median resection of the palate
3. Lateral resection involving approximately half of the soft palate.

The prosthetic treatment does not include surgical obturators, but a temporary intermediate prosthesis is usually constructed in the initial phase postoperatively. The definitive obturator is designed dependent upon the type of soft-palate defect. In the case of a total soft-palate resection, an obturator is placed on the posterior aspect of the patient's denture which extends into the pharynx, thus separating the oral and nasal cavities. At rest there will be a space posteriorly to allow for nasal breathing. When the patient swallows or speaks, muscular activity will close the defect.

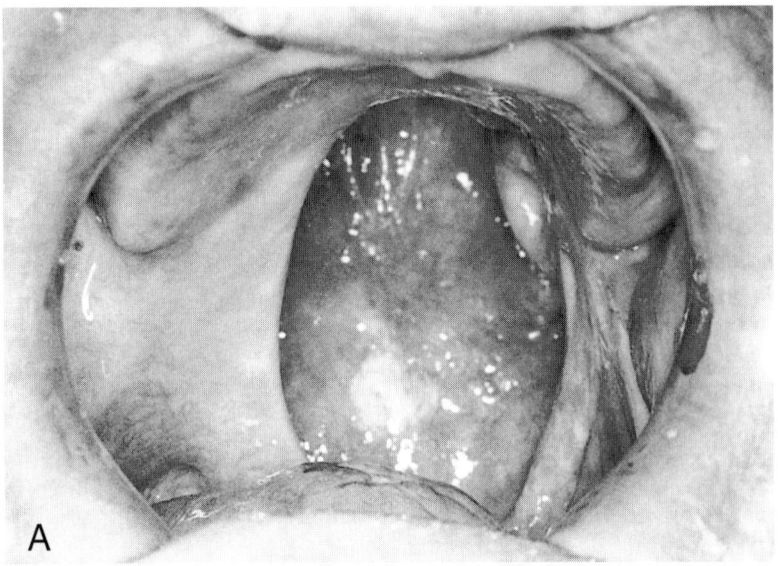

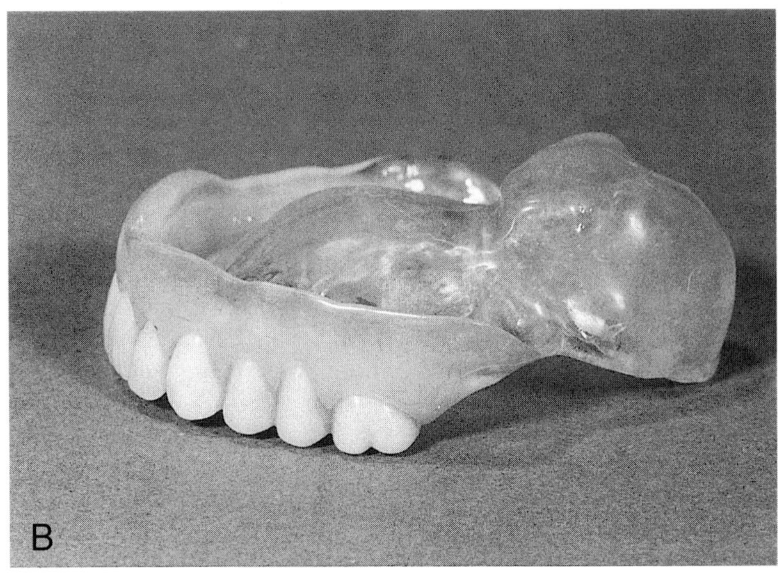

Fig. 8.7

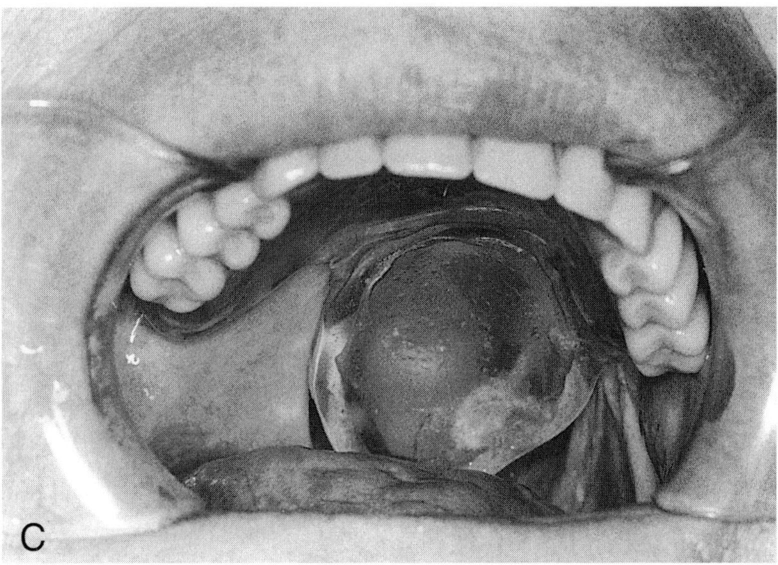

Fig. 8.7 **A.** Soft palate defect. **B.** Upper denture carrying soft-palate obturator. **C.** Soft-palate obturator in situ. The space around the obturator closes during function.

A prosthesis constructed for a median palatal defect is constructed from a functional impression. The obturator extension passes through the defect, and at rest there is a space between the prosthesis and the posterior margin of the defect (Fig. 8.7). Muscular activity during speech or swallowing will close the defect. Lateral soft-palate defects are the most difficult to restore prosthodontically. Often, advanced tumours seen in the faucial/retromolar/soft palate area will require large resections which can produce severe functional disability. Many of these patients are edentulous, which adds to the difficulties.

It has been suggested that the presence of a prosthesis will stimulate muscle function with time as some patients seem to regain the ability of velopharyngeal closure without the use of a prosthesis. However, it is most important that patients with larger defects — and especially those that have been restored with large flaps — are made aware prior to commencement of prosthodontic therapy of the difficulties that are likely to be encountered.

MANDIBULAR DEFECTS

The prosthetic management of mandibulectomy patients is difficult and the results can be extremely variable. The degree of success achieved depends on the site of tumour and the amount of bone and soft tissue that has been removed. The effects of radiotherapy will add to the problem. It is convenient to group mandibular defects into those where tumour surgery has resulted in removal of a portion of mandible but where the lower border is intact (mandibular continuity defect), and those where a section of mandible has been completely removed (mandibular discontinuity defect) (Desjardins & Laney 1979). Resection of the floor of

the mouth and tongue will also affect the prognosis for the prosthesis. The functional disabilities produced by these operations will include impairment of speech, difficulty in swallowing, drooling of saliva and deviation of the mandible towards the resected side, the latter causing occlusal discrepancies, poor masticatory capability and cosmetic deformity. The level of impairment of speech is dependent on the amount of tongue resected and on whether the remainder of the tongue has been used to close the wound. This coupled with sensory and motor nerve defects will lead to speech difficulties. Drooling of saliva occurs due to oral incompetence and the lack of sensation and poor tongue muscular control.

The mandibular continuity defect

The continuity defect usually includes loss of mandibular teeth and alveolar bone. Frequently, if flaps or grafts are used, or even in cases of primary closure, there is a loss of lingual, labial or buccal sulci (Fig. 8.8). All these will serve to reduce the denture-bearing area and can therefore limit the available support for the prosthesis. This would lead to concentration of stress on the residual structures which may lead to loss of teeth and ulceration of mucosal areas. There may be also some lack of lip and cheek support which must be restored by prosthesis.

Prosthodontic aims, in these cases, would include the replacement of lost alveolar bone and teeth to provide lip and cheek support and proper occlusal contact for mastication. In view of the reduced denture-bearing area it is often necessary to perform minor surgical procedures such as vestibuloplasty to increase the denture-bearing area. This may provide sufficient support for a removable prosthesis.

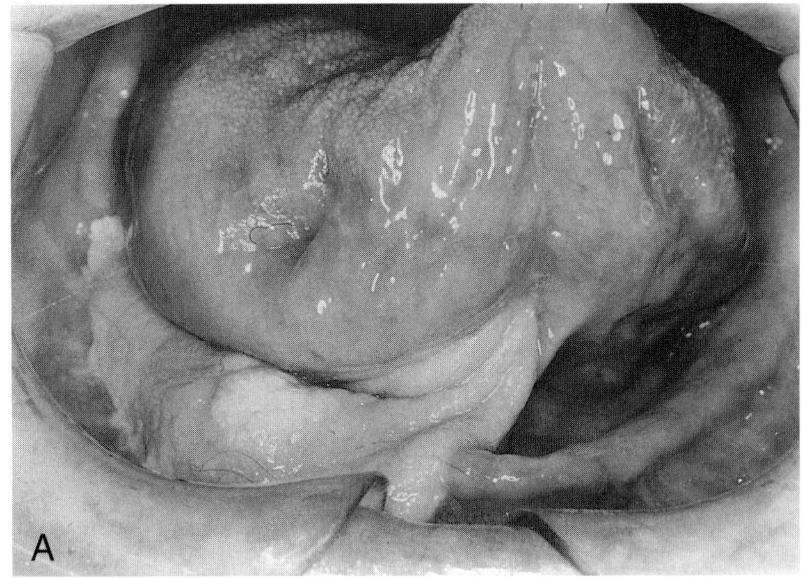

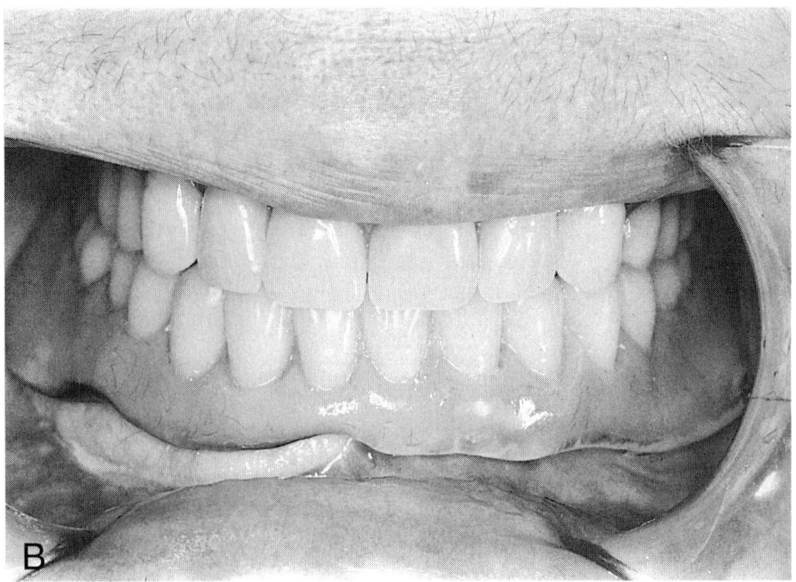

Fig. 8.8 A. Normal alveolar anatomy replaced by a free radial forearm flap. **B.** The denture rests on the mobile skin of the flap.

Support and retention for the prosthesis can be gained from natural teeth in the dentate patient and by the residual alveolar ridge. In the edentulous patient it is essential to extend the base correctly and develop good border seal to contribute to retention and stability. Close attention should also be paid to the occlusion in order to obtain maximum stability of the prosthesis.

Mandibular discontinuity defect

In addition to loss of teeth and alveolar bone, the deviation of the mandible to the defect side causes great problems when considering restoration by a prosthesis. The extent of the deviation is variable and is dependent upon loss of tissue and scar contracture. Some patients can retrain their mandibular movements into a reproducible useful occlusion by simple pressure towards the non-affected side. More commonly, however, the mandible must be retrained using a guide flange prosthesis. If the patient can attain an acceptable occlusion with manual manipulation of the mandible but is unable to consistently repeat this position, a mandibular guide flange prosthesis is appropriate. This consists of a partial denture with a metal or acrylic flange which extends vertically from the buccal aspect to engage the buccal side of the maxillary second premolar and first molar areas on the non-resected side. The depth of the guide flange is determined by the depth of the maxillary buccal sulcus but it should allow adequate opening without disengagement of the flange itself. It would be wise to consider a maxillary prosthesis to counteract any lateral forces placed on the maxillary teeth by the buccal flange. The maxillary appliance could be incorporated into a maxillary partial denture. If the patient does not need a maxillary denture, a temporary palatal retainer could be used. Once the patient can successfully reproduce an acceptable occlusion, the guide flange can be discontinued.

An alternative is to design a maxillary prosthesis, usually constructed in acrylic with the guidance area being placed palatally on the non-defect side. The prosthesis then guides the mandibular teeth into an acceptable occlusion. It has been suggested that this therapy is most successful when the resection involves bony structures with minimal sacrifice to the tongue and floor of mouth. The prognosis for this type of therapy is also improved in patients who have not been irradiated or received a neck dissection (Beumer et al 1982).

Mandibular retraining prostheses can be used only in dentate patients. It is not possible to construct a guide flange prosthesis for edentulous patients due to the instability of complete dentures. Some patients will never be able to assume a correct mandibular position even with training, and for these patients — and for all edentulous patients — the deviated mandibular position must be accepted. For improved masticatory efficiency the prosthodontist must provide two opposing occlusal surfaces. It is perhaps most practical to provide an occlusal table, palatal to the maxillary teeth, with which the mandibular teeth can occlude. The maxillary occlusal table can easily be included in a removable prosthesis which provides palatal coverage. This type of prosthesis can be made for any patient irrespective of how many teeth they have. Support and retention is gained by following normal prosthodontic principles.

Mandibular resection frequently involves the removal of a portion of the floor of mouth and tongue. Suturing often leads to the loss of lingual and/or buccal sulci. This results in the denture resting on mobile tissue and being subject to displacing forces produced by tongue or cheek or lip movements. Additionally, because of the mobile denture-bearing area, no border seal can be achieved, thus leading to decreased retention. The amount of tongue tissue removed during surgery will determine the degree of difficulty the patient experiences postoperatively. The tongue performs several important functions, and in addition to speech being affected the ability to move the food bolus around the mouth and stabilize the complete lower denture will be adversely affected. Many patients, having lost a proportion of tongue tissue, will be unable to wear a lower prosthesis during function. For these patients, a palatal reshaping appliance can be considered which may assist with swallowing and speech. This prosthesis is basically a maxillary denture, the palatal surface of which is constructed from a functional impression taken with the patient swallowing. The denture palate then corresponds to the tongue position which can be achieved during swallowing and may assist the patient to function.

Finlay et al (1992), in a review of 255 patients who had undergone treatment for oropharyngeal cancer, reported that 92% of these patients were edentulous postoperatively. This included a group who had received a dental clearance prior to radiotherapy due to dental decay or periodontal disease. Some 61% were wearing complete upper and lower dentures provided after surgery, 15% were completely edentulous but could wear only the complete upper denture and 16% of these edentulous patients could wear no prosthesis at all. These latter two groups presumably represent patients having undergone surgery to the tongue, oropharynx and floor of mouth. This reflects the difficulties encountered by the prosthodontist following ablative surgery to the intra-oral region.

FACIAL PROSTHESES

Occasionally, extensive surgical procedures are required for advanced tumours of the facial region. In addition to intra-oral defects, the surgery may have included loss of extra oral structures, e.g. nose, ear, lip or orbital contents and associated soft tissue. The functional difficulties may be severe, and in combination with the often gross cosmetic disfigurement will lead to significant psychological problems for the patient and his family. It is therefore imperative that these patients be quickly rehabilitated with surgical means or a prosthesis. Surgical reconstruction may be contraindicated, and the surgical reconstruction of some defects is always inferior to its prosthetic counterpart, e.g. the ear (Fig. 8.9). A prosthesis offers advantages in that it is relatively simply made and does not involve further anaesthesia for medically compromised patients; additionally, the prosthesis can be removed to allow the surgeon to inspect the underlying tissues. Clearly, the success of any prosthesis will depend upon the extent and location of the defect and also on the attitude of the patient. It has been found that patients who have worn dentures successfully prior to surgery often cope better than those who have no denture experience. The prosthesis may replace a missing extra oral portion or may be made in conjunction with an intra-oral prosthesis, e.g. a hemimaxillectomy defect with an orbital exenteration may require an intra- and extra-oral prosthetic component (Fig. 8.10). The replacement of facial tissue by prosthetic means is not a new concept. Indeed, Ambrose Pare, whose work with prostheses in the sixteenth century is well reported, significantly advanced the development of maxillofacial prosthetics. In the eighteenth century, Pierre Fauchard described the replacement of natural teeth using prostheses and described a maxillary obturator. Modern advances in synthetic materials have allowed for significant improvement in the aesthetics of facial prostheses. Modern elastomers and polymers include methylmethacrylate, polyvinylchloride, silicones and polyurethane and these materials are frequently used in the production of facial prostheses.

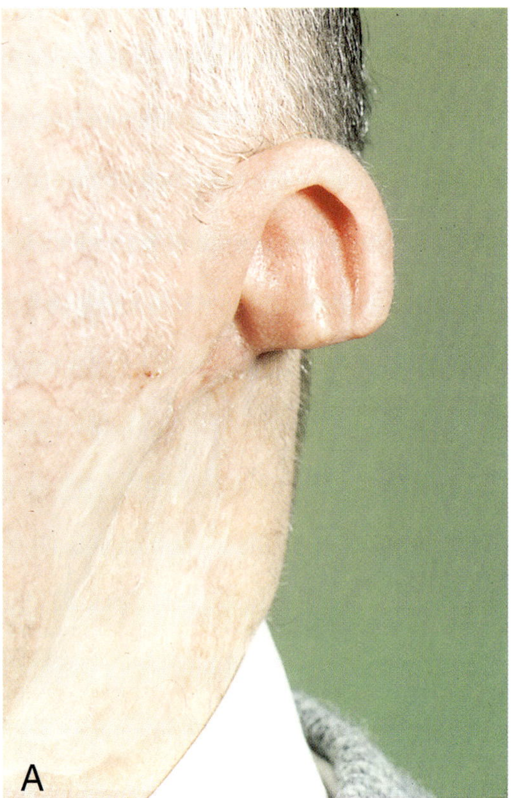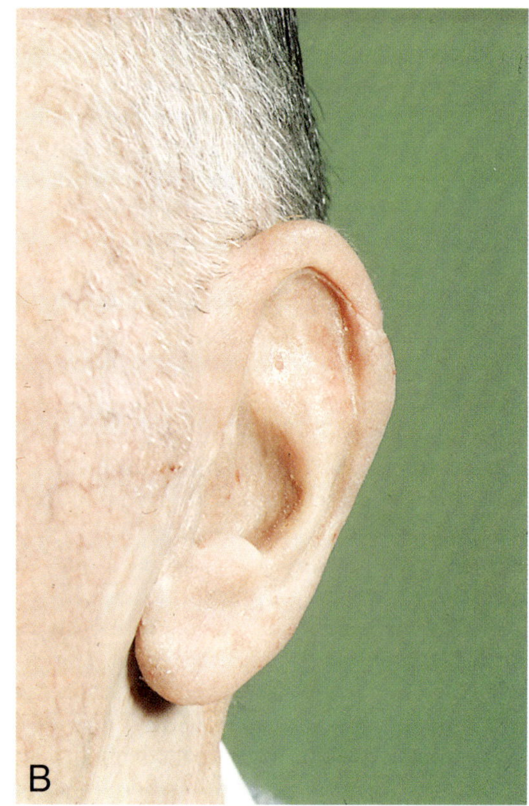

Fig. 8.9 A. This patient refused to have the upper remnant of his ear removed to facilitate a total ear prosthesis. **B.** Modern techniques, however, enabled a satisfactory prosthesis to be fashioned. An excellent colour match can be achieved using silicone elastomers.

Criteria for materials used in facial prostheses

The major requirement is biocompatability but there are a number of other criteria which should be fulfilled. The prosthesis must resemble skin in appearance and touch. The ideal material would be translucent and have the texture and colour of skin and be soft to touch. The material should be heat- and light-stable and should have some strength in thin section to prevent tearing. The material must not irritate the surrounding tissue. It would also be advantageous if the material were easy to work with and inexpensive to produce. There is no absolutely ideal material for the construction of facial prostheses and all have advantages and disadvantages. Many prosthodontists now favour the silicone rubbers for the fabrication of facial prostheses. There are two types, room-temperature-vulcanizing silicone and heat-vulcanizing silicone. Heat-vulcanizing silicone produces a very good colour and is stronger than room-temperature-vulcanizing silicone. However, more equipment is required. Each operator will have his own preference for material (Conroy 1985).

The facial prosthesis is fabricated from an impression or facial moulage. The material of choice is usually an alginate. A working cast is made from this impression on which the prosthesis can be sculpted in wax. The wax pattern is converted to silicone and the prosthesis coloured. The retention of the prosthesis can be accomplished in one of several ways:

1. An orbital or nasal prosthesis can be attached to spectacles. The spectacles will help to hide the margin of the prosthesis and they will provide the sole form of retention. The major disadvantage of this technique is that the prosthesis is removed with the spectacles.
2. The prosthesis may be attached by medical-grade adhesive. There are several suitable adhesives available. Use of adhesive obviates the necessity for spectacles or other carrier but can be messy, and elderly patients may find it difficult to apply.
3. Orbital prostheses have been retained by magnets attached to a silicone shell engaging undercuts within the orbit. The silicone shell may also be attached to a maxillary obturator.
4. Current trends are favouring implant-retained prostheses. Titanium implants are placed within bone in strategic positions. These are left for a 3-month period for osseo-integration to take place. After this period they are uncovered and abutments are attached to the intraosseous implants which will support fixation for the prosthesis. This can take the form of a bar onto which

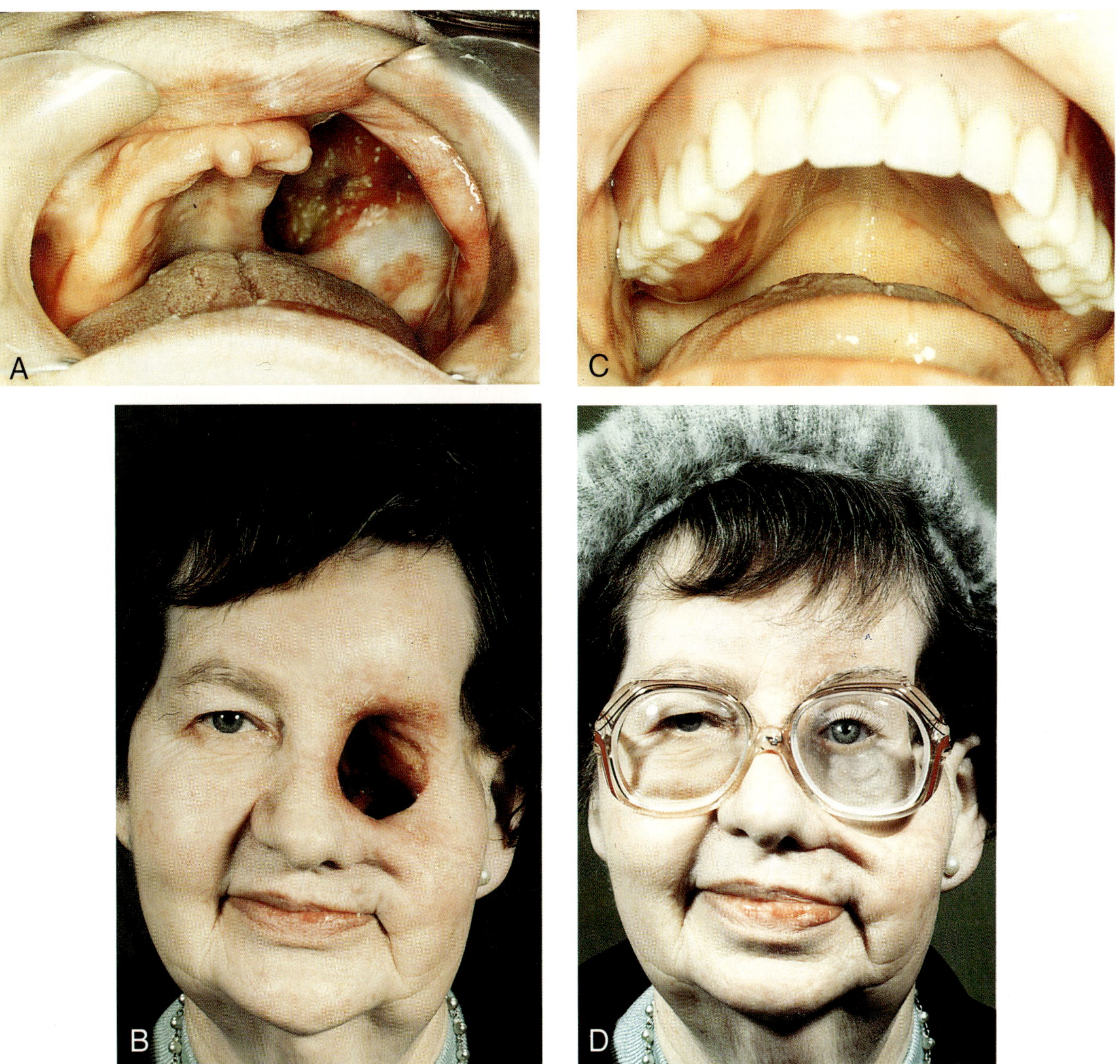

Fig. 8.10 **(A, B)** Defect following radical maxillectomy. **C** A dental obturator closes the intra-oral defect. **D** A separate prosthesis mounted on a spectacle frame is used to obturate the orbital defect.

the prosthesis clips or an acrylic plate which will carry magnets. Implant techniques are suitable for nasal, auricular and orbital prostheses. Occasionally more complicated facial prostheses are constructed covering larger areas of the face. Osseo-integration is defined as a direct structural and functional connection between ordered, living bone and the surface of a load-carrying implant (Branemark et al 1985). The advent of im-

plantology may make the provision of facial prostheses and intra-oral prostheses for difficult cases more successful. It is said that irradiated bone can take implants after one year has elapsed postradiotherapy.

The patient and his relatives must be made aware that however good a facial prosthesis is made the margins will be detectable on close scrutiny. Acceptance of this at an early stage will prevent future disappointment.

MAINTENANCE

All patients who have received any type of prosthesis should be maintained on long-term follow-up. This is especially important for patients who have undergone radiotherapy. It is imperative that the condition of the remaining oral structures be maintained in optimal condition, and the patients should be regularly recalled for evaluation. Patients who have recently acquired an obturator should be very closely followed-up. The patient should be assessed with reference to his adjustment to the prosthesis and its function. Patients never having worn dentures before surgery are especially at risk and should be closely monitored. These patients may require a long period of adjustment and constant reassurance from the prosthodontist that their prosthesis will restore function and aesthetics to near-normality. It is well recognized that oral hygiene standards may fall if patients are not closely monitored. To this end they should be seen by the hygienist regularly in order to maintain high standards of oral hygiene. Since the prosthesis may be gaining support and retention from remaining teeth it is important that these be retained. Therefore, patients who have received an obturator should be reviewed every 3 to 6 months.

CONCLUSION

Maxillary and mandibular or facial defects following surgical removal of neoplastic lesions of the maxilla, mandible and adjacent structures may have a detrimental effect on the patient both functionally and psychologically. Rehabilitation of these patients following surgery is mandatory if they are to be restored to their usual way of life. Rehabilitation can include surgical or prosthetic reconstruction.

Many intra-oral defects affect the normal functions of mastication, deglutition and speech. If a direct communication between the oral and nasal cavity exists in addition to the problems mentioned above, there is also nasal regurgitation of fluids and food. In addition to the functional disabilities, the patient may also be left with a distorted facial appearance.

The aims of prosthodontic rehabilitation of these patients can be summarized as follows:

1.   restoration of mastication and deglutition
2.   restoration of speech
3.   the preservation and maintenance of remaining oral tissues
4.   improvement of appearance
5.   the return of the patient to his normal activities.

The degree to which the appearance and function can be restored depends on the size of the surgical defect and the attitude of the patient. For optimal rehabilitation the prosthodontist should have the opportunity of meeting the patient and being involved in treatment planning from the initial phases. The prognosis for prosthodontic treatment depends upon a number of complicated factors, including the amount and condition of oral tissue remaining, the severity of mandibular deviation, the presence of natural teeth, lip and tongue control and mobility, radiotherapy, and the amount and mobility of remaining tongue. Another most important factor is the emotional and psychological state of the patient. It should be anticipated that the patients will experience difficulty in coping with the functional and cosmetic deficit and their fear of the disease process itself. The patient must be prepared for the prosthodontic treatment and have realistic expectations of the level of rehabilitation achievable. Following discussion with the prosthodontist, the surgeon may be able to modify slightly the surgical excision, thus preserving structures which will greatly enhance the success of the prosthesis.

Never has the need for maxillofacial prosthodontic treatment been greater. Improved treatment regimens mean that an increasing number of patients are surviving disfiguring tumour surgery. Maxillofacial prosthetics has become an essential part of the treatment of head and neck cancer patients and the prosthodontist is an integral part of the team of health care professionals involved in the treatment of these patients.

REFERENCES

Aramany M A, Myers E N 1978 Prosthetic reconstruction following resection of hard and soft palate. Journal of Prosthetic Dentistry 40: 174

Beumer J, Curtis T A, Morrish R B 1976 Radiation complications in edentulous patients. Journal of Prosthetic Dentistry 36: 193-203

Beumer J, Korrasch M, Kagawa T Prosthetic restoration of oral defects secondary to surgical removal of oral neoplasms. 1982 Journal of the Canadian Dental Association 3: 47

Branemark P-I 1983 Osseointegration and experimental background. American Journal of Prosthetic Dentistry 50: 399-410

Branemark P-I, Zarb G A, Albrektsson T 1985 Tissue integrated prostheses. Quintessence Publishing Co, Chicago

Brown K E 1970 Clinical considerations improving obturator treatment. Journal of Prosthetic Dentistry 24: 461

Chalian V A, Drane J B, Standish S M 1972 Maxillofacial multi-disciplinary practice. Williams & Wilkins, Baltimore

Conroy B 1985 Maxillofacial prosthetics. In: Rowe L, Williams J L. (eds) Maxillofacial injuries. Churchill Livingstone, Edinburgh

Desjardins R P 1978 Obturator prosthesis design for acquired maxillary defects. Journal of Prosthetic Dentistry 39: 424-435

Desjardins R P, Laney W R 1979 Typical clinical problems and approaches to treatment. In: Laney W R (ed) maxillofacial prosthetics. PSG Publishing, Littletown, M A

Finlay P M, Dawson F, Robertson A G, Soutar D S 1992 An evaluation of functional outcome after surgery and radiotherapy for intra-oral cancer. British Journal of Oral and Maxillofacial Surgery 30: 14–17

Harrison R 1979 Prosthetic management of the maxillectomy patient. Head and Neck Surgery 1: 366-369

Jacobs J R, Marunick M T 1988 Surgical considerations in maxillofacial prosthetic rehabilitation of maxillectomy patient. Journal of Surgical Oncology 37: 29–32

Shaefer W G, Hine M K, Levy B M 1963 A textbook of oral pathology. W B Saunders, Philadelphia

Section 2

9. The oral cavity

Andrew Batchelor

INTRODUCTION AND HISTORICAL REVIEW

For half a century, following its general introduction in the 1920s, radiotherapy was the gold standard in the management of oral cancer. However, when the results of radiation in the therapy of major oral cancers are examined it is clear that radiotherapy did not hold its position because of its efficacy in attaining long-term cure (Robertson et al 1985). For T3 and T4 lesions, and in any node-positive situation, reported cure rates were clustered around the 10% level. It is only in the last two decades that surgical excision has once again found favour, and this is due to improvements in antibiotics, anaesthesia, excisional technique, oncological thought and, by far most importantly, reconstructive technique.

Before radiotherapy was available surgery offered the only hope of cure. At the end of the last century excisional techniques in relation to oral cancers were well described (Crile 1906). Tumours tended to be advanced, and the excisions extremely ablative. In the absence of reconstruction, direct closure or suture of skin to lining was all that was available (Blair et al 1941). The ensuing deformity and loss of function was often horrific (Steckler et al 1974) and excisions would often be compromised. Reconstruction became possible in the early part of this century after the development of endotracheal anaesthesia, which was probably the greatest single advance in head and neck surgery. The reconstructive techniques were developed from those used for the huge load of traumatic defects caused by the Great War. The technology of the time dictated complex, indirect, multi-staged reconstructions which were very prolonged, frequently taking months (Blair et al 1941).

The cure rate of surgery alone for major tumours was not then, as now, high. Prolonged reconstructive plans would use up the apparent disease-free interval before the clinical recurrence of persistent disease. The tumour would frequently recur during or soon after the completion of the repair (Ewing 1954). This led, not unnaturally, to the concept of delayed reconstruction allowing as much as 2 years after direct closure to select only those patients who

had attained excisional cure. This draconian regimen is still, sadly, persisting nowadays in the practice of some ill-informed clinicians. It is hardly surprising that, in such a background, radiotherapy with modest morbidity and occasional superb results gained popularity in the absence of complete patient group audit.

The situation remained unchanged until the 1960s when more rapid and, more importantly, more reliable techniques of repair became available. The role of surgical excision in the management of oral cancer has been re-examined constantly in the light of the rapidly changing reconstructive technologies since that time. Surgical excision has an important part to play in the modern therapeutic arsenal and its role continues to develop.

The development of excisional technique

It is rather artificial to consider tumour excision entirely separately from reconstruction because the former has usually been modified by the latter. However, as has been alluded to above, excision predated any attempt at reconstruction. Initially, surgical ablation was directed at the primary tumour. Local excision was rapidly found to be ineffective in all but very small tumours. For more advanced disease, which formed the bulk of experience 100 years ago, more and more radical excision was performed with limited success. This lead to whole organ or regional resections rather than the more tumour-directed, clearance margin dictated resections described below.

The Halstedian model of cancer spread, which dictated organ involvement with lymphatic permeative spread to nodes in a stepwise, predictable and ordered way, dictated thinking. Radical excision were designed in terms of normal anatomical blocks rather than with due consideration of how a tumour may spread locally and which specific tissue might or might not be involved. As more conservative excisions were tried the concept of permeation of lymphatics was still maintained and so primary excision and nodal clearance were designed 'en bloc' (Carroll 1952). Before the era of antibiotics the defects so caused frequently provided fearsome septic complications as the intra-oral defect was continuous with the neck, allowing massive infection (McGregor 1993). This 'en bloc' concept is without practical pathological basis for the majority of oral cancers but has been pursued by some up to the present day.

To a large extent patterns of resection have been dictated by the surgeon's reconstructive thought. For smaller tumours the surgeon kept his eye on a method of direct intra-oral closure, usually employing the tongue. As primary reconstruction was not possible, and infection a major risk then, large excisional volumes were frequently resected to allow skin to mucosal closure and produce a controlled salivary fistula. As limited reconstruction became possible, surgeons were often guilty of tailoring the excisional pattern to the limits of the reconstruction available to them. It is only in relatively recent times that a spectrum of flexible, powerful and reliable reconstructive techniques have allowed the development of rational excisional patterns based purely in pathological and therapeutic grounds.

The excision of the mandible

En bloc excisional thinking has caused much difficulty with management of the mandible. If a large regional resection is to be designed and performed in continuity with the lymphatic drainage then the mandible can be argued to be lying in the lymphatic path and require resection (Carroll 1952). This argument was followed right up to the last decade. Those who initially chose to conserve the mandible in more recent times stripped all soft tissue from the bone, risking its necrosis. In the circumstances, osteotomy to improve surgical access further increased the incidence of necrosis — so it was left intact.

Excisions of tumours within the mandibular arch were therefore performed in the 'pull through' manner. The surgical exposure in such technique is poor for all but mobile tongue tumours and this further encouraged surgeons to have a low threshold for mandibular resection. Once potentially involved it was thought that the whole bone was potentially at risk. Mandibular resections were therefore radical and segmental, usually including a complete hemimandible or complete arch from angle to angle (McGregor & McGregor 1986). This was usually the most disabling and disfiguring aspect of the surgery. Attempts to conserve the mandible were based on anatomy and not pathological studies of patterns of tumour invasion or consideration of the bone's nutrition (McGregor & McDonald 1989). Local excisions, localized segmental excision and preservation of inner or outer table of the mandible are not based on sound pathological principle and are subject to high rates of complication (Ch. 3).

It has become clear that, in patients who have not received previous radiotherapy, the mandible is much less likely to be involved by tumour, and, when it is, the pattern of involvement is safely predictable. In most instances the mandible can be partly or totally conserved (McGregor & McGregor 1986).

The management of nodes

During the last century it was clear that even if the primary lesion could be controlled a significant proportion of patients developed nodal disease either before presentation or after primary management. Initially, local nodal excision was practised. Crile rationalized nodal ablation with his description of radical neck dissection (1906). At the time, this was a formidable undertaking without modern anaesthesia, blood transfusion or antibiotics. This was particularly so when it was combined with primary intra-oral resection in an en bloc pattern as this allowed the oral cavity to communicate with the neck. Neck dissection was initially reserved for clinically positive necks and often performed as a staged procedure when the oral cavity was healed. As radiotherapy gained popularity in the management of primary disease, neck dissection was frequently used alone as higher rates of control could be attained by surgery. In some centres neck dissection was reserved for postradiotherapy persistent disease.

During the 1940s and 50s surgery enjoyed the beginnings of its resurgence, and the efficacy and place of radical nodal clearance was confirmed by Martin (Martin et al 1951). Little changed until the 1960s when increasingly frequent surgery underlined the long-term morbidity of the operation, particularly when bilateral. Sub-total operations, such as supra-hyoid and supra-omohyoid (Hanley 1980) clearances, sprang up in an attempt to be anatomically correct but less ablative. Bocca recognized the importance of the loss of the accessory nerve and sternomastoid muscle in the morbidity of the neck dissection and designed and popularized his 'functional' neck dissection (Bocca 1975) which dealt with the crucial anterior triangle nodes reliably and decreased morbidity. Since then a mixture of variously named, modified or conservative operations have been described, some eponymous, along the same lines, almost one for every author on the subject.

The development of reconstruction

The excision of an intra-oral cancer produces, then as now, either an entirely intra-oral defect or full-thickness loss with potential salivary fistula. As stated above, intra-oral defects were closed directly, usually employing the residual tongue. If the mandible precluded easy closure then it was resected —which, as I have said, was in keeping with contemporary oncological thought. This had the effect of increasing deformity by unnecessary mandibular resection and increasing disability by tying down the remaining tongue. The technique is limited, so the temptation to compromise excision margins was always there. The results were poor.

The full-thickness defect was dealt with by closure of skin to mucosa. The ensuing and disabling salivary fistula was closed at interval with flaps from the neck and forehead surgically delayed and prepared during this interval (Blair et al 1941). There were two main conceptual problems. First, the long-term salivary fistula was intolerable, and indeed, life-threatening. The distortion of remaining anatomy engendered by the closure and subsequent shrinkage and scarring further disable the patient. With low local control rates then, clinical persistence often supervened and many patients either never completed reconstruction or had the whole of their clinically disease-free period used in repeated surgery punctuating constant drooling. It is small wonder that surgery was not popular.

In the 50s some groups in the USA started to apply the principles of reconstruction to primary repair. Edgerton (1951) used skin grafts in the buccal and tonsillar areas, difficult sites for this technique. Defects inside the mandibular arch were reconstructed using neck flaps in two stages (Zovickian 1958, DesPrez & Kiehn 1959). This was condemned by many because of the propensity for the neck to be involved in disease.

The real watershed occurred in the early 60s with the description of the powerful and reliable forehead flap (McGregor 1963) and the powerful, versatile if slightly less reliable deltopectoral flap (Bakamjian 1965). These two-stage techniques, which, with appropriate manipulation of the excisional defect, could be made to deal, alone or in combination, with both intra-oral and full-thickness defects. The speed with which these techniques were accepted and spread is a measure of the therapeutic void they filled, despite their disadvantages. Both these techniques are two-stage and they require temporary salivary fistula for 2 to 4 weeks. Retrospective analysis shows a disturbing rate of major secondary haemorrhage in this period. The forehead flap, being a facial donor site, further disfigured the patient. The delto-pectoral flap needed a prior delay procedure if loss of the critical part of the flap was to be avoided in 10% of patients. Even so, they may still have a minor secondary role in exceptional circumstances today.

The next important step was the description of the nasolabial flap on intra-oral reconstruction (Cohen & Edgerton 1971)—a technique, which, although two-stage, is so reliable and useful that it still holds its place today (see below). McGregor (1975) rationalized the technique and role of split-skin grafting in the mouth and, after some initial over-enthusiasm, it, too, has found its place in today's reparative spectrum (see below). This occurred in the early 1970s while the description and acceptance of the axial flap principle (McGregor & Morgan 1973) turned reconstructive surgery on its head and laid the ground for the development of today's large and versatile extra-regional flaps.

The musculocutaneous principle (Orticochea 1983), the fasciocutaneous principle (Ponten 1981) and the emergence of reliable microsurgical tissue transfer (Daniel & Taylor 1973, Macleod & Robinson 1982) happened rapidly in the period around 1980. These gave the head and neck surgeon a toolbox of reparative techniques which have allowed us to re-examine the role and nature of surgical excision and re-assess the quality of results attainable in the last decade.

EXCISIONAL TECHNIQUE – THE PRIMARY

Pathology

Squamous-cell carcinoma accounts for more than 90% of primary cancers in the oral cavity. The majority of the rest are represented by the spectrum of malignant salivary tumours. Rarer tumours, such as mucosal malignant melanomas, are seen. Extrinsic cancers not truly arising from the oral cavity—such as lymphomas, sarcomas and secondary malignancies – form a small part of the differential diagnosis.

Squamous-cell carcinoma

If a squamous-cell carcinoma is grown in tissue culture in a homogeneous gel then it takes the form of a regular expanding sphere. However, in vivo, although it will exhibit this propensity to expand in all directions, it will encounter different tissues and planes which will modify its behaviour (McGregor & McGregor 1986). Malignant lesions spread by local infiltration, lymphatic permeation, perineural permeation and embolic metastasis, either lymphatic or blood-borne (Willis 1973). It appears that, in these cancers, local, perineural and embolic lymphatic spread vastly predominate (McGregor & McGregor 1986). Excisional practice must therefore be designed with this in mind. A general

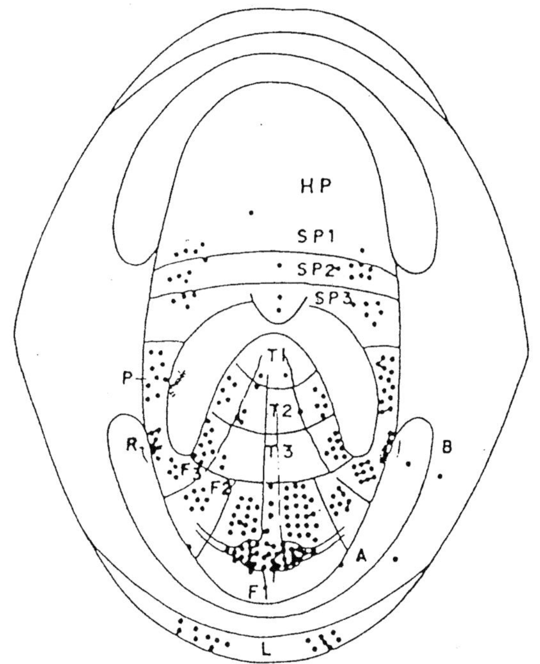

Fig. 9.1 Scattergram of subdivided sites of 222 asymptomatic lesions. T, ventrolateral tongue; F, floor of mouth; SP, soft palate proper; P, anterior pillar; R, lingual aspect of retromolar trigone. (1, 2, 3 refer to anterior, middle, and posterior thirds respectively). L, lip; A, alveolus; B, buccal; and HP, hard palate (by permission of Dr Mashberg and the Editor of Cancer).

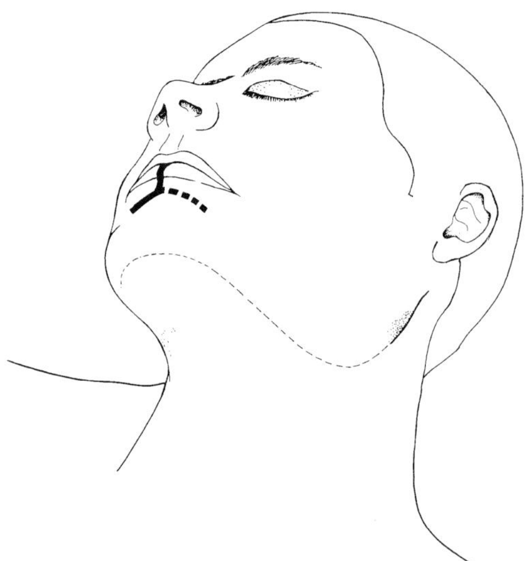

Fig. 9.2 The central lip split can be extended unilaterally or bilaterally to improve access to the oral cavity.

approach to rational decision making is shown in the flow chart Figure 9.5.

Surgical approach

Small, T1 and most T2, lesions in most sites can be accessed directly through the mouth. As the lesions get bigger and, in particular, cause a scirrhous response, producing fixity, some sort of access surgery is necessary to visualize the tumour well. Unless good access provides clear tumour visualization and allows ready tumour palpation then incomplete or misdirected excision will be performed needlessly, risking increased persistence or morbidity.

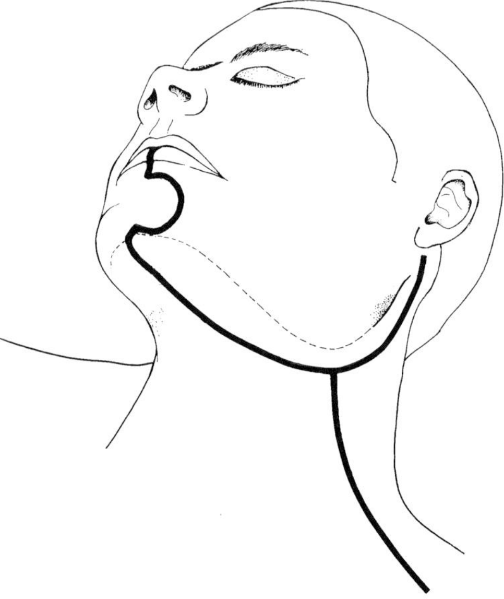

Fig. 9.3 A C-shaped incision skirting the chin and extending into a line continuous with the neck dissection gives access to the mandible, either to perform a parasagittal mandibular osteotomy or by incising the buccal mucosa to raise an innervated cheek flap.

Lesions in the floor and walls of the oral cavity predominate (Fig. 9.1) and can be approached through an extensile pattern of lower lip and, if necessary, mandible splitting incisions. The lip, if not being resected, should be split in the mid-line to the lower buccal sulcus to preserve sensation and motor control. The incision can be extended in either direction if the lesion is lateral, or both if central (Fig. 9.2). The cheek may be reflected by skirting the chin pad and extending the incision across the upper neck so that, by incision of the lower buccal sulcus, an innervated cheek flap is raised giving perfect access to the buccal surface and the outer surface of the mandible (Fig. 9.3). This upper neck incision can be used as part of the pattern of incisions for nodal dissection if indicated.

If the lesion lies within the mandibular arch then a parasagittal mandibular osteotomy carried out anterior to the mental foramen allows excellent exposure of lesions in the tongue, floor of mouth, retromolar trigone/faucial region and lateral soft palate. The precise nature and rationale of this approach are discussed in Chapter 3.

Lesions of the maxilla and hard palate which cannot be visualized through the mouth can be further exposed by some part of the modified Weber–Fergusson incision (Fig. 9.4) which, again, can be used on one or both sides and can be extended to expose the whole maxilla if need be (see Ch.19).

Tumour resection

The surgical approach should allow clear visualization and ready palpation of the tumour. In practice, the approach incision, where used, at some point blends into the excisional incision. It may not be possible to see and feel all excision margins initially but a start can be made and the access developed as the excision proceeds. It is important to stop the excision periodically and re-appraise the pattern of the disease volume and its excision in three dimensions so as to

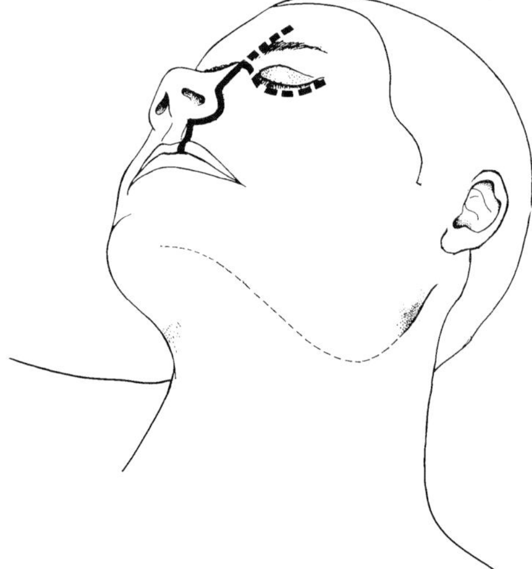

Fig. 9.4 The modified Weber–Fergusson incision can be extended either superiorly or laterally to improve access to the maxilla.

proceed in the most logical way as the precise extent and nature of the cancer is revealed.

Excision margins

The extent of the resection is determined by the tumour volume and the excision margins chosen. Absolute rules as to excision margins are difficult to define as this is the aspect of head and neck cancer surgery that requires most experience and is never mastered even by the most prolific surgeons. Some general observations can be made. It is important to take note of the extent of the tumour carefully. There is often coexisting adjacent early or in situ change which is rather overshadowed by the main tumour bulk. Loupe magnification will be valuable in examining surrounding mucosa as leaving in situ change at the margin invites early recurrence. However, in a field change situation this is sometimes inevitable.

The macroscopic pattern of the tumour should be considered. A clearly mobile exophytic tumour is easier to define and excise with modest excision margins than an ulcerated, indurated, deeply infiltrated, relatively fixed tumour. It should be recognized that the tumour mass is a combination of cancer growth and host inflammatory reaction. Some tumours, rarely, seem to excite very little host response and these are extremely difficult to predict and therefore excise cleanly. This is more difficult in the patient who has previously received external beam radiotherapy as the host response will have been modified by that treatment.

The parent tissue in which the tumour is infiltrating should be considered. As has been said, in vivo cancer will infiltrate preferentially along specific tissue planes and structures, in particular, the submucosa, muscle fibres and nerves. Where these planes have been involved the excision should be extended in an appropriate direction. Modifying the excision in the light of anatomy is also valuable. When an apparently normal and clear tissue plane is encountered this should be followed so long as this is not done so slavishly, compromising good clearance. The principle that the excised specimen should contain one normal structure on all surfaces holds some merit but will lead to needlessly ablative excision in some sites. In general terms, in solid tissue blocks an excision margin at least 1 cm (in practice the author's left index finger tip) of completely normal tissue is advised in loose mobile areas such as the floor of mouth or buccal surface. This margin should rise to 2 cm or more in infiltrative tongue lesions, particularly following radiation therapy.

Perineural spread

Nerves deserve special consideration. Squamous-cell carcinoma of the oral cavity has a particular propensity to perineural spread. This has led to disease persistence at apparently distant sites until it was fully recognized (Dodd et al 1970). The so-called pterygoid fossa recurrence is really persistence or perineural disease of the lingual or, more importantly, inferior dental nerves. If any nerve is encountered in the tumour volume it should be divided as far as technically possible from the tumour, preferably at the skull base. The surgical approach may need modification or extension to achieve this but it is worthwhile as pterygoid fossa recurrence and skull base extension can be virtually eliminated by this practice.

The management of the mandible

Consideration should also be given to the mandible as the majority of advanced tumours will abut and potentially involve or actually involve the bone. In fact, in the unirradiated patient, the mandible is a remarkably efficient tumour barrier. It can be conserved wholly or partially in the vast majority of patients. Patterns of spread, surgical approaches, methods of conservation and reconstruction are described in detail in Chapter 3 and should be examined alongside this description.

Incomplete excision and frozen section control

The overriding principle of surgical excision is that 'If in doubt, excise more widely'. This is because postoperative radiotherapy will not salvage a significant number of patients with histologically incomplete clearances despite evidence to show improved survival in patients undergoing postoperative radical radiotherapy when histological clearance is complete. The finding of incomplete excision should encourage re-excision if the patient be fit and the site and nature of the remaining disease can be defined. This is not always the case.

In the light of the foregoing it is tempting to rely on frozen section to avoid this difficult circumstance. It has been my experience that frozen section control is depressingly unhelpful in the large, complex, multi-tissue and multi-plane clearances dictated by this disease. The problem is simply that often the surgeon does not know which part of the excision to suspect as incomplete, and if he did he would excise it. Frozen section control may be of value in the event of there being specific concern about the involvement of tissue in a particular critical site, e.g. the divided end of a nerve.

Rarer pathologies

Malignancy of salivary origin

There is a spectrum of these tumours but, in general, the smaller the gland of origin the more likely the salivary tumour is to be malignant and the higher the grade of this malignancy. As only the minor mucosal and sublingual glands could be rationally included in the oral cavity then it can be seen that salivary tumours in the mouth are in most cases malignant, with a predominance of medium and high-grade muco-epidermoid and adenoid cystic carcinomas (Batsakis 1979).

In general, the comments made above apply to these tumours. The adenoid cystic cancer must be treated with great caution. This is because it characteristically excites very little host reaction and can therefore be underestimated as alluded to above. This absence of host response invalidates the concept of tissue barriers as the tumour can infiltrate silently through normally resistant structures, for instance the mandible can be freely invaded without radiological change. The most worrying aspect of these tumours is their aggressive perineural spread, often discontinuous, with skip lesions present, which makes clearance of all involved or potentially involved nerves to the absolute limits of practicality imperative.

Mucosal malignant melanoma

This is a very rare condition. As in other sites on the body this is an essentially superficial disease until it is very advanced and probably incurable. Early lesions should therefore be dealt with by clear marginal excision and stripping the lesion off the underlying tissue plane.

Sarcomata

A sarcoma impinging on the oral cavity should be managed as with sarcomata elsewhere. Combination therapy coordinating radiotherapy, chemotherapy and surgical excision needs to be individualized to the patient, site, extent and pathological grade of the cancer. In general, surgical excision will be valuable if complete anatomical clearance can be attained in a survivable, reconstructible way which includes all of every structure involved, including one adjacent normal structure. This is a considerable undertaking in some tumours in some sites. However, there is evidence to suggest that bone sarcomas of the facial skeleton, if managed in this way, carry a more favourable prognosis than those seen in long bones (Carron et al 1971).

EXCISIONAL TECHNIQUES – THE NODES

Intra-oral squamous-cell cancers commonly demonstrate embolic spread to the locoregional lymph nodes. This is along well recognized patterns and most frequently to the ipsilateral nodal group of first drainage but will progress to other groups in either side of the neck in the aggressive or neglected tumour. The frequency of, or risk of, nodal spread increases with primary tumour size – T stage (Myers 1991). The prognosis in oral cancer is more nearly related to nodal stage—N stage—than T stage (Kalnins et al 1977). This spread is embolic so there is no rational basis for ablating nodes in continuity with the primary as in the 'en bloc' principle; conversely, in continuity excision can be perfectly well used if convenient and helpful to the surgical approach.

Indications for neck dissection

Neck dissection is the therapeutic manoeuvre with the highest rate of local control of clinically apparent lymph node metastases (Whafif 1989). In general, all patients with clinically suspect lymphadenopathy in the presence of a primary oral cancer should have nodal clearance in combination with the management of their primary. If real doubt as to the nature of the disease in the neck exists because of concomitant pathology then fine-needle aspiration cytology may be helpful if it makes a positive alternate diagnosis. Usually, such doubts are unfounded and it is wise to treat the neck nodes. It should be remembered in the patient who refuses, or who is not fit for node surgery, that radiotherapy is nearly as effective in nodal control provided that no nodal mass exceeds 3 cm in diameter (Schneider et al 1975).

Prophylactic neck dissection is more contentious. Clearly, small primary disease (T1) need not have associated nodal clearance in the clinically negative neck as only a small proportion will go on to develop nodal disease. More advanced tumours present more of a problem as the rate of eventual nodal involvement is high, even in patients with clinically uninvolved necks on presentation. In advanced disease (T3 and T4) my personal preference is to combine primary and nodal resection in the first procedure because clinically positive nodes are very likely to develop and do so only a short time after primary resection, requiring re-admission to hospital which interrupts the patient's hoped-for recovery from primary management. It is recognized that this means some patients will have unnecessary neck dissection. The difficult line to draw is in relation to how advanced the primary need be before prophylactic nodal excision be performed. It is my view that the T2 stage presents a problem as it includes superficial mobile tumours and deeply infiltrative lesions penetrating nearly 4 cm which represents very advanced and dangerous disease. In this stage it is wise to decide on node management on an individual tumour basis.

Newer scanning techniques showing clinically undetectable disease have further complicated the issue as most data relate to palpable lymphadenopathy. However, it would take a brave surgeon and patient to ignore a positive CAT or MRI scan.

Most contentious of all is the situation where the surgical approach will include opening tissue planes in some part of the neck dissection field. There are those surgeons who feel they should dissect the neck if they are forced to enter it at any time. The evidence to support this view is weak. However, tumours of the mouth of sufficient size to warrant an extensive surgical approach—such as mandibular osteotomy—will usually need consideration for neck dissection as described above. In the small group of patients who need neck surgery as part of the primary resection or reconstruction with low risk of nodal disease an expectant policy on the neck is acceptable.

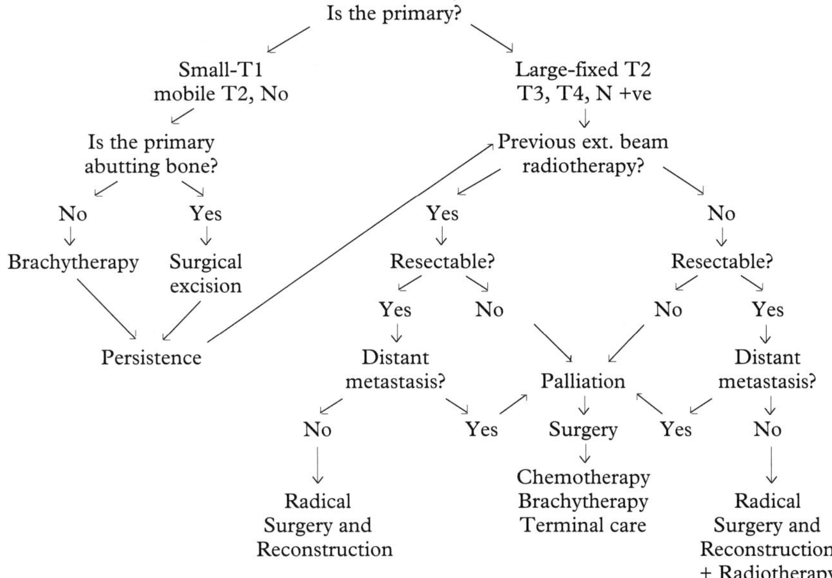

Fig. 9.5 A therapeutic algorhythm for intra-oral cancer.

Pattern of neck dissection

Choosing between a radical or modified (functional) neck dissection should be examined. Radical neck dissection as described by Crile (1906) and Martin et al (1951) is the gold standard in nodal resection in suppressing subsequent neck disease. It should still be employed for a neck with palpable disease greater than 3 cm, inferring extranodal rupture as the rate of persistence in the neck in such circumstances is significant. It is wise to irradiate the necks of such patients following the excision. Radical neck dissection is also recommended in patients developing neck disease following radiation therapy as patterns of spread in such patients are sometimes unpredictable.

If the likely node of first involvement is in or close to the posterior triangle of the neck then radical dissection is advised. As the primary presents further back in the mouth then radical dissection is appropriate. I would certainly choose the radical procedure for primaries in the retromolar trigone and faucal areas.

Functional neck dissection (Bocca 1975) should be employed when the primary is anterior, the nodes are small, or prophylactic dissection is being performed. This is an operation to be avoided by the occasional dissector of necks as it is more difficult than a radical procedure to perform and should be performed on a background of confident familiarity with the more traditional operation. With the advent of functional dissection, reducing cosmetic deformity and morbidity in relation to division of the accessory nerve, there is no longer any justification in performing less than a complete nodal clearance in the bilateral case. Operations such as suprahyoid dissections should disappear (Whafif 1989).

A flow chart of the decision-making process in relation to the management of neck disease is shown in Figure 9.6.

RECONSTRUCTIVE TECHNIQUES

What the surgeon removes from the mouth will determine the patient's chances of survival; what tissue the surgeon replaces it with, and how, will determine the level of function attained for the given volume of ablation dictated by the original tumour. The choice of reconstruction is all-important to the patient in his overall management plan. When considering the choice of reconstructive technique the surgeon should carefully assess the likely defect pre-operatively. He should be aiming to restore all uninvolved anatomy to the position in which it would have been before the cancer, allow the structures to move freely in the way they would have done, and match the missing tissue for surface area, volume and function as closely as possible. This is a pretty tall order and compromises will necessarily have to be accepted. The surgeon must also be prepared to change his

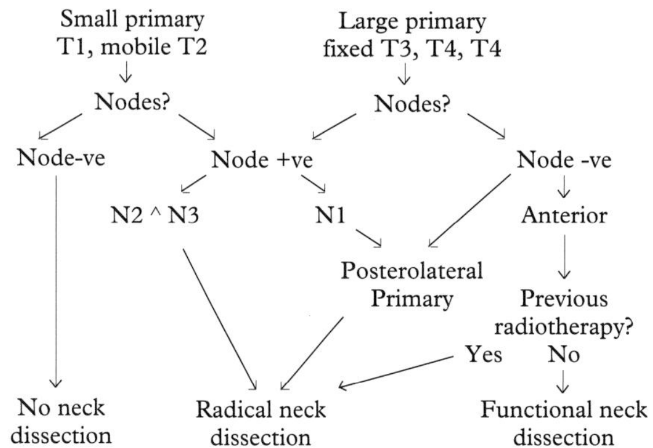

N. B. If neck dissection is not safe/acceptable use radiotherapy for N1 or less.

Fig. 9.6 A therapeutic algorhythm for management of ipsilateral neck disease in oral cancer.

plan intra-operatively as the true nature of the defect is revealed. However, as it is the revolution in reconstruction which has made surgical control of oral cancer a rational option, it behoves the surgeon to have a reconstructive repertoire which will allow him to try. The time should have passed when the only aim is to match the surface area of the reconstruction with the defect to attain healing alone.

The time, in terms of the patient's life, the reconstruction takes is important too. The number of stages required and the overall reliability of the technique chosen determines this. Time is important because only about half the patients presenting with oral cancer will survive the disease (depending on an individual surgeon's pattern of referral). The model of failed cancer therapy is that, after initial management, the patient experiences a variable apparently disease-free interval before symptomatic persistence supervenes, indicating the terminal phase. It is not good medicine to use up this disease-free interval by a protracted, multistage or repeatedly unreliable reconstructive plan. Furthermore, there is increasing evidence that, in advanced disease, postoperative radical radiotherapy confers survival advantage and that this is greatest if the radiation is given in the immediate postoperative period (Robertson et al 1985). It follows, therefore, that the technique chosen should not unduly delay commencement of radiation in these patients. It also follows that any reconstruction chosen in one of these patients should be robust enough to tolerate full-dose radiotherapy in the early postoperative period.

Assessment of the defect and reconstructive choice

When he considers a given defect, the surgeon should look to the qualities the normal tissue which would have been in the defect have. The surface area is most obvious but some thought should be given to the shape of the surface. In other words, a complex folded surface, such as is seen in the lateral floor of mouth, alveolar, retromolar trigone region should be replaced by a repair capable of being folded in an appropriate way. Volume is important. If the reconstructive volume is too low then the defect will collapse, drawing in surrounding structures to an abnormal position. A reconstruction that is too bulky will simply behave as a large foreign body in the mouth, which is surprisingly limited in size, particularly inside the mandibular arch.

The degree of elasticity required of the new surface is, in my view, of greatest importance. If the surrounding structures need to move then they must not be splinted by a rigid, fixed repair. The floor of the mouth, ventral surface of the tongue, faucial, soft palate, retromolar trigone and buccal surfaces require elasticity to avoid tethering of the tongue or trismus. The dorsum and edges of the tongue are an intermediate area requiring rather less elasticity, and the hard palate and both alveoli require a rigid immobile surface.

In general, higher volume defects in mobile elastic areas

need to be replaced by a flap closure, the choice of which depends on the area-to-volume ratio needed. The lower volume defects in more inelastic areas are suitable for skin grafting with the proviso that the walls of the defect are vascularized sufficiently to allow successful grafting. Defects which communicate with the neck, or which are full-thickness, including skin, will require flap closure, but these occur only in elastic areas and are of high volume. It is my view that full-thickness defects are usually better dealt with by using two separate flaps rather than by folding a single flap with a de-epithelialized segment.

Reconstructive options and their roles

No reconstruction

The simplest reconstructive decision is to decide not to excise the primary tumour at all. It is my personal preference to advocate implant radiotherapy (brachytherapy) for all T1 and low-volume T2 lesions in the mouth which do not abut bone and therefore risk osteoradionecrosis. The control rates are similar, and the results in terms of function superior. External beam radiotherapy is not an option as a proportion of cancers will recur. These persistent cancers need to be treated as advanced tumours and will require surgery and radiotherapy in combination, which is no longer available, if external radiotherapy has already been applied.

Direct closure

Defects that are less than 1.5 cm and, on occasion, larger in size, can be closed directly. It is clear from the discussion of excision margins that this will be applicable to only very small superficial lesions—perhaps on the dorsum of the tongue or buccal surface. Occasionally a small lesion on the alveolus, usually the lower, will require a relatively modest mucosal excision but significant alveolar rim excision. In such a situation, the loss of bone height allows direct closure without local advancement of tissue and extra tissue is not required.

Skin grafts

Quilting and fenestrating split-thickness skin grafts (McGregor 1975) made them a reliable one-stage method of attaining healing in some sites. They have been rather over-used by surgeons with a limited reconstructive range. They are useful, however, for superficial defects on the dorsum and edge of the tongue where they tend to take reliably and not to contract and distort the mouth. The graft possesses enough elasticity for tongue movement in that area. The technique should not be used, as it has been, in the floor of the mouth or the buccal surface. The tendency for grafts, which are not splinted, to contract will allow tethering in these elastic sites.

Skin grafts are by far the best form of reconstruction for

defects limited to the hard palate or the low partial maxillectomy defect produced by excision of an intra-oral cancer involving the maxilla from below. However I would no longer recommend skin graft and obturation as the first choice reconstruction of the total maxillectomy defect. (Ch.19).

Local flaps

The use of local flaps from within the mouth is not based on sound oncological or functional reconstructive principles and such flaps are included only to be condemned as a poor, dated and ill-informed practice.

Facial flaps

The nasolabial flap (Cohen & Edgerton 1971), used either unilaterally or bilaterally, is the only two-stage technique that should be considered part of mainstream reconstruction nowadays. This is because it is reliable, predictable and useful. Used singly, the flap will deal with defects up to 3 cm wide and 6 cm long in the buccal surface or anterolateral alveolus. The temptation to de-epithelialize the base of such a flap for buccal use to allow a one-stage reconstruction should be resisted as this renders the normally reliable flap much less so.

Bilateral flaps sewn edge-to-edge will very satisfactorily deal with a defect 5 cm by 5 cm in the mid-line of the anterior floor of the mouth. It is the reconstruction I would choose for a suitably sized defect in the floor of the mouth, ventral surface of the tongue or transalveolar region. It cannot be used to cover two of these regions without tethering the tongue as the reconstruction is not big enough. Nasolabial flaps are difficult to place inside the arch of the dentate mandible; this is partly because the floor of the mouth is such a long way down from the occlusal plane, limiting reach, and also because the pedicle is at risk of being bitten.

Although the nasolabial flap is a two-stage technique it is still tenable because it is so reliable. Flap loss at the first stage is very rare, and the pedicles can be divided and returned safely between 2 and 3 weeks afterwards, the patient having been at home in the intervening period. The second stage can be readily accomplished under local anaesthesia. True, there are temporary salivary fistulae but these are not in a dependent part of the mouth, and they cause little trouble. One of the positive features is the tendency for the reconstruction to suspend the tongue between stages, helping with the postresection airway (McGregor & Mcgregor 1986).

The forehead flap (Mcgregor 1963) is only of historical significance because of the deforming visible donor site and the unexplained but observed propensity for major haemorrhage between transposition and return.

Pedicled flaps from the trunk

The delto-pectoral flap (Bakamjian 1965) certainly changed head and neck reconstruction. Because of its poor reliability without surgical delay, and its relatively limited reach, it is rarely used today. It still has a place in resurfacing the neck and can be arranged as a one-stage transposition for this. The preferred technique for raising the pectoralis major flap (q.v.) surgically delays the deltopectoral flap so that it could be used as a fall back option, although I have not had cause to use this in 7 years.

The pectoralis major musculocutaneous flap (Ariyan 1979) is a most useful one-stage technique which can be used to reach the whole mouth. The reach can be extended, the pedicle bulk reduced and the donor morbidity limited by raising it as a true island flap (Palmer & Batchelor 1990). Enormous flaps can be raised but these are not applicable to the mouth. The size of flap useful in the mouth will allow primary closure of the donor site. The limitation of this flap is the bulk and stiffness necessarily conferred by its musculocutaneous composition. It should only be chosen for defects of appropriately high volume. It is my preferred flap in high-volume tongue defects and defects including the mandible where the mandible is not being replaced. The indication for this flap increase in the very thin male patient when it becomes a rational alternative to the fasciocutaneous free flaps (q.v.). Conversely, the obese patient may preclude the use of any musculocutaneous flaps and require the thinner free flaps.

Analysis of my own consecutive series shows this flap to be completely reliable, although occasionally subject to minor edge necrosis of no therapeutic importance. However, when this patient group was compared to a matched group of patients who had limb flap donor sites, clinically important chest infection was significantly more common following the chest donor site. This may be because of pain causing atelectasis. It may be due to a tendency to favour a pedicled flap over a free flap in patients with poorer cardiopulmonary reserve, although this was not demonstrable on scoring the patients.

The latissimus dorsi (Olivari 1976, Quillen et al 1978) and trapezius (Bertotti 1980) musculocutaneous flaps are one-stage alternatives popular with some. I do not use the former in the mouth because it does not confer specific advantages over the pectoralis major flap and requires dissection of the axilla to raise. Quite extensive dissection is required before it will match the anterior reach of the pectoralis major but this is possible. It is not necessary to turn the patient on his side to raise the flap. I tend to reserve the flap for larger defects which may include some part of the mouth.

The lateral trapezius flap is interesting because it has the ability to provide bone, but other than that it has no features to particularly commend its use. The arc of rotation can be limited by variable anatomy of the venous drainage. The fact that the pedicle needs to be dissected from the lower neck is thought by some potentially to compromise clean neck dissection. The patient will need to be turned partially or repositioned from supine to raise the flap. Raising the flap requires division of the accessory nerve which increases the shoulder morbidity considerably in a patient suitable for a functional neck dissection. In my limited experience with this flap it has not proved as reliable as the two already mentioned.

Free flaps

There are some properties of the free flap in general which are attractive when choosing an intra-oral reconstruction. The variability of design is almost infinite allowing a much better match of reconstruction to the defect. The donor site is separated from the resection with the potential for synchronous surgery shortening the procedure. They are all one-stage and, in expert hands, as reliable and robust as any alternative already mentioned.

Very few patients are unsuitable for microsurgical transfer. In general, if the patient is fit for the tumour resection they will tolerate the reconstruction. Very severe generalized arteriopathy is a relative contraindication but a more local problem can be overcome. In particular, in our own series of 500 consecutive flaps previous radiotherapy had no bearing on flap survival. Jehovah's Witnesses will not accept free transfer as the act of disconnection renders the flap 'not self' in their creed.

Free flaps do demand microsurgical expertise, patient management skills and appropriate anaesthetic technique to make them reliable. An appropriate level of equipment in monitoring, instrumentation and magnification is a prerequisite as is a high-care postoperative unit staffed with suitably experienced personnel. These things are, in my view, necessities for any head and neck service these days anyway. It is likely that the occasional micro-surgeon will experience an unacceptably high failure rate and it is better to avoid free flaps than do them rarely.

The radial forearm fasciocutaneous flap (Soutar et al 1983) is the workhorse of intra-oral flap reconstruction in my practice for moderate and advanced disease. It provides thin, if necessary, flexible, elastic tissue which can be increased in area without major increase in volume. Conversely, by moving the donor site proximally in the forearm it is possible to produce the bulk necessary for most defects except those left by major tongue resection. The pedicle is very long, very reliable anatomically and contains vessels of good calibre which match those in the neck.

The radial flap is also a source of vascularized bone strut and is therefore particularly applicable to compound defects, including mandibular segments (Ch. 5). In terms of surface cover it is excellent in the floor of mouth, ventral and lateral tongue, retromolar trigone, faucial and lateral pharyngeal, palatal and buccal regions. This covers almost the whole mouth apart from the body of the tongue and the maxilla.

The flap may be used as a fascia-only flap which can be skin grafted where a very low volume stable flap is required, as in hard palate fistulae (Batchelor & Palmer 1990).

Some surgeons object to the donor site scarring produced by the radial flap. It is possible to substitute the lateral arm flap (Katsaros et al 1984) in many cases. The pedicle which, in the original description, is of limited length can be extended by approaching it though an additional triceps splitting counter incision usually associated with exploration of the radial nerve (Henry 1973). The lateral arm flap is rarely as thin as the radial, the vessels are smaller and occasionally absent in their distal course.

Volume defects can be filled by musculocutaneous free flaps such as the rectus abdominis flap, but this seems illogical when good reliable pedicle flaps could be perfectly substituted.

The free jejunal transfer is used by some to resurface the mouth by opening the transferred gut along the antemesenteric border. It is particularly thin, flexible and elastic. A long pedicle of good vessel size can be developed. However, the donor site requires laparotomy and small-bowel anastomosis which seems an unnecessary risk when safer good alternatives exist and should be positively avoided in the patient who has a chequered history of abdominal surgery or poor respiratory reserve.

PROBLEMS AND COMPLICATIONS

General

The airway is at risk in the surgical management of oral cancer. Swelling, destabilization of the tongue, bleeding into the airway or closed haematoma all put the airway at risk. As resections get more major and reconstructions get more complex, the surgeon should have a very low threshold for performing tracheostomy. Many will argue that nasotracheal intubation is as good. It is my preference to use tracheostomy for two reasons. Should a patient suffer displacement of an endotracheal tube postoperatively then replacement may be very challenging, even for the most experienced anaesthetist. A tracheostomy provides time in the early postoperative period with an alert cooperative patient to make the transition to a normal airway.

Perioperative nutrition and hydration is also disrupted by poor oral function. Mouth rest and hygiene make a period without food prudent. This can be managed by naso-gastric feeding. The fine bore tubes available cause few symptoms but require to be swallowed—so need to be in place preoperatively and remain through the procedure. If a very prolonged period of tube feeding is anticipated for any reason then it is useful and easy to place a percutaneous transpharyngeal tube at the time of neck dissection as these cause no symptoms and are cosmetically most acceptable. A dietitian will be of help, particularly in the difficult time when a patient is making the transition back to oral feeding when they are so sensitive to the consistency and volume of food.

Infection was the major enemy of head and neck surgeons historically. It no longer presents serious risk, provided that prophylactic antibiotics are used and include a specific drug such as metronidazole, to deal with anaerobes (Sweeney et al 1984).

A head and neck resection is a hammer blow to a patient's well-being, particularly following the new knowledge that he has a major cancer. This can be made much easier for the patients if there is specialist help in the form of a counsellor/psychologist to deal with issues of consent, control, self-image and mortality. A group of patients who have had the spectrum of procedures can help considerably with patient counselling. A social worker to deal with the practicalities is also a great help.

Speech will be rendered less intelligible to a greater or lesser degree either peri-operatively or permanently. A specialist speech therapist with experience in this area is essential. It is important for the speech therapist to be involved before the operation. The choice of reconstruction is important as it is unusual for a patient to be rendered unintelligible by surgery provided that the tongue remnant is mobile, innervated and remains in its normal position at rest.

Problems related to access

The mandibular osteotomy to provide access is a source of difficulty, particularly in the irradiated case or the patient who receives early postoperative radiotherapy. Non-union of the mandible can be quite symptomatic if it is significantly mobile. The fixation is all important. My preference is for rigid internal mini-plate fixation. This should be with titanium plates and be placed without striping of the periosteum, both of which reduce osteo-radio-necrosis of the mandible. Should this or infection occur the plate should be removed and all dead bone excised. If it occurs at time interval then it is essential to look for and close the fistula into the mouth and biopsy the area to rule out persistence.

Problems related to excision

In the oral cavity, with such good access available or attainable, it is possible to avoid unnecessary damage to normal structures. The problems and morbidity are therefore predetermined by the pattern of disease and the excision dictated. It must be remembered that the worst problem in the surgical management of oral cancer is incomplete excision. The surgeon *must not compromise complete excision to conserve function.*

The tongue is a structure supplied by a pair of end arteries, the lingual arteries. If both are damaged in the resection, usually of mid-line floor of the mouth tumour, then the tip of the tongue will often, but not always, necrose. If this be a risk then it is better to await the necrosis and treat this conservatively with continued antibiotics until separation occurs as this allows survival of the maximum amount of tongue; spontaneous healing follows and fistulation is rare.

Bilateral neck dissection will cause considerable swelling. This is reduced but not abolished by leaving one or both internal jugular veins intact during the dissection. This is entirely possible even with a radical pattern neck dissection. It is my habit to dissect the more involved side first as if that jugular is spared then the second side is more relaxed, and, if not, particular attention can be paid to jugular preservation. Even so considerable facial swelling will occur in a proportion of patients. To help with this I administer a single large dose of steroid. However I am not sure how effective or important this is.

The radical neck dissection causes considerable long-term morbidity. The shoulder posture changes and arm elevation is limited. Patients complain of nagging discomfort in the arm. This can frequently be improved with physiotherapy to the shoulder girdle. Neuroma pain, with trigger points, in relation to the cut cervical plexus roots, is not uncommon and is a difficult problem. Referral to a specialist pain service will be valuable. This problem does not occur in the functional dissection presumably because severed nerves are isolated from the skin by sternomastoid.

Problems related to reconstruction

It is essential to have agreed with the patient the freedom to change the reconstructive plan during the procedure. If not, then he may be committed to an inadequate reconstruction. It is essential to be able constantly to reappraise the surgical plan during the procedure.

Loss of the reconstruction either partial or total will occur in a small group of patients. First, it should be noted that this is not the disaster one imagines. Anti-anaerobe antibiotics give the surgeon time to allow the patient to recover from the primary operation and take stock of the defect with its attendant loss of function. Small area losses will heal by secondary intent. Larger losses, usually of complete flaps, will require to be reconstructed but not immediately if the patient is unfit. Provided the external skin is healthy then fistulation is rare. In general, the right thing to do is replace the lost flap with the same or as nearly the same flap as is possible.

Microsurgical failure requires special mention as it results in early total reconstructive loss which may be reversible. Most flaps that fail do not do so because of poor microsurgical technique but because of poor patient management or poor operative design. The patient needs to be kept warm, sedated, pain-free, hypervolaemic and with a hyperdynamic peripheral circulation in the all-important postoperative period. Flaps should be observed by expert staff every 15 minutes for circulatory difficulty. If doubt exists then surgical exploration not medical manipulation is advised. In our series, 8% of the flaps were explored for incipient failure with only 3% failing as 5% were salvaged.

In the event of irretrievable vascular thrombosis the flap must be discarded and another reconstruction performed. Do not be afraid to repeat the free flap from the contralateral donor site as, if it was the correct choice of repair the first time, then it still will be as the defect has not changed.

The exposed carotid, being washed with saliva, is also worth special attention. In the unirradiated unrepaired vessel then this need not cause undue concern as blow-out is not a risk (Marchetta et al 1967). Further repair can proceed as necessary. Conversely, if the carotid has been irradiated or subject to surgical damage or repair then its exposure should be dealt with as a matter of urgency by further flap cover to prevent blow-out. In all this it must be remembered that exposure in the mouth and contact with saliva are just as, if not more, dangerous than the more obvious external exposure of the vessel.

Most transferred flaps become very swollen and stiff regardless of their ultimate characteristics and so oral function will take months to recover. Continued surveillance and rehabilitative help will be required from both the speech therapist and the dietitian during this period — which is made worse and extended by postoperative radiotherapy.

Postoperative radiotherapy itself will not specifically cause difficulties with modern reconstructions, especially free flaps. Patients will, of course, suffer the usual spectrum of radiation reactions, some major, but this is not related to the excision or reconstructive pattern.

Donor site morbidity

This is often a neglected area. In fact, donor site problems are really uncommon as a symptomatic feature. The scars from the nasolabial flaps are often not as good as one would like usually at the area of re-inset after division. This may be due to the inflammation caused by the salivary fistula. I have found that interval revision often produces pleasing improvement.

The radial flap donor site has been criticized by many and has produced a large literature, but critical examination of the donor site shows low morbidity (Bardsley et al 1990). It can be reduced further by direct closure (Elliot et al 1988) or, in the event of skin graft being used, complete take can be assured by meshing the graft (Davison et al 1986), covering the flexor carpi radialis tendon with muscle (Fenton & Roberts 1985) and appropriate splintage (McGregor 1987). With these measures, loss of this graft is minor and uncommon. Occasionally, painful neuromata on the proximal edge of the graft in relation to the radial nerve can be a troublesome and difficult-to-treat problem.

FUTURE DEVELOPMENTS

Management

There are solid retrospective data to demonstrate that a combination of surgery and radiotherapy assembled in quick succession improve local control rates in oral cancer (Robertson et al 1985). This has been made rationally possible only by the improvements in reconstructive technique. The improvement is now being studied prospectively by randomized trial.

There are changes in radiotherapy techniques which are also being studied prospectively. Continuous, hyperfractionated, accelerated, radiotherapy (CHART), a technique of external beam radiotherapy where three small fractions are given each day, without rest days to shorten the overall treatment span, again looks promising enough to justify randomized trial. This may be included in combination therapy in the future to effect.

Brachytherapy can be used in combination with surgical excision also by placing the implant tubes at the time of surgery. The tubes can be placed directly on or in the tissue at risk (Vikram et al 1985). This has been used for palliative resections principally but may develop a more general application.

Chemotherapy has not found a clearly useful or defined role as yet despite extensive investigation. There is early evidence that combinations of radiotherapy and chemotherapy may be beneficial in terms of complete remission rates and possibly survival. The evidence for this is not yet strong, and chemotherapy remains in a doubtful role in solid tumours of the head and neck.

Reconstruction

It is unlikely that there will be enormous changes in reconstruction over the next few years simply because we have just experienced a two-decade reconstructive revolution. The next period is, logically, one in which we will refine and more suitably apply the new techniques. It behoves us constantly to question the established methods of treatment for a given tumour site and to apply the new technology in any way that suggests itself.

Tumour behaviour

The pattern of disease in the mouth is changing. Ratios of affected males to females vary widely from country to country, but in almost all, sexual difference is diminishing. Patterns of smoking change, and the proportion of tumours in non-smokers rises. It remains to be seen whether this indicates a genuine change in disease or behaviour but it seems likely as younger patients without predisposing factors appear to do badly as a group.

As rates of local control rise we are seeing two things emerge. There is increasing concern that systemic metastasis will be a more major problem. Crile (1906) described this as potentially affecting a mere 1% of patients whereas more recent and complete post-mortem studies show 39% of patients to have disseminated disease, frequently occult

(Willis 1930). It is clear that, historically, poor local control rates in advanced disease have masked the clinical impact of metastasis. If we are in any way successful in improving local control then the potential problem of central spread is obvious. Furthermore, as more people survive one oral cancer the rate of second primary tumours or other smoking-related cancers will increase in this group. Close surveillance is necessary but, more importantly, we must look for ways of modifying the patient's biology to reduce the chance of new disease in such an at-risk population.

REFERENCES

Ariyan S 1979 The pectoralis major myocutaneous flap. Plastic and Reconstructive Surgery 63: 73

Bakamjian V Y 1965 A two stage method for pharyngoesophageal reconstruction with a primary pectoral skin flap. Plastic and Reconstructive Surgery 36: 173

Bardsley A F, Soutar D S, Elliot D, Batchelor A G 1990 Reducing morbidity in the radial flap donor site. Plastic and Reconstructive Surgery 86: 287

Batchelor A G, Palmer J P 1990 A novel method of closing a palatal fistula: the free fascial flap. British Journal of Plastic Surgery 43: 354

Batsakis J G 1979 Tumours of the head and neck, 2nd edn. Williams & Wilkins, Baltimore, p78

Bertotti J A 1980 Trapezius musculo-cutaneous island flap repair of major head and neck cancer. Plastic and Reconstructive Surgery 65: 16

Blair V P, Moore S, Byars L T 1941 Cancer of the face and mouth. Henry Kimpton, London

Bocca E 1975 Conservative neck dissection. Laryngoscope 85: 1511

Caron A S, Hadju S I, Strong E J 1971 Osteogenic sarcoma of the facial and cranial bones; a review of 43 cases. American Journal of Surgery 122: 719

Carroll W W 1952 Combined neck and jaw resection for intra-oral carcinoma. Surgery, Gynecology and Obstetrics 94: 1

Cohen I K, Edgerton M T 1971 Transbuccal flap for reconstruction of the floor of mouth. Plastic and Reconstructive Surgery 48: 8

Crile G 1906 Excision of cancer of the head and neck; with special reference to the plan of dissection based on 132 operations. Journal of the American Medical Association 47: 1780

Daniel R K, Taylor G I 1973 Distant transfer of an island flap by microvascular anastomosis. Plastic and Reconstructive Surgery 52: 111

Davison P M, Batchelor A G, Lewis-Smith P 1986 The properties and uses of non-expanded machine meshed skin grafts. British Journal of Plastic Surgery 39: 462

DesPrez J D, Kiehn C L 1959 Methods of reconstruction of the anterior oral cavity and mandible for malignancy. Plastic and Reconstructive Surgery 23: 238

Dodd G D, Dolan P A, Ballantyne A J, Ibanez M L, Chan P 1970 The dissemination of tumours of the head and neck via the cranial nerves. Radiological Clinics of North America 8: 445

Edgerton M T, 1951 Replacement of lining to oral cavity following surgery. Cancer 4: 110

Elliot D, Bardley A F, Batchelor A G, Soutar D S 1988 Direct closure of the radial flap donor site. British Journal of Plastic Surgery 41: 358

Ewing M R 1954 Surgical treatment of oral cancer. British Journal of Plastic Surgery 7: 108

Fenton O M, Roberts J O 1985 Improving the donor site of the radial forearm flap. British Journal of Plastic Surgery 38: 504

Hanley D J 1980 Supraomohyoid neck dissection. British Journal of Plastic Surgery 33: 136

Henry A K 1973 Extensile exposure. Churchill Livingstone, London, p18

Kalnins I K, Leonard A G, Sako K 1977 Correlation between prognosis and degree of lymph node involvement in carcinoma of the oral cavity. American Journal of Surgery 134: 450

Katsaros J, Shusterman M, Beppu M, Bannis J C, Ackland R D 1984 The lateral arm flap: anatomy and clinical applications. Annals of Plastic Surgery 12: 489

McGregor I A 1963 The temporal flap in intra-oral cancer. British Journal of Plastic Surgery 16: 318

McGregor A D 1987 The free radial forearm flap: the management of the secondary defect. British Journal of Plastic Surgery 40: 83

McGregor I A 1975 'Quilted' skin grafting in the mouth. British Journal of Plastic Surgery 28: 100

McGregor I A 1993 The pursuit of function and cosmesis in managing oral cancer. British Journal of Plastic Surgery 46: 22

McGregor A D, McDonald D G 1989 Patterns of spread of squamous cell carcinoma within the mandible. Head and Neck Surgery 11: 457

McGregor I A, Mcgregor F M 1986 Cancer of the face and mouth. Churchill Livingstone, London, pp 399, 452

McGregor I A, Morgan R G 1973 Axial and random pattern flap. British Journal of Plastic Surgery 26: 202

MacLeod A M, Robinson D W 1982 Reconstruction of defects involving the mandible and floor of mouth by free osteocutaneous flaps derived from the foot. British Journal of Plastic Surgery 35: 239

Marchetta F C, Sako K, Maxwell W 1967 Complications after radical head and neck surgery performed through previously irradiated tissues. American Journal of Surgery 114: 835

Martin H, Del Valle B, Ehrlich H, Cahan W G 1951 Neck dissection. Cancer 4: 441

Mashberg A, Meyers H 1976 Anatomical site and size of 222 early asymptomatic oral squamous carcinomas. Cancer 37: 2149

Myers E M 1991 Head and neck oncology. Little, Brown & Co., Boston, p 120

Olivari N, 1976 The latissimus flap. British Journal of Plastic Surgery 29: 126

Orticochea M 1983 The history of the discovery of the musculo-cutaneous flap method as a universal and immediate substitute for the method of delay. British Journal of Plastic Surgery 36: 524

Palmer J P, Batchelor A G 1990 The pectoralis major musculocutaneous true island flap. Plastic and Reconstructive Surgery 80: 365

Ponten B 1981 The facsiocutaneous flap: its use in soft tissue defects of the lower leg. British Journal of Plastic Surgery 34: 215

Quillen C G, Shearin J C, Georgiade N C 1978 Use of the latissimus dorsi myocutaneous flap for reconstruction in the head and neck area. Plastic and Reconstructive Surgery 62: 113

Robertson A G, McGregor I A, Flatman G E, Soutar D S, Boyle P 1985 The role of radical surgery and postoperative radiotherapy in the management of intra-oral carcinoma. British Journal of Plastic Surgery 38: 314

Schneider J J, Fletcher G H, Barkley H J Jr 1975 Control by irradiation alone of nonfixed clinically positive lymph nodes from squamous cell carcinoma of the oral cavity, oro-pharynx, supraglottic larynx and hypopharynx. American Journal of Radiotherapy 123: 42

Soutar D S, Scheker L R., Tanner N S B, McGregor I A 1983 The radial forearm flap: a versatile method of intra-oral reconstruction. British Journal of Plastic Surgery 36: 1

Steckler R M, Edgerton M T, Gogel W 1974 'Andy Gump'. American Journal of Surgery 138: 545

Sweeney G, Watson J D, McGregor I A, Sleigh J D 1984 Successful prophylaxis with tinidazole of infection after major head and neck surgery for malignant disease. British Journal of Plastic Surgery 37: 35

Vikram B, Strong E W, Shah J P 1985 Intraoperative radiotherapy in patients with recurrent head and neck cancer. American Journal of Surgery 150: 485

Whafif R H 1989 Thirty year experience with 457 radical neck dissections in cancer of the mouth, pharynx and larynx. American Journal of Surgery 158: 303

Willis R A 1930 Epidermoid carcinoma of the head and neck, with special reference to metastasis. Journal of Pathology and Bacteriology 33: 501

Willis R A 1973 The spread of tumours in the human body, 3rd edn. Butterworth, London

Zovickian A 1958 Preservation of facial contour after resection of the mandible using cervical skin flaps. Plastic and Reconstructive Surgery 21: 433

10. Total glossectomy with laryngeal preservation

Rammohan Tiwari

INTRODUCTION AND HISTORICAL REVIEW

The incidence of cancer of the tongue varies significantly in different parts of the world (Ali et al 1986, Jayant & Notani 1991). Because of its importance in the functions of speech and swallowing, surgical interventions have traditionally been fraught with the problem of rehabilitation (Terz et al 1973, Harrison 1983). Earlier attempts at surgical ablation for larger tumours were therefore decried (Cade & Lee 1957). The outlook for long-term survival was also poor. A decade later, significant improvement in survival was reported in a large series (Harrold 1967). In the series, larynx was preserved in nearly 50% of cases. The 5-year survival was 21%, and nearly three-fourths of the survivors returned to full-time work. This was undoubtedly a significant achievement at the time. Soon after, Donaldson reported on a small personal series of total glossectomy with laryngeal preservation and with marked improvement in survival (Donaldson et al 1968). He pointed out the importance of preservation of the superior laryngeal nerve in preventing aspiration. Nearly 50% of his patients achieved speech and were able to swallow liquids. Similar reports of larger series appeared from India (Kothary et al 1974, Pradhan et al 1980).

Although radiotherapy was used initially in the treatment of large tongue cancer its use declined in the fifties (Harrold 1967). Radiotherapy techniques have improved in the meantime, and the increased use of external radiotherapy in combination with brachytherapy has since been reported (Lusinchi et al 1989, Jaulerry et al 1991). These were important studies which showed the limitation of radiotherapy as a single-modality therapy in larger tumours. The long-term survival remained poor despite high doses of radiation. Quality of life was not mentioned. Meanwhile, it had been observed that single-modality treatment of larger tumours in general was not showing any improvements in results. Consequently, combination in the form of surgery and radiotherapy was advocated (Geofert et al 1975, Hamberger et al 1976, Marcus et al 1979, Vikram et al 1980).Controversies as to which modality should be

used first did erupt, but died down with the publication of studies comparing results with pre- and postoperative radiotherapy and showing superior results with the latter (van den Brouck et al 1979). Our own experience at the Free University Hospital in Amsterdam with radiotherapy and brachytherapy for carcinoma of the base of the tongue for nearly a decade was disappointing and led to the policy of treating these lesions with a combination of surgery and radiotherapy (Tiwari et al 1989). Radiotherapy with salvage surgery is however still used in some centres. Recent studies on the efficacy of postoperative radiotherapy suggest that tongue cancer responds poorly to postoperative radiation (Zelefsky et al 1990). It has long been realized that management of the larynx is a key factor in the therapy of larger tumours of the tongue and tongue base (Whicker et al 1972). Edgerton & McKee first drew attention to the 'balanced suspension' of the normal larynx, and although their work was not directed to total glossectomy, they had laid the basis for laryngeal suspension which was to have a significant effect on the future of this surgery (Edgerton & McKee 1959).

Swallowing without aspiration after complete resection of the hyomandibular complex, utilizing a simple technique for laryngeal suspension, was reported by Jabaley & Hoopes (1969). This has since been reported in relation to various other head and neck surgical procedures, and its application after segmental mandibular resection has also been described (Calcaterra 1971, Goode 1976, Hillel & Goode 1983). The development of modern imaging techniques has been a significant step in the evaluation of these cancers and has helped in selecting patients whose larynx can be preserved (Larsson et al 1987, Einspieler et al 1991).

In the last decade reports have appeared from different parts of the world which indicated that, with good preoperative evaluation and selection of cases, total glossectomy in combination with radiotherapy plays a significant role in the treatment of larger cancers of the tongue–tongue base and the quality of life can be preserved (Pradhan et al 1980, Effron et al 1981, Biller et al 1983, Sultan & Coleman 1989, Tiwari et al 1989, Weber et al 1991).

INDICATIONS

Five categories of patient may be considered for total glossectomy. These include:

1. patients with large primary tumours (T3–T4) with or without neck node metastases
2. recurrence after initial radiotherapy and/or chemotherapy
3. recurrence following earlier microscopic radical excision and radiotherapy
4. double primary tumours
5. second or third primary tumours.

PRETHERAPEUTIC EVALUATION

Total glossectomy includes the sacrifice of the mobile tongue as well as the base of the tongue with preservation of the vallecular mucous membrane. A careful preoperative assessment is essential to delineate the exact extent of the disease. The natural tendency for the disease is to spread caudally to the vallecula and from there to the pre-epiglottic space. It can also spread caudally via the hyoglossus muscle to the hyoid.

Spread laterally and anteriorly is to the floor of the mouth and eventually to the periosteum on the inner surface of the mandible. Further posteriorly, the tumour tends to spread via the tonsillolingual sulcus to the periosteum at the angle of the mandible and more posteriorly to the tonsil and the lateral pharyngeal wall.

Examination under anaesthetic and careful palpation is essential to determine the fixity to the hyoid, the mandible and submucosal spread. Soft-tissue extension is clearly demonstrated on magnetic resonance imaging, by using T1 SE images (Fig. 10.1). MRI also provides sagittal views which are not obtained by other imaging techniques and visualizes the caudal extension more clearly. CT scans are also helpful, but are not needed if MRI is utilized. Occasionally, the examiner is unable to reach the vallecula with his fingers, because of its distance, but more often because of the tumour. Imaging, especially MRI, is then invaluable. Imaging also visualizes suspicious lymph nodes which may not be palpable (Stevens et al 1985, Feinmesser et al 1987, van den Brekel et al 1990). CT scanning here is equally informative (Larsson et al 1987).

A pretherapeutic evaluation must be followed by a discussion of the results with the patient and his/her family and an assessment of his/her motivation. A visit by a previously operated and rehabilitated patient helps in answering the many questions that patients have and restores his/her confidence in the surgical team. The nursing staff should be included in this discussion.

At the end of this evaluation a clear picture emerges as to whether the patient is a suitable candidate for total glossectomy. One is also informed whether it would be possible to save a part of the tongue and whether this is likely

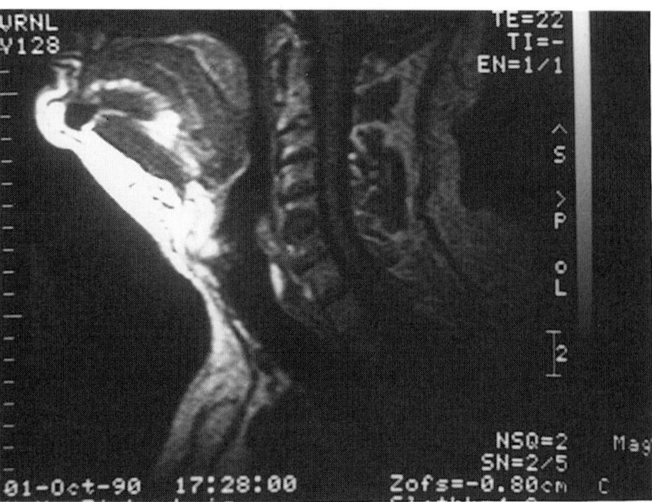

Fig. 10.1 Magnetic resonance imaging showing tumour on the dorsum of the tongue–tongue base. The epiglottis and valleculae were free. This was a second primary tumour. The patient is alive and well 3 years after total glossectomy.

to be viable and functional. This is a question which is foremost in the mind of the patient and the surgeon alike. It is stated that if more than half of the organ is involved then a total glossectomy should be performed (Donaldson et al 1968). The question that needs to be answered is whether the lingual artery and the hypoglossal nerve can be preserved on the 'uninvolved side' without compromise of the surgical margins. There are two factors which influence this decision. One is the course of the lingual artery itself which comes close to the median line at the base of the tongue and is thus vulnerable. Secondly, cancers of the tongue and tongue base tend to have satellite metastases within the organ and show a strong tendency to perivascular and perineural spread. This necessitates a wider margin of excision than is normally the case at other localization of squamous carcinoma. There are occasions when a final answer to the question of preservation may have to be answered only by exploring the contralateral lingual artery and hypoglossal nerve as the first surgical step in the operation. The other question is whether total glossectomy must also include the larynx or the floor of mouth or the lateral pharyngeal wall, the tonsil and a part of the mandible. Each additional excision inflicts physical defects. It is observed that when the cancer involves the larynx, the older group of patients tend not to consent to surgery, while the relatively younger patients are keen on preserving a part of the tongue. This is important, for while extensions elsewhere can be excised and reconstructed within reasonable limits the loss of larynx is a serious handicap when combined with total glossectomy. Partial excisions of the larynx with total glossectomy have been sporadically reported, but the number is small, the follow-up short, and complications not uncommon (Weisberger & Lingeman 1983).

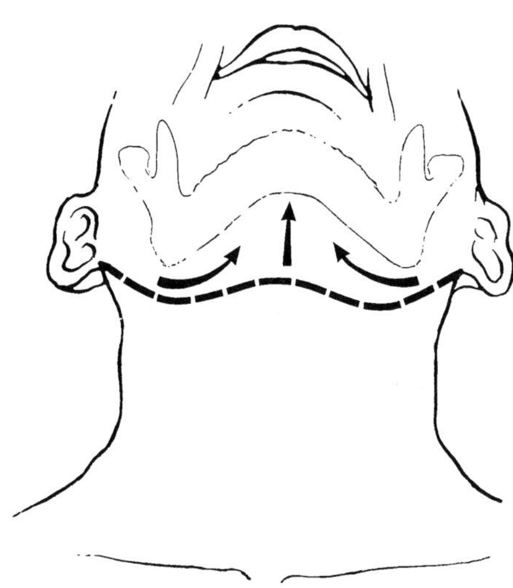

Fig. 10.2   Incision for preparation of a visor flap.

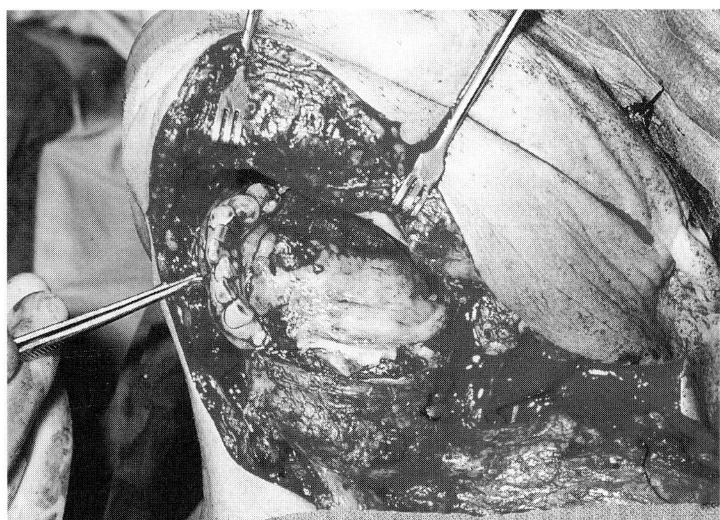

Fig. 10.3   Total glossectomy with marginal mandibular resection. The specimen is being delivered into the neck while the intact mandible is retracted upwards. (See also colour plate section)

EXCISION TECHNIQUES

Total glossectomy combined with total laryngectomy entails an extension of the total laryngectomy incisions along the lateral floor of the mouth on either side. On the other hand, laryngeal preservation with total glossectomy requires judgement and precision. Several surgical approaches are available for this purpose. Although the choice of the approach depends to some extent on the presence or absence of extension of the disease to the floor of the mouth or the tonsillar region, there are a few general principles worthy of mention. Whenever possible, the integrity of the lower lips should be preserved. If the nerve supply to the lower lip can be preserved then it is still better to keep the lips intact. This helps the patient later to learn to articulate. Preservation of the integrity of the mandible, though desirable, is not imperative. A tumour close to the mandible may need a marginal or occasionally a segmental mandibulectomy. When the tumour does not involve the lateral or anterior floor of the mouth, the tongue can be approached from below, the mandible retracted upwards, and the tongue can then be removed via a pull-through approach. Access to the oral cavity can then be obtained through a visor flap, preserving the integrity of the lips. Loss of the mental nerve on both sides in such cases produces anaesthesia of the lower lips. Although a paramedian transmandibular approach offers better access, it is not desirable to split the lip. It may however be possible to combine this approach with a visor flap (Fig. 10.2).

The incidence of neck node metastases is high in lingual carcinoma (Leipzig & Hokanson 1982, Ali et al 1986). The neck nodes must be included in all cases. The operation is begun with contralateral neck dissection. A comprehensive neck dissection with preservation of the accessory nerve on both sides whenever possible and preservation of the internal jugular vein on the less involved side of the primary tumour is performed through an incision that extends from the tip of one mastoid to the other at the level of the upper border of the thyroid cartilage. A vertical 'S' type extension is added on the ipsilateral side, and a modified McFee incision may be used on the contralateral side. This provides additional protection for the preserved internal jugular vein. The specimens of neck dissections are left attached to the lower border of the mandible. Of late, supra-omohyoid dissection has been advocated as a therapeutic measure for carcinoma of the oral cavity and oropharynx (Medina & Byers 1989, Shah 1990). On the other hand it is well documented that the incidence of regional recurrence is appreciably higher with supra-omohyoid dissections (Spiro et al 1988). Supra-omohyoid dissection is a good staging procedure, but in large aggressive tumours, like those of tongue and base of tongue, it is better to perform a comprehensive dissection. This is confirmed by significantly lower regional recurrences in comprehensive neck dissections (Leemans et al 1990). If the disease is predominantly unlateral, or if involvement of the opposite neck is in doubt, then a supra-omohyoid dissection is performed. Any suspicious nodes are subjected to frozen section, and should this reveal tumour then a comprehensive dissection is carried out.

If the disease does not extend to the floor of the mouth, intra-oral incisions are placed along the lateral floor of the mouth on both sides and the mobile tongue is delivered into the neck by completing the incision anteriorly through the floor of the mouth. Both lingual arteries and veins are ligated and divided, and the base of the tongue is cut away from the hyoid with a diathermy. If the floor of the mouth is involved on one side and marginal mandibular resection is needed, this is performed and delivered with the floor of the mouth and the tongue in the neck, the opposite lateral floor of the mouth being preserved (Fig. 10.3). In case a segmental mandibular resection is needed—for instance, in extension

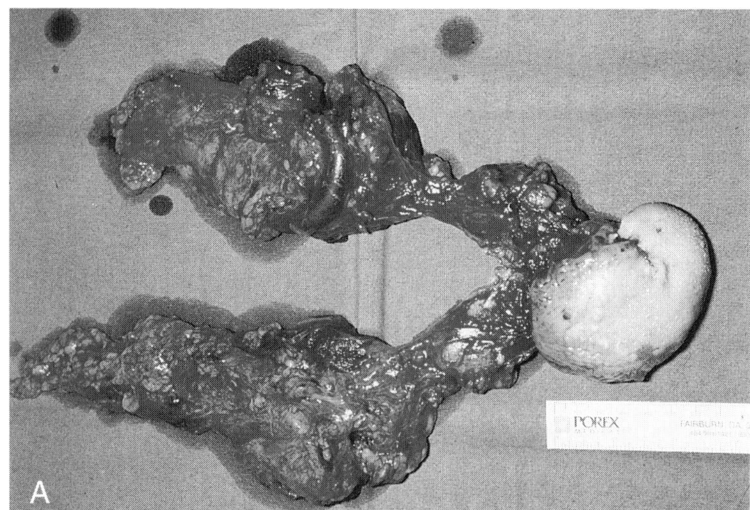

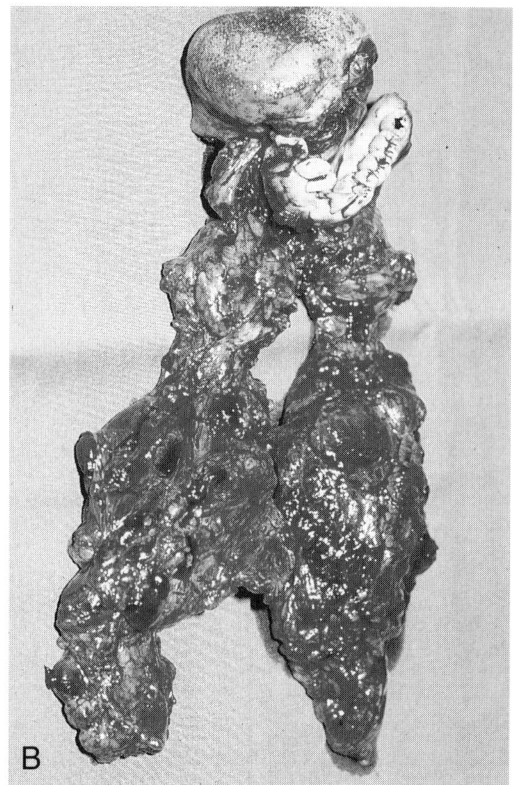

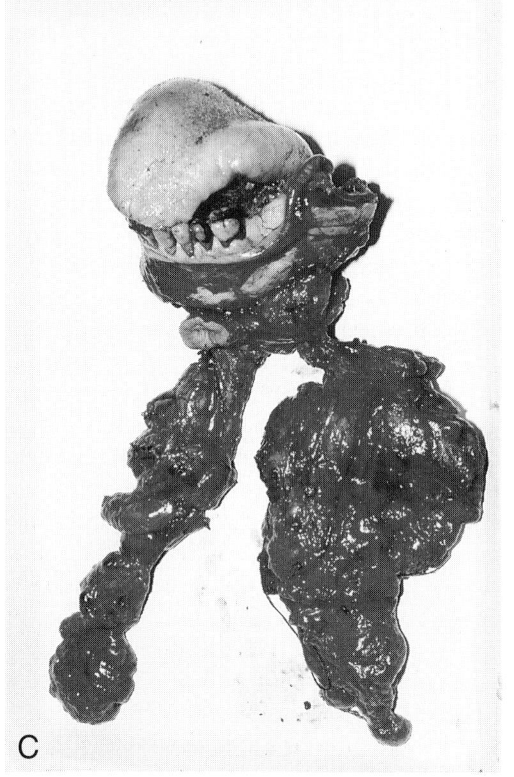

Fig. 10.4 **A.** Specimen of total glossectomy with bilateral en bloc comprehensive neck dissections. **B.** Total glossectomy with marginal mandibular resection and en bloc comprehensive neck dissections. **C.** Total glossectomy with segmental mandibular resection, right supra-omohyoid and left radical neck dissections.

of the tumour to the oropharynx or in the event of an extension on the lateral floor of the mouth in a patient with adentulous narrow mandible—then this is performed and the whole tongue sectioned from the hyoid (Fig. 10.4). The base of the tongue at its attachment to the hyoid is carefully examined during resection. Caudal extension of the disease can often be seen and palpated. If the tumour is fixed to the hyoid, half or whole of the hyoid bone is removed. Frozen section control of the margins of excision is carried out.

RECONSTRUCTION

The reconstructive choice after total glossectomy lies basically between myocutaneous flaps and free vascularized flaps. In addition, use is made of the remaining local tissues such as the floor of the mouth, usually on the contralateral side.

Laryngeal suspension is an essential step, and preparations are first made for this procedure. When the mandible is intact, burr holes are made with a fine burr through the body of the mandible about 2 cm lateral to the mental foramen and approximately 1 cm from the lower border, just large enough to allow a 5 '0' stainless steel wire to pass through. The wires are picked up and passed under hyoid bone on both sides, and the two ends of the wires are held together with a Kocher artery clamp (Fig. 10.5). The larynx and trachea are mobilized by blunt dissection on either side and the infralaryngeal muscles are divided. While an assistant supports and gently pulls the larynx cranially, the stainless steel wires are pulled taught but not tied. This elevates the larynx, and it is at this moment that the distance between the outer border of the mandible in the midline and the epiglottis is measured. The distance between the two horizontal rami of the mandible just in front of angle is also measured. A flap 1 cm larger than these dimensions is then marked. The wires are not tightened at this stage and

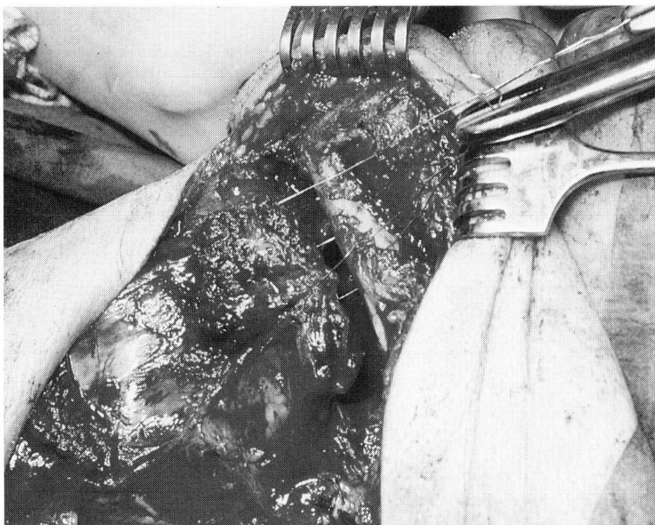

Fig. 10.5 Steps in laryngeal suspension. The specimen has been removed. Stainless steel wires for laryngeal suspension are in place. Infralaryngeal muscles have been sectioned, and the larynx and trachea have been mobilized. (See also colour plate section)

tracheotomy is deferred until the very end of the procedure. The pectoralis major myocutaneous flap has been used personally on 23 consecutive patients with good results. The flap is raised in the usual fashion and brought into the defect. Sutures are placed in one layer through the muscle and the skin of the flap on the one hand and the pre-epiglottic mucosa or whatever vallecular mucosa is left. Usually there is just enough space for about five sutures. Laterally, one of these sutures must include the lateral pharyngeal wall to close the three-point junction. The sutures are placed and held on a clamp and not tied. Anteriorly, the muscle and skin

of the flap can be closed in two layers to the orbicularis oris and the mucosa of the lower lip. Two sutures placed between the muscle of the flap and the periosteum help to prevent retraction of the lip. Laterally, the flap is approximated to the buccinator if the patient is edentulous. In a dentate patient the choice is dependent upon the state of dentition. In the presence of desolate dentition, extraction is carried out and the alveolar mucosa is removed. The bone is smoothed with a polishing burr and the flap is stitched to the buccinator muscle and the buccal mucosa in two layers. In the rare event of this procedure being carried out in a patient with good dentition, the flap has to be anchored to the gums on the inner surface in one layer. It is better to use a paramedian mandibulotomy approach in such cases to ensure stable suturing of the flap. When the flap is in place, osteosynthesis of the mandible is carried out. The site of placement of the osteosynthetic plates should have been marked and burr holes made before mandibulotomy is actually performed so that the flap is least disturbed and not handled during osteosynthesis.

Once the flap is in place, the undersurface is examined and possible leaks sutured and sealed. The muscle of the flap is anchored to the soft tissues under the jaw to overcome any downward drag. The larynx is now gently brought up manually and the stainless steel wires are tightened and laryngeal suspension completed (Fig. 10.6). Should a segmental resection of the mandible have been necessary then the larynx is suspended to the cranial end of the cut mandibular bone (Fig. 10.7). A feeding tube is left.

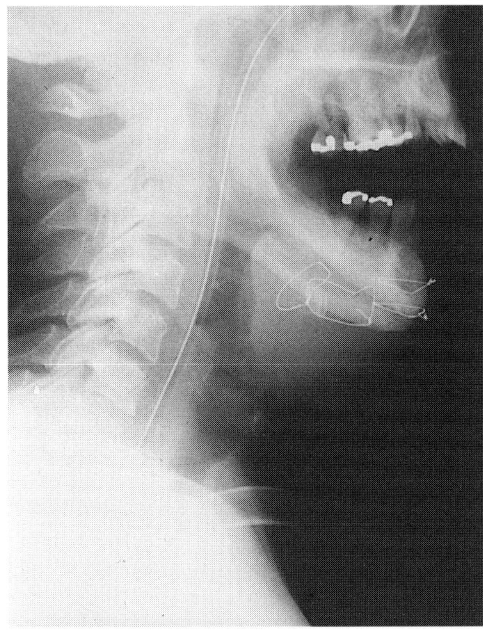

Fig. 10.6 Median laryngeal suspension with intact mandible.

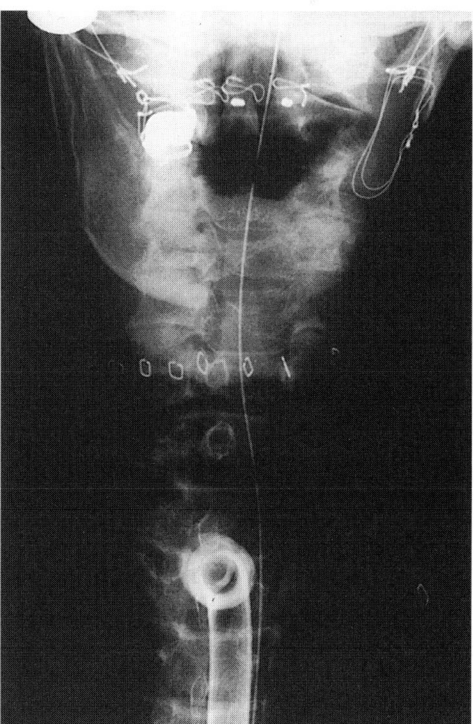

Fig. 10.7 Lateral laryngeal suspension after segmental mandibular resection.

Tracheotomy is performed and incisions are closed with vacuum drain.

A free vascularized skin-flap alone offers no significant advantage. It provides only a single layer closure. A composite flap with muscle is better. A vascularized sensory flap would be ideal. However, this is possible in very few centres. The complication rate reported with such reconstructions in large series is high (Keyserlingk et al 1989). In addition, these patients must receive prompt postoperative radiotherapy which retards the restoration of sensation in such flaps. When possible, a nerve graft of the mental nerves is helpful. Laryngeal suspension brings the larynx upwards and forwards. This manoeuvre reduces the pressure in the PE segment and assists in the resumption of swallowing (Sultan & Coleman 1989). It also brings the hypopharyngeal mucosa towards the defect, thereby reducing the size. Approximately 2 weeks later patients can be decannulated, and once the wound has healed they learn to swallow (Figs 10.8 and 10.9). This is surprisingly easy with a little guidance, and most patients resume swallowing pulverized food and liquids by the end of 4 or 5 weeks. In the author's own series this has been possible in all cases (Table 10.1). Patients are often pleasantly surprised to find themselves speaking without the tongue. This helps to restore confidence and improves communication. The guidance of an experienced speech therapist and a successfully rehabilitated patient is invaluable at this stage. In the author's own series, speech was acquired postoperatively by all patients (Tiwari et al 1993). Postoperative radiotherapy often holds back recovery, and patients need to be given an explanation and guided through this difficult phase.

When the larynx has been sacrificed as well, a large defect ensues. This is broad anterosuperiorly in the region of the floor of the mouth and long and narrow posteriorly and caudally. Closure of such defects is achieved by a myocutaneous flap from the pectoralis major. The flap is shaped almost like a tennis racket. Wound healing is usually smooth and complete at the end of 3 weeks.

PROBLEMS AND COMPLICATIONS

A thorough preoperative evaluation will prevent intra-operative encounter of tumour extensions, especially those caudally towards the hyoid and the pre-epiglottic space.

Table 10.1 Total glossectomy with laryngeal preservation: functional results

Authors	Number of patients	Year of publication	Mortality (%)	Speech (successful %)	Aspiration (Yes / No)	Swallowing (successful %)
Donaldson et al	14	1968	NIL	50	Yes	57
Korthary et al	26	1974	15	NS	no?	NS
Effron et al	24	1981	NIL	100		100 (two patients used tube feeding)
Sultan & Coleman	7	1989	6	80	yes	93
Weber et al	27	1991	NIL	92	yes	67
Tiwari et al	21	1993	NIL	100	no	100

NS=not specified. (With kind permission of Archives of Otolaryngology Head and Neck Surgery.)

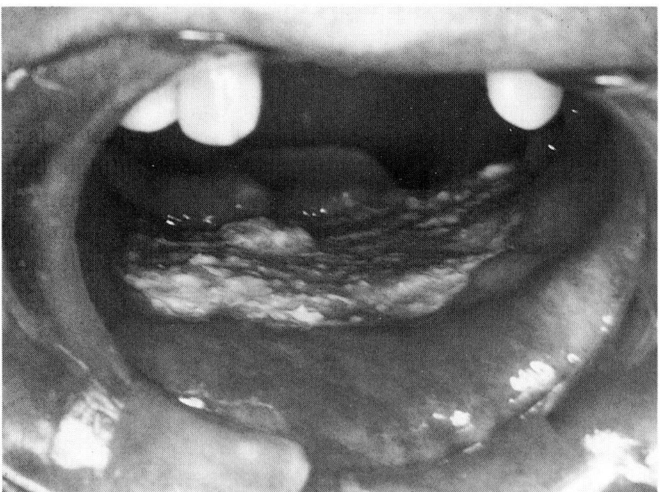

Fig. 10.8 Total glossectomy reconstruction with pectoralis major muscle and split skin graft. Note the epiglottis in the background and its high position because of laryngeal suspension. (See also colour plate section)

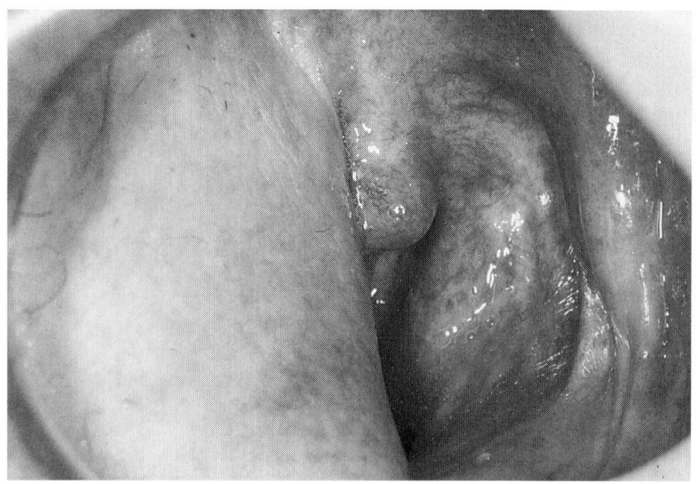

Fig. 10.9 Reconstruction after total glossectomy and segmental mandibular resection with laryngeal preservation. The contralateral floor of the mouth has been used along with the myocutaneous flap from pectoralis major. The epiglottis is not seen. (See also colour plate section)

Patients have difficulty in appreciating why a part of the tongue cannot be saved. Once a carcinoma of the tongue has spread to the contralateral side, it is better to be prepared to take a decision intraoperatively to go ahead with total resection of the tongue. There has been no mortality related to this procedure, and the morbidity is relatively low. Patients need guidance to learn to swallow. The flap is insensitive, but laryngeal suspension helps to restore swallowing. Aspiration, if present, is temporary only in the first week or two. Whenever the mental nerves are cut, as is often the case, the ensuing insensitivity of the lower lip causes inconvenience in drinking warm beverages. Rehabilitation of these patients and their return to normal social activities can be achieved by regular contact with the patients by the surgeon, radiotherapist, speech therapist and the nursing staff. Occasionally, the lower lip may be indrawn and a vestibuloplasty may be needed. Patients need to be educated to use the orbicularis oris and articulate. Some patients experience mild trismus. While the problem of

development of distant metastases still remains, total glossectomy with laryngeal preservation offers good locoregional control with preservation of a reasonably good quality of life. When the larynx, too, is removed, patients can swallow, but have no speech and rely on a vibrator. Attempts to establish speech with the help of a voice prosthesis are usually not successful in these cases as there is very little pharyngeal mucosa left.

FUTURE PROSPECTS

It is possible that free vascularized sensate composite flaps will be used in the future for reconstruction after total glossectomy. Computerized analysis of the speech of successfully rehabilitated patients has already been done at our centre. It is possible that electronic devices may be developed which will help patients to pronounce those vowels and consonants which they miss in their speech. The fitting of a dental prosthesis with such devices is a possibility.

REFERENCES

Ali S, Tiwari R M, Snow G B, Van der Waal I (1986) Incidence of squamous cell carcinoma of the head and neck. Journal of Laryngology and Otology 100: 315–327

Biller M F, Lawson W, Baek S M (1983) Total glossectomy. A technique of reconstruction eliminating laryngectomy. Archives of Otolaryngology 109: 69

Cade S, Lee E S (1957) Cancer of the tongue. A study based on 653 patients. British Journal of surgery 44: 433

Calcaterra T (1971) Laryngeal suspension after supraglottic laryngectomy. Archives of Otolaryngology 94: 306

Donaldson R C, Skelly M, Paletta F X (1968). Total glossectomy for cancer. American Journal of Surgery 116: 585–590

Edgerton M, McKee D M (1959) Reconstruction with loss of the hyomandibular complex in excision of large cancers. Archives of Surgery 78: 425–436

Effron M Z, Johnson J T, Myers E N, Curtin H, Berry Q, Sigler B. (1981) Advanced carcinoma of the tongue. Archives of Otolaryngology 107: 694

Einspieler R, Ebner F, Posanetz W, Ranner G, Fluckiger F, Lammer J (1991) MR imaging with GdDTPA in carcinoma of tongue, oro- and hypopharynx. European Journal of Radiology 13: 21–26

Feinmesser R, Freeman J L, Nojek A M, Birt B D (1987) Metastatic neck disease. A clinical radiographic, pathologic correlative study. Archives of Otolaryngology—Head and Neck Surgery 113: 1307–1310

Friedman M, Shelton V K, Mafee M, Bellay P, Grybauskas V, Skolnik E (1984) Metastatic neck disease. Evaluation by computed tomography. Archives of Otolaryngology 110: 443–447

Goefert H, Jesse R H, Fletcher G B, Hamberger A 1975 Optimal treatment for the technically resectable squamous cell carcinoma of the supraglottic larynx. Laryngoscope 85: 14–32

Goode R L 1976 Laryngeal suspension in head and neck surgery. Laryngoscope 86: 349

Hamberger A O, Fletcher G H, Guillamondegui O M, Byers R B 1976 Advanced squamous cell carcinoma of the oral cavity and oropharynx—treatment with irradiation and surgery. Radiology 119: 433–438

Harrison D 1983 The questionable value of glossectomy. Head and Neck Surgery 6: 632

Harrold C C 1967 Surgical treatment of cancer of the base of the tongue. American Journal of Surgery 114: 493–497

Hillel A D, Goode R L 1983 Lateral laryngeal suspension. A new procedure to minimize swallowing disorders following tongue base resection. Laryngoscope 93: 26–31

Jabaley M C, Hoopes J E 1969 A simple technique for laryngeal suspension after partial or complete resection of the hyomandibular complex. American journal of Surgery 118: 685

Jaulerry C, Rodriguez J, Brunin F, Mosseri V, Pontvert D, Brugere J, Bataini J P 1991 Results of radiotherapy in carcinoma of the base of the tongue. Cancer 67: 1532

Jayant K., Notani P 1991 Epidemiology of oral cancer. In: Rao R S, Desai P B (eds) Oral cancer. Professional educational division. Tata Memorial Hospital, Bombay, pp 1–17

Keyserlingk J R, Francesco J D, Breach N, Rhys Evans P, Stafford N, Motta A 1989 Recent experience with reconstructive surgery following major glossectomy. Archives of Otolaryngology—Head and Neck Surgery 115: 331

Kothary P M, Paymaster J C, Potdar G G 1974 Radical total glossectomy. British Journal of Surgery 61:209

Larsson S G, Hoover L A, Julliard G J F 1987 Staging of base of tongue carcinoma by computed tomography. Clinical Otolaryngology 12: 25–31

Leemans C R, Tiwari R M , Van der Waal I, Karim A B M F, Nauta J J P, Snow G B 1990 The efficacy of comprehensive neck dissection with or without postoperative radiotherapy in nodal metastases of squamous cell carcinoma of the upper respiratory and digestive tracts. Laryngoscope 100: 1194

Leipzig B, Hokanson J A 1982 Treatment of cervical lymph nodes in carcinoma of the tongue. Head and Neck Surgery 5: 3

Lusinchi A, Eskandari J, Son Y, Gerbaulet A, Haie C, Mamelle G, Eschwege F, Chassagne D 1989 External irradiation plus curietherapy boost in 108 base of tongue carcinomas. International Journal of Radiation Onocology Biology and Physics 17: 1191

Marcus R.B, Million R R, Cassisi N J 1979 Postoperative irradiation for squamous cell carcinoma of the head and neck. Analysis of time dose factors related to control above the clavicles. International Journal of Radiation Oncology Biology and Physics 5: 1943

Medina J E, Byers R M, 1989 Supraomohyoid neck dissection. Head and Neck 11: 111

Pradhan S A, Rajpal R M, Kothary P M, 1980 Surgical management of postradiation residual recurrent cancer of the base of the tongue. Journal of Surgical Oncology 14: 201

Shah J P 1990 Cervical lymph mode metastases. Diagnostic, therapeutic and prognostic implications. Oncology 4: 61

Spiro J D, Spiro R H, Shah J P, Sessions R B, Strong E W 1988 Critical assessment of supraomohyoid neck dissection. American Journal of Surgery 156: 286

Stevens M H, Harnsberger R, Mancuso A A, Davis R K, Johnson L P, Parkin J L 1985 Computed tomography of cervical lymph nodes staging and management of head and neck cancer. Archives of Otolaryngology 111: 735

Sultan M R, Coleman J J 1989 Oncologic and functional considerations of total glossectomy. American Journal of Surgery. 158: 297

Terz J J, King R E, Lawrence W 1973 Primary rehabilitation after total glossectomy. Surgery Gynecology and Obstetrics 136: 227–278

Tiwari R M, Greven A J, Karim A B M F, Snow G B 1989 Total glossectomy reconstruction and rehabilitation. Journal of Laryngology and Otology 103: 917

Tiwari R M, Karim A B M F, Greven A J, Snow G B 1993 Total glossectomy with laryngeal preservation. Archives of Otolaryngology—Head and Neck Surgery 119: 945–949

Vikram B, Strong E W, Shah J, Spiro R H 1980 Elective postoperative radiation therapy in stages III and IV epidermoid carcinoma of the head and neck. American Journal of surgery 140: 580–584

Van den Brekel M W M, Stel H V, Castelijns J A, Nauta J J P, Van der Waal I, Valk J, Meyer C J L M, Snow G B 1990 Cervical lymph node metastases: Assessment of radiologic criteria. Radiology 177: 379–384

Van den Brekel M W M, Castelijns J A, Croll G A, Stel H V, Valk J,

Van der Waal I, Golding R P, Meyer C J L M, Snow G B 1991 Magnetic resonance imaging versus palpation of cervical lymph mode metastases. Archives of Otolaryngology—Head and neck Surgery 117: 666–673

Van den Brouck C, Sancho H, Le fur R, Richard J M Cachin Y 1977 Results of a randomized clinical trial of preoperative irradiation versus postoperative in treatment of tumours of the hypopharynx. Cancer 39: 1445

Weber R, Ohlms L, Bowman J, Jacob R, Goepfert H 1991 Functional results after total or near total glossectomy with laryngeal preservation. Archives of Otolaryngology—Head and neck Surgery 117: 512

Weisberger E C, Lingeman R E 1983 Modified supraglottic laryngectomy and resection of lesions of the base of tongue. Laryngoscope 93: 20

Whicker J H, De Santo L W, Devine K D 1972 Surgical treatment of squamous cell carcinoma of the base of the tongue. Laryngoscope 82: 1853

Zelefsky M J, Harrison L B, Fass D E, Armstrong J, Spiro R H, Shah J P, Strong E W 1990 Postoperative radiotherapy for oral cavity cancers. Impact of anatomic subsite on treatment outcome. Head and Neck 12: 470

11. The oropharynx

William R. Panje   Michael R. Morris

INTRODUCTION

The goals of this chapter are to advise the reader on the different techniques of oropharyngeal tumour exposure and to provide a thorough discussion of reconstructive principles highlighting proven options. No comments will be made regarding the applicability of radiation therapy and/or chemotherapy as an alternative or adjunct in the management of these tumours.

The surgical ablation of any oropharyngeal cancer must be aggressive and complete. Limited experience or preconceived notions about tumour extent and/or reconstructive options can influence a surgeon's aggressiveness, which may compromise excision and have an adverse effect on the patient's survival and quality of life. Once the final surgical defect is apparent, the surgeon will appreciate the extent of functional impairment and aesthetic insult his ablation has created. Most patients can functionally overcome the loss of up to 50% of any single swallowing region; however, the problem with oropharyngeal resection is that oftentimes adjoining regions are excised and a significant debility can occur. The finest, state-of-the-art reconstruction will not recreate the complex neuromuscular interactions necessary for normal swallowing. The surgeon and patient must realize that rehabilitation and practice are of paramount importance to the ultimate success of restoring quality to day-to-day living after major head and neck cancer surgery.

The surgical approach and reconstructive option chosen will be influenced by a variety of factors. The general health and mental stamina of the patient will have a profound impact. A vibrant 70 year old should have several more years of productive living and he should be managed with that in mind. Conversely, a 50 year old with significant cardiac disease, diabetes, and malnutrition will have a greatly increased perioperative risk, and anaesthetic time should be minimized. The presence of metastases and the local extent of the primary tumour will also have an influence. Recurrent tumours, especially those in irradiated fields, generally require a wider resection. Patients with poor self-esteem and limited mental fortitude will not accept any significant

cosmetic or functional deformity well. It may be beneficial to delay an elaborate reconstruction on such patients to gain the appreciation and motivation needed to rehabilitate successfully.

Any surgeon involved with the ablation and reconstruction of these defects must have a clear understanding of the donor-site morbidity for various reconstructive options. For example, if the patient is a golfer or plays tennis then he is going to require shoulder strength and mobility to maintain these hobbies postoperatively. If the surgeon disregards these needs and cripples a shoulder for the sake of using a certain reconstructive technique, then he is doing that patient a grave disservice. Surgeons must know a variety of reconstructive options so that their level of skill and understanding are not the limiting factors in providing quality care.

Once the surgical defect has been finalized the more subtle aspects of the reconstruction can be analysed. The oropharyngeal component of swallowing is involuntary and consists of the tongue base moving posteriorly and the velopharynx closing off. The hyoid is pulled anteriorly, causing the laryngeal complex to move forward and up under the base of tongue. The surgeon should recognize the need to recreate tongue base bulk, velopharyngeal competence, and laryngeal position as part of the reconstruction so that aspiration and dysphagia are minimized.

SURGICAL APPROACHES

Transoral approach

This approach causes the least morbidity for patients and with the advent of lasers can be applied to many of the small tumours of the oropharynx (Panje et al 1989). The limited thermal injury and oedema caused by lasers reduces the need for tracheotomy and minimizes the patient's discomfort postoperatively.

A Crochard or Dingman mouth gag provides attachable cheek retractors to facilitate exposure. Alternative methods include the use of a bite block or Denhart Gag. A towel clamp or stitch can be placed in the tongue if necessary to improve access. The operating microscope is often used to provide magnification and lighting. When dealing with field cancerization, as is often the case with the soft palate, toluidine blue is used. The mucosa is washed with a 1% acetic acid solution, blotted dry, and a 0.25% dye solution is applied. The area is then copiously irrigated with saline after 1–2 minutes. Areas of cellular atypia will stain a violet colour because of increased nucleic acid/cytoplasm ratio and greater intercellular distance. The CO_2 and KTP lasers have been extremely useful in providing a precise resection in a relatively bloodless field. Once the excision is started the specimen is stabilized by passing a large silk suture through the incision margin. These sutures also provide retraction and prevent sliding of the specimen. Oropharyngeal tumours as large as 3–4 cm can be excised with this approach; however, the surgeon must be cautious in applying it to larger tumours (>2 cm) or whenever significant neck metastases are present. Transoral removal of a primary tumour means managing the neck in a discontinuous fashion, which may have an adverse affect on the patient survival (Leemans et al 1991).

The close support of a skilled pathologist is also mandatory since orientation can be complex and precise margin information is required for success.

Pull-through approach

The pull-through approach offers excellent exposure for removing smaller tongue base and/or tonsil/anterior pillar lesions without mandibulotomy. This method also allows for an en bloc excision of primary tumour and neck contents. An upper horizontal cervical skin incision is placed from the mastoid tip to the contralateral submentum (Fig. 11.1) Access to the neck can be accomplished either by dropping

a vertical limb or using a MacFee approach (MacFee 1960). Once the submandibular triangle has been completely excised, attention is turned intra-orally. A mucosal incision is made through the floor or the mouth close to the lingual surface of the mandible from the contralateral Wharton's orifice, around to the anterior margin of planned tumour excision. Depending on the exact site of the tumour, the anterior, lateral, palatal and medial mucosal margins can all be incised. Attention is then turned to the neck where the mylohyoid muscle is cut, laterally to medial. The tongue is then delivered into the neck below the mandible. By utilizing silk retraction sutures on the specimen and adjacent tongue, enough mobility can be obtained to complete any mucosal cuts and subsequently remove the specimen.

Visor flap approach

Another method of accessing oropharyngeal tumours is with the visor flap (Fig. 11.2) (La Ferriere et al 1980). This technique is useful when a lateral mandibulotomy or composite resection is planned. An incision is placed from the tip of the mastoid extending horizontally 3–4 cm below the mandibular border into the contralateral submental area. If additional neck exposure is needed for lymph node dissection a vertical limb can be added to the visor incision or a MacFee type of approach can be used. The neck contents are dissected superiorly and left attached to the jaw segment that will be removed (composite resections). The patient is then given a paralytic agent to allow full relaxation. A gingivolabial/buccal incision is then made extending from the contralateral canine to the mental foramen on the tumour side. Care is taken to leave a good cuff of alveolar mucosa attached to the jaw to facilitate closure. Elevation of the mentum on a supraperiosteal plane will allow connecting the intra-oral incision with the neck. The visor flap is then dissected posteriorly by elevating the masseter off of the

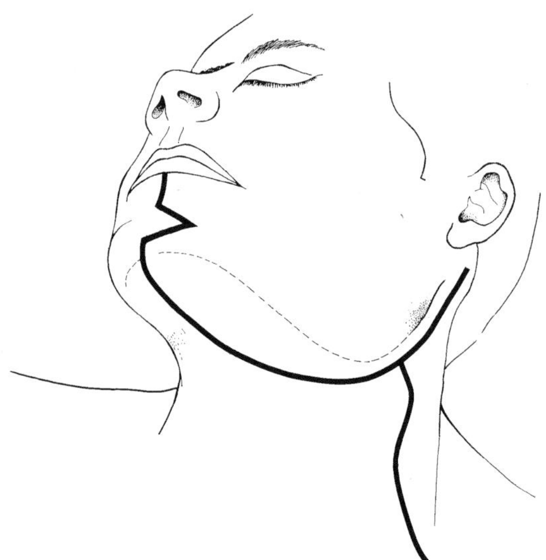

Fig. 11.1 Incision for access to the oropharynx and en bloc neck dissection.

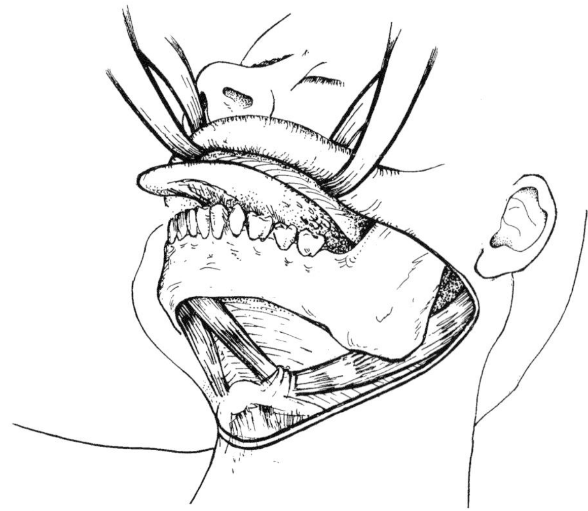

Fig. 11.2 Visor flap. Integrity of the lower lip is preserved.

angle and ramus of the jaw. This will allow retraction of the 'visor' flap superiorly and provide for wide exposure. The exact site of the initial mandibulotomy will dictate where the gingivolabial/buccal incision will cross over the alveolus into the floor of mouth and continue posteriorly to the planned tumour resection margin. It is important not to have the alveolar incision directly over the mandibulotomy site so a short flap is usually elevated proximally or distally (mandibulotomy versus mandibulectomy). Great care must be taken to avoid injuring the contralateral mental nerve otherwise the patient will awake with an insensate lower lip.

Cheek flap approach

The cheek flap combined with mandibulotomy offers the very best visualization and is recommended for operators with limited experience (Fig. 11.3). The upper horizontal limb of the neck incision is carried up over the mentum to the midline of the lower lip. A short horizontal 'stair-step' cut is made in the vermillion and the lip is split. The gingivolabial/buccal incision is just as was described for the visor approach unless a symphyseal osteotomy is planned. The cheek is rapidly elevated on a supraperiosteal level back to the masseter or the osteotomy site. Further reflection of the masseter off of the lateral jaw allows for wide exposure of the oral cavity/oropharynx. The mental portion of the incision can be altered as dictated by the facial structure of the patient. For example, if a protuberant chin is present the incision can curve around its contour for a more aesthetic scar.

Median labiomandibular glossotomy approach

This approach has applicability limited to the management of T1 and small T2 cancers of the posterior pharyngeal wall and very small midline base of tongue tumours (Tollefsen et al 1971). A midline incision is made from the midline of the lower lip (vermillion stair-step) down to the hyoid. Both sides of the mentum are dissected a short distance to allow exposure of the symphysis. A midline mandibulotomy is performed and gentle retraction of the jaw segments allows for a sagittal floor of mouth cut between Wharton's orifices. The tongue is then rapidly split down the midline all the way to the hyoid and the two halves retracted laterally. This allows for good exposure of the posterior pharyngeal wall (Fig. 11.4A). If this approach is used for a small tongue tumour then the midline excision is carried posteriorly on as far as the anterior margin of the planned excision. Reconstruction following this approach is usually not necessary. Posterior pharyngeal wall excision sites are left to granulate and the tongue, floor of mouth and mandible closed primarily (Fig. 11.4B).

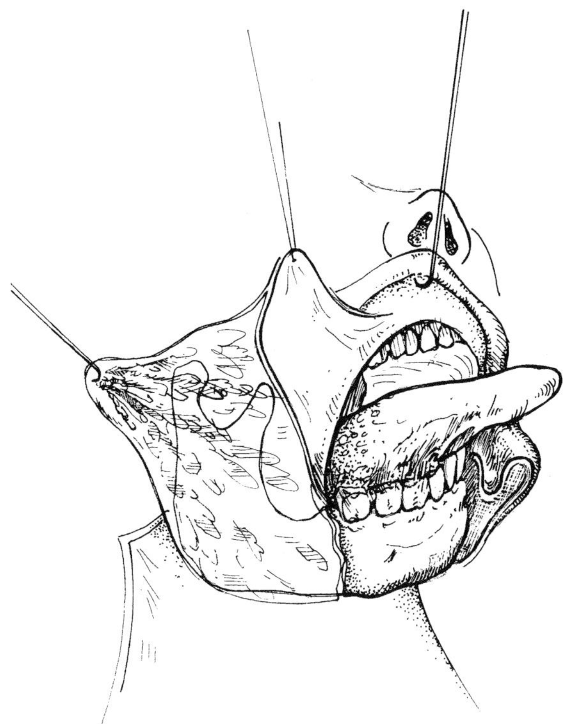

Fig. 11.3 Cheek flap; it provides good access to the oral cavity as well as the oropharynx.

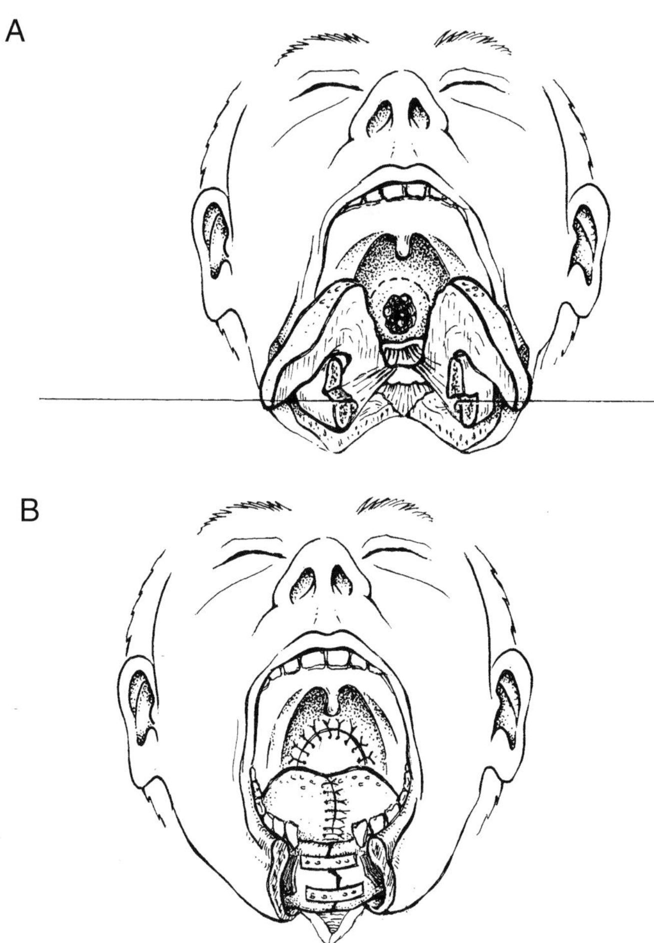

Fig. 11.4 A, B. Median labiomandibular glossotomy approach to posterior pharyngeal wall.

Transhyoid pharyngotomy approach

This technique is also quite limited in its application. Small base of tongue tumours that do not extend to the vallecula can be adequately exposed with this approach thereby avoiding a mandibulotomy. An upper cervical incision is made and carried down to the hyoid bone. The length of the incision depends on the need for simultaneous neck surgery. Once the hyoid is identified the superior muscle attachments are sharply separated. Dissection proceeds until the vallecula is entered. This pharyngotomy is opened horizontally allowing for retraction and exposure of the tongue base (Fig. 11.5).

MANDIBLE AND MANDIBULOTOMY

The mandible or its periosteum is often the lateral margin of resection with oropharyngeal tumours. The decision of whether or not to remove mandible in conjunction with the tumour can be confusing in a non-radiated mandible, the periosteum offers a significant resistance to tumour penetration (Marchetta et al 1971). Tumours can seem quite close to and even abut the jaw but not invade the periosteum. Preoperative evaluation must include a panorex, and if the tumour/mandible relationship is in question a bone scan and/or MRI scan will help delineate invasion. In nonradiated patients without obvious invasion, the plane between the lingual surface of the mandible and the periosteum can be carefully elevated. If no adhesions are encountered it is unlikely any invasion is present and the periosteum serves as the lateral margin. If the tumour is bulky and/or abuts the jaw a marginal resection of the jaw can be done to provide the operator a safer lateral margin while preserving jaw continuity. This type of marginal resection should be done only if there is at least 1 cm of bone height above the mental foramen. If mandibular invasion is suspected by preoperative

work-up a segmental resection is generally necessary to avoid tumour transgression (Fig. 11.6). The most common site for a non-radiated mandible to be invaded by carcinoma is through the alveolus (McGregor & MacDonald 1988). Any involvement of alveolar mucosa overlying an edentulous segment of jaw should be managed as though invasion was present. Invasion of the alveolar nerve can readily occur in senile jaws because the loss of vertical height brings the nerve in close proximity to the oropharynx.

In patients who have been previously radiated, other factors must be taken into account. There is no consistent pattern of tumour invasion and the periosteum loses its barrier quality. There is usually little fibrous stromal reaction with tumour spread, and the plane between bone and periosteum can be relatively non-adherent even though invasion is present (McGregor & MacDonald 1988). Moreover, problems with osteoradionecrosis must be considered. Marginal resections are generally not recommended for managing radiation failures. Another confusing situation is with a patient who has already had a mandibulotomy for access during a previous cancer surgery. Whenever a mandibulectomy is needed it should encompass any previous osteotomy site and include a coronoidectomy. The condyle portion is usually removed as well to avoid subsequent problems with osteoradionecrosis of this segment. This problem has been encountered and can cause delayed wound breakdown and great worry about tumour recurrence for both the doctor and the patient.

When only a mandibulotomy is necessary, the surgeon must decide where to place it. The midline osteotomy site allows retention of muscle attachments and generally heals very well. It also allows for maximum exposure with retraction and is recommended for less experienced surgeons (Spiro et al 1981). The major drawback is that if the tumour has been underestimated, a composite resection will require a hemimandibulectomy. A cheek flap is generally required if utilizing a symphyseal osteotomy and a lower central

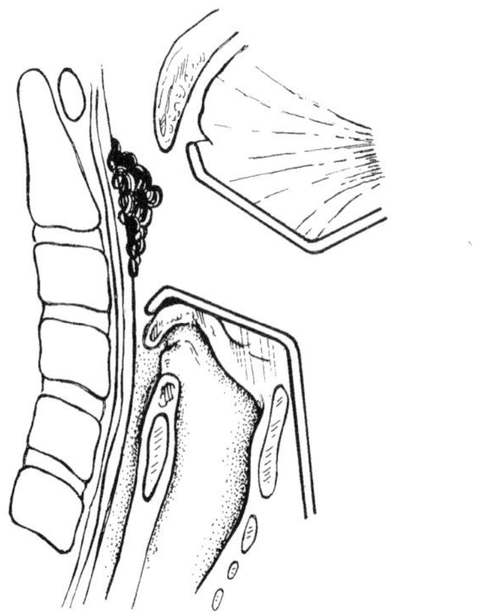

Fig. 11.5 Transhyoid approach to posterior pharyngeal wall. The base of tongue has been retracted upwards.

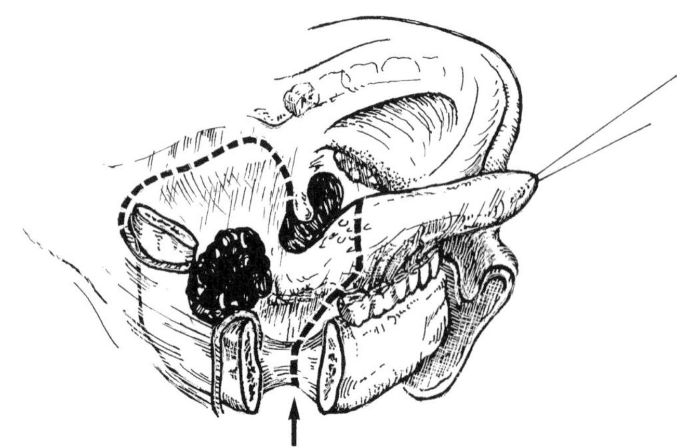

Fig. 11.6 Segmental mandibulectomy for tumours abutting against the angle of the mandible.

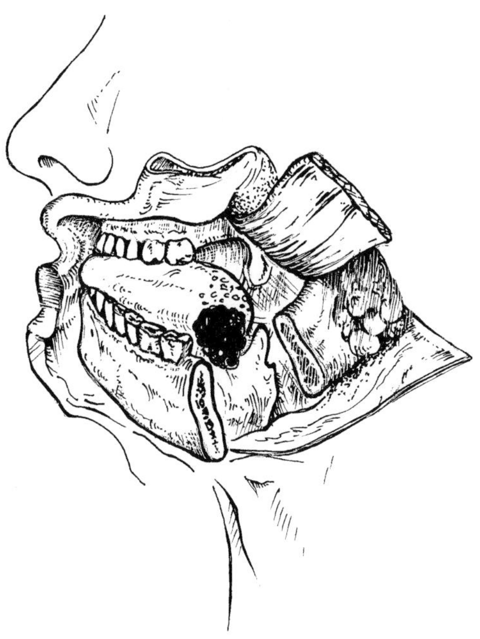

Fig. 11.7 Lateral mandibulotomy. The inferior alveolar artery and nerve have to be sacrificed. The approach provides good access to the base of the tongue.

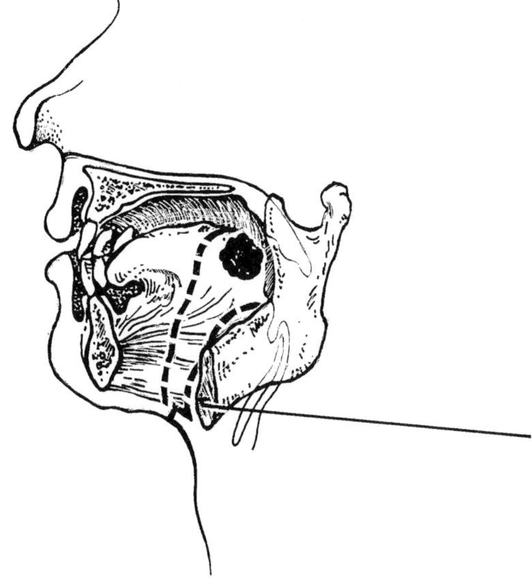

Fig. 11.8 Paramedian mandibulotomy (McGregor)

incisor must be pulled (if present) to allow enough room for the bone cut.

The lateral osteotomy is preferred in radiation failure patients and whenever there may be a chance a composite resection would be needed. The exact site of the cut will vary depending upon the tumour extent and the patient's dentition. Healing is generally very good and a visor flap can be used, thereby avoiding a lower lip scar (Fig. 11.7).

An alternative osteotomy site is just lateral to the digastric insertion (McGregor & MacDonald 1983) (Fig. 11.8).

The touted advantage is an improvement in postoperative deglutition by preserving the integrity of the digastric, genioglossus, geniohyoid insertions. I have not found this to be of much significance.

Once the position for the cut has been decided, a titanium or vitallium (cobalt–chromium alloy) mandibular reconstruction bar is bent to adapt to the contour of the adjacent mandible. A minimum of three holes are drilled on each side of the planned osteotomy. Bone drilling is always done at low speeds (25–50 r.p.m.) under constant copious cool saline irrigation. Each hole is then manually tapped and the depth measured so that screw will be bicortical. The osteotomy is either a stair-step or notch design and the cuts are made with a pneumatic saw under copious saline irrigation. Care must be taken when retracting the mandible following osteotomy because the floor of mouth/alveolar mucosa can easily tear into the tumour. Through and through intra-oral cuts are made, and the mandible retracted gradually until the needed exposure is obtained or the margin of planned excision encountered. Once reconstruction has been completed and the mandible re-approxi-

mated, the metal bar is repositioned and secured to provide rigid fixation of the segments. The osteotomy defect can be filled with bone dust collected during the initial cuts. The surgeon should avoid having the mucosal, periosteal and bone cuts all in the same place. By having an overlap there is less chance of salivary contamination with possible infection, breakdown and malunion.

PRINCIPLES OF EXCISION

Oropharyngeal tumours are often much larger than appreciated on visual examination. Tumours originating in one area will often involve adjacent areas, necessitating a rather radical ablation for cure. Trismus and pain pre-operatively signal deep pterygoid involvement. An insensate lip or portion of the face or other cranial nerve deficit (IX,X,XI,XII) denotes an aggressive tumour with possible base of skull involvement. General anaesthesia with paralysis allows for bimanual palpation, an orderly endoscopy, and mapping of the tumour. This is combined with CT scan and/or MRI scan to help develop the approach and general operative plan.

The goal of surgery will be to complete an en bloc resection of the cancer with at least 1–2 cm normal tissue completely surrounding. The one exception to this 1–2 cm normal tissue cuff is when utilizing the mandibular periosteum as the lateral margin.

Frozen sections should be reserved for diagnosing cryptic areas of tumour (nerve invasion). Mucosal margins can be looked at with frozen sections by sampling tissue circumferentially around the defect. If there is any doubt about the validity of margins, as in densely irradiated tissue, reconstruction should be delayed. The excised specimen must be precisely oriented for the pathologist so there is no confusion.

The tongue base is particularly problematic because of the deep invasion commonly present. Excisional cuts need to be made squarely and deep to avoid tumour transgression. The surgeon must prepare himself and the patient for the possibility of losing both hypoglossal nerves. This could require additional laryngeal surgery for airway protection.

The posterior cuts with oropharyngeal tumours will be in close proximity to the internal carotid artery. Surgeons must always be aware of the location of this vessel. The pterygoid cuts should be the last ones made so that the specimen can be rapidly removed and the usually encountered brisk bleeding tamponaded. The deep dissection of posterior pharyngeal wall tumours should be in the prevertebral space. Cancer encroachment into this area is a grave prognostic sign.

Patients who have received preoperative chemotherapy or radiation and radiation failure cases can create significant problems for a surgeon. The dimensions of the tumour before preoperative therapy or before the radical radiation is what dictates the margins of excision. Even though the area of tumour involvement is visually smaller or even absent, the entire tumour bed is involved and must be removed. Surgeons utilizing induction chemotherapy and/or radiation therapy must carefully stage and map cancers before therapy is begun to avoid an incomplete ablation.

Ablation must proceed without consideration for reconstruction. Only after a complete tumour removal can formal plans for reconstruction begin.

PRINCIPLES OF RECONSTRUCTION

In rebuilding a large oropharyngeal defect the surgeon must understand the intricate relationships of the various areas during swallowing. Most oropharyngeal resections will not impair lip seal; however, when the ablation includes a hemimandibulectomy (or greater) there may be ipsilateral lower lip incompetence due to the lack of bony support. This must be anticipated and the lip suspended to avoid problems. The bolus preparation and transport phase is often affected with radical resections. Contact of tongue to hard palate and tongue mobility are the key items for this action. In general, the tongue and floor of the mouth are reconstructed as separate structures attempting to maximize tongue mobility, maintain a lingual vestibule, and restore sufficient height to the floor. Tongue bulk is most important posteriorly to help with the oropharyngeal phase of swallowing. The use of inferiorly pedicled musculocutaneous flaps to rebuild the base of tongue can result in increased tethering over time as the pedicle contracts. This can actually reduce a patient's function and require additional surgery.

The involuntary aspects of the swallow occur once the bolus reaches the oropharynx. The hyoid is pulled anteriorly and superiorly to contact the posterior pharynx and force the bolus down. The larynx follows the pull of the hyoid and the velopharynx seals off to prevent nasal regurgitation. With the larynx tilted up under the base of tongue and its tiered sphincter systems closed, the cricopharyngeus relaxes and the upper oesophagus opens to allow the bolus to pass (Shaker et al 1990). Oropharyngeal resections may alter velopharyngeal competence which can be addressed with a palatal or pharyngeal flap to narrow the area and reduce nasal regurgitation. The base of tongue contact with the posterior and lateral pharynx can be lost causing an inefficient transport of the food bolus which will create coordination and timing problems with upper oesophageal sphincter relaxation and laryngeal closure. This will cause pharyngeal pooling and aspiration and will tremendously frustrate patients. The surgeon should attempt to replace the soft-tissue defect with a comparable amount of tissue, try to rebuild base of tongue bulk, and address the larynx if a significant impact is expected. Laryngeal suspension and/or a cricopharyngeal myotomy (Goode 1975) will often help considerably in these situations.

This chapter will not discuss options for reconstruction of the jaw following a composite resection. There are several methods currently employed that provide excellent and dependable vascularized bone (Urkin 1991) for primary reconstruction. Metal bars/plates also work well to maintain the contour and occlusion (Shockley & Weissler 1990). The surgeon must decide whether rebuilding the jaw is in the patient's best interest. Restoring the contour of the jaw does improve cosmesis; however, a functional swallow is usually of greater concern for patients. The reconstruction of ramus/lateral body defects common with oropharyngeal composite resections can lead to increased trismus and limited jaw motion postoperatively. If the lateral defect is reconstructed with adequate tissue bulk (myocutaneous flap) and care taken to avoid malocclusion, then mandibular drift is usually insignificant. The surgeon should use internal maxillary fixation and/or active isometric exercises postoperatively until proper healing is well established to maximize results. Jaw opening and swallowing is generally better in these patients and the aesthetics are acceptable (Komisar 1990).

Small defects (up to 3–4 cm) created with a laser during a transoral approach can simply be left to heal by secondary intention. The limited thermal damage in surrounding tissue limits tissue infection and necrosis which greatly reduces pain. Defects of the tongue, tonsil, soft palate and posterior pharyngeal wall have all been managed successfully. Patients are allowed to eat as soon as is tolerable, and meticulous hygiene is stressed.

A skin or dermal graft can be used to resurface any of these small defects and can be applied to larger resection areas as well. With larger areas there is usually a partial loss of the graft with resultant scarring and reduction in function. Anytime raw bone is exposed these grafts will probably be inadequate.

Primary closure is also an alternative for many of the defects encountered. This is always the best option provided the postoperative function will not be significantly compromised. The larger the defect, the more likely primary reconstruction will tether tongue mobility, reduce the patient's ability to articulate and swallow and increase aspiration. Primary closures in previously operated or radiated patients tend to have more problems with wound breakdown and fistula.

RECONSTRUCTION TECHNIQUES

Defects of the lateral oropharynx with an intact mandibular arch

The actual dimensions of the defect and the involvement of the adjoining base of tongue and soft palate will certainly influence the applicability of the various options. Generally, musculocutaneous flaps will have much too much bulk for

these defects. The very best options are the temporalis muscle or musculofascial flap (Shagets et al 1986, Koranda & McMahon 1988), the superiorly based sternocleidomastoid flap (Tiwari 1990, Charles et al 1987) and the temporoparietal fascial flap (Panje & Morris 1991). Other useful options are the pectoralis muscle or musculofascial flap (Ariyan 1979), the masseter crossover flap (Tiwari & Snow 1989), the laterally based tongue flap (DeSanto et al 1975) and and the hard palatal island flap (Gullane & Arena 1979). Numerous free flaps have been applied to this area, the most significant being the split jejunal flap (Reuther et

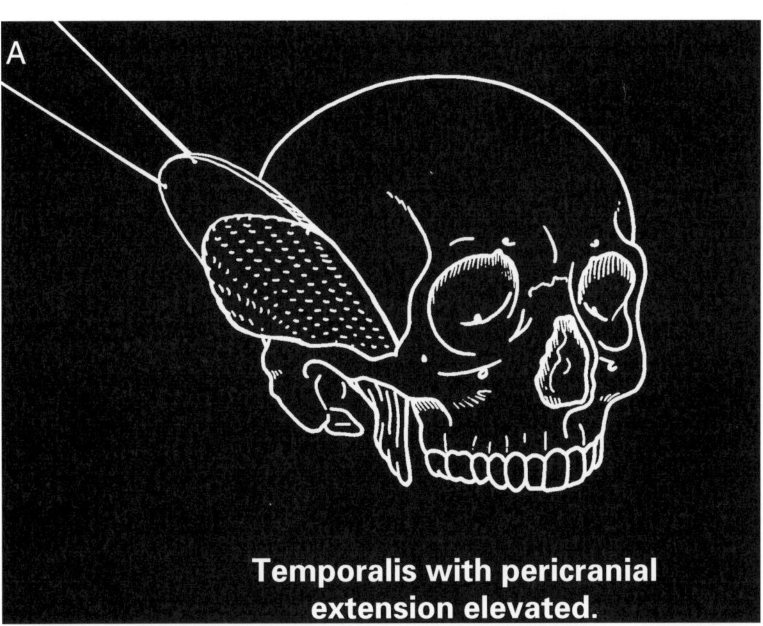

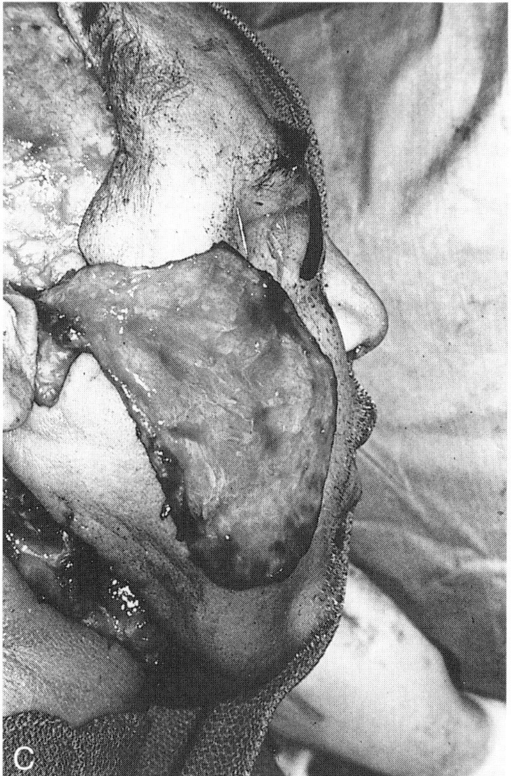

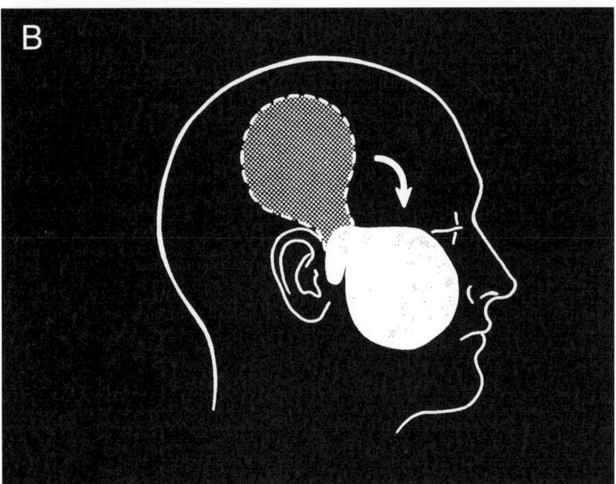

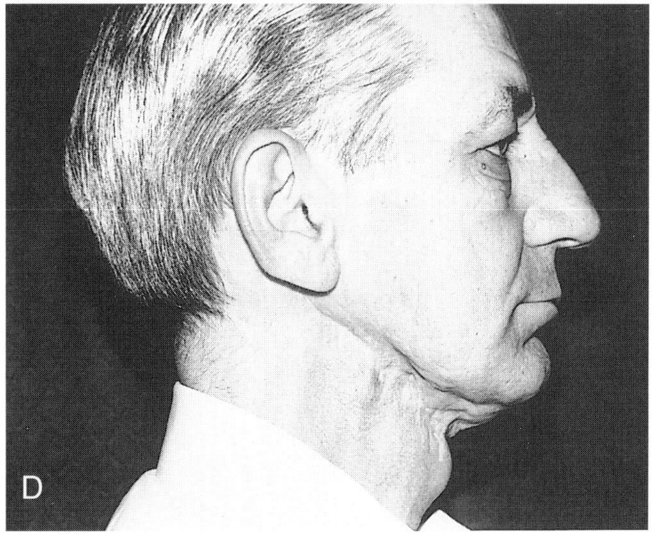

Fig. 11.9   A, B. Schematic representation of temporalis flap. **C.** Intraoperative photograph showing temporalis flap harvested and ready for transfer. **D.** Postoperative clinical photograph of patient.

al 1984, Buckspan et al 1986), the gastro-omental flap (Panje et al 1987) and the radial forearm flap (Soutar et al 1983). Each of these method will be discussed in some detail.

Temporalis flap (TF) (Fig. 11.9).

The vascular supply of the temporalis muscle arborizes in a manner that allows the muscle to be split coronally into separate anterior/posterior portions or sagittally into medial/lateral portions. The deep temporal fascia which can be harvested with the muscle actually has an axial blood supply of its own. A curvilinear incision is made from the helical base superiorly onto the lateral scalp. This is carried down through superficial layers to the deep temporal fascia. Scalp clips are useful to control bleeding. After gaining exposure, incisions are made through fascia and temporalis muscle circumferentially down to calvarium, except for the area of the zygomatic arch. The muscle is rapidly elevated from its fossa down to the arch area attachments. An incision is made through the fascia above the arch allowing a subfascial dissection over the arch for lateral exposure. A small incision is placed at the lateral canthal area and carried down to the malar eminence. A medial subfascial tunnel is developed and connected with the earlier dissection to allow full exposure of the arch. The bony zygomatic arch is removed to provided the necessary space to reflect the muscle. If a coroniodectomy is performed great care must be taken in separating the temporalis attachments posteriorly to avoid injury to the vascular supply. A tunnel is easily developed through the infratemporal area and the flap delivered into the defect area. The remaining mucosal edges are sewn to

the fascial or muscle surface so that a vest-over-pants overlap is created. This provides a more reinforced anastamosis and a better barrier to salivary penetration.

The advantages of the flap are its local availability, reliability, minimum donor morbidity, superiorly oriented pedicle and capacity to form two relatively independent components to 'regionalize' the reconstruction. The zygomatic arch can be rewired into place after reflecting the muscle; however, this is usually not cosmetically necessary.

Superiorly based sternocleidomastoid flap (SBSF) (Fig. 11.10)

When the management of the neck metastases so frequently present with oropharyngeal tumours permits a modified approach with preservation of the sternocleidomastoid (SCM), then this muscle can provide an ideal source of reconstructive tissue. The sternal/clavicular attachments of the muscle are separated and dissection proceeds superiorly only as far as needed to provide the necessary arc of rotation into the defect. The spinal accessory nerve (if preserved) may restrict the superior rotation. Preservation of the superior thyroid artery contribution should be attempted to improve the flap's vascular supply.

The mucosal edges of the defect are sutured to the muscle so that there is plenty of overlapping (vest-over-pants). The exposed muscle surface heals beautifully; however, a skin graft can be used if desired.

Temporoparietal fascial flap (TFF)

The temporoparietal fascia is a 2–4 mm thick, very vascular tissue in the lateral scalp that is in continuity with the galea/epicranius muscle/SMAS. The first step in developing this axial pattern flap is to verify and locate its arterial pedicle, the

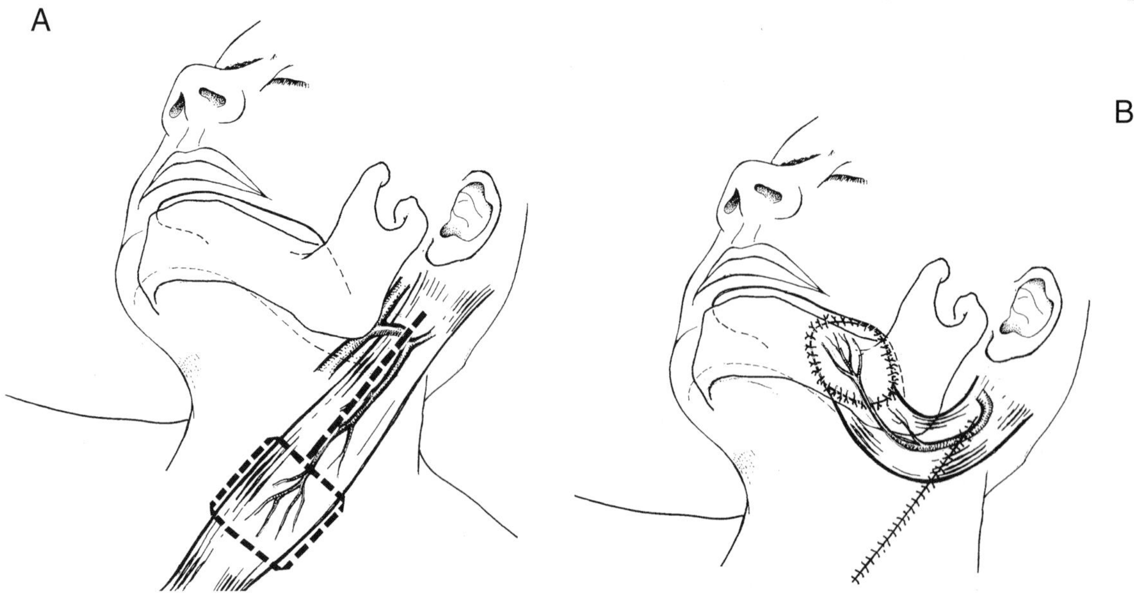

Fig. 11.10 A & B. Diagrammatic representation of the superiorly based sternomastoid myocutaneous flap.

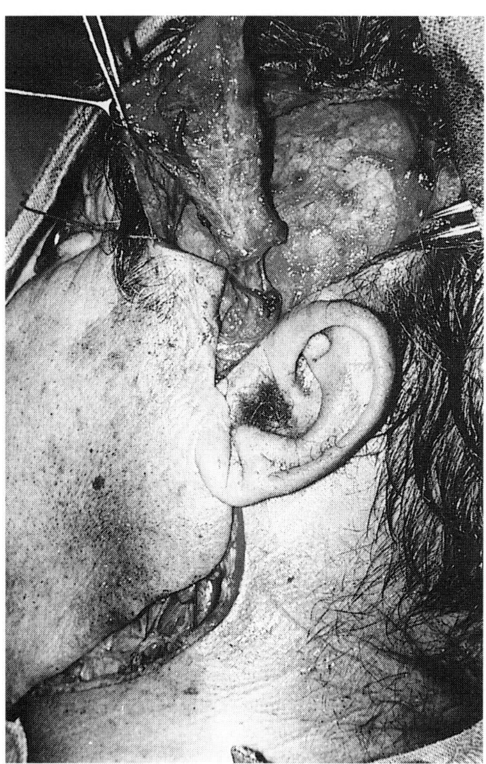

Fig. 11.11 Intraoperative photograph of temporoparietal fascial flap raised and ready for transfer. The vascular pedicle is visible.

superficial temporal artery. A curvilinear incision is made in the lateral scalp as was described for the temporalis flap; however, it is carried down only through the skin. The plane between the superficial fascia and subcutaneous scalp is easy to identify just above the ear. It becomes much more difficult to develop as dissection continues superiorly. Bipolar cautery is essential for the control of haemorrhage to avoid excessive damage to hair follicles. Once the desired amount of fascia is exposed it is circumferentially incised down to the deep temporal fascia (or pericranium) preserving the area of the vascular pedicle (Fig. 11.11). The pedicle is then carefully narrowed and dissected proximally over the zygoma. A tunnel is then developed bluntly from below the zygoma into the oropharynx to allow passage of the flap. The zygoma can be temporarily removed, if necessary to facilitate exposure and delivery and then rewired into place at the conclusion of the case. The workability and versatility of this tissue allows it to conform to complex defects. Mucosal edges are sewn to the tissue with the overlap previously described. The exposed surface of the flap is left to granulate.

Pectoralis muscle flap (PMF)

The pectoralis major is the workhorse flap for most head and neck surgeons. The musculocutaneous flap is ideal for reconstructing lateral composite resections; however, it is

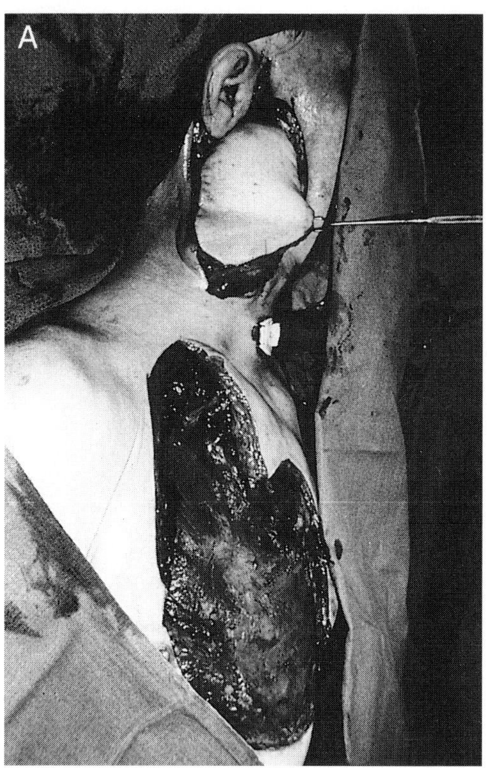
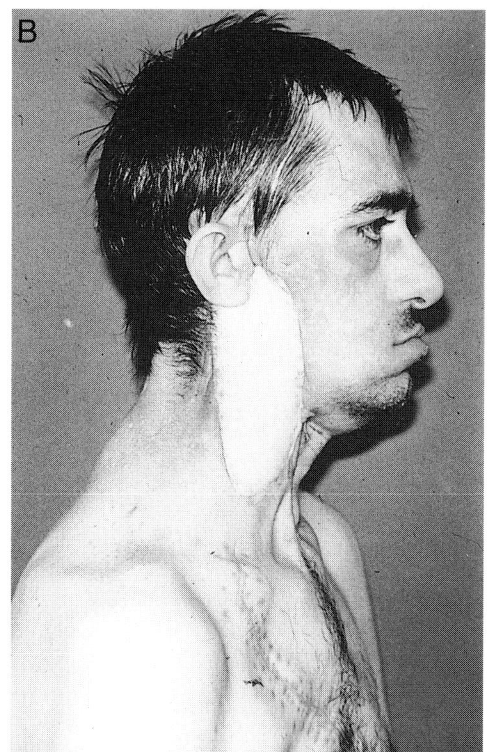

Fig. 11.12 A, B. Pectoralis major myocutaneous flap.

usually too bulky for repairing defects with an intact mandible (Fig. 11.12). The bulk problem is avoided by utilizing a muscle only or a myofascial flap (Fig. 11.13). An incision is placed along the anterior axillary line and carried down to the lateral edge of the muscle. The anterior surface of the muscle is quickly exposed by elevating on a subfascial plane. The avascular plane between the pectoralis major and minor is bluntly developed and the thoracoacromial pedicle identified. The medial, inferior and lateral margins of the muscle are then separated distally to proximally, providing a broad attachment. The pedicle is narrowed (but never skeletonized) as the clavicular portion of the muscle is separated. Dissec-

tion proximally should proceed only as far as needed to provide for rotation into the defect. The flap is reflected over the clavicle up into the defect. The mucosal edges of the defect are sewn to the muscle with as much overlap as possible. A skin or dermal graft can then be secured and quilted to the exposed surface of the muscle.

Masseter cross-over flap (MCF)

This flap is suitable for defects in the tonsillar fossa/pillar area (Fig. 11.14). A visor or cheek flap is necessary to expose the masseter. The muscle is detached from the visor or cheek flap subfascially (if not already elevated) and freed from the mandible and parotid. The tissue is next rotated over the jaw under any buccal/alveolar mucosa remaining. Some bony contouring of the superior medial aspect of the retromolar trigone region will be necessary. The masseter is anastamosed with the tongue base creating a sling arrangement (Fig.

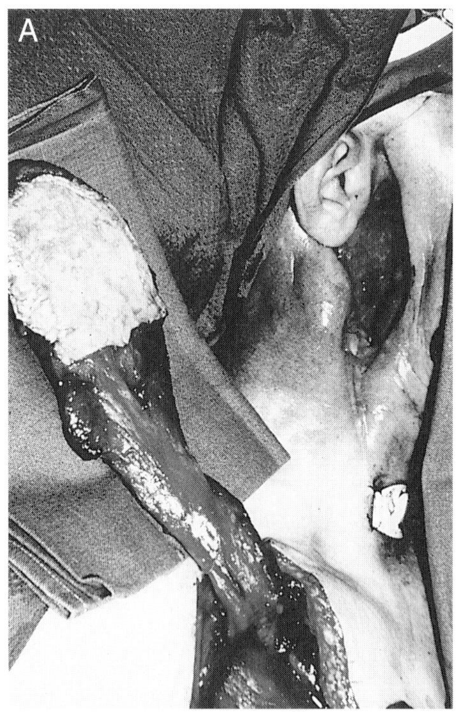

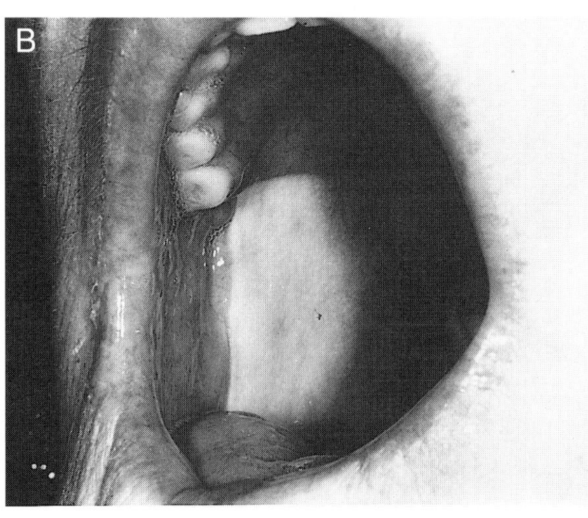

Fig. 11.13 **A.** Pectoralis major myofascial flap with dermal graft. Ready for transfer. **B.** Postoperative intra-oral view of the healed graft.

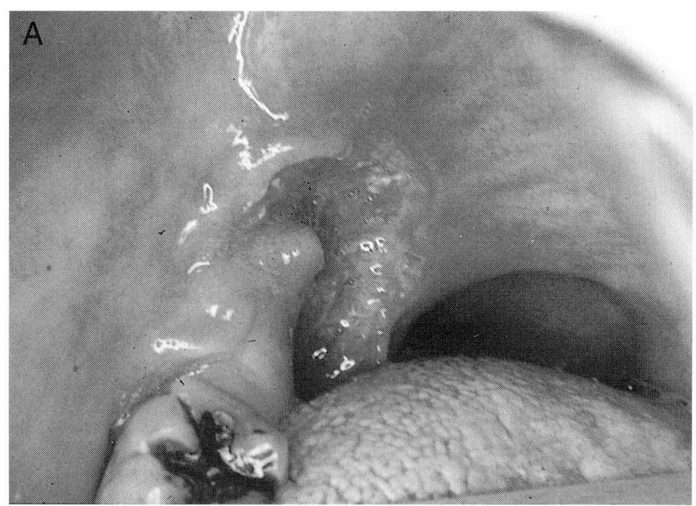

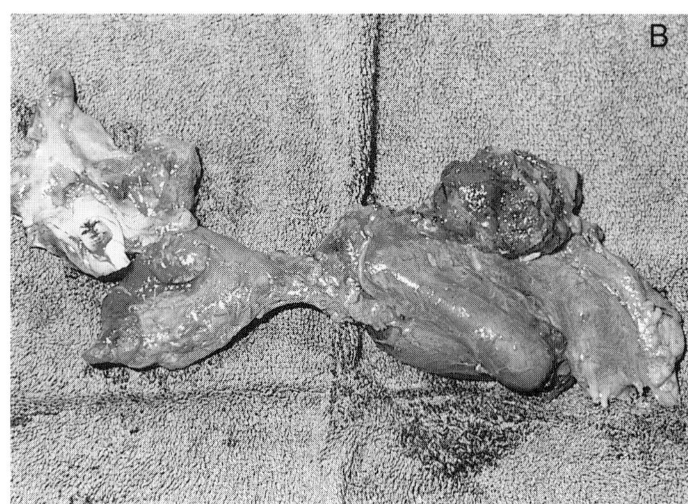

Fig. 11.14 **A.** A T2 squamous-cell carcinoma of the anterior pillar of the tonsil. **B.** Operative specimen, showing excised tumour with marginal mandibular resection and en bloc neck dissection.

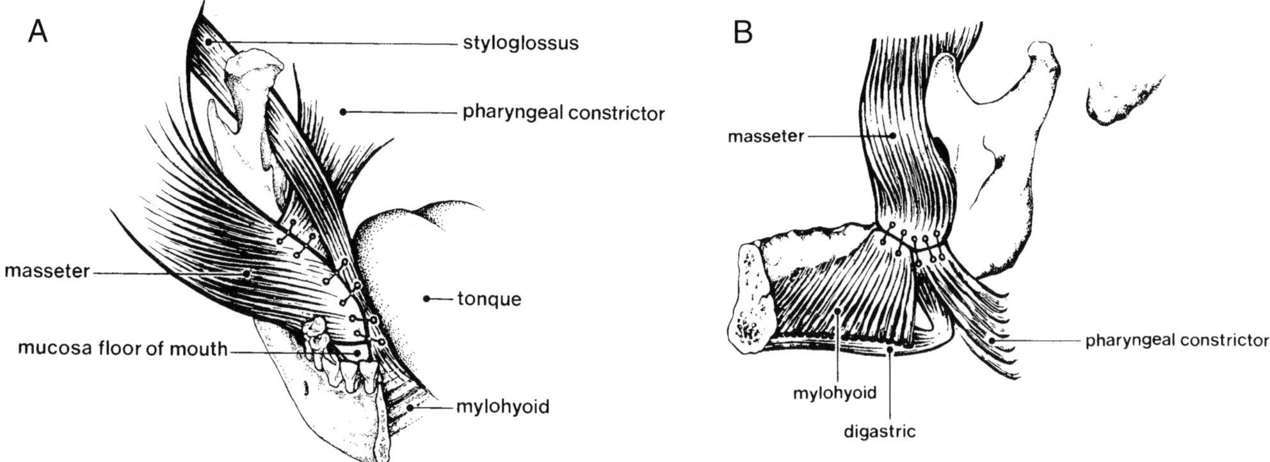

Fig. 11.15 A, B. Diagrammatic representation of masseter muscle transfer for oropharyngeal–oral reconstruction. (Reproduced with permission from John Wiley & Son Inc. Head and Neck Surgery.)

11.15). The elevated buccal/alveolar mucosa is usually of sufficient quantity to close the defect primarily. This provides the patient with a sensate mucosal surface and very functional swallow (Fig. 11.16).

Laterally based tongue flap (LBTF)

The tongue offers a good source of tissue for rebuilding oropharyngeal defects. The tissue is reliable, locally available, and quickly dissected; however, one must remember that the goal of the reconstruction is to maximize the function of the tongue. Sacrificing the tongue for reconstruction may be detrimental to patient function and for this reason the surgeon should consider other options before selecting an LBTF. The flap is based on the lateral floor of mouth attachments. A midline incision is made through the mucosa of the tongue and into the intrinsic musculature for

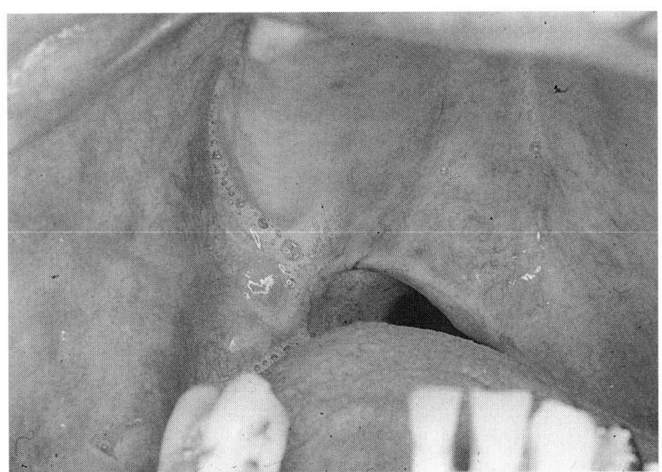

Fig. 11.16 Postoperative intra-oral photograph of the same patient as in Fig. 11.14A.

1–2 mm. A myomucosal flap is developed by unrolling the lateral tongue sharply. This tissue can then be rotated into the defect and secured. The remaining tongue is closed on itself.

Hard palatal island flap (HPIF)

The mucoperiosteum of the hard palate can be pedicled on a single greater palatine vascular pedicle and reflected into the retromolar trigone, anterior tonsil, or soft palate area for reconstruction. The tissue is somewhat stiff and should be avoided in previously radiated patients. It is fairly well vascularized, reliable and locally available making it a valuable alternative for these defects.

The palatal mucosa is incised sharply (laser is useful) from the greater palatine foramen of the contralateral side around to just adjacent to the ipsilateral foramen. About 1 cm cuff of mucosa is left on the pedicle to avoid skeletonizing. The tissue is bluntly elevated off the palate and rotated into the surgical defect. The donor site is left to granulate or a palatal prosthesis can be inserted to cover the denuded bone until it heals.

Split jejunal flap (SJF)

This method of reconstruction offers the advantage of reconstituting an oropharynx with a vascularized mucosal surface. The harvesting of the jejunum is done by a general surgeon concomitant with the cancer ablation. A segment of jejunum is located that can be isolated on a single vascular pedicle. Once the ablation is complete, the jejunum still desired, and recipient vessels identified and prepared, the jejunal segment (12–15 cm) is detached and the pedicle dissected and separated as proximally as possible. The jejunum is split along the antimesenteric border after the cervical reanastamosis is completed. The revascularized mucosa is then inserted into the defect and the mucosal edges sewn. A feeding jejunostomy is placed before the abdomen is closed and a jejuno-jejunostomy is performed. The morbidity of an intra-abdominal operation to obtain tissue must be carefully considered. There is no question that for circumferential pharyngeal defects a revascularized jejunum is the Mercedes repair, but for simply resurfacing the oropharynx it seems a bit extreme. When compared with reconstruction with a gastric patch, the jejunum has other drawbacks. The jejunal mucous is very scant and not of much significance, mucosal folds are often quite pronounced and can actually trap food, and the tissue has limited bulk for reconstituting any soft tissue loss. The gastric patch (see below) flattens out over time and secretes an abundant amount of mucous that can have a profound impact on a patient's xerostomia and dysphagia problems. A large volume of omentum can be included with the gastric patch satisfying any need for bulk and reinforcing the mucosal closure.

Gastro-omental flap (GF)

The GF replaces the resected tissue with a secreting mucosal surface. The mucosa of the greater curvature is secreting, supple and pliable allowing it to conform to complex defects and significantly help with xerostomia if present preoperatively. The harvesting of the flap is done by a general surgeon and can proceed simultaneously with the ablation. A GIAR stapler is used to remove the necessary amount of the greater curvature (up to 144 cm^2). A large omental flap can be left pedicled along with the gastric patch. The right gastro-epiploic artery is the usual pedicle and it can be traced proximally to provide a long (10–12 cm) length. The feeding vessels are not separated until the ablation is complete and the surgeon has identified good recipient vessels for a micro-re-anastamosis. Once the transfer and revascularization are complete the gastric patch is secured to the mucosa surrounding the defect and the omentum fills in any dead space. This is one of the finest methods available to resurface an oral cavity or oropharyngeal defect in a xerostomic patient providing adequate recipient vessels can be located. A feeding jejunostomy is placed before the abdomen is closed.

Radial forearm flap (RFF)

This flap is relatively quick and easy to harvest and provides for a very long pedicle. The tissue is quite pliable and ideally suited for resurfacing the complex contours of the oral cavity and oropharynx. These facts underscore the immense popularity of this tissue in reconstruction; however, one significant drawback must be stressed: albeit only rarely reported, a contracture of the hand can occur as a result of using this tissue. This potentially devastating donor morbidity must

be considered in the light of the vast number of other excellent options available for oropharyngeal reconstruction.

The donor area also provides cutaneous nerves that can bridge a motor nerve gap or be re-anastamosed to the lingual nerve to make a sensate cutaneous flap. Patients gain sensory information from this technique that has proven to be of value in their functional rehabilitation postoperatively. A preoperative Allen test is essential, and the results are documented in the chart. The flap design is centred over the radial artery on the volar aspect of the forearm. The vessels are located and marked out as well. The first incision is made inferiorly in the area of the cosmic snuffbox allowing for positive identification of the radial artery. Medial and lateral incisions are then made and the skin reflected toward the septum between the bracheoradialis and flexor carpi radialis. The sensory nerves (medial/lateral antebrachial) are found on top of the brachioradialis. The surgeon should carefully watch for a good vein during elevation of the flap. Usually the cephalic vein is the best option, and it, along with the radial artery, is tracked superiorly to provide good pedicle length. Only the inferior one-half of the flap is attached to the vessels. The donor tissue is left in situ until the recipient site has been prepared. When ready to transfer, the vascular pedicle is severed as proximally as possible. After revascularization (and re-innervating) the flap is used to fill the defect.

The donor site is closed with a split thickness skin graft. It is important to preserve Tenon's capsule over the tendons so that the graft will take. The forearm is then splinted in a neutral position. Alternative management of the donor area is to close primarily with a local transposition flap or to tissue expand pre-operatively.

Defects of the base of tongue (BOT)

Tumours in this area must be widely resected and occasionally both hypoglossal nerves will be sacrificed. If only one-half of the tongue base is lost and there is good contralateral function the best option would be a tongue set-back flap (Komisar & Lawson 1985). This will recreate the BOT bulk and maintain anterior tongue mobility. Other alternatives are the superiorly based sternocleidomastoid (SCM) muscle flap or the re-innervated SCM musculocutaneous flap (Mikaelian 1984). Inferiorly pedicled muscle or musculocutaneous flaps tend to have substantial contraction over time and this can lead to tethering and compromise of function. Free flaps avoid the problem of pedicle contraction and can be applied to this situation; however, it should be understood that patients can generally tolerate the loss of one-half of the base of the tongue and retain adequate function with minimal aspiration. This fact, coupled with the added time, expense and operative risks involved with regional and free flaps, seems to make them an inappropriate choice for managing this defect.

When the function of both hypoglossal nerves is lost

along with the total or near-total bulk of the tongue base, the operator is faced with a major league problem. It is important to maintain any anterior tongue if possible and incorporate it into the reconstruction since it provides valuable sensation information for initiating a swallow. The decision of how to protect the airway will be based on several factors. In medically unstable, debilitated, mentally handicapped or alcoholic patients it is probably best to remove the larynx to avoid the devastating aspiration that is sure to occur. The total/near-total glossectomy defect with laryngectomy can be reconstructed with a trapezius island flap (Netterville et al 1987), a pectoralis major, or latissimus dorsi musculocutaneous flap, as well as the previously described free flaps.

With motivated and healthy patients, the tongue reconstruction can be coupled with laryngeal suspension/cricopharyngeal myotomy (Goode 1975) and/or epiglottoplasty/laryngo-plasty (Biller et al 1983) to retain a lung-powered voice. The tongue bulk must be maintained and a very active rehabilitation effort is essential to succeed with these people. The best method for reconstruction in this situation seems to be the re-innervated latissimus dorsi musculocutaneous free or pedicled flap (Haughey & Fredrickson 1991). The re-innervated SCM musculocutaneous flap (Mikaelian 1984) can succeed in a less than total defect. The lateral thigh (Hayden 1991) and radial forearm neurofasciocutaneous free flaps have been applied with success as well.

Tongue set-back flap (TSF)

This flap is the very best method for reconstructing a hemi-base of tongue defect from the vallecula to the circumvalate papilla. It is locally available, extremely easy to develop and satisfies the requisites of maintaining anterior tongue motility and posterior tongue bulk. The patient will function excellently following this reconstruction. After the ablation is complete and good margins are obtained, the anterior tongue is split down the midline all the way to the level of the hyoid. The remaining anterior tongue is then set back into the base defect pedicled on lateral floor of the mouth and anterior/inferior muscle attachments. The contralateral anterior hemitongue is closed on itself (Fig. 11.17).

Re-innervated SCM musculocutaneous flap (RSF)

The 11th nerve innervation of the SCM muscle is routinely identified during head and neck surgery. It can be easily transected and re-anastamosed with the ipsilateral hypoglossal nerve if necessary to prevent muscle atrophy. The transferred muscle is pedicled superiorly, thus avoiding the tethering problem previously discussed. The bulk of the tissue is also very compatible with the tongue base defect requirements. The overlying skin, if transferred, has little intervening fat, which is ideal for oral reconstruction.

The myocutaneous flap must be planned for before making any neck incisions. The amount of skin that can be transferred is limited to the width of the muscle, and a 1–2 cm random extension over the clavicle can be added. An island type of pedicle is not very reliable and is discouraged, especially in previously radiated patients. The skin over the entire muscle is mobilized with the muscle and great care is taken to identify and preserve the superior thyroid artery contribution. The excess skin and any overlying the portion of muscle being tunnelled into the defect is de-epithelialized. The muscle is secured to the tongue musculature, and the cutaneous tissue secured to the mucosal edges of the defect. The neck skin can be closed primarily.

A

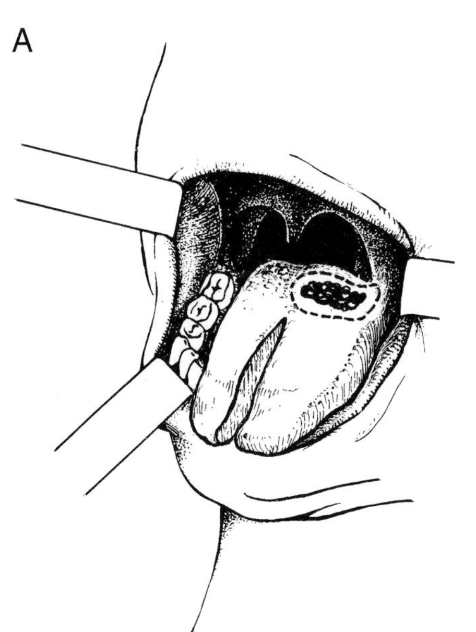

B

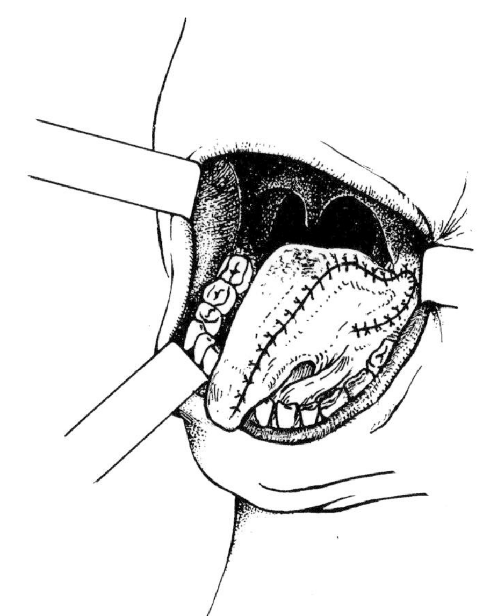

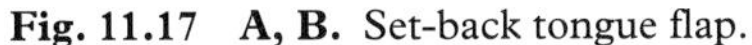

Fig. 11.17 A, B. Set-back tongue flap.

Trapezius island flap (TIF) (Fig. 11.18)

The island flap is based on the transverse cervical vessels so the integrity of this pedicle must be ascertained before committing to this flap. The course of the transverse cervical vein will usually dictate the available arc of utilization of the flap. Once the artery and vein have been clearly identified and felt to be anatomically suited, the flap can be designed. The cutaneous island is generally centred on the acromion and up to 40% of the area can be located over the deltoid. This will provide a two-level flap, one section composed of skin, subcutaneous tissue, and muscle, and one section composed of only supple skin and subcutaneous tissue. As can be imagined, this is an ideal arrangement for base of tongue defects with the bulky part filling posteriorly and the supple part resurfacing anteriorly.

The deltoid portion of the flap is incised and elevated up to the scapular spine. The remainder of the paddle is incised down to the underlying trapezius muscle. The posterior and superior muscle cuts are made utilizing a finger under the muscle protecting the pedicle. The flap is developed in a posterior-to-anterior direction with care to look for the ascending branch of the dorsal scapular artery. When encountered, it can be dissected inferiorly for a short distance and ligated. This will provide a site for re-anastamosis, if needed, during the reconstruction. The final muscle cuts along the spine are facilitated by placing a finger along the levator scapulae down to its insertion. The muscle is divided superficial to this plane. The flap is then rotated into the surgical defect, sewing muscle to muscle and cutaneous tissue to the mucosal edges. The vascular supply to this flap is not protected by a muscular cuff like in the pectoralis major, so that the surgeon must be careful not to skeletonize the vessels when developing the pedicle. He must also ensure that there is no tension on the vessels when the flap is in place; otherwise, complications will arise. The donor area can be closed primarily or skin grafted.

The accessory nerve should not be denervated for the sake of using a trapezius flap in the reconstruction. Conversely, use of the island flap does not necessarily require interfering with the innervation of the muscle. In other words, this flap can be elevated and still retain the function of the remaining, undisturbed trapezius. It is generally best to avoid this flap unless the 11th nerve has been cut during the ablation.

As with the pectoralis major, this flap provides for an excellent closure of a lateral composite defect.

Re-innervated latissimus dorsi musculocutaneous flap (RLDF)

This musculocutaneous flap is the distal extent of a vascular pedicle that gives rise to the serratus anterior muscle/musculocutaneous flap, the parascapular/scapular fasciocutaneous flaps, and the lateral scapula bone flap. The reconstructive potential of this combination of flaps is remarkable. The nerve supply to the latissimus can also be harvested with the flap and re-anastamosed to the hypoglossal

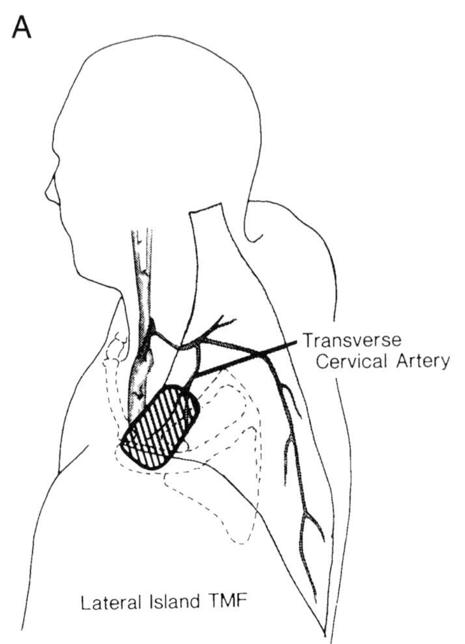

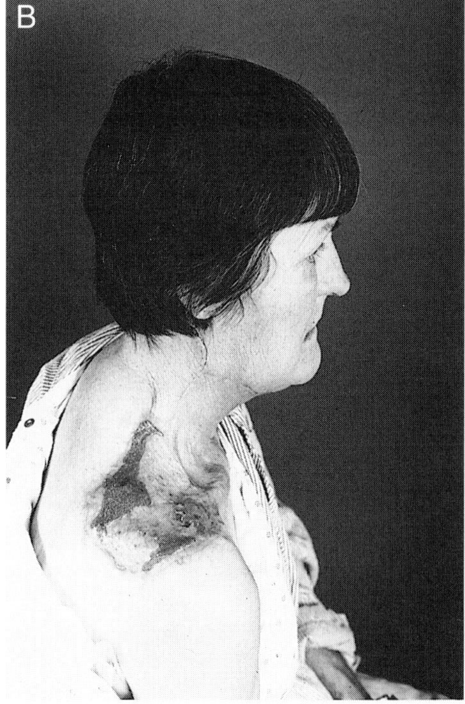

Fig. 11.18 A. Lateral trapezius island myocutaneous flap. **B.** Clinical photograph of patient showing donor area after split skin grafting.

nerve. This will prevent the normal muscle atrophy secondary to the denervation that occurs during flap elevation and delivery. The bulk of this musculocutaneous flap is ideal for rebuilding lateral composite defects. The morbidity of losing this muscle involves trunk rotation and will have a limited affect on shoulder strength. Latissimus function is of prime importance for golfers and skiers so be sure to question patients about their hobbies and recognize the impact of your reconstructive choice.

For total glossectomy defects the free flap design is preferred to avoid the tethering inherent with an inferior pedicle. The cutaneous portion of the flap is centred over the midpart of the muscle where there is a greater density of perforators. Its design should correspond with the dimensions of the oral defect. The island is incised circumferentially down to the underlying muscle and tacked down. An incision is placed to run along the posterior axillary line (anterior border of latissimus) superiorly into the axilla. The vascular pedicle runs longitudinally about 2–3 cm inside the anterior border of the muscle. The latissimus–serratus junction is located and bluntly dissected to separate the latissimus. The inferior and medial muscle incisions are made away from the island to provide good overlap for the reconstruction. The flap is reflected superiorly and the pedicle identified and traced proximally. The vessels separate from the muscle 6–8 cm from its insertion into the humerus, so that dissection in this area must be careful. A pedicle with good length and relatively large vessels is easy to develop. Once revascularization and re-innervation have been successfully completed the reconstruction begins. The flap is suspended at the tonsillar fossa area providing an anterior-horizontal portion and a posterior-vertical portion just as with the tongue. The flap is actually sewn to the superior constrictors with the tonsillar fossa and to the remaining pterygoids to form a sling configuration at the oropharyngeal inlet. The flap must have enough height to just contact the hard palate at rest. Patients have successfully regained swallowing function with minimal aspiration. Even supraglottic laryngectomy patients have been rehabilitated with this technique. The ability to maintain a lung-powered voice is great for the patient's well-being; however, one must not overapply this technique. Debilitated, alcoholic and mentally impaired patients will have great problems with rehabilitation and may develop significant aspiration-related sequelae. It is these people who would probably be best managed with a total laryngectomy following a total glossectomy.

The major drawback with utilizing the latissimus flap is that the patient must be in a lateral decubitus position. Most cancer ablations in the head and neck can be easily accomplished with the patient in a lateral decubitus position so that all it takes is to have good prior planning.

Lateral cutaneous thigh neurofasciocutaneous flap (LCTF)

This flap is quite useful for total glossectomy reconstruction. It is a neuro(fascio)-cutaneous flap so that no atrophy will occur, and a branch of the lateral femoral cutaneous nerve can be harvested with the donor tissue, allowing for re-innervation. The sensory information provided can be helpful to a patient's postoperative rehabilitation. The 3rd perforating branch of the profunda femoris perfuses a large amount of lateral thigh skin. A line is drawn from the greater trochanter to the lateral limit of knee to form an axis on which to design the flap and locate the perforators. The 4th perforator is a continuation of the profunda and can be incorporated into the flap to improve perfusion. A long flap design should always be done so that no perforators are missed and closure is easier. The anterior incision is made down to the tensor fascia lata and the tissue folded back on itself until the fascial septum is identified. The perforators travel within this septum and great care must be taken to avoid inadvertent injury. The septum should be initially incised below the perforators which are visible, relatively small and subject to easy spasm. Proximal dissection will identify the linea aspera which must be separated from the underlying femur. The 4th perforator should be preserved if possible but all muscular branches encountered are ligated. The pedicle will travel through the short head of the biceps so a cuff of this muscle is taken to avoid skeletonization. The pedicle should be followed only as proximally as the junction of the 2nd perforator. This vessel must be preserved as it is the key supply to the femur and surrounding musculature. Once the pedicle dissection has been completed the posterior flap is incised and elevated and the flap is left in situ until the ablation is completed and the recipient site prepared. This will allow for re-evaluation of the flap's perfusion and confidence in its design. The harvesting of this flap can be done at the same time as the cancer ablation. The cutaneous supply to the skin is relatively hyperperfused by the dissected pedicle. When transfer is ready, the pedicle is separated close to the 2nd perforator. The cutaneous nerve is re-anastamosed to the lingual nerve. Once revascularization of the flap has been successfully completed, the tissue is contoured to recreate a tongue shape with careful attention to obtain enough height so that good contact with the hard palate is achieved. The flap is of fairly uniform thickness so that it can be quite mouldable. The donor area can be closed primarily or with a split thickness skin graft. The donor morbidity is relatively limited. There is a potential for hair growth and the cutaneous tissue is dry but people have the potential to swallow without aspiration. Proper patient selection and aggressive rehabilitation are the keys to success.

Laryngoplasty

Another method of retaining a lung-powered voice following a total glossectomy and providing a patient with significant protection from aspiration is to perform a laryngoplasty. An incision is made down each aryepiglottic fold, over the arytenoid, and into the interarytenoid area. An inner and outer flap are created with limited dissection and the two sides of the supraglottis are closed in an inner then outer layer. The entire laryngeal inlet will be obliterated except for a small opening at the tip of the epiglottis. The glossectomy defect can then be closed with virtually any of the musculocutaneous or free flaps described. Patients are maintained with a tracheostomy but do well with speech. This closure can be reversed partially or totally if it is felt that patients have regained adequate control of their secretions. It seems a better alternative to a diversion because it allows for a lung-powered voice while being a reversible procedure.

Defects secondary to pharyngo-cutaneous fistula

Fistulas can be early/acute, occurring in the immediate postoperative period, or delayed/late. Infection and poor wound healing are usually the culprits with postoperative fistulas. These are managed initially by opening the neck to allow debridement and provide for controlled salivary egress. Aggressive local wound care and good nutrition will usually allow healing by secondary intention.

Delayed fistulas or non-healing early fistulas should cause concern for recurrent or cryptic tumour and/or osteoradionecrosis. Significant diabetes or hypothyroidism can also predispose a patient to develop this problem. Several factors will force surgical intervention in managing a fistula and include exposure of vital structures (carotid artery), need to initiate radiation therapy within an appropriate time (6 weeks postoperatively), patient desires (job, desire to eat), and significant patient morbidity (pain from radionecrosis, maceration of adjoining skin). The surgeon must remove all contaminated and diseased tissue and then reconstruct the defect in three layers if possible: an internal cutaneous or mucosal layer, an intervening layer of well-vascularized tissue, and an outer cutaneous layer. The vest-over-pants principle is essential to prevent recurrence of the problem. Any musculocutaneous flap and many free flaps will work nicely; however, the superiorly based trapezius flap (Netterville et al 1987) and the omental free flap (Panje & Pitcock 1989) deserve special mention.

Superiorly based trapezius flap (STF)

This flap is supplied primarily by the paraspinous perforators (usually only 3–4) and secondarily by the occipital artery so that it is available even after a radical neck dissection. It provides excellent cutaneous coverage for defects of the lateral neck up to the buccal area. An incision is made along the anterior border of the trapezius muscle down to the level of the acromion. The posterior incision runs roughly parallel to the anterior one travelling toward the midline at the C5–6 level. After crossing over the midline it turns cephalad for

a short distance. The caudal incision is placed along the scapular spine. Random deltoid extensions of skin have been successfully employed. The plane deep to the trapezius is bluntly developed and the dissection started inferiorly to superiorly. A finger along the levator scapulae helps define the proper level over the superior scapula. The posterior incision through the muscle is carried only as far as necessary to provide the necessary arc of rotation into the defect. Once adequate rotation has been achieved the fistula site is debrided. With old chronic fistulas turn-in flaps can be developed to provide the internal layer of closure. An alternative would be to skin graft the undersurface of the muscle. The outer skin margins of the defect are undermined for 2–4 cm so that the muscle can be tucked in and good overlapping created. This will make it hard for saliva to leak out and reinforces the internal and external closures with well-vascularized muscle. The donor defect may be closed primarily; however, a skin graft is frequently needed. This flap is very reliable, and nearly always immediately available, and it provides an excellent option for managing fistula with carotid exposure.

Omental free flap (OF)

The omentum is the best reparative tissue the body has. It can conform to complex defects just as water in a cup. The rich lymphatic network within the omentum combined with its vascularity allow it to heal just about any wound encountered in the head and neck. On occasion, the stagnant lymphoedema that accompanies our patients following aggressive surgery/radiation therapy is actually improved with an omental flap as it provides bridging lymphatic channels that help reduce the oedema. The omentum is harvested by a general surgeon through an upper midline incision. Work on the fistula site can be done simultaneously with the abdominal dissection. The recipient site must be thoroughly debrided of all necrotic tissue and bone and vessels for re-anastamosis must be located. The omental flap is developed by incorporating two to three vessel arcades down to the distal take-off from the gastroepiploic. The pedicle usually consists of the right gastroepiploic vessels and can be dissected proximally for several centimetres. Once the transfer is ready, the pedicle is separated and the re-anastomosis is performed. Omentum is unique in that it can just fill in the defect and there is no need for a mucosal or skin covering. The omentum is tucked around the mucosal edges so that a vest-over-pants arrangement is created and the exposed surfaces are left to granulate. A skin graft can be used if desired. A feeding gastrostomy or jejunostomy is created before closing the abdomen. This tissue is unmatched in its reparative ability and the surgeon should remember it whenever faced with a difficult head and neck wound.

REFERENCES

Ariyan S 1979 The pectoralis major myocutaneous flap. Plastic and Reconstructive Surgery 63: 73–81

Biller H F, Lawson W et al 1983 Total glossectomy. Archives of Otolaryngology 109: 69–73

Buckspan G S, Newton E D et al 1986 Split jejunal free-tissue transfer in oropharyngoesophageal reconstruction. Plastic and Reconstructive Surgery 77: 717–726

Charles G A, Hamaker R C et al 1987 Sternocleidomastoid myocutaneous flap. Laryngoscope 97: 970–974

DeSanto L W, Whicker J H et al 1975 Mandibular osteotomy and lingual flaps. Archives of Otolaryngology 101: 652–655

Goode R L 1975 Laryngeal suspension in head and neck surgery. Laryngoscope 85: 349–355

Gullane P J, Arena S 1977 Palatal island flap for reconstruction of oral defects. Archives of Otolaryngology 103: 598–599

Haughey B H, Fredrickson J M 1991 The latissimus dorsi donor site. Archives of Otolaryngology—Head and Neck Surgery 117 : 1129–1134

Hayden R 1991 Symposium on reconstruction of the tongue. Presented at the American Academy of Facial Plastic and Reconstructive Meeting, Kansas City, Mo, September 1991

Komisar A 1990 The functional results of mandibular reconstruction. Laryngoscope 100: 346–373

Komisar A, Lawson W 1985 A compendium of intraoral flaps. Head and Neck Surgery 8: 91–99

Koranda F C, McMahon M F 1988 The temporalis muscle flap for intraoral reconstruction: technical modifications. Otolaryngology—Head and Neck Surgery 98: 315–318

LaFerriere K A, Sessions D G et al 1980 Composite resection and reconstruction for oral cavity and oropharynx cancer. Archives of Otolaryngology 106: 103–110

Leemans C R, Tiwari R et al 1991 Discontinuous vs in-continuity neck dissection in carcinoma of the oral cavity. Archives of Otolaryngology—Head and Neck Surgery 117: 1003–1006

MacFee W F 1960 Transverse incision for neck dissection. Annals of Surgery 151: 279–284

McGregor I A, MacDonald D G 1983 Mandibular osteotomy in the surgical approach to the oral cavity. Head and Neck Surgery 5: 457-462

McGregor A D, MacDonald D G 1988 Routes of entry of squamous cell carcinoma to the mandible. Head and Neck Surgery 10: 294–301

Marchetta F C, Sako K et al 1971 The periosteum of the mandible and intraoral carcinoma. American Journal of Surgery 122: 711–713

Mikaelian D O 1984 Reconstruction of the tongue. Laryngoscope 94: 34–37

Netterville J L., Panje W R et al 1987 The trapezius myocutaneous flap. Archives of Otolaryngology—Head and Neck Surgery 113: 271–281

Panje W R, Morris M R 1991 The temporoparietal fascia flap in head and neck reconstruction. ENT J 70: 311–317

Panje W R, Pitcock J K 1989 Free omental flap reconstruction of complicated head and neck wounds. Otolaryngology—Head and Neck Surgery 100: 88–93

Panje W R, Little A G et al 1987 Immediated free gastro-omental flap reconstruction of the mouth and throat. Annals of Otolaryngology, Rhinology and Laryngology 96: 15–21

Panje W R, Scher N et al 1989 Transoral carbon dioxide ablation for cancer, tumours, and other diseases. Archives of Otolaryngology—Head and Neck Surgery 115: 681–688

Reuther J F, Steinau H U et al 1984. Reconstruction of large defects in the oropharynx with a revascularized intestinal graft: an experimental and clinical report. Plastic and Reconstructive Surgery 77: 717–726

Shagets F W, Panje W R et al 1986 Use of temporalis muscle in complicated defects of the head and face. Archives of Otolaryngology—Head and Neck Surgery 112: 60–65

Shaker R, Dodds W J et al 1990 Coordination of deglutitive glottic closure with oropharyngeal swallowing. Gastroenterology 98: 1478–1484

Shockley W W, Weissler M C 1991 Immediate mandibular replacement using reconstruction plates. Archives of Otolaryngology—Head and Neck Surgery 117: 745–749

Soutar D S, Scheker L R, et al 1983 The radial forearm flap : A versatile method for intra-oral reconstruction. British Journal of Plastic Surgery 36: 1–8

Spiro R H, Gerold F P et al 1981. Mandible 'swing' approach for oral and oropharyngeal tumours. Head and Neck Surgery 3: 371–378

Tiwari R M 1990 Experiences with the sternocleidomastoid muscle and myocutaneous flaps. Journal of Laryngology and Otolaryngology 104: 315–321

Tiwari R M, Snow G B 1989 Role of masseter crossover flap in oropharyngeal reconstruction. Journal of Laryngology and Otolaryngology 103: 298–301

Tollefsen H R, Spiro R H et al 1971 Median labiomandibular glossotomy. Annals of Surgery 173: 415–420

Urkin M L 1991 Composite free flaps in oromandibular reconstruction. Archives of Otolaryngology—Head and Neck Surgery 117: 724–731

Urkin M L, Weinberg H et al 1990 The neurofasciocutaneous radial forearm flap in head and neck reconstruction: a preliminary report. Laryngoscope 100: 161–173

12. The hypopharynx

Jatin P. Shah   Dennis H. Kraus

Jatin P. Shah   Dennis H. Kraus

INTRODUCTION AND HISTORICAL REVIEW

Carcinoma of the hypopharynx is a challenging problem for the head and neck oncologist. By anatomical site, the hypopharynx offers the worst prognosis among all epithelial cancers arising in the upper aero-digestive tract. This is largely related to a majority of patients presenting with advanced disease at the time of diagnosis. Although radiation therapy had been employed in the past, the overall control rate with external irradiation was disappointing (Lederman 1967). Surgical resection, on the other hand, provided complete removal of the tumour and an improvement in overall survival (Shah et al 1976). Surgical planning must however ensure adequate resection with satisfactory margins and, whenever feasible, a single-stage procedure for reconstruction. Historically, most pharyngeal carcinomas were treated by surgical extirpation incorporating a total laryngectomy. Ogura championed the concept of partial laryngopharyngectomy for carcinomas of the pyriform sinus which were localized in selected patients. (Ogura et al 1980). Similarly, resection of early tumours confined to the lateral wall and posterior wall of the pharynx was feasible with preservation of the larynx. However, more advanced lesions did require total laryngectomy with either partial pharyngectomy or total pharyngectomy.

Field cancerization is a phenomenon described by Slaughter which is most prevalent in pharyngeal carcinomas (Slaughter et al 1953). Submucosal extension of pharyngeal cancer into the cervical oesophagus is not uncommon. Similarly, multifocal carcinomas involving the pharynx and oesophagus are also fairly common. For these reasons, pharyngeal carcinomas with extension into the cervical oesophagus require a total pharyngolaryngo-oesophagectomy with appropriate reconstruction.

One of the biggest challenges facing the head and neck surgeon is reconstruction of the hypopharynx to establish continuity between the oral cavity and the oesophagus. In the past, pharyngostomes were created at the time of pharyngolaryngectomy for subsequent secondary reconstruction. Closure of the pharyngostome required a multiple staged operative procedure using either skin from the neck or a tubed pedicle graft transferred from the pectoral skin in multiple stages. The simplest closure of the pharyngostomes was performed by the Wookey procedure using cervical skin in a trapdoor fashion (Wookey 1942). Due to the poor vascularity of the cervical skin used in repair of the pharyngostome, the Wookey procedure often failed to achieve the desired goal of restoration of the continuity of the alimentary tract in one operation.

Bakamjian popularized the medially-based delto-pectoral flap in reconstruction of the pharyngo-oesophageal surgical defect (Bakamjian 1965). Although the delto-pectoral flap could be used without delay, it did require creation of a controlled salivary fistula at the initial stage of the reconstruction of the pharyngeal conduit. Approximately 6 weeks following the initial procedure, the pedicle of the delto-pectoral flap was severed and the lower end of the newly created pharynx was closed to establish the continuity of the alimentary tract. Although, ideally, two stages were required to accomplish reconstruction of the pharynx over a period of 6 to 8 weeks, this was seldom achieved in most instances (Shah et al 1984). On an average, four operations were required to complete reconstruction of the pharynx using the delto-pectoral flap and often the reconstruction effort was complicated by wound breakdown with development of fistulae, and stenosis at the junction between the delto-pectoral flap and cervical oesophagus requiring repeated dilatations or revision surgery.

Introduction of the pectoralis major myocutaneous flap was a significant advance over previously employed reconstructive methods. The pectoralis major myocutaneous flap permitted reconstruction of pharyngeal defects in a single stage at the time of surgical resection of the pharyngeal cancer. The flap served admirably for partial pharyngeal defects but was inadequate when circumferential defects required reconstructive effort (Shah et al 1990). Technically, it is difficult to form a tube from the pectoralis myocutaneous flap, particularly in obese patients or in females, and the reconstructed pharynx had an unacceptably high rate of pharyngocutaneous fistula.

For circumferential defects of the pharyngo-oesophageal region, the currently available methods of reconstruction are transfer of a free segment of jejunum with microvascular anastomosis in the neck or a transthoracic transposition of the stomach with pharyngogastrostomy. For pharyngo-oesophageal defects which do not extend into the thoracic oesophagus, the microvascular free jejunal transfer remains the ideal choice. It must however be borne in mind that this method of reconstruction has at least two vascular anastomoses and three visceral anastomoses to include pharyngojejunostomy, jejuno-oesophagostomy in the lower part of the neck and jejunojenunostomy in the abdomen. An admirably high success rate using free jejunum has been reported by several authors (Coleman et al 1987). However, it must be borne in mind that utilization of a free segment of jejunum requires the expertise of a microvascular surgeon. When the pharyngo-oesophageal defect extends into the thoracic region, a total oesophagectomy is desirable with reconstruction using the transposed stomach. The advantage of the transposed stomach is a single visceral anastomosis between the pharynx and the fundus of the stomach. The morbidity of the operative procedure is reported to be significant, and therefore stringent pre-operative case selection is necessary to keep the morbidity and mortality to an irreducible minimum (Spiro et al 1991).

EXCISION TECHNIQUES

The hypopharynx is the lowermost part of the pharynx beginning at the level of the tip of the epiglottis and ending at the level of the lower border of the cricoid cartilage (Fig. 12.1). The pyriform sinuses on each side, the posterior pharyngeal wall, and the post-cricoid region form the three designated anatomical sites within the hypopharynx. Their boundaries however overlap as their demarcation is somewhat arbitrary. Physiologically, the hypopharynx is a critically important anatomical site as it is a component of the upper aero-digestive tract contiguous with the supraglottic larynx. Thus, surgical treatment of any tumour arising in the hypopharynx will, of necessity, produce disturbance in the mechanism of swallowing with resultant aspiration in the respiratory tract.

The cervical oesophagus begins where the hypopharynx ends at the level of the lower border of the cricoid cartilage. The lower border of the cervical oesophagus is somewhat arbitrary. It is generally accepted that the cervical oesophagus ends at the thoracic inlet. Primary tumours of the cervical oesophagus are, however, infrequent. Because of its continuity with the post-cricoid region cephalad and its contiguity to the larynx and proximal trachea anteriorly, surgical treatment of cancer of the cervical oesophagus requires consideration of resection of the larynx and proximal trachea along with primary tumour.

Involvement of cervical lymph nodes by metastases is very common and occurs early in the course of the disease. If the cervical lymph nodes are grossly involved by metastatic disease, then a comprehensive radical neck dissection is undertaken. However, if the regional lymph nodes are not grossly enlarged, then clearance of the lymph nodes at levels II, III and IV in the deep jugular chain on the ipsilateral side for a lesion of the pyriform sinus is undertaken. However, if the lesion involves the postcricoid region and extends to both sides of the midline, then clearance of lymph nodes at levels II, III and IV on both sides of the neck is recommended. Surgical treatment of regional cervical lymph nodes therefore is an integral part of surgical treatment planning for resection of hypopharyngeal carcinomas.

Pre-operative work-up for pharyngo-oesophageal lesions should include a detailed head and neck examination with appropriate televideoscopic equipment. Radiographic evaluation of the lesions with a barium swallow is required for all lesions whose lower extent is not readily visible. This is

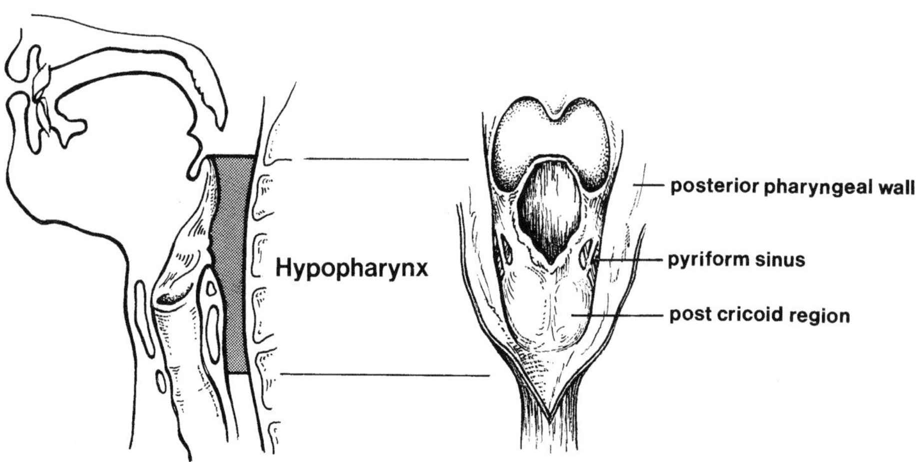

Fig. 12.1 Surgical anatomy of the hypopharynx.

particularly valuable if the patient presents with obstructive symptoms or there is clinical suspicion of extension of a pharyngeal lesion into the oesophagus. Endoscopic evaluation of the primary lesion immediately preceding surgical intervention is vitally important and should not be omitted. Satisfactory endoscopic assessment will greatly enhance the capability of the surgeon in assessing local extensions of the tumour to facilitate appropriate surgical approach and in assessing the extent of surgical resection. Due to the inherent nature of pharyngeal carcinoma exhibiting submucosal extension beyond what is seen on the surface, it is imperative that frozen section examination is performed from the margins of the surgical defect to ensure adequacy of satisfactory surgical resection.

PARTIAL LARYNGOPHARYNGECTOMY FOR EARLY CARCINOMA OF THE PYRIFORM SINUS

Early primary carcinomas of the pyriform sinus and pharyngeal wall are amenable to surgical resection with preservation of the larynx or in conjunction with partial laryngectomy. However, several important criteria must be met before a particular lesion or patient is considered for partial laryngopharyngectomy.

The following are important tumour factors to be considered for selection of a patient for partial laryngopharyngectomy for pyriform sinus or pharyngeal wall carcinoma: (i) the primary tumour must be confined to the anatomic site of origin within the hypopharynx, that is, either pyriform sinus or pharyngeal wall; (ii) the tumour must not extend to the apex of the pyriform sinus; (iii) the tumour must be limited to the pyriform sinus with no significant extension to the base of the tongue; (iv) the ipsilateral hemilarynx must be mobile; (v) the tumour may extend to involve the supraglottic larynx but should not involve the larynx in a transglottic fashion.

Amongst the patient factors, it is vitally important that the patient is able to understand the nature of the disease and its treatment. He should have the understanding and the capability to participate in a vigorous postoperative recovery effort in terms of pulmonary clearance of aspirated secretions. Pulmonary functions should be satisfactory to tolerate small amounts of chronic aspiration. There should not be any previous treatment—such as radiation therapy—for the hypopharynx cancer, and the patient must understand that a total laryngectomy may be necessary, depending on the extent of the tumour found at the time of surgery or, in the case of chronic symptomatic aspiration, in the postoperative period.

A preliminary tracheostomy is performed under local anaesthesia prior to induction of general anaesthesia to establish a safe airway. Translaryngeal endotracheal intubation is best avoided to minimize trauma to the lesion during intubation and to facilitate endoscopic evaluation and surgical manipulation during the operative procedure.

A transverse incision at the level of the thyrohyoid membrane is employed for exposure of the supraglottic larynx and hypopharynx. The skin incision is deepened through the platysma and upper and lower skin flaps are elevated to expose the hyoid bone and the suprahyoid musculature cephalad and the thyroid cartilage caudad. (Fig. 12.2) The strap muscles are detached from the undersurface of the hyoid bone and are retracted laterally for subsequent closure. Similarly, musculature of the base of the tongue on the ipsilateral side of the hyoid bone is detached with an electrocautery to bare the superior surface of the hyoid bone on that side. The hyoid is divided in the midline with a bone cutter.

Using a power surgical saw, the upper end of the thyroid cartilage on the ipsilateral side is divided from the midline up to its posterior margin. Approximately 3–5 mm of the upper edge of the thyroid cartilage is divided. At this point, entry is made into the oropharynx via the mucosa of the glosso-epiglottic fold in the midline. (Fig. 12.3) The tip of the epiglottis is visualized through this opening in the oropharynx. The epiglottis is grasped with a toothed forceps, and, using an electrocautery with a needle tip, it is divided through its full thickness in the midline from its tip down to its infrahyoid portion. The cut in the epiglottic cartilage now meets with the cut through the thyroid notch.

The vertical cut in the midline is connected to the transverse cut of the thyroid cartilage on the same side. This will now permit rotation of the surgical specimen to the same side, giving a view of the primary tumour of the pyriform sinus (Fig. 12.4). Using an electrocautery or angled scissors, the specimen of that half of the supraglottic larynx in conjunction with the pyriform sinus is resected with adequate mucosal and soft-tissue margins around the primary tumour under direct vision. Brisk haemorrhage from the branches of the superior laryngeal artery is to be expected but this is easily controlled with appropriate haemostasis.

The surgical defect following removal of the specimen shows the remaining larynx, including the left half of the glottic larynx (Fig. 12.5). A large raw area remains at the left lateral pharyngeal wall from where the primary tumour is removed. Frozen sections are obtained from the margins of the surgical defect to ensure satisfactory resection of the tumour. No attempt is made to obtain mucosal closure of the surgical defect, which is allowed to granulate.

A nasogastric feeding tube is inserted and pharyngeal closure is performed with re-approximation of the musculature of the base of the tongue to the detached strap muscles of the ipsilateral side using interrupted chromic catgut sutures (Fig. 12.6). No mucosal or skin flaps are necessary to provide lining to the lateral pharyngeal wall. The raw area usually epithelializes spontaneously over the next few weeks. After satisfactory muscular closure is obtained, a Penrose drain is inserted and the remaining incision is closed in two layers.

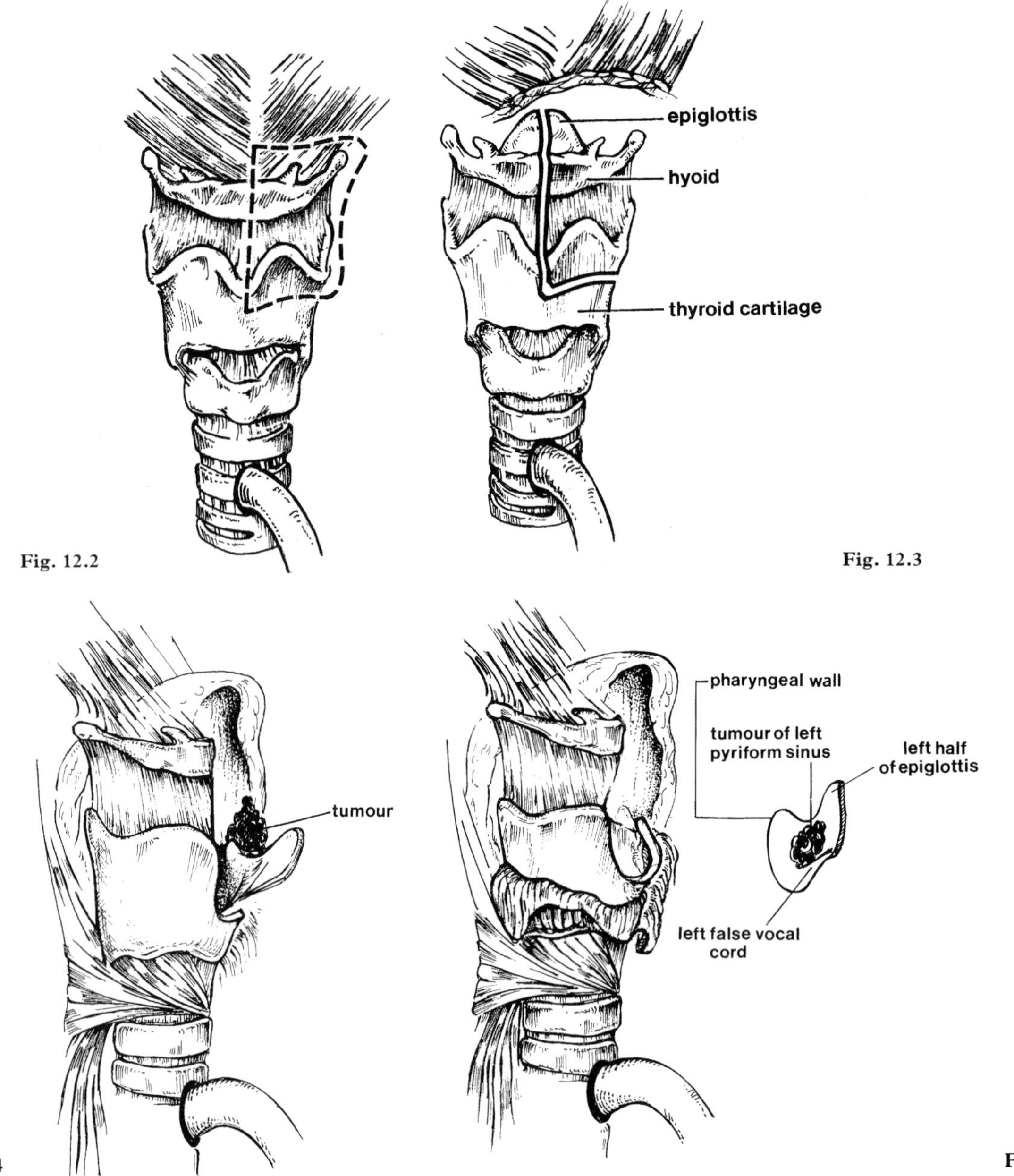

Fig. 12.2–12.5 Excision of a small tumour of the left pyriform sinus.

RESECTION OF CARCINOMA OF THE POSTERIOR PHARYNGEAL WALL

Tumours of the posterior pharyngeal wall of limited extent are amenable to posterior wall pharyngectomy via several approaches depending upon the location of the tumour, its surface dimensions, and the depth of infiltration of the lesion through the musculature of the pharyngeal wall. Small superficial tumours of the posterior pharyngeal wall in the upper part of the pharynx, particularly those which extend into the oropharynx, can be excised through the open mouth. The surgical defect may be left open to granulate and epithelialize. If such a procedure is undertaken, it is desirable that the mucosal edges of the surgical defect be tacked down to the prevertebral fascia with interrupted chromic catgut sutures. Alternatively, a skin graft can be applied to the surgical defect. If a split thickness skin graft is used, then it is tacked to the mucosal edges with interrupted chromic catgut sutures and is retained snug with the prevertebral fascia by several quilting sutures of chromic catgut to maintain adherence between the prevertebral fascia and the split skin graft.

Similar limited tumours of the lower part of the posterior pharyngeal wall can be excised through a transhyoid

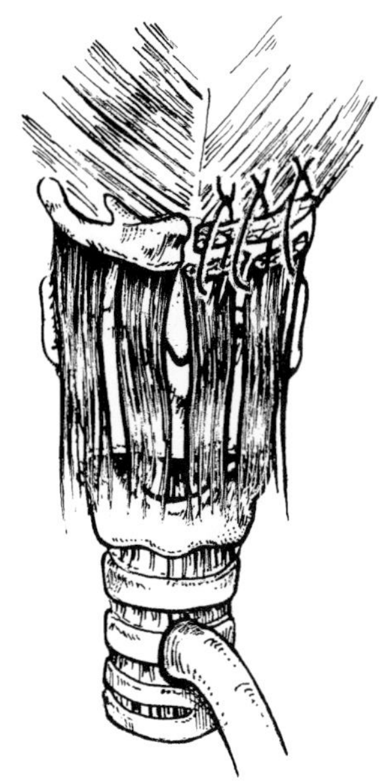

Fig. 12.6 Reconstruction following excision of left pyriform sinus tumour. The strap muscles are approximated to the musculature of the base of the tongue. No mucosal approximation or skin grafts are used.

pharyngotomy. (Fig. 12.7) In that situation, a transverse incision is employed through the region of the thyroid membrane to expose the suprahyoid musculature. After division of the platysma and elevation of upper and lower skin flaps, the suprahyoid musculature is detached from the superior surface of the hyoid bone using an electrocautery. (Fig. 12.8A) Entry is made into the hypopharynx through the mucosa of the glosso-epiglottic fold and valleculae on each side (Fig. 12.8B). Generous exposure of the posterior pharyngeal wall can be obtained through this approach for a limited tumour which can be directly excised using an electrocautery (Fig. 12.9 A and B). The surgical defect thus created is either left open to granulate and epithelialize or, alternatively, it can be covered with a split-thickness skin graft. The edges of the mucosal defect are tacked down to the prevertebral fascia, and if a skin graft is employed it is sutured to the edges of the mucosal defect with interrupted chromic catgut sutures. Quilting sutures are taken between the skin graft and the prevertebral fascia to retain it in its position. A nasogastric feeding tube and a tracheostomy are both essential until such time that the patient is able to swallow by mouth.

Larger defects of the posterior pharyngeal wall require a more substantial reconstructive effort. Partial pharyngectomy of the entire posterior pharyngeal wall extending from the oropharynx down to the lower border of the cricoid cartilage supero-inferiorly and from the lateral wall of the pyriform sinus on one side to that on the other can be undertaken, still preserving the larynx. However, under these circumstances, more elaborate reconstructive methods are required to repair the surgical defect. The ideal choice of reconstructive

surgery in this setting is the radial forearm microvascular free flap. The surgical technique of extensive posterior wall partial pharyngectomy and reconstruction with a radial forearm flap is described as follows. Most patients requiring this extent of posterior wall pharyngectomy will have either clinically apparent cervical lymph node metatasis, requiring a radical neck dissection, or an elective dissection of regional lymph nodes involving levels II, III and IV on one or both sides of the neck. The surgical procedure can be accomplished with a single transverse incision extending from the anterior border of the trapezius muscle on one side of the neck to that on the other side of the neck at the level of the thyrohyoid membrane. The patient is usually placed under general anaesthesia through a preliminary tracheostomy done under local anaesthesia to avoid any trauma to the lesion due to orotracheal intubation. After adequate assessment of the lesion has been performed by endoscopy, the surgical procedure begins through the transverse incision as described above.

The skin incision is deepened through the platysma, and the upper and lower skin flaps are elevated. Neck dissection of the appropriate side is completed in the usual fashion. If a radical neck dissection is necessary for clinically apparent cervical lymph node metastasis, then a vertical component of a single trifurcate incision is taken on the ipsilateral side of the neck extending from just posterior to the carotid bifurcation along the transverse incision up to the mid-clavicular point in a curvelinear fashion. The specimen of the excised lymph nodes through a radical neck dissection is removed from the surgical field before resection of the primary tumour is undertaken. Alternatively, if the neck is clinically negative, then clearance of cervical lymph nodes at levels II, III and IV on both sides of the neck is indicated. This is accomplished in a meticulous fashion encompassing all the lymph nodes from levels II, III and IV in a monobloc fashion from each side. After both the specimens are removed, the excision of the primary tumour is undertaken.

A lateral pharyngotomy is made on the side opposite to the dominant side of the lesion to avoid entry through tumour-bearing pharyngeal wall. The inferior constrictor muscle along the posterior border of the thyroid cartilage is incised and entry is made into the mucosa of the apex of the pyriform sinus on the contralateral side (Fig. 12. 10). Mucosal incision in the lateral pharyngeal wall is then extended cephalad up to the lower pole of the tonsil and caudad down to the cervical oesophagus. This permits entry into the hypopharynx and provides a generous view of the surface extent of the tumour to facilitate subsequent excision which is accomplished under direct vision (Fig. 12.11). The larynx is retracted anteriorly; this puts mucosa of the opposite pharyngeal wall under tension, providing adequate exposure of the remaining peripheral extent of the tumour. Mobilization of the posterior pharyngeal wall musculature is now undertaken by digital dissection between the preverterbral fascia and the musculature of the posterior

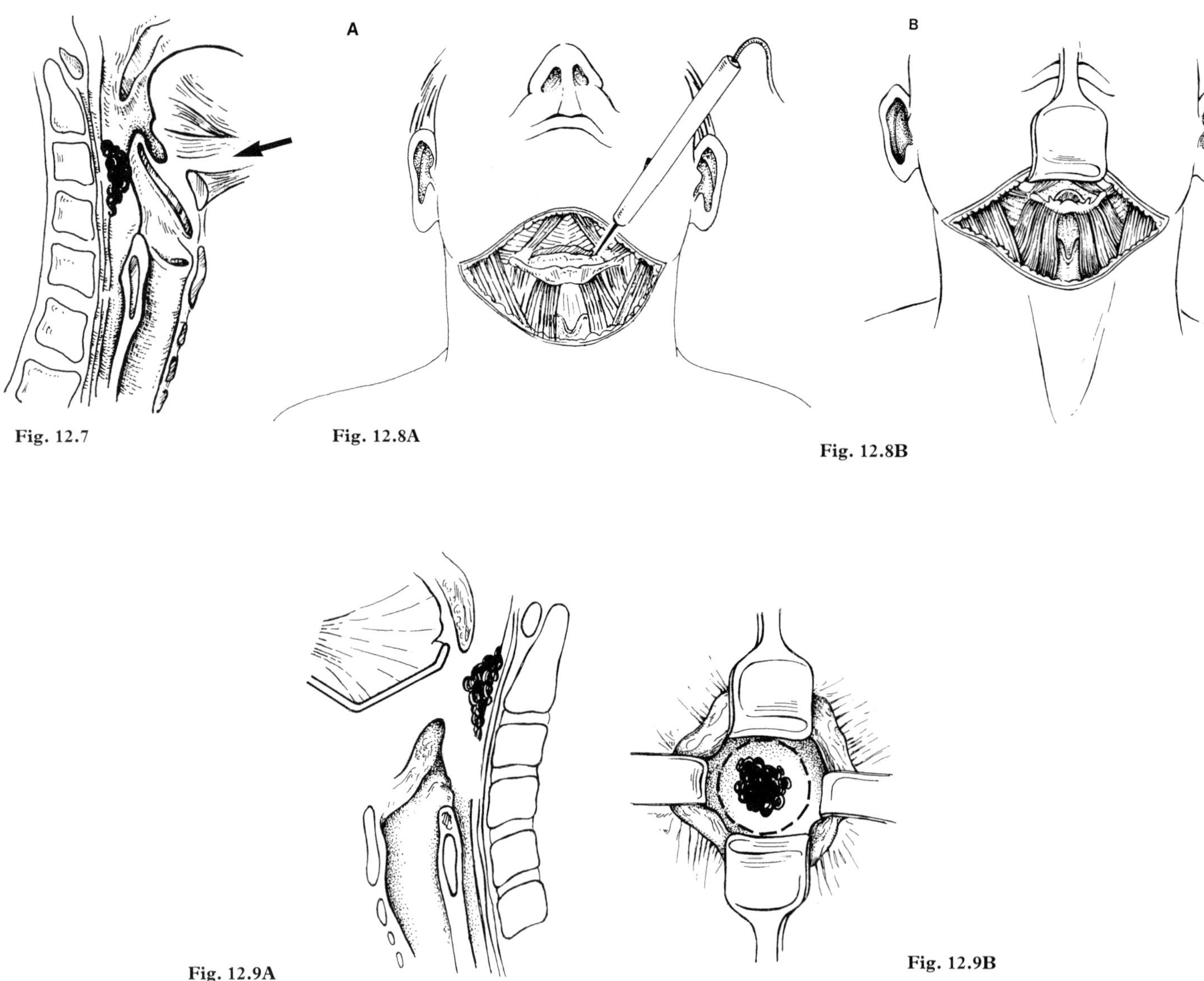

Fig. 12.7   **Fig. 12.8A**

Fig. 12.8B

Fig. 12.9A   **Fig. 12.9B**

Fig. 12.7–12.9 Transhyoid pharyngotomy approach for excision of small tumours in the posterior pharyngeal wall.

pharyngeal wall. The entire posterior pharyngeal wall is mobilized beyond the surface extent of the tumour cephalad and caudad. Under direct vision now, using a Mayo scissors, full-thickness resection of the posterior pharyngeal wall is undertaken with satisfactory mucosal margins circumferentially around the primary tumour. Care is taken to avoid dissection along the anterior aspect of the pyriform sinuses on each side so as to preserve the continuity of mucosa along the pharyngo-epiglottic fold and at the valleculae on both sides. Thus, a full-thickness resection of the posterior pharyngeal wall is accomplished preserving the anterior attachment of the soft palate and base of the tongue to the larynx (Fig. 12.12). Similarly, all the suprahyoid muscles remain intact without any disturbance to the supports to the larynx. Adequate hemostasis is obtained by controlling the bleeding points from the cut surfaces of the pharyngeal wall.

A radial forearm microvascular free flap of appropriate dimensions is now developed on its vascular pedicle and brought to the surgical field. Microvascular anastomoses of the flap is completed using the facial artery and one of the branches of the internal jugular vein as the donor vessels. After satisfactory completion of the vascular anastomosis, closure of the pharyngeal defect is begun (Fig. 12.13).

The flap is inset into the surgical defect and closure begins at the opposite side using interrupted absorbable sutures. The skin edges of the flap are sutured to the mucosa and musculature of the pharyngeal wall defect, beginning at the nasopharynx and continuing along the lateral pharyngeal wall up to the cervical oesophagus. The closure of the flap to the margins of the defect in the posterior pharyngeal wall continues until a water-tight closure is accomplished. A nasogastric feeding tube is inserted. Suction drains are placed in the neck wound, and the skin incisions in the neck are closed in routine fashion.

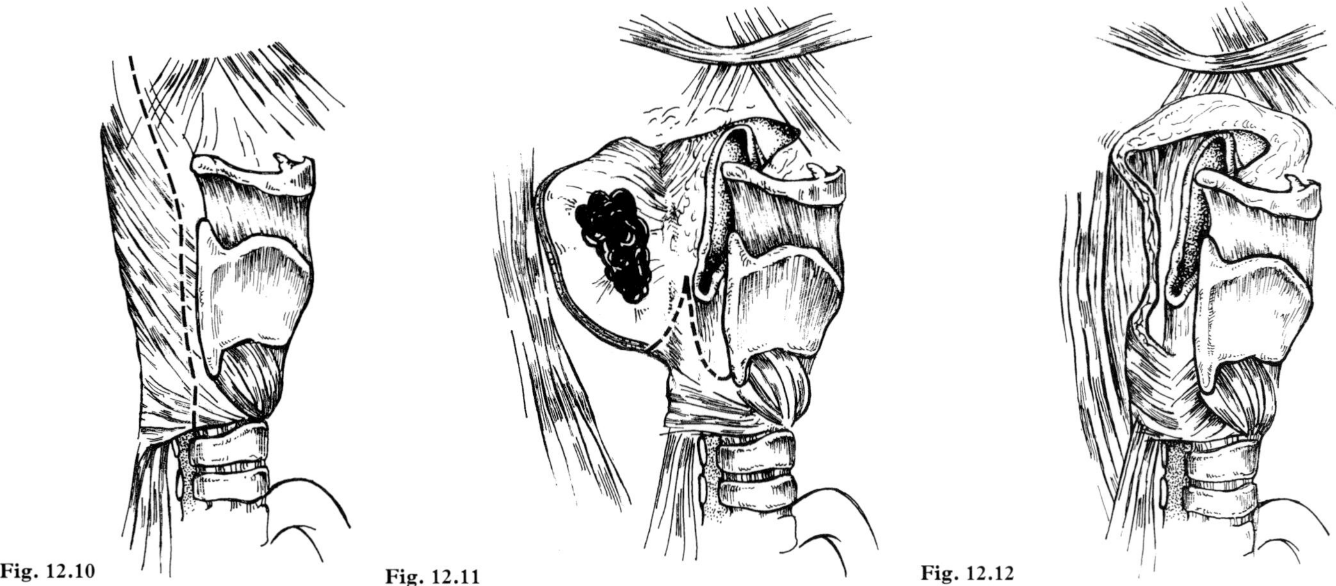

Fig. 12.10   **Fig. 12.11**   **Fig. 12.12**

Fig. 12.10–12.12   Lateral phryngotomy approach for excision of larger tumours of the posterior pharyngeal wall.

TOTAL LARYNGECTOMY WITH PARTIAL PHARYNGECTOMY

The vast majority of lesions of the hypopharynx arise in the pyriform sinus and present with advanced (T3 and T4) disease. Surgical management of these lesions generally requires total laryngectomy and partial pharyngectomy. Indications for total laryngectomy include involvement of

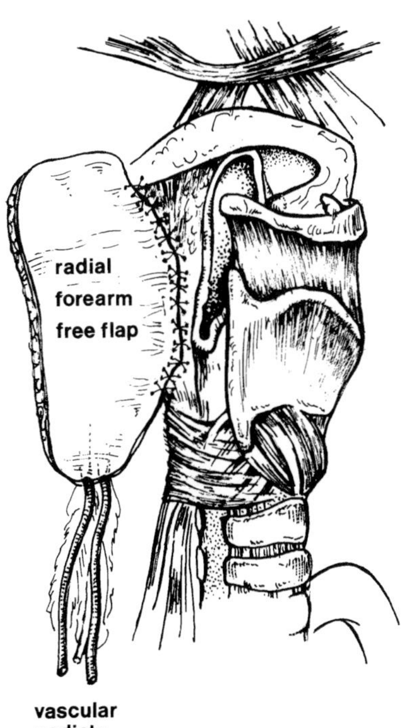

Fig. 12.13   Reconstruction of the posterior pharyngeal wall using a free radial forearm flap.

the apex of the pyriform sinus, mucosa of the postcricoid region, paralysed hemilarynx or invasion of the cartilagenous framework of the larynx.

After induction of general endotracheal anaesthesia via an orotracheal intubation, an endoscopy is performed to assess adequately the extent of the tumour. Following endoscopy, the patient is prepped and draped in the usual fashion and a modified T-shaped incision is taken, beginning at the tip of the mastoid process and following an upper neck skin crease at the level of the thyrohyoid membrane up to the contralateral sternocleidomastoid muscle. A vertical curvelinear component of this incision begins posterior to the carotid bifurcation and ends at the midclavicular point.

An appropriate neck dissection is completed, leaving the contents of the dissected neck attached at its medial edge to the soft tissues in the central compartment of the neck.

The lower anterior skin flap is elevated up to the contralateral sternoclavicular joint to expose the entire central compartment of the neck. The site of the proposed tracheostome is marked out prior to beginning the operative procedure in the suprasternal notch. A generous permanent tracheostome is desirable. The tracheostome should be of an oval shape measuring at least 3 cm in its supero-inferior dimensions and 2 cm in its side-to-side dimensions. A disc of skin of the dimensions mentioned above is removed for creation of the permanent tracheostome.

Following completion of neck dissection, mobilization of larynx begins by dividing the strap muscles in the suprasternal notch as low as possible. Both the sternohyoid and sterno-thyroid muscles are divided with the use of the electrocautery, freeing up the inferior muscular attachments of the larynx. An ipsilateral thyroid lobectomy is usually performed to encompass tracheo-oesophageal groove lymph nodes on the side of the primary tumour. Therefore, mobilization of the thyroid isthmus is undertaken and, using two straight Halstead clamps, the isthmus is divided. The stump of the isthmus on the side of the thyroid lobe that is to be preserved is suture-ligated with a continuous interlocking 3-0 chromic catgut suture. This thyroid lobe is then detached from the tracheo-oesophageal groove and the cricothyroid membrane using an electrocautery, carefully preserving the posterior fascia of the thyroid lobe and the superior and inferior blood supply to the thyroid lobe. Adequate haemostasis is secured as this mobilization of the thyroid lobe proceeds. Once the thyroid lobe is detached from the laryngotracheal complex, it is retracted laterally to expose the cervical trachea. An appropriate level of the trachea is chosen for creation of the permanent tracheostome. However, the trachea is not divided at this point.

Attention is now focused to superior and lateral mobilization of the laryngopharynx. The suprahyoid musculature of the tongue is detached using an electrocautery. (Fig. 12.14) The entire superior surface of the hyoid is completely bared of its muscular attachments. Following this, the neurovascular bundle entering the interior of the larynx through the thyrohyoid membrane is isolated on each side, carefully dissected, divided between clamps, and ligated. This neurovascular bundle contains the superior laryngeal artery and the superior laryngeal nerve and blood vessels traversing with the nerve. The superior thyroid artery on the ipsilateral side of the tumour is divided and ligated. Similarly, the inferior thyroid artery on the ipsilateral side is also divided between clamps and ligated. At this point, the larynx is nearly completely devascularized of its dominant blood supply. Attention is now focused on the creation of the permanent tracheostome. Using an electrocautery, the proposed line of transection of trachea is outlined in an oblique fashion with the incision in the anterior wall of the trachea lower than that in the membranous trachea. This then permits creation of an oval-shaped tracheostome. The trachea is then transected using either an electrocautery or a scalpel. The orotracheal tube is removed and anaesthesia is continued using a flexible endotracheal tube passed through the permanent tracheostome into the distal trachea. The distal trachea is mobilized from the cervical oesophagus through the tracheo-oesophageal plane to provide sufficient mobilization for anastomosis of the stump of the trachea to the skin margins at the permanent tracheostome. Interrupted nylon sutures are used to create the permanent tracheostome. This begins with four corner sutures dividing the circumference of the transected trachea into four equal quadrants and then several interrupted sutures are taken in each quadrant to complete creation of the permanent tracheostome.

At this point, the laryngopharyngeal specimen is ready to be mobilized for delivery. Entry is made into the hypopharynx through the contralateral vallecula by dividing the mucosa of the glosso-epiglottic fold. Incision into the mucosa of the

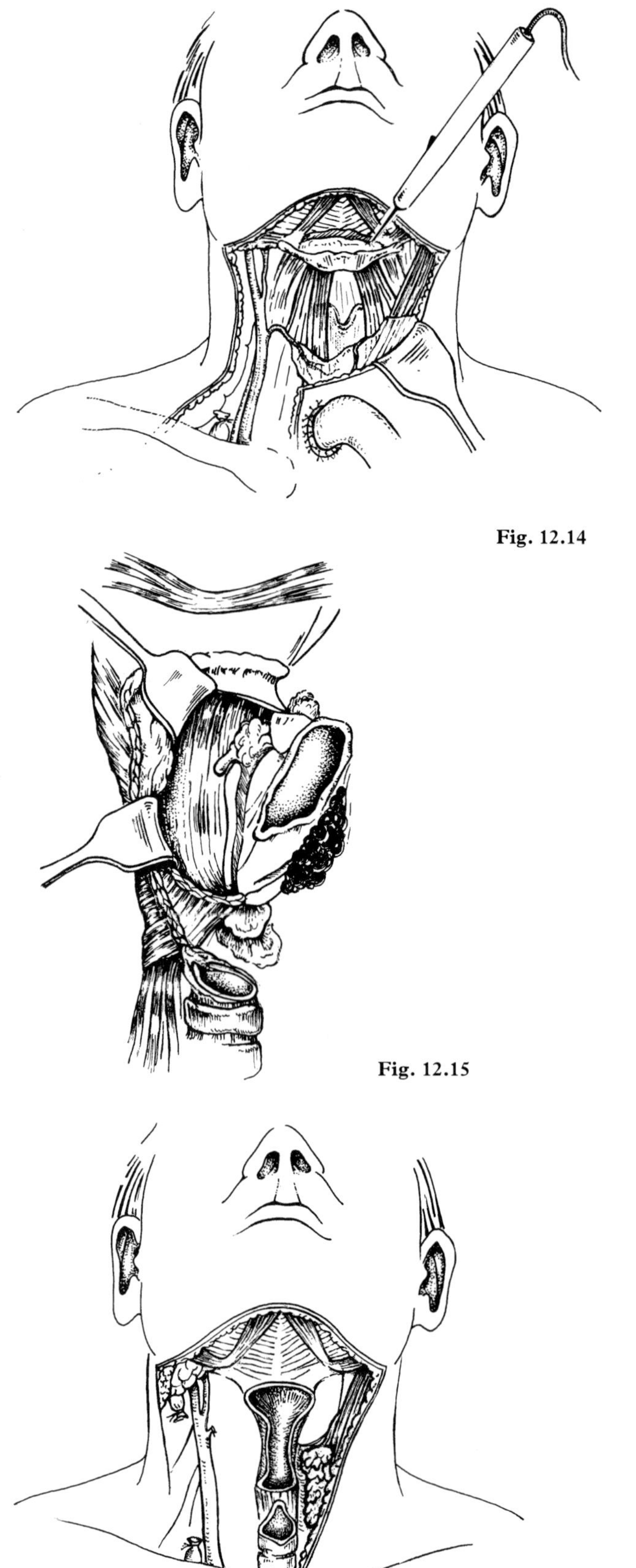

Fig. 12.14

Fig. 12.15

Fig. 12.16

Fig. 12.14–12.16 Total laryngectomy (Figs. 12.14, 12.15) with partial pharyngectomy (Fig. 12.16) for advanced (T3–T4) tumour.

base of the tongue continues on both sides providing generous entry into the hypopharynx. A Richardson retractor is now introduced through this pharyngotomy to retract the base of the tongue and provide a view of the interior of the hypopharynx (Fig. 12.15). Using an electrocautery, the inferior constrictor muscle of the ipsilateral side is divided along the posterior margin of the thyroid cartilage. Now under direct vision, a mucosal incision is made into the contralateral pyriform sinus up to the postcricoid region separating the laryngo-pharyngeal complex from the contralateral pharyngeal wall. This manoeuvre now permits the specimen to be rotated externally on the ipsilateral side exposing the tumour in toto. Under direct vision, the remaining mucosal and muscular attachments of the pharyngeal wall are divided to deliver the specimen containing the larynx, the hypopharyngeal cancer, the ipsilateral thyroid lobe and the contents of the ipsilateral side of the dissected neck (Fig.12.16). Bleeding points from the transected edges of the muscular wall of the pharynx are controlled by ligation or electrocautery. Tissue samples are obtained from the pharyngeal wall defect which are considered to be closest within the proximity of the primary tumour for frozen section examinations. Once satisfactory

resection is accomplished by confirmation of negative frozen section margins, reconstruction of the surgical defect is begun.

If the excision of the primary tumour has resulted in resection of approximately a third or less of the circumference of the pharynx, then primary closure of the surgical defect is feasible. Primary closure of the defect is undertaken in a single layer using 2-0 chromic catgut interrupted inverting sutures (Fig. 12.17A). While a transverse closure is desirable it is often not feasible and a T-shaped closure is achieved (Fig. 12.17, B and C). Inasmuch as a water-tight closure is obtained, satisfactory healing should be anticipated. A nasogastric feeding tube is inserted prior to completion of the closure for maintenance of nutrition in the immediate postoperative period. The wound is irrigated again after closure of the pharynx and suction drains are introduced and the skin incisions are closed in two layers in the usual fashion. Alternatively, if the pharyngeal resection results in excision of 50% or more of the circumference of the pharynx, then a primary closure of the surgical defect is not feasible (Fig. 12.17D). Under these circumstances, appropriate reconstructive methods are employed to restore the continuity of the alimentary tract. Partial pharyngeal

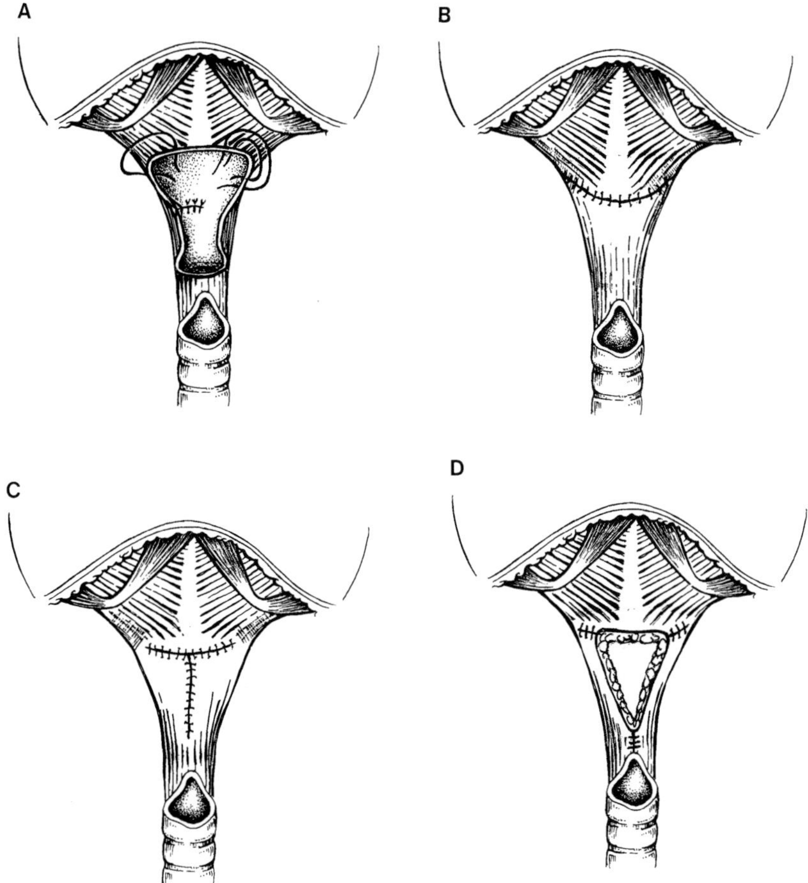

Fig. 12.17 Primary closure of the pharyngeal defect. **A–C.** Excision of more than 50% of the circumference of the pharynx leaves a defect where primary closure is not feasible **(D).**

defects resulting from this surgical procedure can be repaired using a pectoralis major myocutaneous island flap, a radial forearm free flap, or a microvascular patch of jejunum split at its antimesenteric border and employed as a patch pharyngoplasty for repair of the surgical defect. Each of these reconstructive methods will be discussed later in this chapter.

TOTAL LARYNGOPHARYNGECTOMY

The need for laryngectomy in conjunction with total circumferential pharyngectomy (total laryngopharyngectomy) or total laryngopharyngo-oesophagectomy is based on the circumferential extent of the tumour and its inferior extent as it pertains to involvement of the cervical oesophagus and/or upper thoracic oesophagus. The shape of the hypopharynx is like that of a funnel with a larger upper circumference which narrows down to a narrower circumference as the pharynx merges with the cervical oesophagus. Thus, lesions of the pharyngo-oesophageal junction and cervical oesophagus require circumferential excision for adequate resection of the primary tumour. Similarly, lesions arising in the postcricoid region or lesions of the posterior pharyngeal wall extending below the level of the cricoid cartilage require circumferential pharyngo-oesophagectomy.

The initial surgical approach for mobilization of the larynx and neck dissection is similar to that employed for total laryngectomy with partial pharyngectomy. The type and extent of neck dissection depends on the presence or absence of palpable cervical lymph node metastasis. Mobilization of the laryngopharyngeal complex is similar up to the entry into the pharynx through the contralateral vallecula.

Therefore, those steps of the operative procedure will not be repeated here.

Once entry is made into the pharynx through the mucosa of the contralateral vallecula, a Richardson retractor is introduced into the pharyngeal opening and the base of the tongue is retracted cephalad to obtain view of the interior of the pharynx (Fig. 12.15). Under direct visualization, the superior extent of the tumour is ascertained and circumferential pharyngeal transection is undertaken, either with an electrocautery or with Mayo scissors (Fig. 12.18A). Adequate mucosal and soft tissue margin of the full thickness of the pharyngeal wall is secured superior to the upper border of the tumour. Once the pharynx is circumferentially transected, the laryngopharyngeal complex becomes detached and is freely mobilized into the surgical defect remaining attached to the patient only at its inferior extent to the cervical oesophagus. At this point, a decision needs to be made regarding the lower border of transection of the surgical specimen, depending upon the inferior extent of the tumour. If endoscopic evaluation of the inferior extent of the tumour was not possible, then the radiographic extent of the tumour is taken as a guide and the pharynx is opened in the posterior midline or through its lateral wall, the longitudinal incision being carried caudad into the cervical oesophagus until a satisfactory lower margin is obtained below the lower border of the tumour. Needless to say, if the radiological extent of the tumour or endoscopic assessment indicated extension of the tumour into the thoracic oesophagus, then gastric transposition is planned pre-operatively. At this point, the cervical oesophagus is circumferentially transected and the surgical specimen is delivered (Fig. 12.18B).

Complete haemostasis is secured with the use of ligatures

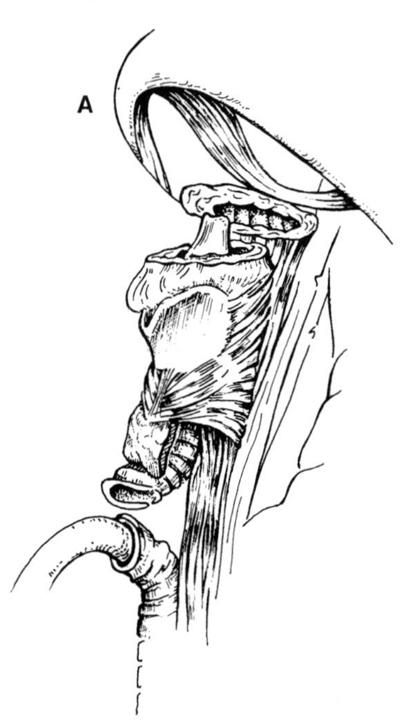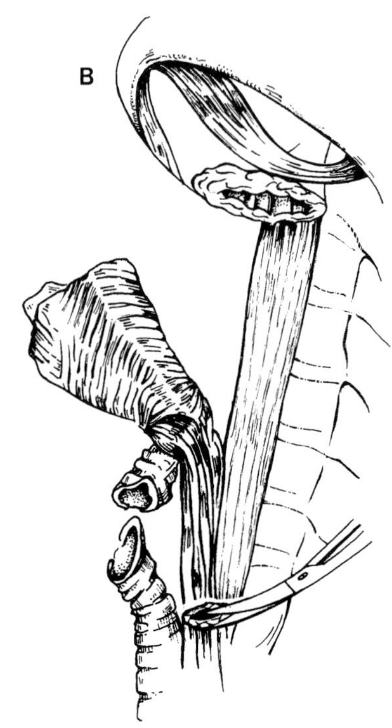

Fig. 12.18   Total laryngopharyngectomy.

or electrocautery at both the cut ends of the pharynx and thoracic oesophagus. Reconstruction of this missing segment to restore the continuity of the alimentary tract requires a tubular replacement. This is ideally done with a free segment of jejunum with microvascular anastomosis. Alternatively, a radial forearm free flap tubed over itself can be employed. In extremely thin patients, a pectoralis major myocutaneous flap can also be employed to provide a circumferential repair, although this is less than ideal and is not the preferred choice of treatment.

PHARYNGOLARYNGO-OESOPHAGECTOMY

When the primary lesion extends to involve the lower part of the cervical oesophagus or into the upper thoracic oesophagus, then a total pharyngolaryngo-oesophagectomy is warranted. This operation, of necessity, requires mobilization of the stomach and transthoracic transposition into the neck to re-establish the continuity of the alimentary tract by a pharyngogastrostomy. The operative procedure is ideally done by two surgical teams working simultaneously. The head and neck surgical team works in the neck and in the superior mediastinum, and a thoracic surgical team works in the abdomen and the lower mediastinum to mobilize the stomach and the lower thoracic oesophagus.

All the previously described steps for mobilization of the larynx, pharynx and cervical oesophagus remain the same except that, after circumferential transection of the pharynx at the upper end, the cervical oesophagus is not divided. Dissection proceeds in the tracheo-oesophageal plane, carefully mobilizing the membranous trachea from the oesophagus anteriorly and laterally to obtain circumferential mobilization of the upper thoracic oesophagus. This is best done under direct vision. A Deaver retractor assists in retracting the trachea from the oesophagus in the tracheo-oesophageal plane. Care must be employed to avoid inadvertent injury to the membranous trachea with the retractor. Use of long instruments and haemoclips greatly facilitates division of the segmental blood supply to the oesophagus coming through its lateral fascial attachments and branches of the bronchial artery. Digital dissection of the oesophagus in the mediastinum facilitates its mobilization (Fig. 12.19). Any fibrous bands containing blood vessels are divided between haemoclips to obtain satisfactory haemostasis. Mobilization of the upper thoracic oesophagus can be accomplished up to the level of the carina through this approach.

The thoracic team performs an upper midline laparotomy and mobilizes the stomach, preserving its blood supply through the gastro-epiploic and right gastric arteries, but transecting all other attachments of the stomach which, of necessity, will require division of the left gastric artery, the short splenic vessels, and the greater omentum (Fig. 12.20).

A pyloromyotomy is performed to provide drainage of the stomach due to the bilateral vagectomy which will result by mobilization of the stomach into the neck. The right crus of the diaphragm is divided and the diaphragmatic hiatus is widened by digital dissection. Mobilization of the distal thoracic oesophagus is accomplished, also under direct vision, with a long flexible light source as well as a specially designed pistol-grip type of long single-arm haemoclip applier. Digital dissection of the distal thoracic oesophagus will aid in its mobilization, carefully avoiding any inadvertent injury to its blood supply or tear into the muscular wall of the oesophagus. In anterior mobilization of the lower thoracic oesophagus, the heart requires retraction with a Harrington retractor, and, during this manoeuvre, the right ventricle is compressed—leading to transient hypotension. Extreme caution should be exercised to monitor the patient's blood pressure and heart rate during this dissection. It may be necessary intermittently to relax the retractor to restore blood pressure and heart rate and then continue dissection.

Once the entire oesophagus has been circumferentially mobilized, the surgical specimen of the larynx, pharynx and cervical oesophagus is pulled from the neck, keeping the remaining oesophagus in continuity, and pulling the fundus of the stomach through the thoracic oesophageal bed into the neck. Assistance by the thoracic surgeon from the abdomen facilitating delivery of the stomach past the mediastinum into the neck makes the delivery of the stomach easy (Fig. 12.21). Once the fundus of the stomach and the oesophagogastric junction is seen in the mediastinum, Babcock forceps are used to deliver the stomach into the neck. An intestinal stapler is used for transection of the oesophagogastric junction. After the oesophagus has been transected at its lower end, the specimen of pharynx, larynx and oesophagus is delivered.

A gastrotomy is made through the fundus of the stomach measuring approximately 4 cm in diameter. Haemostasis is secured at the cut edges of the stomach. A single-layered anastomosis between the transected pharynx and the gastrotomy is made using 2-0 interrupted chromic catgut sutures (Fig. 12.22). A water-tight closure must be secured. Prior to completion of this pharyngogastric anastomosis, a nasogastric tube is inserted which is passed through the stomach up to the pyloric end to provide for drainage of the gastric contents in the immediate postoperative period. After completion of the pharyngogastric anastomosis the neck incision and the abdominal incision are closed in the usual manner. A permanent tracheostomy is created in the manner described before.

RECONSTRUCTION

When pharyngeal resection requires laryngectomy, special considerations must be given to closure of the pharynx. The discussion that follows will therefore address the issue of pharyngeal repair where laryngectomy has been performed. For lesions which require resection of less than one-third of the circumference of the pharynx, no special reconstructive

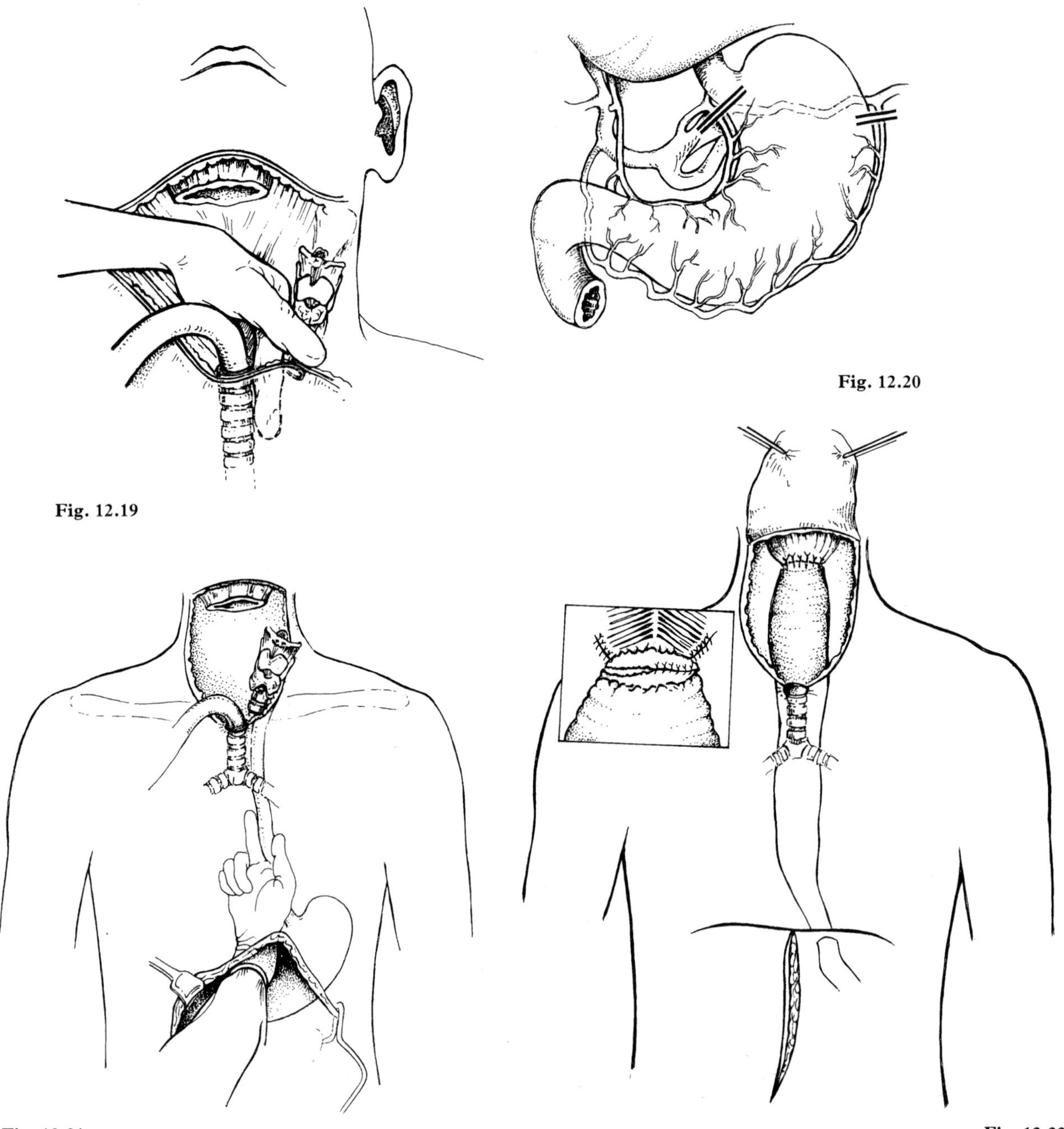

Fig. 12.19

Fig. 12.20

Fig. 12.21

Fig. 12.22

Fig. 12.19–12.22 Laryngopharyngo-oesophagectomy reconstructed by gastric pull up and pharyngogastric anastomosis

techniques need to be employed. Primary closure of the surgical defect is the method of choice for restoration of the continuity of the alimentary tract. Whenever feasible, the pharyngeal closure is performed in a single transverse suture line. Our preference is to employ interrupted inverting sutures with either chromic catgut or similar absorbable suture material. The sutures take a generous portion of the soft tissues of the musculature of the pharynx and the base of the tongue but include only the edge of the mucosa on each side to provide for satisfactory inversion of the suture line. The knots are placed inside the lumen to ensure adequate inversion. In some instances, a transverse closure may not be feasible and a T-shaped closure is performed. However, this particular type of closure has the disadvantages of creating a trifurcation point where two horizontal limbs of the suture line meet the vertical limb, leaving a weak point in the suture line which is at greatest risk for wound breakdown and fistula formation.

In instances where between one-third and 70% of the pharyngeal circumference has been resected, the optimal means of reconstruction of this surgical defect is by utilizing a pectoralis major myocutaneous flap. The flap is raised with an island of skin on the muscle paddle which is used as a patch pharyngoplasty to restore the continuity of the alimentary tract. The skin island is designed over the muscle paddle after appropriate measurements are taken from the island pedicle of the flap using that as the pivot over an arc of rotation in such a fashion that the distal portion of the skin island easily reaches the superior edge of the pharyngeal wall defect (Fig. 12.23). The details of elevation of the pectoralis major myocutaneous flap are not discussed here since they are covered elsewhere in the book. The proximal part of the vascular pedicle of the myocutaneous flap is dissected and overlying pectoralis major muscle is excised to keep the flap attached through only its feeding vascular pedicle. Interrupted absorbable sutures are employed to anastomose the skin of the flap with the pharyngeal mucosal defect. A watertight closure is performed to ensure complete restoration of the continuity of the alimentary tract. Care must be exercised in avoiding any tension or kink on the vascular pedicle of the flap as it traverses the clavicle onto the neck. Any tension on the flap must be avoided or else venous drainage will be compromised leading to loss of the flap.

When more than 70% of the circumference of the pharynx has to be resected, it is desirable to proceed with a circumferential pharyngectomy. When the circumferential pharyngeal defect extends to include the cervical oesopha-

gus and thoracic oesophagus, then gastric transposition is the optimal choice of reconstruction.

However, when a circumferential pharyngo-oesophageal defect does not extend into the chest, then the short segment circumferential defect is best repaired using a free segment of jejunum on its vascular pedicle with microvascular anastomosis. An appropriate segment of jejunum with satisfactory vascular arcades is isolated by a laparatomy, preferably by a second surgical team. The length of the segment of jejunum depends on the length of the surgical defect. After the jejunal segment has been isolated, its mesentery is divided carefully, preserving the vascular arcades leading to its vascular pedicle (Fig. 12.24). The feeding artery and draining vein are divided and the free segment of jejunum is transferred to the neck for restoration of its blood supply. End-to-end anastomosis at the site of the resected segment of jejunum is accomplished in the usual manner in the abdomen following which the mesenteric defect is also closed with interrupted chromic catgut sutures. The laparotomy wound is closed in the usual fashion.

After transfer of the jejunal segment into the neck, vascular anastomosis is carried out first, carefully laying the jejunal segment in the defect in a satisfactory fashion. Excessive length of the jejunum should be trimmed off to provide a segment which would snugly fit into the defect without any kinks at the site of pharyngojejunal or jejuno-oesophageal anastomosis. The donor blood vessels for anastomosis may be either the facial artery, the superior thyroid artery or the transverse cervical artery and their accompanying veins. Standard microvascular techniques are employed with optical magnification using a microscope to accomplish the vascular anastomoses. Once vascular anastomoses have been completed and circulation to the jejunal segment is restored, haemostasis is essential at the cut ends of the jejunum which is secured prior to anastomosing the jejunum with the pharyngeal defect. The jejunum is split

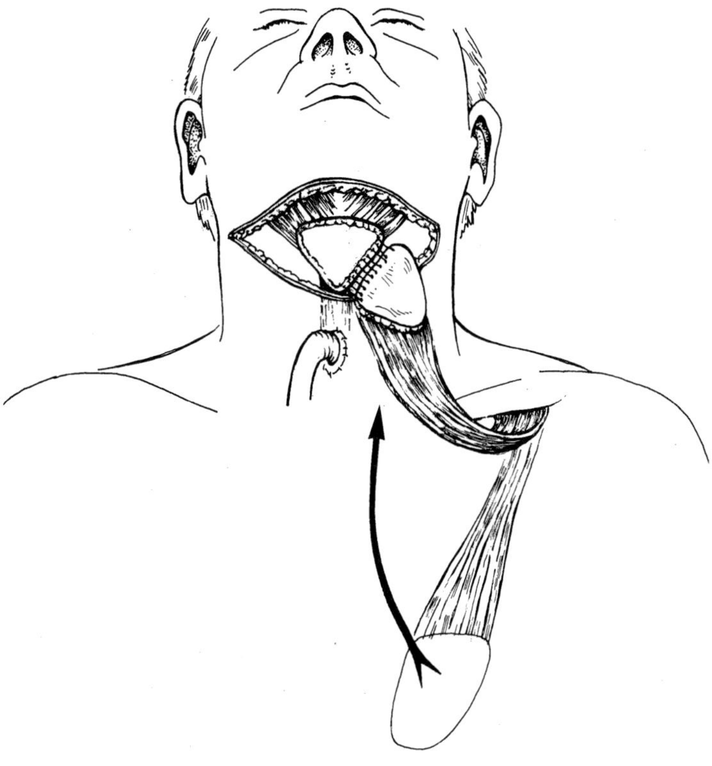

Fig. 12.23 Pectoralis myocutaneous flap for reconstruction of partial pharyngeal resections.

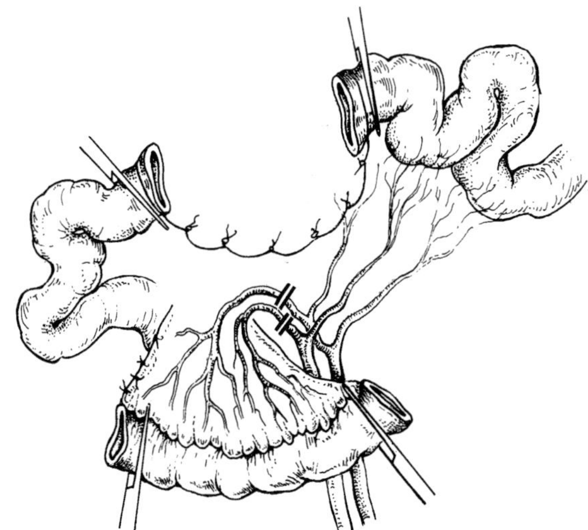

Fig. 12.24 Harvesting a free jejunal transfer.

through its antimesenteric border at its upper end to enlarge the circumference of the upper end to match the pharyngeal circumference. Interrupted absorbable inverting sutures are employed to secure a water-tight pharyngojejunal anastomosis (Fig. 12.25). A nasogastric feeding tube is passed through the pharynx, past the jejunum, into the distal oesophagus and into the stomach. After completion of pharyngojejunal anastomosis, jejuno-oesophageal anastomosis is performed with interrupted inverting absorbable sutures. A water-tight closure must be secured. Following completion of this anastomosis, the wound in the neck is closed in the usual fashion with suction drains. Care must be employed to avoid placement of the suction drains in the vicinity of the vascular anastomosis.

PROBLEMS AND COMPLICATIONS

Individuals undergoing partial laryngopharyngectomy require significant preoperative counselling to help them to understand the physiology of deglutition and the rigorous effort necessary on the part of the patient to participate in postoperative care. In spite of adequate preoperative counselling, postoperative care can be complicated by difficulties in deglutition due to aspiration. As noted before, individuals with poor cardiopulmonary reserve— and particularly those with chronic obstructive pulmonary disease— are not good candidates for this procedure. Postoperative instruction in supraglottic swallowing technique is essential to assist in the return of swallowing function. In the early postoperative period, patients require adequate pulmonary hygiene

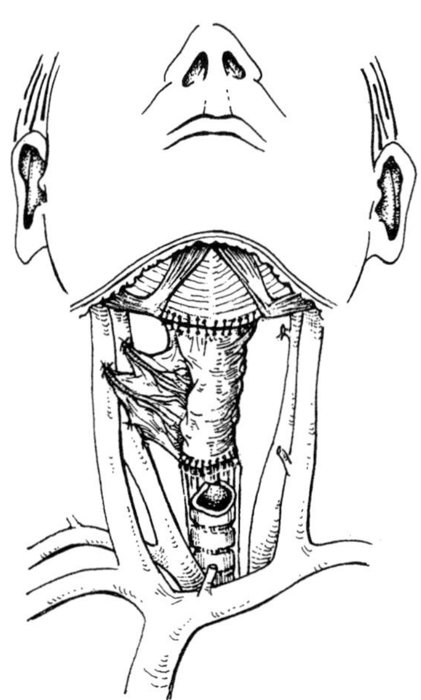

Fig. 12.25 The jejunum is inset into the neck and anastomosed to the oropharynx proximally and the oesophagus distally, and the tissues are revascularized by microvascular anastomosis to major vessels in the neck.

to prevent pneumonia. Patients must be monitored on a long-term basis to assure that they are not suffering from chronic aspiration pneumonia. Individuals with repeated bouts of life-threatening aspiration pneumonia may require completion laryngectomy. In our experience, cricopharyngeal myotomy does not play a significant role in the return of swallowing function. For this reason, we do not employ this technique routinely in individuals undergoing this procedure.

For individuals undergoing resection of the larynx as part of management of hypopharyngeal cancer, the single most significant complication of treatment is the development of a pharyngocutaneous fistula. In general, the more elaborate the repair, the higher the incidence of fistula. Moreover, the rate of fistula increases in individuals who have undergone previous radiation therapy. Fistula rates for individuals undergoing primary closure are relatively low, in the range of 5–10%. On the other hand, the frequency of fistula formation increases with the use of pectoralis major myocutaneous flap, particularly in those individuals who undergo circumferential reconstruction with a tubed pectoralis major myocutaneous flap. The incidence in our experience was in excess of 80% and has led us to abandon this procedure for circumferential reconstruction of the pharynx with pectoralis myocutaneous flap (Vetto et al in press). Finally, the incidence of pharyngocutaneous fistula in either gastric transposition or free microvascular transfer of jejunum is related to the viability of the tissue transferred. Particularly with the transposed stomach, it is the most distal portion of the stomach which serves as the anastomotic site with the pharynx. Breakdown of the pharyngogastric anastomosis places the patient at significant risk for life-threatening mediastinitis. Similar concerns exist for fistulae with the transplanted jejunum although the absence of mediastinal dissection puts the patient at less risk for mediastinitis.

Regardless of the form of reconstruction, all patients must be closely monitored in the first 10 postoperative days for signs of fistula formation. Patients who have received previous chemotherapy or previous radiation therapy often develop pharyngocutaneous fistula quite late, up to a period of 4 to 6 weeks following surgery. The early detection of fistula treated by diversion of the fistula tract with mechanical debridement and frequent irrigations with saline solution and packing changes provides optimal care for this situation. Although commonly used, antibiotics are secondary to the drainage of the pharyngeal contents trapped in the soft tissues of the neck.

Injury to the trachea is a life-threatening condition in patients undergoing pharyngolaryngo-oesophagectomy and transthoracic gastric transposition. Necrosis of the membranous trachea by over-manipulation is usually the cause. Interruption of the segmental tracheal blood supply can also result from contamination of the mediastinum and mediastinitis. If the membranous trachea is perforated or torn during mobilization of the oesophagus, then every precaution must be taken to minimize the length of the tear until the stomach has been transposed. Ideally, a #10 endotracheal tube should be introduced into the distal trachea prior to mobilization in the tracheo-oesophageal plane, and the balloon on the endotracheal tube should be deflated to avoid any stretch on the membranous trachea. Pulmonary ventilation is maintained with adequate pressure held on the respirator, keeping in mind the air leak that will result due to lack of inflation of the balloon. In spite of these precautions, if the tear does take place, then attempts to repair this by suture are usually unsuccessful. Allowing the serosa of the stomach to rest against the membranous trachea usually provides adequate soft-tissue support to permit epithelialization over the serosa of the stomach. Tracheal intubation in the postoperative period should be avoided to prevent further pressure necrosis. Spontaneous healing with epitheliatization over the serosa of the stomach should be anticipated over the next several days.

One of the late sequelae of multi-modality treatment of hypopharyngeal cancer is the development of hypothyroidism and occasionally hypoparathyroidism. Patients who have received previous radiotherapy or those who undergo partial thyroidectomy as an integral part of hypopharyngeal resection and receive postoperative radiation therapy are particularly at higher risk of hypothyroidism. The onset of hypothyroidism is usually insidious. It is therefore desirable to monitor thyroid hormone levels in the postoperative period and appropriate replacement administered when indicated. Patients who have undergone near total thyroidectomy as an integral part of the pharyngeal resection require close monitoring of serum calcium levels in the postoperative period. Appropriate replacement may be indicated if hypocalcemia is symptomatic in the postoperative period.

Restoration of voice is an important consideration in patients undergoing laryngectomy. In the initial postoperative period, patients are trained to communicate with the use of an electrolarynx. With satisfactory healing and restoration of satisfactory swallowing oesophageal speech training is started within 3–4 weeks following surgery. All patients are given a trial of oesophageal speech and only those individuals who are exceptionally motivated are considered candidates for tracheo-oesophageal puncture. Alternatively, individuals who have failed oesophageal speech may be considered on an individual basis for tracheo-oesophageal puncture and voice prosthesis. Patients undergoing pharyngeal reconstruction with a pectoralis major myocutaneous flap, transposed stomach, or microvascular segment of jejunum are considered poor candidates for tracheo-oesophageal puncture speech rehabilitation. Complications resulting from tracheo-oesophageal puncture in any of these patients with the above-mentioned reconstructive procedures can lead to disastrous consequences.

Postoperative swallowing is usually not a problem in patients undergoing total laryngectomy compared to those in whom partial laryngectomy is performed. Patients manifesting difficulty in swallowing, either in the early postoperative period or as a delayed phenomenon, require the use of barium swallow to ascertain the status of patency of the anastomosis and development of stricture or recurrent disease. Anastomotic stricture can usually be managed by repeated dilatations but will often require either an internal stent or secondary repair.

FUTURE DEVELOPMENTS

A number of issues need to be considered as priorities in the management of cancer of the hypopharynx. Submucosal spread of primary tumour complicates the adequacy of surgery for hypopharyngeal carcinomas. More adequate preoperative criteria need to be developed for identifying those patients who would be candidates for larynx-sparing surgical procedures, and more appropriate criteria need to be developed for ascertaining the ability of patients to tolerate larynx-sparing pharyngeal resections. In the field of reconstructive surgery, the use of microvascular sensate fasciocutaneous or skin flaps needs to be investigated to restore the sensations of the replaced pharyngeal lining which may aid in the ability to swallow. Methodology needs to be developed for quantification of the impact on speech impairment and the impairment in deglutition following hypopharyngeal resections. Specific criteria need to be developed regarding the applicability of gastric transposition versus free microvascular transfer of a jejunal segment.

The role of combined treatment with adjuvant radiotherapy in the management of hypopharyngeal carcinoma remains unquestioned. There appears to be some benefit with postoperative radiotherapy compared to preoperative radiation. Clearly, control at the primary site and the neck has improved but improvement in survival has not been reported. The role of multimodality treatment in the management of advanced hypopharyngeal cancer needs to be addressed, particularly with a view to preserving the larynx. To this end, the employment of induction chemotherapy utilizing Cis-platinum and 5-FU has produced complete responses in a significant number of patients with laryngeal and hypopharyngeal carcinomas, avoiding the need for laryngectomy. Sustained remissions are observed using post-chemotherapy external irradiation as definitive treatment. On a short follow-up in a randomized series of patients with laryngeal cancer studied at the Veterans' hospitals in the United States, the survival rates with the chemotherapy/radiotherapy group were comparable to those treated by conventional surgery requiring laryngectomy followed by postoperative radiotherapy (Wolf et al 1991).

A significant number of patients with hypopharyngeal cancer presenting with advanced disease are at a risk of distant metastasis. Early detection and effective prevention or management of distant metastasis should be an important future goal. Similarly, patients with hypopharyngeal carcinoma are at a significant risk of development of a subsequent new primary carcinoma in the upper aero-digestive tract.

Prevention of such subsequent primary tumours is also a vitally important goal for the overall control of squamous carcinomas of the upper aero-digestive tract.

REFERENCES

Bakamjian V Y 1965 A two-stage method for pharyngoesophageal reconstruction with primary pectoral skin flap. Plastic and Reconstructive Surgery 36: 173

Coleman J J III, Searies J M, Hester T R et al 1987 Ten years experience with free jejunal autograft. American Journal of Surgery 154: 394

Lederman M 1967 The role of irradiation in the treatment of cancer of the hypopharynx, post-cricoid and cervical oesophagus. In: Conley J (ed) Proceedings of the International Workshop on Cancer of the Head and Neck. Butterworths, London, p 347

Ogura J H, Marks J E, Freeman R B 1980 Results of conservation surgery for cancers of the supraglottis and pyriform sinus. Laryngoscope 94: 591

Shah J P, Shaha A R, Spiro R H et al 1976 Carcinoma of the hypopharynx. American Journal of Surgery 132: 439

Shah J P, Shemen L, Spiro R H et al 1984 Selecting variants in pharyngeal reconstruction. Annals of Otolaryngology, Rhinology and Laryngology 93: 318

Shah J P, Haribhakti V, Loree T R et al 1990 Complications of pectoralis major myocutaneous flap in head and neck reconstruction. American Journal of Surgery 160: 352

Slaughter D P, Southwick H W, Smejkal W 1953 'Field cancerization' in oral stratified squamous epithelium: clinical implications of multicentric origin. Cancer 6: 963

Spiro R H, Bains M, Shah J P et al 1991 Gastric transposition for head and neck cancer: a critical update. American Journal of Surgery 162: 348

Vetto J, Shah J P, Haribhakti V et al Pectoralis major myocutaneous flap in pharyngeal reconstruction (in press)

Wolf G T, Fisher S G, Wong W K et al 1991 Induction chemotherapy plus radiation compared with surgery plus radiation in patients with advanced laryngeal cancer. VA Laryngeal Cancer Study Group. New England Journal of Medicine 324: 1685

Wookey H 1942 The surgical treatment of carcinoma of the pharynx and upper oesophagus. Surgery, Gynecology and Obstetrics 75: 499

13. Laryngeal cancer

David E. Schuller   Keith M. Wilson

INTRODUCTION AND HISTORICAL REVIEW

Laryngeal cancer represents one of the most common head and neck malignancies. In spite of its common occurrence within the realm of neoplasms arising in the head and neck, it still accounts for only approximately 1.3% of all new cancers, and 0.8% of cancer deaths in the United States (Silverberg 1984). Laryngeal cancer is similar to other head and neck malignancies in that it is primarily a disease of men in the sixth and seventh decades (Rothman et al 1980). Although it is still a disease primarily involving men, the ratio of men to women has been decreasing in the last twenty years (Wynder et al 1956, 1976). There does appear to be an increased prevalence among blacks in the last few years.

There is a strong relationship of cancer of the larynx with certain risk factors. A percentage of laryngeal cancers may be preventable disease if there was total cessation of some of the risk factors. Tobacco represents the primary factor. There is an abundance of epidemiological data which supports the correlation between tobacco and laryngeal cancer (Wynder et al 1956, 1976, Hammond 1966, Kahn 1966, Wynder & Stellman 1977, Burch et al 1984). There also appears to be an increase in risk with the quantity of cigarettes smoked. The risk ratios for laryngeal cancer range anywhere from 6 to 15 in smokers versus non-smokers. The risk with cigar and pipe smoking is considerably less (Sasaki & Carlson 1986). There is also an increased incidence of cancer in people who consume alcohol (Wynder et al 1956, 1976, Flanders & Rothman 1982). There appears to be a potentiation between tobacco and alcohol so that the combination of the two does increase the risk by 50% above that predicted by adding the risk of alcohol with tobacco usage (Sasaki & Carlson 1986).

As mentioned previously, cancer can be considered almost a preventable disease with the avoidance of tobacco and alcohol usage. In the smoker, cessation can also decrease the smoker's risk of laryngeal cancer development. Wynder et al (1976) demonstrated that the risk diminishes dramatically after 6 years of cessation and approaches that of a non-smoker after 15 years of cessation.

Information about occupational risks and laryngeal cancer is somewhat confusing. There was previously some concern about asbestos and laryngeal cancer (Burch et al 1981). Other literature suggests that asbestos is not much of a risk factor (Rothman et al 1980).

It is important to recognize that a variety of therapeutic options exist for laryngeal cancer. Radiation therapy remains a mainstay of treating laryngeal cancer in many parts of the world. Chemotherapy used concurrently with irradiation or subsequent to radiotherapy represents a potential regimen for locoregional and distant control. However, surgery has been and continues to be a common mode of treating laryngeal cancers and will be emphasized in this chapter.

The role of surgery in the treatment of laryngeal cancers dates back more than 100 years. In a textbook by Burnett published in 1893, surgical options for managing laryngeal cancer included: '(a.) endo-laryngeal attempts at removal, (b.) endo-laryngeal cauterizations, (c.) tracheotomy, (d.) complete extirpation, and (e.) partial extirpation or resection' (Burnett 1893). This same textbook describes total laryngectomy being performed by Patrick Watson of Edinburgh in 1866. The procedure was not repeated until 1873 when Billroth performed his much publicized operation. The literature includes reports of total laryngectomy during this time period, again by Watson, Heine and others. One of these groups of early total laryngectomy patients died with recurrence in 6 months, and all the others died within a few days. However, Bottini in 1875 performed a total laryngectomy for a sarcoma, and this patient was alive and functioning normally after ten years.

Partial laryngectomy in the form of removing half of the larynx in the vertical plane was even described in the late 1800s. Hahn reported successful removal of a portion of the larynx in 1885. It is interesting that Burnett (1893) described the indication for partial laryngectomy for 'unilateral and intra-laryngeal epithelioma, and in recent non-infiltrating sarcoma'. His clinical assessment has proven to be accurate 100 years later, and it accurately characterizes the primary indications for this particular version of conservation laryngeal surgery.

EXCISION TECHNIQUE

The larynx is both embryologically and anatomically compartmentalized into the supraglottic, glottic, and subglottic regions. This fact, coupled with the tight adherence of laryngeal mucosa to submucosal structures, provides certain opportunities for surgical resection of laryngeal cancers that do not exist with cancers arising in the oral cavity, oropharynx or hypopharynx. In these areas, the numerous structures in the submucosal tissue, such as vessels and nerves, as well as the fascial planes, seem to facilitate submucosal extension of disease that is not routinely observed with laryngeal cancers. Accordingly, it is technically feasible and oncologically sound to resect laryngeal cancers with relatively small margins of non-cancerous tissue around the disease. This ability to resect cancer with narrow cuffs of normal tissue represents the basic rationale for conservation laryngeal surgery. Whereas margins of 2–2.5 cm around the clinically detectable borders of oral cavity and pharyngeal cancers are necessary in order to obtain a safe cuff, conservation laryngeal surgery can be performed safely with margins of resection which are only 3–4 mm away from clinically detectable laryngeal cancers.

Regional cervical lymphatics

There is no question that nodal metastases do occur with laryngeal cancer for all sites, excepting tumours involving only the glottis. Nodal dissections are recommended either for diagnostic and/or therapeutic reasons. It is also important to remember obviously that non-surgical therapeutic options do exist, primarily in the form of radiation therapy, for the treatment of metastatic cervical adenopathy with laryngeal cancer. The literature certainly supports the idea that radiation therapy has curative potential for microscopic N1 and even some N2 disease.

Surgery also has therapeutic effectiveness. The debate continues about the appropriateness of radical versus some type of modified neck dissection. Both nodal dissections are useful. Both types of operation create morbidity, including shoulder dysfunction. Patient selection becomes critically important in terms of which nodal dissection is recommended. The authors have some concern about whether a modified neck dissection adequately deals with the potential for extracapsular histological nodal disease. Soft-tissue extension from neck nodes is the most ominous prognostic sign in head and neck cancer (Goffinette et al 1984). Extracapsular spread most commonly involves skeletal muscle and the adventitia of the internal jugular vein, which are both structures that are routinely preserved during modified neck dissection (Carter et al 1985). It certainly has been well documented that extracapsular disease de-

Table 13.1 Staging

	RND	MND	Supra-omohyoid
N0	No	Poss	Yes
N1	Some	Yes	No
N2A	Yes	No	No
N2B	Yes	Poss	No
N3A	Yes	No	No
N3B	Yes ... but	Poss	No
N3C	Yes ... but	Yes ... but	No

creases the survival (Snow et al 1982, Johnson et al 1985, Snyderman et al 1985). Considering the reality of the frequency of nodal matastases coupled with the negative impact of extracapsular spread on prognosis, the authors have developed certain generalized recommendations regarding the types of nodal dissection recommended for the variety of clinical situations relative to laryngeal cancer. These recommendations are listed in Table 13.1. This table demonstrates that radical neck dissection really is not recommended for N0 disease. It is possible that some type of modified neck dissection can be used for N0 disease. However, the authors do prefer supra-omohyoid nodal dissection as a diagnostic staging approach which will ultimately determine whether postoperative radiation therapy is recommended. N1 disease can at times require radical neck dissection if it is found to be clinically invading structures routinely preserved with a modified neck dissection. However, the majority of N1 disease can be treated with modified neck dissection. Supra-omohyoid neck dissection is not utilized for N1 disease because of the inadequacy of cervical lymphatic removal with this diagnostic procedure. The authors recommend using radical neck dissection for N2A and N2B disease. It is possible that modified neck dissection can be utilized for N2B disease. Once again, supra-omohyoid neck dissection has no role in the treatment of advanced neck nodal disease. It is recommended that neck nodal disease which is classified as N3A be treated with radical neck dissection. Radical neck dissection is recommended also for N3B and N3C disease. However, it is plausible that N3B disease can be considered to be more of a manifestation of systemic rather than anatomical spread of disease, and there are times when this clinical situation may be treated with modified neck dissection in combination with systemic chemotherapy.

The authors perform radical neck dissection as described in several texts. If feasible, incontinuity dissections with the primary tumour resection are performed. However modified neck dissection can involve preservation of structures that are routinely preserved with this approach as described in the literature. The authors primarily preserve only the spinal accessory nerve with modified neck dissection, and sometimes the internal jugular vein. The increased morbidity with removal of the submandibular salivary gland, sternocleidomastoid muscle, and cervical sensory lymphatics is questioned by the authors and consequently they are not routinely preserved with modified neck dissection. There is no hesitancy on the part of the authors to resect either the internal jugular vein and/or the spinal accessory nerve if the disease is found to be involving them during the course of the modified neck dissection, subsequently converting the procedure into a radical neck dissection.

A supra-omohyoid neck dissection represents a diagnostic sampling of tissue to base the decision regarding postoperative radiation therapy on microscopically analysed tissue rather than on clinical impression. The procedure involves removal of the submandibular triangle as well as the lymph nodes throughout the anterior jugular compartments in addition to some of the posterior inferior neck compartments.

Preoperative planning

Conservation laryngeal surgery is now a proven oncologically safe surgical approach which has obvious positive results on the psychosocial health of the patient. It is mandatory for the head and neck oncological surgeon to have skills in diagnostic and surgical extirpative procedures as well as reconstructive techniques to maximize this opportunity for the patient which can have a profound impact on not only their survival but also the quality of their survival. It is imperative to obtain as much information about the extent of disease preoperatively as possible. This is done primarily with physical examination. Indirect laryngoscopy provides useful information about the superior and lateral extent of disease but limited information about the inferior border. It also provides critically important information about true vocal cord mobility. However, the indirect and even direct laryngoscopical examination is limited in its ability to assess inferior extent. Imaging studies, whether thin-sliced computed tomography and/or magnetic resonance imaging, does provide useful information about inferior extent of disease which is difficult to obtain with any other approach. After indirect laryngoscopical and imaging studies have been completed the next step is to proceed with direct laryngoscopy in the operating room where an even more thorough examination can be performed that, once again, helps to determine as thoroughly as possible the extent of the disease as well as to obtain biopsies to establish histopathology. The authors also continue to perform bronchoscopy and oesophagoscopy at the time of direct laryngoscopy to rule out the existence of concurrent secondary neoplasms. It is not uncommon in the United States for the laryngoscopy and biopsy with frozen section analysis, bronchoscopy and oesophagoscopy to be performed as the initial phase prior to the resection in an effort to reduce health care costs by avoiding the need for multiple anaesthetics and hospitalizations created by separating the diagnostic from the extirpative procedures.

Vocal cord immobility implies invasion of the neoplasm into the vocalis muscle which represents an ominous clinical situation. However, there is evidence that some impaired vocal cord mobility can result from bulky exophytic superficially invasive disease. It is imperative for the head and neck oncological surgeon to be aware of this possible physical limitation in vocal cord movement that does not have the same serious prognostic ramifications as the patient who has infiltrative neoplasm into the vocalis muscle. There are no techniques which precisely enable the surgeon to make this distinction except for having an awareness of this clinical fact and of having the experience and expertise to make a determination about the actual aetiology of cord immobility. It is imperative that the surgeon communicates with the surgical pathologist in terms of the planned resection so that the surgical pathologist understands the clinical significance of his assessment of the frozen section. If the pathologist does not have a comfort level with diagnosis on the frozen section, the resection needs to be deferred until definitive histopathology is determined using permanent sections.

Primary tumour site(s)

Supraglottic laryngeal cancer

When laryngeal cancers involve the supraglottic portion of the larynx, horizontal partial (i.e., supraglottic) laryngectomy is feasible. The primary essential feature which permits supraglottic laryngectomy is a relative freedom of involvement of the glottic larynx. There are modifications of the standard surgical approach which permit resection of some of the glottic larynx in association with supraglottic laryngectomy, and this will be discussed later. The neck skin incision which is used for supraglottic laryngectomy is determined by two factors: (i) that which will provide good exposure to the supraglottic larynx, and (ii) access to one and/or both sides of the neck for some type of nodal dissection either at the time of resection of the primary or subsequent to the primary site surgery. The horizontal T incision with the adjustment of the plane of the horizontal limb provides excellent access to the primary site as well as current or future access to the neck for nodal dissection. Surgical exposure is achieved by releasing both the suprahyoid and infrahyoid extrinsic laryngeal muscles. Electrocautery is frequently utilized to release the suprahyoid musculature. However, it is advisable to use scissors to release the muscle attachments around the greater cornu in an effort to minimize injury to the hypoglossal nerve whose course may be close to the greater cornu of the hyoid bone. All of the infrahyoid strap muscles are released with a single incision at about the level of the superior border of the thyroid cartilage and reflected inferiorly with the deep plane of dissection being adjacent to thyroid cartilage perichondrium. This continuous muscular sheet provides a second layer of closure following resection and it is important not to separate it into the separate muscles. The thyroid cartilage perichondrium is incised along the superior border of the

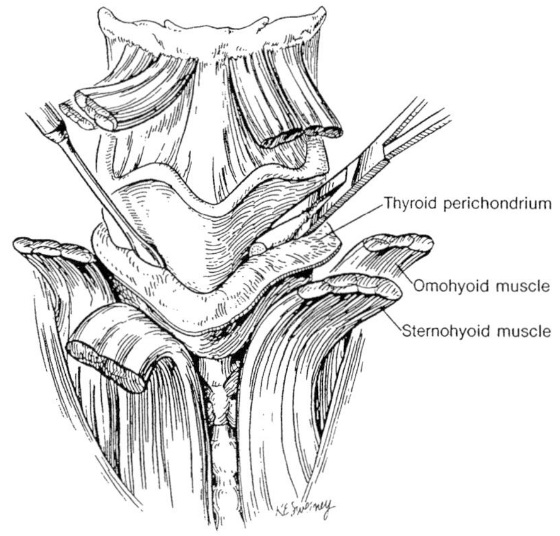

Fig. 13.1 In supraglottic laryngectomy, strap muscles are cut just above the thyroid cartilage, and the perichondrium is incised along the superior border of thyroid cartilage.

cartilage and reflected inferiorly using a freer elevator for this subperichondrial dissection (Fig. 13.1). The perichondrium is invariably thinner in the midline, especially at the level of the thyroid notch. Elevation of the perichondrium over each of the bodies of the thyroid cartilage and then connecting these two areas with subsequent elevation in the midline facilitates this manoeuvre and minimizes the possibility of perforating the perichondrium. The perichondrial eleva-

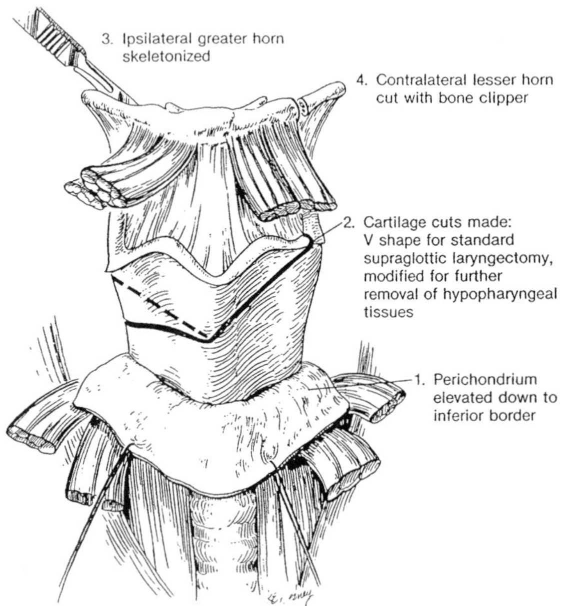

Fig. 13.2 Thyroid cartilage perichondrium elevation is completed to just slightly beyond the inferior border of the planned resection, and then cartilage cuts are made. This may be modified for further removal of hypopharyngeal tissues according to the size of lesion. Ipsilateral greater horn is skeletonized.

tion should not extend much beyond the horizontal plane where one intends making the thyroid cartilage cuts. Elevating the perichondrium removes the cartilage's blood supply, and accordingly it is important to maintain this contact with the cartilage except in the areas where it must be elevated.

The thyroid cartilage cuts are made with a high-speed oscillating saw. These saws, which have sharp disposable blades of differing sizes and angle, provide excellent precision for this phase of the operation that did not exist with previous cartilage-cutting techniques. If the supraglottic laryngeal cancer involves one side of the larynx, the thyroid cartilage resection on the non-involved side can be less and is usually performed by angulating the cartilage cut so that the superior cartilage cornu on the non-involved site is preserved (Fig. 13.2). The thyroid cartilage cut is placed at the horizontal plane which is just slightly superior to the point of attachment of the true vocal cords to the thyroid cartilage. The hypopharynx is entered through the vallecula, and the tongue base is released from its attachments to the supraglottic portion of the larynx at the level of the vallecula (Fig. 13.3). The pyriform sinus mucosal incisions are made in an inferior direction retaining as much non-involved mucosa as is safe. These initial lateral hypopharyngeal incisions do facilitate exposure. It is advisable for the surgeon to stand at the head of the operating table looking over the patient's face which provides improved visual access to the supraglottic larynx. The exposure can be improved by having the surgeon place a bone-biting instrument on the hyoid bone and retracting it superiorly at the same time that the anaesthesiologist makes sure that the patient is paralysed for maximal tissue relaxation.

The initial incision of the endolaryngeal mucosa is made

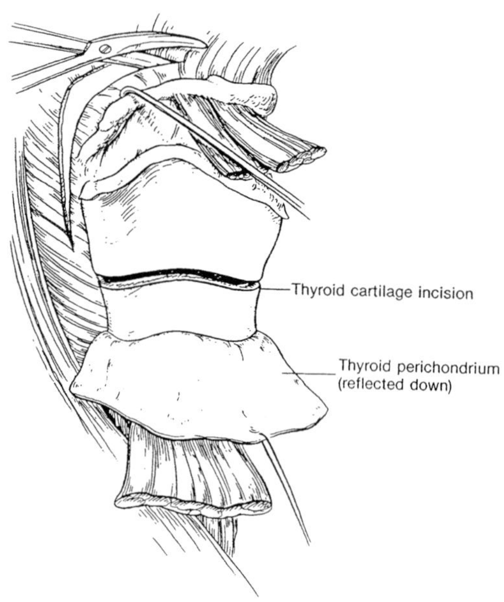

Fig. 13.3 Pyriform fossa and vallecula are entered on the side of lesion, while greater horn of hyoid bone is retracted for exposure.

with curved scissors over the body of the arytenoid on the non-involved side. This incision is carried into the laryngeal ventricle. The curved-scissor is then rotated 180° so that the tip is pointing upward, hopefully as a safeguard against the possibility of inadvertently incising the true vocal cord, and an incision is then made through the laryngeal ventricle on the uninvolved side to the anterior commissure. The mucosal incision is accompanied by incising the submucosal tissues through the horizontal planes established previously by the thyroid cartilage cut on that side. After the tissues have been incised on the uninvolved side to the anterior commissure, there is marked improvement of the exposure. It is at this point that a scalpel is used to incise sharply the mucosa around the disease with a preferred margin of 3–4 mm. However, sometimes even smaller margins are feasible. After the mucosal incisions have been made with the scalpel, the submucosal tissues are incised using a curved scissors until the lesion is amputated (Fig. 13.4).

Small samples of tissue from true vocal cords and other areas of concern are submitted for frozen section analysis to provide some component of security that the disease has been completely resected. Assuming that the frozen sections are clear of microscopic neoplastic disease, closure begins by inserting a nasogastric tube followed by closure of the lateral hypopharyngeal extensions with inverting Connell type sutures using 3-0 silk followed by approximation of the thyroid perichondrium to stitches placed deeply into the tongue musculature adjacent to the mucosal border of the tongue base. All of the stitches are placed before tying them. After the initial layer has been completed and the sutures are tied, the second layer of closure is achieved with the approximation of the infrahyoid strap muscles to the tongue

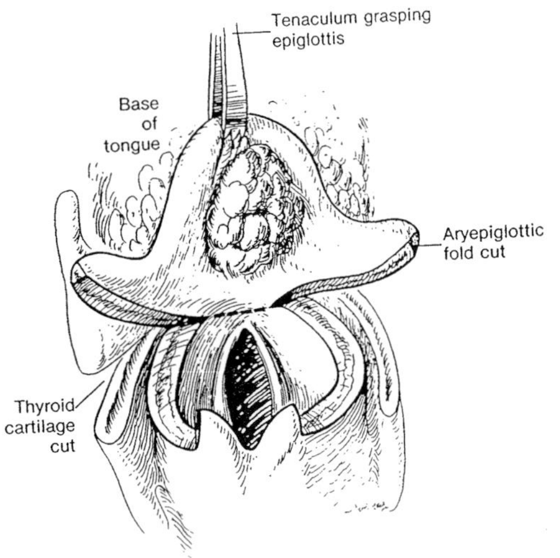

Fig. 13.4 Epiglottis is grasped with tenaculum, and scissors are used to cut through the aryepiglottic fold in front of the arytenoid and down into the ventricle. Once both supraglottic incisions have been made through the aryepiglottic folds, the intervening tissues are incised to join the thyroid cartilage cuts.

musculature and lateral neck musculature. The wound is irrigated with copious amounts of saline and active drainage tubes are inserted. The neck flaps are subsequently closed in layers to provide an air-tight closure.

A tracheotomy is obviously inserted as the initial phase of this surgery and is kept in place usually for 7 to 9 days postoperatively. It is usually about the eighth to the tenth postoperative day that oral feedings are begun.

Oral feedings do not begin until both the tracheotomy and the nasogastric tubes have been removed. Patients are given a booklet which explains a new swallowing technique prior to beginning oral feedings. This technique is directed at trying to minimize the potential for aspiration and involves initial inspiration followed by swallowing a bolus of semi-solid food three times without taking a breath. After the third swallow, the patient is instructed to cough forcefully and then to breathe. The forceful cough tends to expel any retained food which may be lying on the superior surface of the true vocal cords. Patients are personally supervised every time they eat for the first few days. Intravenous fluids are maintained during this time to assure against dehydration. If there is no improvement apparent with oral feedings after a few days, a nasogastric tube is inserted and the patient is discharged on nasogastric feedings to be given more time for resolution of laryngeal and/or pharyngeal oedema before making another attempt at oral feedings. This approach has been successful, with only a relative handful of patients not being able to resume satisfactory oral swallowing function.

There are times when lesions which are primarily supraglottic do extend inferiorly to involve a portion of the true vocal cord. This involvement of the glottic larynx is usually in the area of the anterior commissure. In this situation, an extended supraglottic laryngectomy is feasible by including the resection of that portion of the glottic larynx which is involved. Once again, narrow margins of resection are oncologically safe. Such resections can involve one or both true vocal cords. If there has just been a small distance of each anterior portion of the vocal cords resected, reattachment to the remaining thyroid cartilage can be achieved by drilling a hole through the thyroid cartilage and passing a suture through this to approximate the true vocal cord(s) to the midline. If primary closure is not possible, reconstruction is feasible and will be discussed in the section on reconstruction.

There are times when supraglottic laryngectomy can be expanded to resect some of the pharyngeal tissue when disease extends into the hypopharynx. It used to be felt that the supraglottic laryngectomy could be performed so as to include some of the medial wall of the hypopharynx. However, the authors have extended those indications to resect neoplasms that involve the supraglottic larynx as well as a substantial amount of both the medial and lateral wall of the hypopharynx, oropharynx, and even tongue base. The major challenge with these types of resection is in reconstruction, which will be discussed later in this chapter.

Glottic laryngeal cancer

Quality of voice is derived from a variety of laryngeal and pharyngeal tissue vibrations as well as air flow through this region. There is no question that alterations at the level of the glottis have the greatest impact on altering voice quality. It subsequently follows that surgical resections of cancers involving the glottic larynx will have more of an adverse impact on quality of voice than those lesions that permit retention of the true vocal cords. There are times when glottic laryngeal cancers can be managed endoscopically. Although the literature abounds with descriptions of endoscopic approaches for T1 and even T2 laryngeal cancers, the authors continue to use endoscopic excision for those lesions which are small and superficially invasive. There is no question that suspension microlaryngoscopy utilizing the carbon dioxide laser attached to the microscope does provide an effective and precise means of resecting superficially invasive laryngeal cancers, especially those involving the glottis where the resection of even a millimetre or two of tissue beyond what is necessary can have a profound impact on the quality of the patient's voice.

The authors' means of extirpation is somewhat different from the standard laser cordectomy where the laser simply becomes a means of incising the tissue around the involved area. The authors vaporize the involved tissue to a plane in the vocalis musculature which clinically appears to be free of disease. After the vaporization has been completed, frozen sections are obtained from the deep margins in the anterior, middle and posterior extent of the area that was vaporized using microlaryngeal cup forceps. If there is no evidence of microscopic disease, the procedure is terminated and the defect involving the upper portion of true vocal cord heals by secondary intention with eventual mucosal migration that ultimately produces a vocal cord, whose appearance is oftentimes clinically indistinguishable from a normal vocal cord. The advantage of this technique is that it does provide a means of preserving the free edge of the vocal cords, admittedly at a plane different from that of the free edge. However, the subsequent healing re-establishes the same horizontal plane with voice quality that appears to be superior to the standard approach of laser cordectomy.

In those glottic laryngeal cancers which are not amenable to endoscopic excision, vertical partial laryngectomy (i.e., hemilaryngectomy) is undertaken. Given the paucity of lymphatics draining the glottic larynx, it is rare to have to consider neck nodal dissections, and the neck incision does not usually have to account for that possibility. A horizontally oriented incision placed over the larynx in a relaxed skin tension line that is equidistant from the midline provides both excellent exposure and aesthetics after healing is completed. Neck flaps are elevated in a subplatysmal plane, and the infrahyoid strap muscles are split in the midline, dissected away from the involved site of the thyroid cartilage, and retracted laterally. A perichondrial flap is developed by

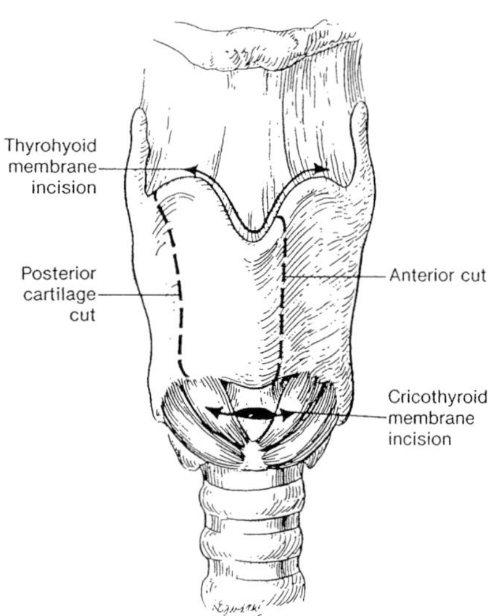

Fig. 13.5 After the posterior cartilage cut is made, the anterior cut is made 2–3 mm away from the midline on the contralateral side. Entry is made just superior to the true vocal cords and extended superiorly into the thyrohyoid membrane.

incising along the superior and inferior borders of the thyroid cartilage on the involved site and connecting them with a vertical incision about 3–4 mm beyond the planned medial cartilage cut, which is usually in the midline, but can extend for any distance across the midline on the contralateral side. The cartilage cut should be at a plane that is decidedly beyond the extent of the disease within the larynx but within 2–3 mm. Once again, the high-speed oscillating saws represent a precise means of making the medial and lateral cartilage cuts. The lateral cut is made about 2–3 mm within the lateral extent of the thyroid cartilage framework (Fig. 13.5). It is advisable to preserve the lateral thyroid cartilage border for support of the retained tissues as well as providing anatomical landmarks for possible future surgical interventions.

The endolarynx is entered by laterally retracting the edges of the medial cartilage cut with single-pronged skin hooks and incising through the soft tissues between the cartilage cuts with a No.11 scalpel, initially incising at a plane above the level of true vocal cords and directed superiorly into the thryo-hyoid membrane and then across the thyro-hyoid membrane on the involved side. The surgeon's exposure is facilitated by using a headlight and having the anaesthesiologist paralyse the patient for maximal tissue relaxation. After this incision has been made through the thyrohyoid membrane there is improved exposure to permit the surgeon to incise precisely through either the anterior commissure or the contralateral vocal cord at a distance 2–3 mm away from the disease, extending that incision inferiorly through the cricothyroid membrane on the ipsilateral side. The lateral mucosal incision is made with a scalpel, and the submucosal incisions are completed with the curved scissors with eventual excision of the lesion (Fig. 13.6). Multiple

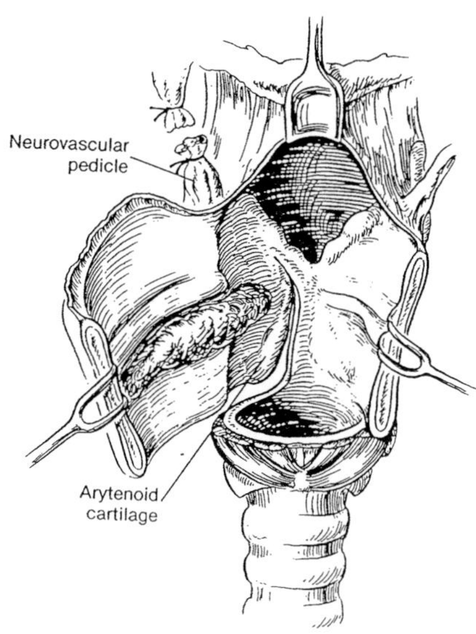

Fig. 13.6   The Posterior margin is incised in front of, through, or including the arytenoid, according to the extent of disease.

frozen sections of the margin are submitted and, if clear, the larynx is then closed. The larynx can be closed without any attempts to reconstruct the cord by approximating the perichondrial flap and the strap muscles as a second layer of closure. This is done after insertion of a nasogastric tube. However, the authors do prefer some type of tissue insertion in the area of the resected vocal cord and this will be discussed in the next section on reconstruction.

The potential for aspiration is considerably less with vertical hemilaryngectomy as opposed to supraglottic laryngectomy. Nasogastric feedings usually persist for 5 to 6 days and then the tracheotomy tube as well as the nasogastric tube are removed and the patient starts oral feedings. No special swallowing techniques are necessary because the retained uninvolved supraglottic portion of the larynx maintains the normal aspiration protective mechanisms.

Transglottic laryngeal cancer

The general recommendation for those cancers that extend from one laryngeal region (supraglottic, glottic, subglottic) into another is to undergo total laryngectomy. Some form of nodal dissection is done usually in conjunction with resection of the primary tumour site. Once again, it is important for the head and neck oncological surgeon to attempt aggressively to preserve enough laryngeal structure, if oncologically safe, to maintain function. The diagnostic approaches described earlier in this chapter are critically important in this situation. It is possible to perform some type of conservation laryngeal surgical procedure with flap reconstruction that ultimately can preserve laryngeal function and avoid the need for permanent tracheostoma. The reconstructive considerations will be discussed in the next session of this chapter. When conservation laryngeal surgery is not feasible, total laryngectomy is performed.

The neck skin incision for total laryngectomy also needs to include the possibility of access to the lateral neck contents for nodal dissection. The apron incision does provide good exposure to the primary tumour site as well as access to one or both sides of the neck. The apron incision is extended posteriorly so that it overlies the direction of the trapezius muscle and then curved across the lower portion of the neck in a relaxed skin tension line that leads to the planned area for the tracheostoma, extending to the anterior border of the contralateral sternocleidomastoid muscle. After elevation of the flaps in the subplatysmal plane, the nodal dissection is initially performed. If there is clinically detectable nodal disease, the neck specimen is left attached to the larynx. The nodal dissection is performed from a lateral to a medial direction. The initial phase of total laryngectomy entails releasing the muscular attachments to the larynx and usually begins with the release of the infrahyoid strap muscles. The ipsilateral thyroid lobe and a portion of the isthmus are included with the resection as a lateral cuff around any disease that may have extended through the larynx. The inferior constrictor muscles are released bilaterally, as are the suprahyoid muscles.

The hypopharynx is subsequently entered at a location that is presumed to be uninvolved with disease. This entrance can be superiorly at the level of the vallecula by separating the tongue base from the supraglottic larynx, laterally through a pyriform sinus pharyngotomy, or inferiorly following tracheal transection. The trachea is transected in a bevelled fashion to increase the circumference which permits a large tracheostoma and decreases the chance for stomal stenosis. After the lesion has been resected, once again, frozen sections of the margins determine histological clearance.

The hypopharynx is subsequently closed using 3-0 silk with inverting Connell type stitches as the primary layer followed by a secondary layer approximating the strap muscles over the mucosal closure. Vocal restoration is performed primarily and will be described in the reconstruction section. Drainage tubes are placed and the flaps are approximated. Oral feedings usually begin approximately 6 to 7 days postoperatively. The routine with oral feedings involves a clear liquid diet for the first feeding to determine that no fistula exists. If negative, the patient proceeds immediately to a regular diet. The volume and consistency of regular food tends to have a dilatory effect on the freshly reconstituted hypopharynx and hopefully acts to minimize the potential for any hypopharyngeal stenosis.

Tracheostomal recurrent cancer

Tracheostomal recurrent cancer occurs in 5–15% of all patients undergoing total laryngectomy. Sisson has developed a classification system for stomal recurrence which is listed in Table 13.2 (Sisson et al 1976). Types 1 and 2 stomal recurrences are localized to the superior aspect of the stoma

Table 13.2 Classification of stomal recurrence

Type I	Localized to superior aspect of stoma No oesophageal involvement
Type II	Localized to superior aspect of stoma With oesophageal involvement
Type III	Originates from inferior aspect of stoma and involves superior mediastinum
Type IV	Extension laterally beneath clavicles and into superior mediastinum

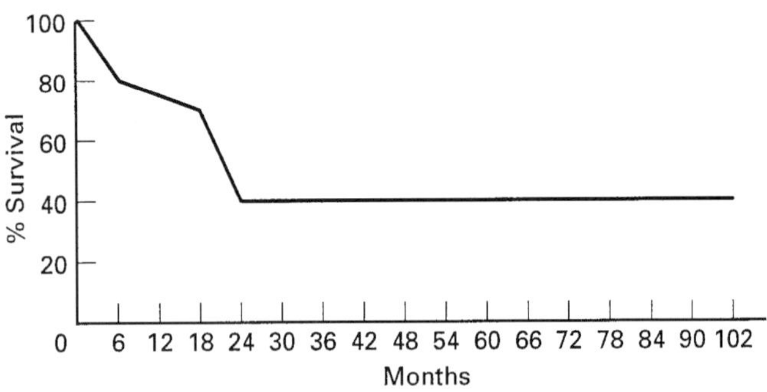

Fig. 13.7 Graph depicting determinant survival for Sisson types 1 and 2 stomal recurrence.

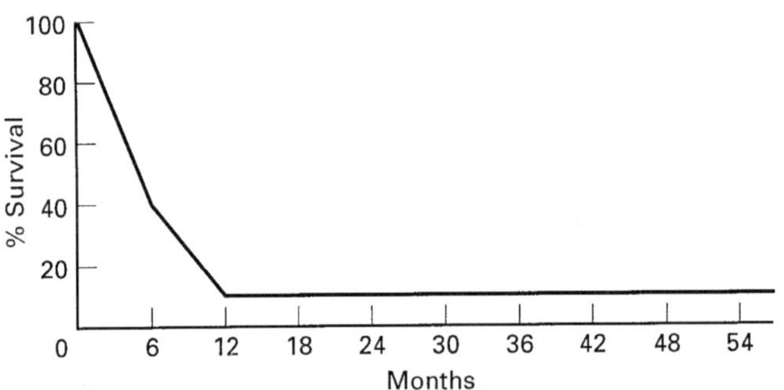

Fig. 13.8 Graph depicting determinant survival for Sisson types 3 and 4 stomal recurrence.

and have a more favorable prognosis (Fig. 13.7) compared to types 3 and 4 stomal recurrences (Fig. 13.8) which involve structures located inferior to the stoma. Their prognosis is much more ominous. Tracheostomal recurrent cancer is treated with mediastinal resection. Schuller et al (1981) and Gluckman et al (1987) have reviewed their collective experience with mediastinal dissection, developed by Sisson (Sisson et al 1976). Both of the reports conclude that the procedure does have curative potential for some patients with stomal recurrences and certainly can improve quality of survival. However, they have also documented that there is morbidity and even mortality with this dangerous operation. However, there are currently no viable therapeutic alternatives to mediastinal dissection.

The procedure involves resection of the surrounding neck and upper chest skin around the disease. The operation is basically a dissection of both carotid artery systems as well as the superior mediastinal structures. The manubrium as well as one or both proximal clavicles are resected primarily as a means of gaining access to the superior mediastinum. A

portion or all of the pharynx and/or cervical oesophagus is included if there is disease involvement. The mediastinal soft tissues from the arch of the aorta superiorly are included as a cuff around the disease. After the resection has been completed, reconstruction of the neck and chest skin, trachea and oesophagus are undertaken and will be discussed in the reconstruction section.

RECONSTRUCTIVE TECHNIQUES

Reconstruction of the larynx is intended to restore the primary physiological function of that organ, which is protection of the airway during deglutition. Phonation is obviously important. However, protection from aspiration represents the primary goal of laryngeal reconstruction. The bulk of tissue flaps, oftentimes mentioned as a disadvantages for their reconstructive capabilities, is frequently an advantage as it pertains to their use in laryngeal reconstruction and the prevention of aspiration.

Another important consideration in laryngeal reconstruction is the maintenance of the airway by the cricoid cartilage. Once again, the high-speed oscillating saws provide increased capabilities for partial cricoid resections which did not exist with earlier means of cartilage incision. Partial resections of the cricoid cartilage are certainly feasible using certain reconstructive techniques and technologies. In short, the reconstructive techniques that relate to tissue transfer and tissue fixation have expanded the capabilities of laryngeal reconstruction which have had a positive impact on the quality of survival of the patient with laryngeal cancer. It is imperative for the contemporary head and neck oncological surgeon to have not only diagnostic and extirpative skills, but also a full reconstructive armamentarium.

Primary tumour site reconstruction

Supraglottic

Most defects following supraglottic laryngectomy can be closed primarily. However, there are times when the supraglottic larynx is resected as a part of a cuff of tissue around a tongue base cancer. There are also times when a supraglottic laryngeal cancer extends to involve a portion of the hypopharynx and even beyond. Whereas these clinical situations often prompted a total laryngectomy in the past, current tissue transfer techniques are feasible with preservation of laryngeal function. The pectoralis musculocutaneous flap is an effective means of reconstructing tongue base defects as well as pharyngeal defects in association with supraglottic laryngectomy. In this situation, the skin island is sutured directly to the remaining thyroid cartilage perichondrium and the lateral walls of the skin island are approximated to the hypopharyngeal mucosa, with the other end of the skin island being sutured to the remaining tongue base. The bulk of this flap provides a protective function for the remaining larynx and minimizes aspiration. Patients who have undergone this type of tongue-base reconstruction with supraglottic laryngectomy actually swallow more easily than those patients who have undergone primary closure without any tissue transfer. The one clinical situation where this technique is not useful occurs when the tongue-base resection is so extensive that it produces bilateral hypoglossal nerve paralysis. The combination of a totally adynamic tongue with an adynamic skin island has produced an unsatisfactory amount of aspiration which necessitated total laryngectomy. Lateral hypopharyngeal and even oropharyngeal as well as tongue defects in conjunction with partial laryngeal resection have been reconstructed with larger pectoralis musculocutaneous flaps. Once again, the bulk of tissue provides protection from aspiration while maintaining an adequate airway.

Sometimes suspension of the remaining larynx following supraglottic laryngectomy also helps to minimize aspiration. The suspension is achieved by drilling holes in the mid portion of each thyroid cartilage body along its superior edge and passing a large non-absorbable suture through this hole and using either the suprahyoid musculature adjacent to the mandible or the mandibular periosteum as the other point to create an anterior–superior traction to pull the larynx under the protective hood of the tongue base. However, the authors do not always use these laryngeal suspension sutures.

Cricopharyngeal myotomy has been advocated as a means of facilitating deglutition following supraglottic laryngectomy. However, there is conflicting information in the literature about its value. A current multi-institutional trial headed by Wayne State University and involving The Ohio State University (Jacobs et al 1985) is prospectively evaluating the efficacy of myotomy on deglutition function. These results will provide clinically useful information.

In those patients who have undergone an extended supraglottic laryngectomy that has involved a portion of the true vocal cords, there are times when primary approximation of the remaining vocal cords to the anterior commissure region is not feasible. In this situation, a portion of one of the strap muscles, usually the superior belly of the omohyoid, can be approximated to the remaining true vocal cords. However, the anterior posterior dimension of the glottic portion of the larynx needs to be maintained with the insertion of a keel at the level of the anterior commissure. This oftentimes produces an effective reconstruction of the glottis that was resected. It has the obvious disadvantage of requiring another procedure to remove the keel after several weeks in order to allow re-epithelialization over the strap muscles that were attached to the remaining true vocal cords.

Glottic

It was mentioned earlier in this chapter that some head and neck oncological surgeons allow healing by secondary intention following hemilaryngectomy. Aspiration is rarely a problem following hemilaryngectomy, most probably because one side of the larynx retains its normal function. However, voice quality is certainly changed after removing one, and possibly a portion, of the other true vocal cord. There are those who feel that voice quality can be improved with attempts to reconstruct that portion of the larynx that was resected. The literature describes a variety of tissue interposition techniques, frequently using a portion of the sternohyoid muscle. However, the fact that a portion has to be utilized means that there is the chance of devascularizing it. An alternative technique involves the use of either all or most of the superior belly of the omohyoid. This can be tunnelled into the endolarynx through a perforation made in the thyroid cartilage perichondrial flap. The end of the omohyoid muscle is attached to whatever remains of the arytenoid on the resected side. Some of the remaining mucosa can be sutured to the omohyoid muscle in an effort to direct the mucosal migration over this muscle. The reader needs to understand that these muscle interposition techniques provide bulk but certainly not a functioning true vocal cord. The hope is that this bulk will facilitate glottic closure by the remaining vocal cord to improve quality and to minimize any chances for aspiration during deglutition. The bulk of the resected side of the larynx can be subsequently augmented following muscle interposition with teflon injections in an attempt to further refine voice quality or to minimize aspiration.

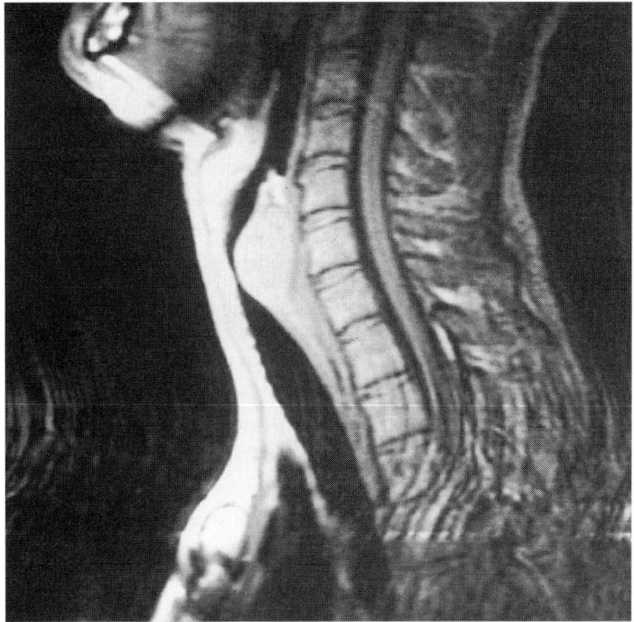

Fig. 13.9 This imaging study demonstrates a chondrosarcoma arising from the cricoid cartilage that was resected and reconstructed without the need for total laryngectomy.

Subglottic

Squamous-cell carcinoma arising in the subglottic region is rare. It is clinically more common to have this region involved by extension from the glottis. However, the subglottic region can be involved with chondrosarcomas arising from the cricoid or arytenoid cartilages (Fig. 13.9). Whereas this entity was previously considered to be treatable only with total laryngectomy, there is some information to suggest that the biological behaviour of chondrosarcomas does not necessitate wide margins of resection. Accordingly, the surgeon can take advantage of the high-speed oscillating saws as a piece of technology that will facilitate partial cricoid resection in an effort to resect adequately the disease but to preserve the continuity of the cricoid arch and the adequacy of the airway. However, there will be times when a chondrosarcoma is resected that involves full-thickness partial cricoid resection. Usually this resection is completed via a midline thyrotomy which provides exposure to the disease. After a portion of the thyroid cartilage is resected, the cricoid can be reconstructed with a composite costal cartilage-perichondrial graft that can even be bent to mimic the normal contour of the portion of the cricoid cartilage that was resected. This composite graft can be held in position with the use of a soft silastic tracheal t-tube to provide internal support using micro-stabilization plates. These micro-stabilization plates appear to have clinical usefulness for some of these specialized laryngeal reconstructions. The tracheal t-tube is left in place for several weeks to provide support of the composite graft and hopefully permit mucosal migration over the perichondrial portion of the graft so that the airway lumen is totally lined with epithelium.

Transglottic

Transglottic laryngeal cancers which extend beyond the confines of the larynx, necessitating a partial pharyngectomy as well as total laryngectomy, can be reconstructed in a one-stage procedure utilizing a pectoralis musculocutaneous flap. The technique for this has been described in other publications (Schuller & Parrish 1988).

Primary vocal restoration has been routinely performed in patients undergoing total laryngectomy for the last 12 years. The advantages of primary vocal restoration include no additional procedures or hospitalizations in addition to being psychologically beneficial. Primary vocal restoration also does not restrict the potential of the patient's vocal rehabilitation with any of the other alternative techniques. In fact, some patients have utilized tracheo-oesophageal speech following primary vocal restoration as a means of learning oesophageal speech with eventual removal of the prosthesis and closure of the fistula and total reliance on oesophageal speech. There have been some reports in the literature describing complications following primary vocal restoration. Reviews of the Ohio State University experience on two different occasions (Trudeau et al 1986, 1988) have provided objective information supporting the continuation of primary vocal restoration. Primary vocal restoration also does not appear to be adversely affected by postoperative radiation therapy (Trudeau et al 1989).

The technique for primary vocal restoration involves the placement of a right angle haemostat through the hypopharyngeal defect following total laryngectomy, using the tip of this to identify the site of the planned tracheo-oesophageal fistula. The posterior tracheal wall mucosa in the midline is incised for a distance of 2–3 mm approximately 5 mm from the tracheocutaneous junction, and the tip of the haemostat is used to push the oesophageal mucosa through this incision where the oesophageal mucosa is then incised. The end of a 14 French red rubber catheter is grasped with the haemostat and pulled through the tracheo-oesophageal fistula. The catheter is then directed inferiorly through the oesophagus into the stomach. The patient is fed through this tracheo-oesophageal tube, avoiding the need for a nasogastric tube and adding to the patient's comfort. The tube is sutured into position and left in place for a period of 3 weeks at which time it is removed and fitting for the prosthesis is performed by the speech pathologist with the commencement of vocal restoration. Vocal restoration training proceeds throughout the patient's period of postoperative radiation therapy.

There is a disadvantage to primary vocal restoration which involves an increased incidence of tracheostomal stenosis. This stenosis seems to be related to an increased amount of manipulation of the healing stoma created by the need for prosthesis replacement and digital pressure over the stoma during vocalization at the same time that postoperative radiation therapy is also being administered to these same tissues. The authors have recently begun to perform primary tracheostomoplasty in an effort to decrease the frequency of stomal stenosis. The stomoplasty is achieved by creating a triangular based advancement flap 180° away from the tracheo-oesophageal fistula from the upper chest skin and advancing this into a vertical full-thickness tracheotomy performed through the tracheal wall for a distance of about 2.5–3 cm. This added circumference, along with the jagged line closure, is intended to minimize the chance for subsequent stenosis development.

Tracheostomal recurrence reconstruction

There can be several defects that need to be reconstructed following mediastinal dissection. If all of the oesophagus is resected, gastric pull-up has been the preferred reconstructive approach because it provides a pharyngeal anastomotic line which is located in the neck rather than in the mediastinum. If there is a partial oesophageal resection, a pectoralis musculocutaneous flap is utilized to reconstruct the partial oesophageal defect. Oftentimes the remaining tracheal stump is only 2–3 cm away from the carina. The authors have used the deltopectoral flap curled in a spiral fashion to reconstruct the trachea and also partially to resurface the neck skin defect. This tracheal reconstruction needs to be supported with some type of a tracheal cannula or tracheotomy tube until there is enough rigidity developed with the underlying fibrous tissue to support the airway circumference. If there is additional neck or chest skin that needs to be resurfaced, that is achieved with a deltopectoral flap from the other side. In spite of numerous defects created by the resection of a tracheostomal recurrence utilizing mediastinal dissection, most of these defects can be recostructed totally at the time of the same procedure.

PROBLEMS AND COMPLICATIONS

Problems and complications can and do occur with resection and reconstruction of any of the laryngeal procedures described in the earlier sections of this chapter. The most important aspect of complications is not how to manage them but rather how to prevent them. Complications associated with this type of surgery are usually related to clinical situations that predispose to the development of infection. It is imperative that there is absolute haemostasis prior to closing these types of wound. It is imperative that all precautions have been taken to ensure that pharyngeal closures are water-tight and that neck flap closures are air-tight so as not to introduce that potential for contamination with either saliva or air. Although neck wound infections in the absence of pharyngeal leakage do occur, they can usually be treated effectively with drainage of the infected fluid and appropriate systemic therapy and local wound care. The complication that can create a life-threatening situation is the development of a pharyngeal fistula, especially if the carotid artery can be contaminated as a result of a concurrent neck nodal dissection.

The first step in the management of a pharyngeocutaneous fistula is early detection. Most fistulae do not begin to show clinically detectable signs until about the fifth to sixth postoperative day. At this time, one should be suspicious of a fistula developing if the neck flaps become oedematous and erythematous and the patient begins to run a low-grade fever. It is important to establish drainage of a fistula as early as possible rather than deferring the drainage procedure until the time when the clinical findings are overwhelmingly consistent with the development of a fistula. If one waits until that stage, there is usually more infection of the neck soft tissue and greater undermining of the tissues by the accumulation of saliva underneath the neck flaps. The delay in proper drainage increases the potential risk to the carotid artery system. The optimal management of a pharyngocutaneous fistula involves draining the fistula via an incision through a stab wound that hopefully will direct the saliva away from the carotid artery system. It is

preferable to make a separate stab incision rather than opening a portion of the neck incision that might predispose the remaining portion of a freshly healing incision to open. This incision provides a means of drainage of saliva as well as subsequent irrigation and packing of the wound. Once again, all local wound efforts are directed at decompression of the fistula and especially decompression away from the carotid artery. Local wound care in the form of regular irrigations, in addition to systemic antibiotics and nasogastric feedings, usually permit closure of the fistula without the need for additional surgical intervention.

There are times when the laryngeal closure will not heal properly so that a laryngeal fistula subsequently develops. This usually occurs in those patients who have undergone a partial laryngeal procedure following persistent or recurrent disease as a result of initial curative radiation therapy. Conservation laryngeal surgery is still feasible in this clinical setting. However, the patient must be apprised of the increased chance of developing a fistula. Once again, proper drainage, systemic antibiotics, and nasogastric feedings are the mainstay of eventual healing.

In those clinical settings where some type of conservation laryngeal procedure is performed in addition to pharyngeal resection with flap reconstruction, there can be instances where some or all of the skin island of the musculocutaneous flap may not survive. It is rare for total flap necrosis to occur with the musculocutaneous flaps. The pectoralis major musculocutaneous flap has an extraordinary blood supply that oftentimes enhances the wound healing capabilities of areas whose healing has been compromised with prior radiation and/or surgery. It is important to recognize that, frequently, all that is necessary is debridement of the non-viable portion of the skin that will subsequently permit epithelialization of the underlying viable musculature of the flap. Systemic antibiotics are usually not necessary for this clinical situation. Nasogastric feedings are advisable to decrease the contamination of food passing over the devitalized tissues with oral feedings.

The most common medical complication following this type of laryngeal surgery usually involves the lungs. Patients with laryngeal cancer have an increased incidence of chronic obstructive pulmonary disease which predisposes them to postoperative pulmonary complications. Whether preoperative pulmonary therapy has a significant impact on the frequency of postoperative pulmonary complications is a matter that is currently being evaluated. However, it is important for the head and neck oncological surgeon to assess preoperatively the magnitude of the pulmonary compromise in patients who are candidates for some type of conservation laryngeal surgery, especially supraglottic laryngectomy. It is the authors' impression that just about all patients following supraglottic laryngectomy will aspirate. The degree of aspiration is the only thing that varies. The other variable is the patient's ability to withstand the aspiration. That ability is obviously linked to their preoperative pulmonary capabilities. There are no laboratory tests which will unequivocally identify those patients who are candidates for this type of surgery. The final decision rests with the experience and expertise of the head and neck oncological surgeon in the total evaluation of the patient and the patient's suitability for this type of surgery.

FUTURE DEVELOPMENTS

The future for the role of surgery in the excision and reconstruction of laryngeal cancers may be changing. These changes may well be in the direction of surgery's role evolving into treating those patients who have failed radiated therapy and chemotherapy. The organ preservation studies recently published (Department of Veterans' Affairs Laryngeal Cancer Study Group 1991) suggest that surgery might be developing a role as the modality for salvage for patients rather than first-line treatment used with previously untreated patients. However, the ramifications of that type of approach involve the potential for increased incidence of postoperative complications owing to the vulnerability of patients whose healing capabilities have been compromised from the previous therapy. Surgical refinements of the basic conservation laryngeal procedure will continue and even expand as reconstructive techniques and technologies advance. We are in the forefront of progress in reconstructive capabilities utilizing some of the newer plating systems. Microvascular surgery and modifications of the musculocutaneous flaps will provide new opportunities in extirpation and reconstruction. All of these surgical as well as nonsurgical therapeutic and reconstructive advancements will hopefully result in significant progress in the improvement of survival as well as the quality of survival for patients afflicted with cancer of the larynx.

Acknowledgements

This publication was made possible in part by Grant No. 2P30CA16058 from the National Cancer Institute and the American Cancer Society, Ohio Division, Inc., American Cancer Society Professorship of Clinical Oncology. The authors acknowledge support for this project from The Ohio State University Comprehensive Cancer Center Head and Neck Oncology Program

REFERENCE

Burch J D, Howe G R, Miller A B, Semenciw R 1984 Tobacco, alcohol, asbestos, and nickel in the etiology of cancer of the larynx: a case-control study. Journal of the National Cancer Institute 67: 1219–1924

Burnett C H 1893 Deformities and morbid growths of the pharynx and the larynx. In: Burnett C H (ed) System of diseases of the ear, nose and throat. Lippincott, Philadelphia PA, vol II, pp 780–787

Carter R L, Bliss J M, Soo K C, O'Brien C J 1985 Radical neck dissections for squamous carcinomas: pathological findings and their clinical implications with particular reference to transcapsular spread. International Journal of Radiation Oncology—Biological Physics 13: 825–832

Department of Veterans' Affairs Laryngeal Cancer Study Group 1991 Induction chemotherapy plus radiation therapy compared with surgery plus radiation therapy in patients with advanced laryngeal cancer. New England Journal of Medicine 324: 1685–1690

Flanders W D, Rothman K J 1982 Interaction of alcohol and tobacco in laryngeal cancer. American Journal of Epidemiology 115: 371

Gluckman J L, Hamaker R C, Schuller D E, Weissler M C, Charles G A 1987 Surgical salvage for stomal recurrences: a multi-institutional experience. Laryngoscope 97: 1025–1029

Goffinette D R, Fee W E, Goode R L 1984 Combined surgery and postoperative irradiation in the treatment of cervical lymph nodes. Archives of Otolaryngology—Head and Neck Surgery 110: 736–738

Hammond E C 1966 Smoking in relation to the death rates of one million men and women. National Cancer Institute Monograph 19: 127

Jacobs J, Cooper J, Longeman J 1985 A phase III study of the role of cricopharyngeal myotomy in the treatment of dysphagia following major head and neck surgery. Radiation Therapy Oncology Group Protocol #85–30

Johnson J T, Myers E N, Bedetti C D, Barnes E L et al 1985 Cervical lymph node metastases: incidence and implications of extracapsular carcinoma. Archives of Otolaryngology—Head and Neck Surgery 111: 523–537

Kahn H A 1966 The Dorn study of smoking and mortality among US veterans. National Cancer Institute Monograph 19: 1

Rothman K J, Cann C I, Flanders D, Fried M P 1980 Epidemiology of laryngeal cancer. Epidemiology Review 2: 195–209

Sasaki C T, Carlson R D 1986 Malignant neoplasms of the larynx. In: Cummings C W, Fredrickson J W, Harker L A, Krause C J, Schuller D E (eds) Otolaryngology—Head and Neck Surgery. Mosby, St. Louis MO, pp 1987-2017

Schuller D E, Parrish R T 1988 Reconstruction of the larynx and trachea. Archives of Otolaryngology—Head and Neck Surgery 114: 278–286

Schuller D, Hamaker R, Gluckman J 1981 Mediastinal dissection: a multi-institutional assessment. Archives of Otolaryngology 107: 715–720

Silverberg E 1984 Cancer statistics. CA: A Cancer Journal for Clinicians 34: 7

Sisson G A, Bytell D E, Becker S P 1976 Mediastinal dissection—1976. Indications and newer techniques. Laryngoscope 87: 751–759

Snow G B, Annyas A A, Van Slooten E A, Bartelink H, Hart A A 1982 Prognostic factors of neck node metastasis. Clinical Otolaryngology 7: 185-192

Snyderman N L, Johnson J T, Schramm V L, Myers E N et al 1985 Extracapsular spread of carcinoma in cervical lymph nodes: impact upon survival in patients with carcinoma of the supraglottic larynx. Cancer 56: 1597–1599

Trudeau M D, Hirsch S M, Schuller D E 1986 Vocal restorative surgery: why wait? Laryngoscope 96: 975–977

Trudeau M D, Schuller D E, Hall D A 1988 Timing of tracheosophageal punture for voice restoration: Primary V. secondary. Head and Neck Surgery suppl 2: 130–134

Trudeau M D, Schuller D E, Hall D A 1989 The effects of radiation in tracheosophageal puncture: a retrospective study. Archives of Otolaryngology—Head and Neck Surgery 115: 1116–1117

Wynder E L, Bross I J, Day E 1956 A study of environmental factors in cancer of the larynx. Cancer 9: 86

Wynder E L, Covey L S, Mabuchi K, Mushinski M 1976 Environmental factors in cancer of the larynx: a second look. Cancer 38: 1591

Wynder E L, Stellman S D 1977 Comparative epidemiology of tobacco related cancers. Cancer Research 37: 4608

14. Near-total laryngectomy

Bruce W. Pearson

INTRODUCTION

In the early 1970s, most surgeons in our medical centre believed that squamous-cell carcinomas that fixed one vocal cord required a total laryngectomy with few exceptions. The implications of total laryngectomy for voice drove some patients to elect primary radiation, but most of these cases also came to total laryngectomy when radiation therapy failed. There were, of course, a few carefully selected patients who were candidates for individualized conservation operations, hemilaryngectomies and frontolateral partial laryngectomies for example. These were patients with T2 glottic lesions, usually limited cord motion but not invasive fixation, whose cancers were mainly exophytic and well demarcated without evidence of cartilage involvement. Except for these, most patients with squamous-cell carcinoma which fixed the vocal cord, seemed to have lesions beyond the reach of any tolerable extension of the usual conservation procedures. To ablate the cancer safely and to achieve reliable swallowing without aspiration, a total laryngectomy was performed (DeSanto 1984).

During the 1980s, in our institution at least, near-total laryngectomy found more and more use in more and more of these patients. This operation had been developed in the late 1970s for lateralized laryngeal (and pyriform) cancers whose chief characteristic was cord fixation (Pearson et al 1980). Serial section studies has shown that fixation meant deep extension and invasion of the paraglottic space. Near-total laryngectomy was simply a way of excising the cancer without compromise and of trying to reconstruct a sphincteric voice passage way with the remaining elements of the larynx, from the side opposite the main focus of cancer. The continuous mucosal strip between the trachea and the pharynx should guarantee a fistula that might permit voice. Preservation of superior and recurrent laryngeal innervation to the residuum of intrinsic laryngeal muscle should enable the prevention of aspiration.

Eventually, near-total laryngectomy took its place in our practice, as it continues to do today, for two reasons: we did not observe an increased incidence of local cancer recur-

rence, and most of our patients talked, without any dependence on a prosthesis (Pearson & Keith 1989). Of course, less extensive (and more conventional) partial laryngectomies, like cordectomy, hemilaryngectomy and supraglottic laryngectomy are still performed in greater numbers. However, this is because T1 and T2 laryngeal cancers are more common in our practice than are T3 and T4 cancers, and our bias towards surgery in limited cancer limits the application of radiotherapy. Moreover, total laryngectomy is still in use and has not been eliminated by near-total laryngectomy. Extensive bilateral laryngeal cancers, particularly ulcerated necrotinizing lesions recurring after radiation therapy, cannot be safely encompassed by anything less. That the local control of T3 and some T4 cancers by near-total laryngectomy has proven to be as good as that obtained with total laryngectomy should not be surprising. Case selection is the reason. The observations we have made with near-total laryngectomy are similar to those made by others for supraglottic laryngectomy. Successful control of a localized laryngeal cancer depends upon complete local excision of the cancer, guided by negative margins. This is not the same as complete local excision of the larynx. It is the cancer, not the organ, that must be extirpated.

It is difficult, of course, to make truly accurate comparisons of the local control rates of near-total laryngectomy as opposed to total laryngectomy. Case selection *is* such an important factor. In general, near-total laryngectomy is used on primary lateralized T3 and T4 cases in our practice. The presence or absence of nodes is not a factor, but the clarity of the extent of the local disease certainly is. Total laryngectomy is more likely to be used on the massively invasive cases, particularly after radiation failure obscures the margins. Post-cricoid involvement or interarytenoid spread excludes near-total laryngectomy, and so does circumferential subglottic cancer. In a sense, then, within a T3 and T4 category, the better cases were more likely to be selected for near-total laryngectomy, and consequently, the less favourable cases will show up in the total laryngectomy groups.

Near-total laryngectomies are not to be considered

'conservation' operations. They extend from the trachea to the tongue base. They do not permit the avoidance of a permanent tracheal stoma. They often require neck dissection. They do not preserve, on the side of the cancer, any portion of the cricoid, arytenoid, or even the overlying thyroid lobe. They sacrifice the entire epiglottis and pre-epiglottic space. Extensive pharyngeal resections, even to the point of requiring flap reconstruction of the hypopharynx, can be combined with the near-total concept. T3/T4 (and a few extensive T2) glottic and transglottic squamous-cell carinomas are candidates (Pearson 1981). So are supraglottic and aryepiglottic fold cancers beyond the reach of a supraglottic laryngectomy (or those in which the patient cannot tolerate the post-operative pulmonary stress of a supraglottic laryngectomy) (DeSanto et al 1989). Pyriform sinus carcinomas with cord fixation, cartilage invasion and pyriform apex involvement (but no spread to the post cricoid or interarytenoid regions) are also candidates; in fact, this has become one of our commoner indications (Dumich et al 1984).

The decision regarding a patient's suitability for near-total laryngectomy can usually be made by office examination. The advent of high-quality video laryngoscopy examinations has extended this capability in recent years. For the first time, office examinations can be stop-action replayed to clarify the issue of cord mobility, and re-studied in consultation with a colleague if necessary. At the time of direct laryngoscopy, the extent and the cell type of the lesion is confirmed by inspection and biopsy. The status of the tissues the surgeon expects to transgress (e.g. the ventricle on the 'good' side) or preserve can be further studied also. Ultimately, microscopic margin confirmation *during* the operative procedure is necessary: the quality control officer during a near-total laryngectomy is an interested, informed and readily available frozen-section histopathologist. His or her findings must confirm your selection before the patient leaves the operating room; a delayed report changing a negative to a positive margin would be unacceptable practice in near-total operations.

Since near-total laryngectomy has not replaced other surgical procedures, where does it fit in the spectrum of operations for laryngeal cancer? Beyond it lies total laryngectomy, which is applied to patients for whom near-total laryngectomy is an inadequate excision. This implies a permanent stoma and an oesophageal mechanism for voice. The air source can be gulping or pulmonary (via tracheo-oesophageal puncture), but the pharyngo-oesophageal segment will be the sound generator, and air must be injected into the oesophagus for this to occur. Before near-total laryngectomies are the classical partial laryngectomies, primarily horizontal supraglottic laryngectomy and/or vertical hemilaryngectomy. These provide voice without the obligation of a stoma, so they are always superior when feasible. Near-total laryngectomy helps surgeons conversant with these procedures avoid surgical brinkmanship in their bor-

derline cases. When a vertical hemilaryngectomy is tenuous because of dysplasia at a surgical margin, or a supraglottic laryngectomy is questionable because of extension into the pharynx, or a partial laryngopharyngectomy is inadequate because of disease extension to the apex of the pyriform, near-total laryngectomy is an appropriate option. A permanent tracheotomy becomes the price of voice, but the risk of local recurrence is greatly curtailed in these cases. Some patients have cancers anatomically suitable for a supraglottic laryngectomy, but they do not have the physiologic capacity. Protection against pulmonary aspiration is much more reliable following near-total laryngectomy than supraglottic laryngectomy. Thus, there are physiological indications for near-total laryngectomy where supraglottic laryngectomy would have been oncologically applicable (DeSanto et al 1989).

Near-total laryngectomy is, in essence, a total laryngectomy with the exception that a very narrow strip of laryngeal tissues connecting the trachea and the uninvolved side of pyriform fossa over one arytenoid are preserved. A shunt diameter of more than 6 mm is necessary for speech to occur at physiological airway pressures. Despite this requirement, the extent of the tumour is the fundamental decisive factor as to how much larynx is excised. Specimens include the entire hemilarynx on one side, the anterior subglottis, a little true cord and the supraglottic larynx of the other side, and as much of the trachea, vallecula, tongue base, pyriform or pharyngeal wall as is necessary. Tumours originating within the larynx (i.e. glottic, supraglottic) when excised in this fashion, leave behind too narrow a strip of residual larynx to form a vocal fistula of adequate diameter. Therefore, some residual pharynx (from the side from which the larynx tumour was excised) is used to augment this strip (Pearson & DeSanto 1990). In cases where the cancer arose in one of the pyriform fossa and invaded the paraglottic space to fix the cord from without, enough larynx, almost a hemilarynx, can be preserved to create a shunt of adequate diameter. No augmentation is necessary. This is fortunate because, in pyriform cases, the pharyngeal excision is extensive. There is nothing in the way of pharyngeal tissue to spare, nothing that can be donated to the speaking shunt to increase its functional diameter.

We believe the indications for near-total laryngectomy are as follows:

1. Lateralized glottic carcinoma where hemilaryngectomy is contraindicated by (i) cord fixation or (ii) limited mobility with subglottic extension
2. Lateralized transglottic carcinoma (with fixation)
3. False cord cancer (i.e. lateralized supraglottic) beyond the scope of a supraglottic laryngectomy
4. False cord cancer beyond the patient's ability to tolerate a supraglottic laryngectomy
5. Aryepiglottic fold cancer
6. Pyriform sinus cancer without : (i) postcricoid spread,

(ii) anterior laryngeal spread to the opposite side, and
(iii) posterior hypopharyngeal spread to the opposite side.

DIAGNOSIS

Most cases of near-total laryngectomy begin with a direct laryngoscopy at which, for the first time, the confirmatory biopsy is obtained. In typical cases, the clinical diagnosis of cancer is evident; the biopsy is taken to exclude a rare granuloma, papilloma, pseudoepitheliomatous hyperplasia, etc. When squamous-cell carcinoma is reported with confidence we are used to proceeding on the basis of the frozen section diagnosis. The tumour extent is mapped out with several specific aids, including the microscope, but the most important accessories are probably the laryngeal telescopes. The 0° scope allows a distal wide-angle view of the tumour (from the tip of the laryngoscope). An outstanding view of the lower edges, beyond the main bulk of the tumour, and a direct assessment of the anterior commissure are obtained with a 70° scope. The 70° also allows precise inspection of the ventricle, which will later become important as one point of division between the tissues resected and tissues preserved.

EXCISION TECHNIQUES

Following the laryngoscopy, don't forget to insert the nasogastric feeding tube. Then prepare and drape the neck in the fashion dictated by your preferences. We usually start with a tracheotomy, entering the neck through the transverse limb of the skin incision and the trachea just below the thyroid isthmus. Then the anaesthesia tubing is switched to this location, and connected to sterile tubing across the chest.

Most cases with tumours invasive enough to require a near-total laryngectomy also merit a neck dissection. In general, a conservation neck dissection seems appropriate in N0 necks, and a more conventional neck dissection (all five areas, plus the sternomastoid muscle and internal jugular vein, but not the accessory nerve) in N1 and 2. The neck dissection is usually performed through an incision which sweeps down from the mastoid and over the sternomastoid muscle, to cross the neck at the level of the cricothyroid membrane. A supraclavicular extension can be extended at right angles from this, if necessary, to increase the exposure of the posterior triangle.

The tracheotomy was performed through the transverse limb of the main surgical incision because that provided excellent early exposure. If the permanent tracheostomy is sited in this incision, however, the crease that extends from either margin may create an air leak when the patient valves the stoma to speak. Therefore we plan to make a lower separate opening in the skin later, and sew the skin margins to the opening in the trachea. The use of 0 chromic catgut will obviate the need to pick sutures from the stoma at a later date. The best edge-to-edge approximation between the opening in the trachea and the opening in the skin seems to occur when a vertical mattress suture is placed with respect to the skin, but just a simple vertical loop is used to capture the edge of the trachea. To reduce interference from the endotracheal tube, tailor the lower margin of the stoma when the endotracheal tube still crosses from the main incision. Then remove the endotracheal tube, re-insert it through the final permanent stoma, and complete the suturing of the upper margin. Bear in mind that the patient cannot learn to speak until the stoma can be finger-valved successfully. Perform the tracheotomy with care and precision and your near-total laryngectomy patients will speak better and sooner.

Begin the laryngeal procedure by sharply dissecting the cervical fascia off the medial edge of the strap muscles to the left of the midline. In this way, the prelaryngeal fascia will be included in the resection with the specimen while the left strap muscles will remain with the patient. Continue your sharp dissection to release the insertion of the left strap muscles from the hyoid bone (only) and peel them back a little from the external surface of the larynx so that the left thyroid ala is visible. Lower down, divide the thyroid isthmus from the left lobe and over-sew the edges with a blanket stitch. The isthmus and right lobe will go with the specimen. The left thyroid lobe will remain in place, covering the left recurrent laryngeal nerve, which we expect to preserve for our shunt.

After these preliminaries, surgery on the right side virtually duplicates the familiar elements of a total laryngectomy. Divide the right strap muscles low, mobilize the thyroid gland under them, and divide the inferior neurovascular

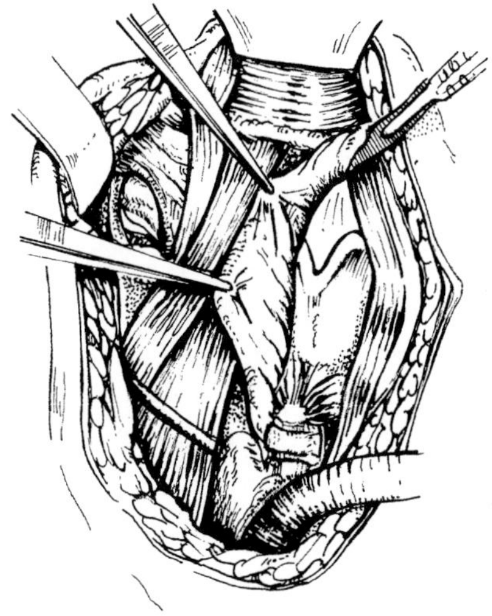

Fig. 14.1 The anterior edge of the strap muscles on the proposed side for the creation of the vocal shunt, is identified. In this case it is the left side. The exposure is obtained by rolling the prelaryngeal fascia and the thyroid isthmus to the opposite side. The tumour in this case is on the right.

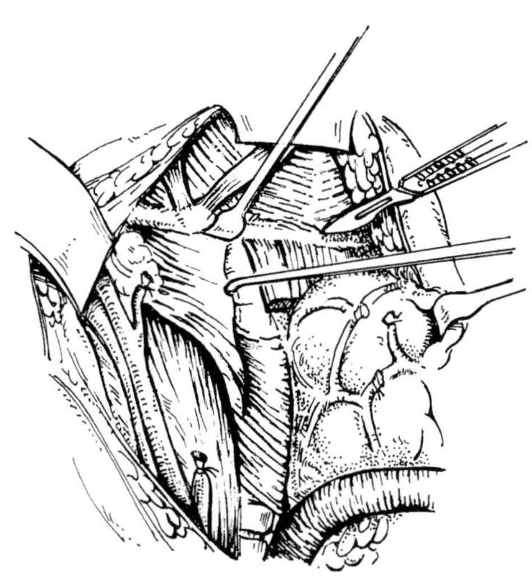

Fig. 14.2 The entire right side is mobilized as if a total laryngectomy was underway. This mobilization is commenced by taking the superior and inferior neurovascular pedicles.

pedicle (the recurrent nerve and inferior thyroid artery). Superiorly on the right, divide the superior neurovascular bundle (the superior laryngeal nerve and the superior thyroid artery), and free the greater horn of the hyoid. Release the suprahyoid muscles from the hyoid bone, at least above the right greater horn and the body. Then incise the inferior constrictor all along the posterior edge of the right thyroid cartilage ala, clearly delineating the superior thyroid cornu above, and the cricothyroid articulation below. This completes the external laryngeal dissection on the tumour-bearing side of the specimen.

Now turn your attention to the left side of the larynx. The

issues you confront are how to enter the larynx without risking contact with the cancer and how to make sure an appropriate division is obtained between what needs to be saved for the speaking shunt and what needs to be resected to ablate the cancer. A good first step is to free the anterior and inferior margins of the left cricothyroid muscle from the cricoid so that this uninvolved element, important to the dynamic functions of the subsequent shunt, can be reflected back and preserved. The next step is to transect the hyoid bone on the left, then the thyroid cartilage. The hyoid can be cut with a Cottle-Kazanjian cutting forceps at the anterior end of the left greater horn. Thus the central body of the hyoid, and with it, the pre-epiglottic soft tissues, will be resected as part of the specimen.

Divide the left thyroid ala by actually removing a vertical wedge from its middle third. This is done with the aid of a saw if the degree of calcification demands it. Otherwise, a simple incision along the superior margin of the thyroid ala allows a curved nasal elevator to be passed downwards in contact with its internal surface. Then the middle third can be removed with the cutting forceps again. Pay particular attention to a clean resection and removal inferiorly; soft-tissue attachments to the inside of the thyroid cartilage by the upper fibers of the cricothyroid muscle are prominent at the lower edge of this dissection. With the removal of this thyroid wedge, you have broken the rigidity of the laryngeal framework and initiated the exposure through which entry to the laryngeal interior can begin.

I prefer to enter the larynx through the saccule. This will be technically unfamiliar unless you rehearse it on a cadaver larynx. Many surgeons prefer to enter through the vallecula, and this is also a valid technique. Whichever entry is chosen, the next part of the operation is very reminiscent of a supraglottic laryngectomy. Using a headlight, carefully observe the soft tissues you have exposed by your removal of

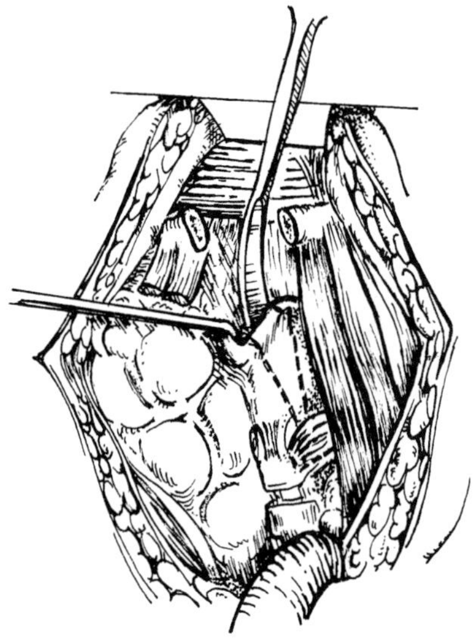

Fig. 14.3 Midalar wedge is mobilized from the thyroid cartilage on the left. The hyoid now has been divided at the junction of the body with the greater horn. At this stage it is important to elevate the cricothyroid muscle off the cricoid cartilage so that it can be preserved with the shunt.

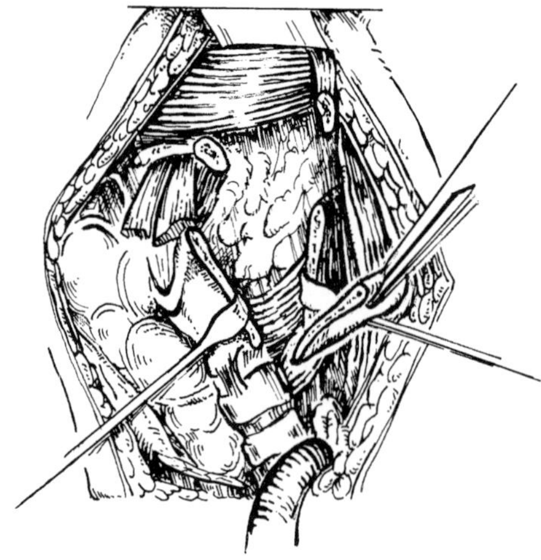

Fig. 14.4 The wedge in the middle third of the left ala of the thyroid cartilage is removed. This exposes the paraglottic soft tissues. The main landmark is the thyro-arytenoid muscle whose outer fibres are visible.

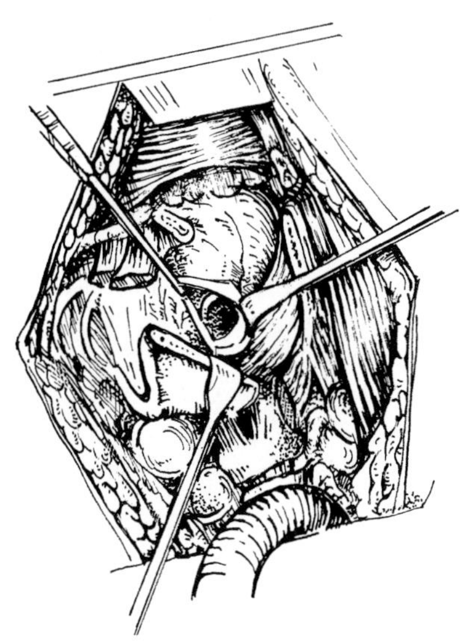

Fig. 14.5 The left ventricle is opened to enter the larynx. The ventricular saccule lies just above the upper fibres of the thyro-arytenoid muscle.

the middle third of the thyroid ala. In the lower half of this field, the transverse muscular elements of the outer surface of the main left glottic musculature are visible. This is the left thyroarytenoid, the muscle on the side opposite the cancer that will later be important in preventing aspiration. The fibro-fatty tissue superior to this is actually the rather vascular submucosal tissue that clothes the left saccule. Occasionally, the saccule has already been opened, at its apex, during the cartilage dissection. More frequently it has to be grasped and opened specifically to enter the lumen of the larynx. Recall that the left ventricle was free of cancer at direct laryngoscopy. Therefore, the relatively 'blind' initial entry here does not jeopardize the oncological result. The

ventricle is not necessary for construction of the shunt either, so that entry here will not diminish the voice result.

With good lighting and meticulous retraction, the lower edge of the left false cord. (i.e. the ventricular band) will be discernable from within the ventricle. With no laryngeal framework to inhibit your progress or your exposure, cut upwards from the ventricle with scissors. In effect, transect the 'good' false cord, leaving the left arytenoid with the patient but isolating the pre-epiglottic space and epiglottis with the specimen. At the level of the vallecula, turn horizontally and, with one scissors blade in the vallecula itself, and the other in the soft tissues above the hyoid bone, cut the larynx free from the base of the tongue. Retract the tongue base with a small Deaver retractor and grasp the epiglottis; fold the specimen outward and to the right. Through the supraglottic entry thus gained, visualize the as yet undisturbed glottic level. The tumour itself should be well exposed at this point, and the remainder of the resection can proceed under direct vision as the glottic, subglottic, posterior and pharyngeal resection lines are planned.

The next step in a near-total laryngectomy consists of releasing the involved right glottic and subglottic elements while, with an adequate margin, preserving the uninvolved laryngeal tissues on the left. By looking down on the left vocal cord from above, the decision regarding where exactly to transect the left vocal cord should be evident. This is determined by gauging the extent of the cancer, which generally involves the anterior commissure and, to varying degrees, the anterior portion of left vocal cord. It is not, of course, the extent of spread onto the left vocal cord that has created the indication for a near-total laryngectomy. It is the extent of deep infiltration of the right hemilarynx. Near-total

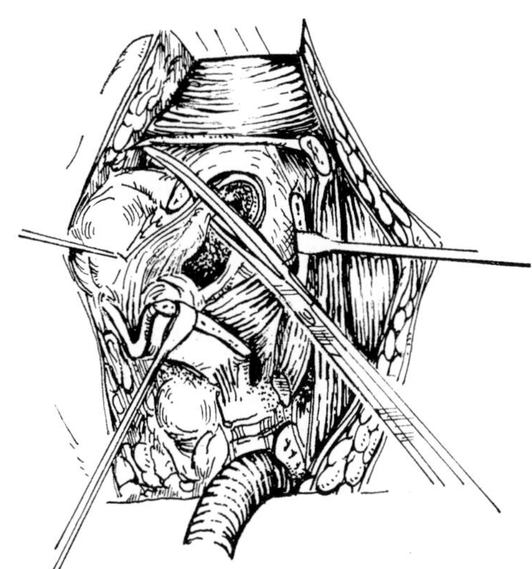

Fig. 14.6 The left false cord has been transected by cutting up from the ventricle alongside the epiglottis. The cut is extended cranially across the vallecula to release the supraglottic larynx from the tongue.

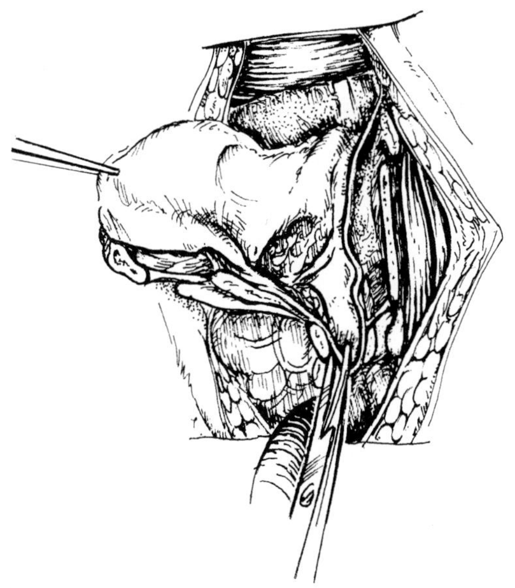

Fig. 14.7 Caudally, the glottic cut is extended downwards through the cricoid avoiding and keeping clear of any tumour on the left vocal cord and anterior commissure under direct vision.

laryngectomy was not designed for 'horseshoe' lesions of the anterior commissure and both vocal cords, but for infiltrative lateralized lesions in which some of the mucosa and much of the musculature of the opposite side is spared.

The glottic and subglottic excision starts with a downwards transection across, roughly, the midportion of the left vocal cord. Proceed down across and through the anterior arch of the cricoid. Continue across the trachea, horizontally, on the right, cutting the right cricoid arch free of the trachea, then drawing the transection line up through the posterior subglottic region near the midline of the posterior cricoid plate. Variations in this general pattern can be made, of course, depending on how much subglottic cancer is present. If the resection has to include a small portion of the upper trachea on the right, this is a perfectly acceptable extension of the operation. On the other hand, there is good reason not to sacrifice subglottic mucosa unnecessarily. The wider the shunt can be made below the glottic level, the more efficient will be the vocal activity of the speaking fistula. One technical problem should also be mentioned. After the anterior arch of the cricoid has been divided, the subglottis still cannot be opened out very far with retractors. The cricoid is a complete ring and the posterior cricoid plate is still intact. Therefore, retract the margins of the anterior cricoid cut with hooks and raise the posterior cricoid plate forward with a finger in the post-cricoid hypopharynx. Now, if an incision is made with a 15 blade into the laryngeal lumen-facing cortex of the posterior cricoid plate, the right near-total laryngectomy specimen will break outward and away from the left laryngeal remnant, exactly as planned, and the final release and delivery of the right near-total laryngectomy specimen can be affected now by completing the resection line upwards, through the wall of the right side of the hypopharynx.

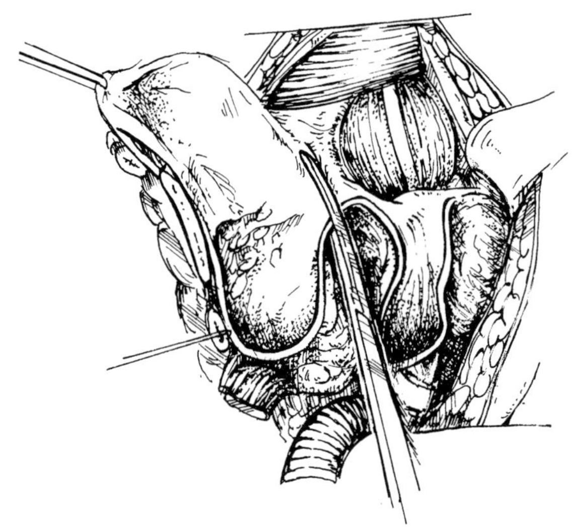

Fig. 14.9 The specimen is removed by taking adequate mucosa of the right pyriform sinus that is considered necessary depending upon the primary tumour. *All* excision margins are controlled by frozen section.

Many cases requiring near-total laryngectomy demand that the right pyriform sinus be included with the specimen. After all, pyriform mucosa lies over paraglottic space; it might be involved, on its under surface, by the tumour.

Once the specimen has been delivered to the pathologist, the stage is not quite set yet for reconstruction. Send the pathologist a few fine slivers of mucosa from the margins of the laryngeal remnant in the patient. Label these carefully so that a meaningful histopathological report will be produced. A vocal shunt is contraindicated unless negative margins are obtained intra-operatively. Complete the haemostasis with a bipolar cautery, check the positioning of the feeding tube in the pharynx, and thoroughly flush the wound with irrigation.

RECONSTRUCTIVE TECHNIQUES

Once the laryngeal cancer (the near-total laryngectomy specimen) is resected, what is left behind? The upper trachea and the left pyriform fossa are connected by a strip of mucosa and muscle, approximately the posterior quadrant of the left hemilarynx. This connecting strip of laryngeal tissue should be widest in the subglottic region (where it may be comprised of half or even more than half of the circumference of the subglottis). At the glottic level it is narrow and more indistensible. Much of what remains at this level is arytenoid, which is rigid, and cord, which is taunt. The width of the remaining larynx at this level is the horizontal length of the arytenoid, plus as much interarytenoid muscle as could be saved, plus as much membranous cord as could be saved, given the anterior resection of the tumour which extended across the anterior commissure onto the 'good' cord. At the highest level, the remaining laryngeal mucosa flows over the corniculate and cuneiform cartilages into the

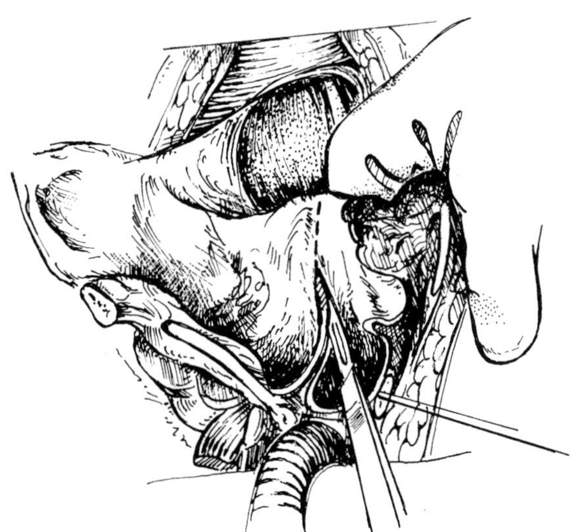

Fig. 14.8 The caudal incision on the specimen is placed at the junction of the trachea and cricoid on the right side. The posterior lamina of the cricoid is cut in the mid-line.

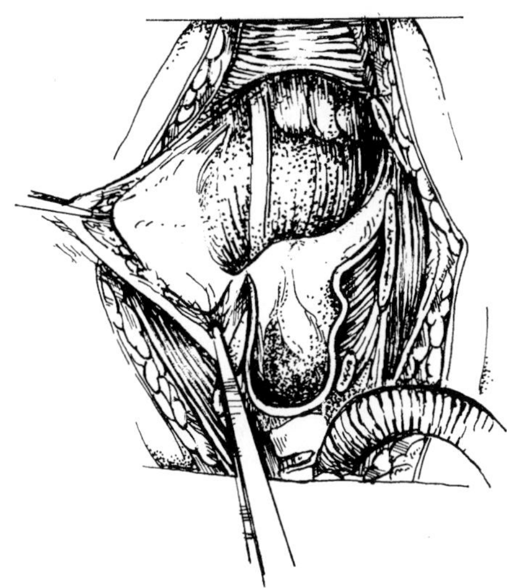

Fig. 14.10 If the remaining strip of tissue joining the left side of the hypopharynx to the trachea is too narrow to form a shunt of adequate diameter it should be augmented with a pharyngeal mucosal flap from the right side.

piriform sinus. The width of the remnant here depends on how much interarytenoid mucosa was preserved, and how much left false cord and aryepiglottic fold remain.

The object now is to make a sphincteric shunt from these remnants connecting the trachea, above the 'anterior wall' stoma, to the pharynx, into which the vocal tones will emerge. A fistulous connection between the trachea and the pharynx is assured, because no suture line of the reconstruction will cross this mucosal connection. Sphincteric activity can be expected only if the left recurrent laryngeal nerve is inviolate, and the left cricothyroid and intrinsic laryngeal muscle has been spared the indignity of excess cauterization or dismemberment.

Making a functioning vocal shunt of this remnant requires fulfilling two conditions. First, enough mucosa must be provided, even if this means donating some from the pharynx, to achieve an adequate fistula diameter. Second, any remaining elements of the future shunt that restrict its flaccidity, or render the laryngeal remnant too rigid to collapse and close on swallowing need to be removed. Thus, while the pathologist studies the margin specimens just sent in, resect the remaining cricoid with a careful submucosal technique. Actually, the subglottic shunt tissues will be well enough mobilized to be tubed before every last bit of the residual left cricoid is resected. Knowing this, we stop when adequate mobilization has been achieved. In practice, this usually means that a small portion of the cricoid on the 'good' side posteriorly, remains. This is usually the part of the cricoid that articulates with the inferior cornu of the thyroid cartilage. This is fortunate, because the recurrent laryngeal nerve passes behind the inferior cornu at this point and thus escapes injury during the dissection.

By the time the cricoid remnant has been resected to render the laryngeal remnant malleable, the pathologist is reporting the margins. Now the shunt can be constructed. To achieve an adequate diameter, a judgement must be made. Should the shunt, particularly at the relatively indistensible glottic level, be augmented with a small myomucosal flap from the remaining pharynx? Or is the amount of larynx remaining sufficient to construct the shunt by itself? Where the lesion was primarily supraglottic, or the larynx was a large masculine specimen, tubing the laryngeal remnant itself will sometimes prove adequate. In a transglottic lesion, such as the one described, with a rather extensive resection, especially in a small or female larynx, an augmentation flap from the pharynx will undoubtedly be required to bring the remnant up to a suitable calibre.

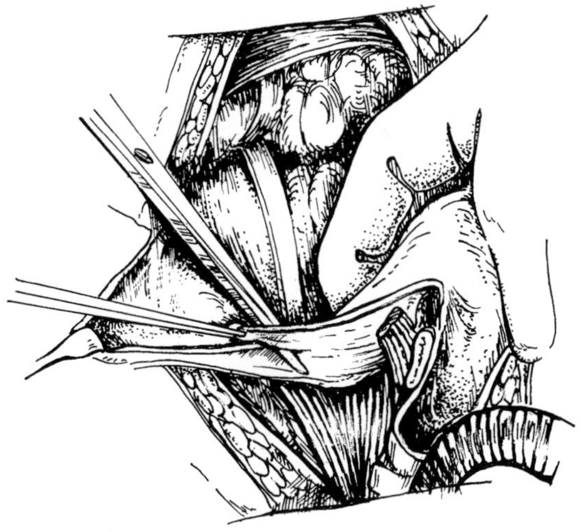

Fig. 14.11 The pharynx is very distensible and only a small inferiorly based flap needs to be cut.

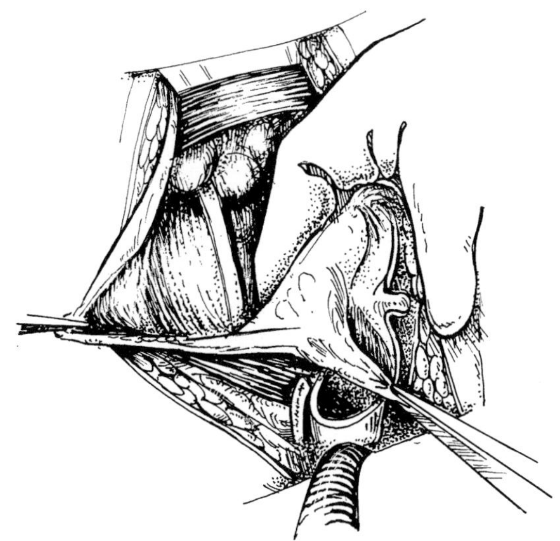

Fig. 14.12 The mucosal flap is swung medially and downwards so that its mucosal surface faces towards the lumen of the vocal shunt.

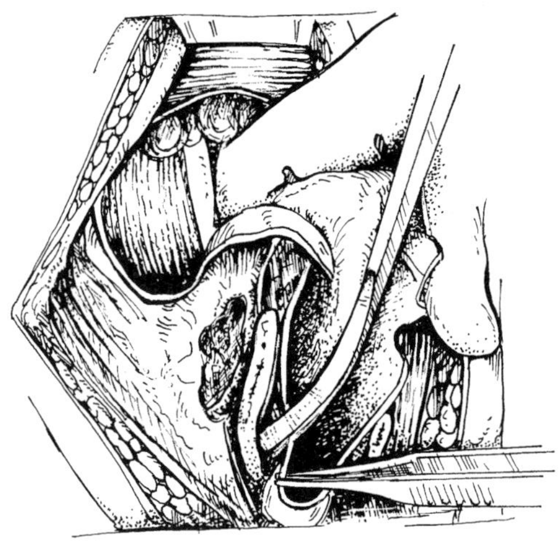

Fig. 14.13 In order that the subglottic portion of the shunt may not be held open by residual elements of the left cricoid cartilage, any excess posterior and lateral cartilage is dissected and removed before the flap is sewn in place.

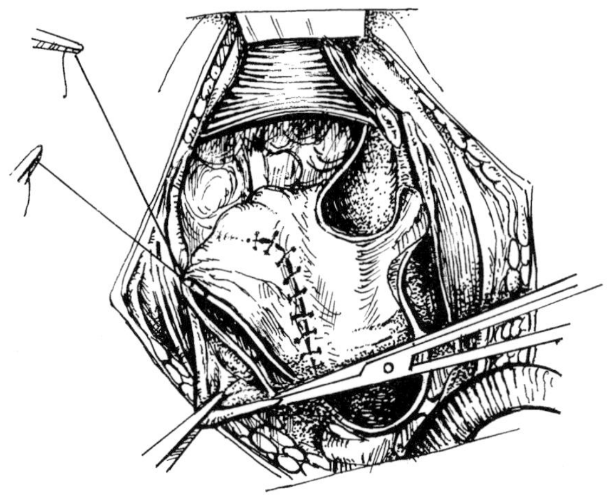

Fig. 14.14 The flap has been placed parallel to the posterior margin of the laryngeal remnant and is sutured to it. The defect on the right pyriform fossa is now carefully repaired before the shunt is tubed.

It is a relatively simple matter to make a short oblique cut in the right edge of the pharyngotomy and to produce a pennant-shaped mucosal flap, based inferiorly. The base should lie roughly on the same horizontal plane as the left corniculate cartilage. Turn this flap, which is technically a local rotation flap of right lateral upper hypopharyngeal wall, forwards and downwards, so that its mucosal surface faces the lumen of the eventual vocal shunt and the base where it folds over becomes part of the lip of the shunt. In position, it lies side-by-side with the laryngeal remnant, to which it should be sewn with 4-0 chromic catgut. Thus, a vertical suture line is created posteriorly in the midline, uniting the flap to the laryngeal remnant. The result is a wider strip of mucosa bridging the distance from the trachea to the hypopharynx, one that can now be tubed, to create the vocal shunt.

Check the dimensions before tubing this tissue with two thoughts in mind. Particularly at the glottic level, you want a shunt that could temporarily accommodate, as an intra-operative gauge only, a no.14 French catheter. You are trying to create a mucosal orifice somewhat similar to, although certainly not as large as, the original glottis. Secondly, you do not want a shunt that is too wide above the glottic level. Otherwise the fistula will be chalice-shaped at its upper end, and this will serve as a passive repository for fluids and saliva. This can result in either aspiration or a bubbly voice, requiring a surgical revision. In narrowing the shunt at its upper end, do not resect mucosa from the flap. This is the base or nutrient end of the flap, and you might compromise circulation to the tip further down. It is perfectly satisfactory, preferable in fact, to narrow the shunt at its upper end, if necessary, by resecting mucosa (only) from the former false cord and aryepiglottic fold. This can be done with no sacrifice of function since the muscular elements in the supraglottic tissues are minimal.

One additional element of shunt construction deserves mention. Try to avoid side-wall diverticulae in the finished shunt. They impede vocalization. The most likely source of a diverticula will be residual mucosa from the left laryngeal ventricle. Try and observe this, and resect it with this concern in mind.

Having achieved the optimum mucosal dimensions, and the flaccidity you want, roll the shunt into a vertical tube and close the anterior seam with chromic sutures. If the rigidity of the first or second tracheal cartilage restricts you, cut out a notch here to overcome this difficulty. Rolling the mucosa together and creating the shunt results in a continuous vertical seam up the front, which eventually rises from the trachea to the level of the pharynx. With this, the shunt is completed. You may wish to confirm the diameter of the lumen with a no. 14 French gauge catheter, but make sure you remove and discard this when you are satisfied. You do

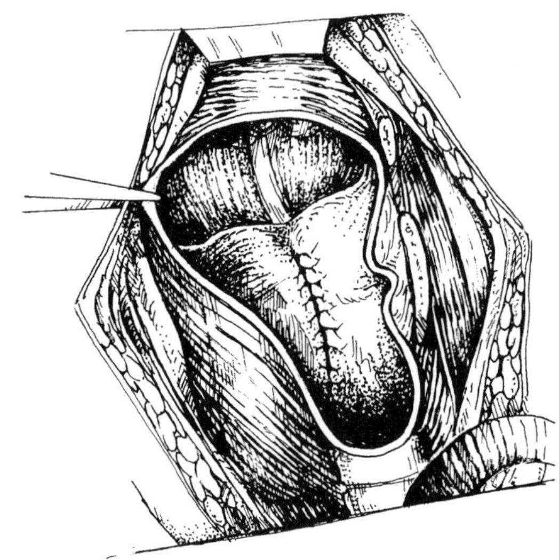

Fig. 14.15 The right pyriform fossa has now been repaired and the flap is in place.

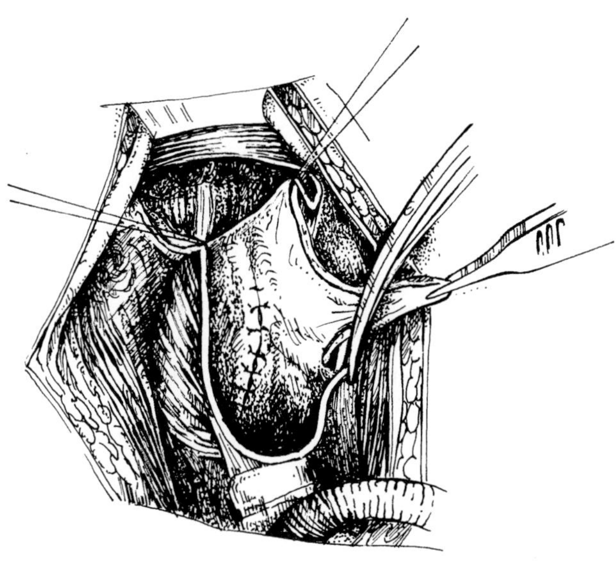

Fig. 14.16 Any redundant mucosa of the left ventricle is trimmed to avoid a blind pouch in the wall of the shunt.

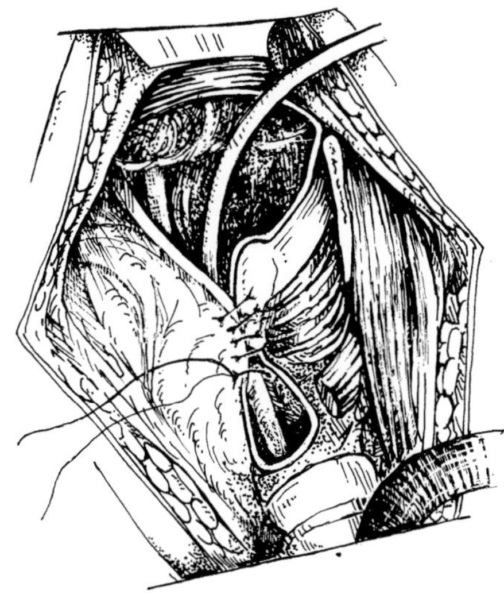

Fig. 14.17 The anterior wall of the tracheopharyngeal vocal shunt is closed. The catheter shown here is only to demonstrate the size which conforms to no. 14 French gauge.

not want to leave a foreign body in the shunt. The concept of a stent does not make sense in this completely mucosalized reconstruction. There now remains a simple pharyngotomy to close an anterior wall defect in the pharynx. This can be closed in a T, just as it is in a total laryngectomy, using a running over-and-over Connell stitch in the mucosa, and interrupted simple suture in the second layer.

In constructing the shunt as described, the surgeon will naturally incorporate the intrinsic laryngeal musculature. This is still united to the mucosa at the glottic level. However, take a moment to find the free anterior end of the cricothyroid muscle, and draw it over the shunt as well. Incorporate it with a few sutures into the reconstruction. These laryngeal muscle remnants cannot, of course, completely surround the shunt or act as a complete 'purse string' sphincter. They can, however, be disposed as widely as possible throughout the walls of the shunt, acting later, perhaps to deform it, perhaps to reneurotize the muscularis layer of the pharyngeal flap. What is clear is that innervation and muscular activity must occur, otherwise patients with this patent and speaking shunt will aspirate.

At the conclusion of the closure of pharynx, the left strap muscles which are still present, still attached to the remaining thyroid cartilage element (the posterior one-third) along the oblique line, might as well be drawn up to a relatively anatomical position. The medial fibres of the left strap muscles, which were released from the hyoid, can now be sewn back to the suprahyoid musculature. This probably increases the chance that the thyrohyoid muscle, which is still innervated, will elevate the laryngeal remnant during deglutition and act to help the shunt occlude during swallowing. After this, repeat the irrigation (peroxide, then saline) and place suction drains in the neck, according to the dictates of the wound. Lead these out through separate stab incisions, perform a running, water-tight subcutaneous closure, then re-approximate the skin in a standard fashion. The tracheal stoma is supported with antiseptic gauze and an appropriate tracheotomy tube.

Nutrition will commence through the nasogastric tube after the first 48 hours, and a period of postoperative management identical to that for a total laryngectomy will begin. The difference will be that when the patient has regained swallowing and the stoma is healed, a speaking connection will exist between the airway and foodway, and the patient will soon be ready to acquire fistula speech without aspiration. As the swelling within the lumen of the shunt abates, the patient will find it possible to occlude the stoma, pass air up into the pharynx and thus generate

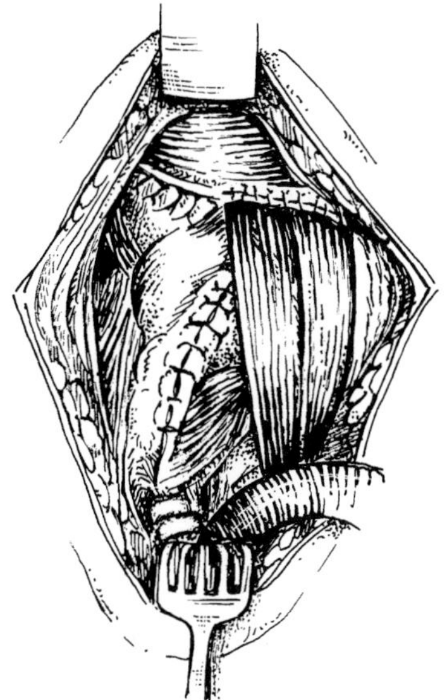

Fig. 14.18 The shunt and pharyngotomy closures are completed and the strap muscles on the left are resutured to the suprahyoid muscles. A permanent tracheostomy is now fashioned.

speech. Interestingly, it appears that the functions of the shunt are inverted. The musculature at the glottic level controls aspiration, and the soft tissues at the supraglottic level are what the patient sets into passive oscillations to produce sound.

The medical care of the tracheotomy site at home must be meticulous. There is no substitute for experienced nursing instruction in changing the tube, cleaning the site, and dealing with the inevitable low-grade infection or topical inflammation that occurs in this region. An anterior wall tracheotomy site always takes longer to heal than the end-on tracheal stoma of a total laryngectomy. Therefore, the rules about how early a patient may be weaned off his tracheotomy tube do not apply. The time scale must be stretched out over a longer period before the stoma itself can go unsupported, or well sealed stomal valving can begin. Each patient must be individualized, and swallowing plus a stable airway must be goals that precede communication.

The options for long-term stomal management are as varied as the patients. Some use a Helsper silicone stoma button because they find they can seat their finger on its trumpet-shaped face-plate more securely and achieve a tighter seal when they valve. This enables a patient to vocalize more efficiently without producing extraneous stomal noises. Some patients can use the Blom—Singer tracheostomy valve after several months, when their voicing pressure comes down, and thus achieve hands-free speech. Other arrangements, such as continued use of a metal tracheotomy tube, which is easy to clean, the long-term use of a silicone laryngectomy tube, which acts as a soft stomal 'keeper' and management of the permanent stoma with no device whatsoever, are also appropriate.

A speech therapist is still the heart of the rehabilitation programme. Shunt speech may change the type of instruction required, but it certainly does not preclude the very valuable aid of the speech therapist's programme. In the course of the relationship, most patients learn their best valving techniques as well as other tricks of articulation. They are often encouraged to slow down, and counselled in optimal stomal management. A speech therapist with experience in laryngectomy voice rehabilitation, including fistula speech and tracheo-oesophageal puncture prosthesis techniques, should talk with the patient before surgery. This prepares them to provide interim communication in the early postoperative period, to tide the patient over until fistula speech is established.

RESULTS

Before reaching its current level of acceptance, near-total laryngectomy has had to overcome several perceptions and attitudes. Initially, there was, of course, the question of adequate margins. Long-term oncological safety has now been established. The difficulty of visualizing the anatomical concepts (it is easier to excise the organ than just the disease) may have inhibited some surgeons as well. The expectation of voice after *total* laryngectomy, with the advent of tracheo-oesophageal puncture techniques, has possibly diminished enthusiasm for an alternative resection too—and there was, of course, the fears of aspiration or voice failure, something for which no surgeon would like to be responsible. The practical justification for near-total laryngectomy is that the paraglottic space can be resected en bloc, with all its neighbouring tissue. The resection and reconstruction are done in one stage. A prosthesis is not required to stent or to valve the vocal shunt. Voice does not have to traverse the pharyngo-oesophageal segment. Rather, it emerges directly into the pharynx, and thus is not constrained by cricopharyngeal spasm or innovative reconstructions of the pharynx.

Classical or extended hemilaryngectomies are not appropriate to the patients we have treated with near-total laryngectomy. It is interesting to note that some serial section studies have shown that 30–50% of T3 lesions are under-staged. Several clinical studies have revealed a propensity for oncological failure when classical conservation procedures are pushed to accommodate the more challenging cases, those with partial limitation of movement.

We have recently reviewed our own Mayo Clinic data. From 1974 to 1991 we performed 178 near-total laryngectomies at all three Mayo Clinic sites. Of these, 159 were available for functional follow-up, 145 with a minimum three-year follow-up for cancer. (The total patient population included 13 near-total laryngectomies for 'laryngeal liability' indications in patients with neurological disease and aspiration. In addition, there were three postoperative deaths unrelated to the cancer or the surgery, and three patients were lost to follow up.)

One-hundred-and-eight patients underwent near-total laryngectomy, 31 underwent near-total laryngopharyngectomy (for pyriform cancer) and six underwent extended near-total laryngopharyngectomy, that is, resections in which the near-total laryngectomy principle was used but pharyngeal reconstruction required a flap. Our data includes nearly equal proportions of glottic/transglottic, supraglottic and pyriform lesions. We analysed the recurrence and mortality due to cancer and found 13 'local' recurrences. This group included seven with stomal, oesophageal or nasopharyngeal recurrences, i.e. only six local recurrences arose from the shunt. An additional 12 patients developed regional and/or distant disease without ever manifesting local recurrence. Thus, nearly 18% of our patients developed recurrent disease, and roughly 14% died of their disease. The difference represents surgical salvage after recurrence. Of the six patients who developed local recurrences *in the shunt*, three had been treated with previous radiation. The recurrences developed at 9, 21, 31, 37, 45, and 81 months. Only one of these cases was glottic. Three were supraglottic and two were pyriform. Of the six local recurrences in the shunt, three patients were salvaged by further surgery.

In the course of our review, we asked ourselves: 'If near-total laryngectomy is performed for suitable indications, what is the chance the patient will talk and what is the chance the shunt will leak?'. Of 159 patients, 14 (9%) developed leakage sufficient to warrant revision. Eleven of these were successfully treated by procedures designed to tighten their shunt or repair side-wall fistulae without sacrificing voice. Three were treated early in our experience by resection of the shunt. Some 86% of our patients (136 of 159) achieved conversational voice with their shunt. To achieve this result, nine patients in this series were treated with successful revision voice procedures, primarily shunt dilatations. An additional 10 underwent similar efforts, but failed.

In summary, based on 15 years' experience, the incidence of significant leakage after near-total laryngectomy is 9%. Successful revision without destruction of the shunt can be performed in the majority of instances where leakage occurs.

Speech acquisition occurs in just over 90% of near-total laryngectomy patients where the operation was performed for a glottic or transglottic carcinoma; it falls to around 80% for the supraglottic and pyriform cases. Speech acquisition is independent of the pharyngo-oesophageal segment, and speech maintenance is independent of prosthesis management.

Near-total laryngectomy appears to be an effective treatment for properly selected patients with invasive laryngeal cancer from glottic, supraglottic and pyriforms sites. It is clear to us that satisfactory functional results are achievable. We would consider radiation failure to be a relative contra-indication to near-total laryngectomy. Total laryngectomy (with and without puncture prosthesis voice rehabilitation techniques) is still required in the overall management of laryngeal cancer, but perhaps not nearly so often as it has been before this technique was available.

REFERENCES

DeSanto L W 1984 T3 glottic carcinoma: options and consequences of the options. Laryngoscope 94: 1311–1315

DeSanto L W, Pearson B W, Olsen K D 1989 Utility of near-total laryngectomy for supraglottic, pharyngeal, base-of-tongue, and other cancers. Annals of Otology, Rhinology and Laryngology 98: 2–7

Dumich P S, Pearson B W, Weiland L H 1984 Suitability of near-total laryngopharyngectomy in pyriform carcinoma. Archives of Otolaryngology 110: 664–669

Pearson B W, Woods R W, Hartman D 1980 Extended hemilaryngectomy for T3 glottic carcinoma with preservation of speech and swallowing. Laryngoscope 90: 1950–1961

Pearson B W 1981 Subtotal laryngectomy. Laryngoscope 91: 1904–1911

Pearson B W, Keith R L 1989 Near-total laryngectomy. In: Johnson J T, Blitzer A, Ossoff R M, Thomas I R (eds) Instructional courses, American Academy of Otology—Head and Neck Surgery, Mosby, St. Louis, vol 2, pp 309–330

Pearson B W, DeSanto L W 1990 Near-total laryngectomy. Operational techniques. Otolaryngology—Head and Neck Surgery 1: 28–41

15. Tracheal resection and reconstruction

Christoph von llberg   Alexander Weber

INTRODUCTION AND HISTORICAL REVIEW

Primary malignancy of the trachea is extremely rare. Lasson et al (1987) counted less than 1 case per million inhabitants in Sweden. The early symptoms of tracheal tumours, if any, are usually most uncharacteristic. For the purpose of diagnosis we nowadays use sophisticated techniques such as flexible endoscopy, ultrasound and computed tomography. We therefore cannot expect to find observations of tracheal malignancy in the early literature before the indirect larynx inspection was discovered by Garcia (1854), Tuerck (1858) and Cermark (1858) (cited by Heymann & Kronenberger 1898) and before the direct endoscopy of the larynx was developed by Kirstein (1896).

The first case of primary trachea carcinoma known from the literature was described by Langerhans (1871) (cited by von Bruns 1898).In his famous book on diseases of the head and neck Mackenzie (1880) mentioned only one case of trachea malignancy, which was diagnosed post mortem by pathologists. Von Bruns (1898) could already collect 31 cases of primary tracheal carcinoma from the literature.

For the first known cases of the primary malignancies of the trachea there existed neither adequate diagnostic nor therapeutic modalities: tracheostomy (Mackenzie 1880), intubation (von Bruns 1898, Killian 1903), T-tubes (Killian 1903) or bouginage (von Schroetter 1876) to overcome respiratory distress were applied in these cases with very limited effect. New techniques for the treatment of tracheal tumours were developed from the experience gained by surgery of the more frequent stenosis due to inflammatory processes such as syphilis, diphtheria, tuberculosis and rhinoscleroma.

Early descriptions of partial resection of the trachea were published at the end of 19th century by surgeons such as König (1886) and Küster (1884). Obviously these techniques were afflicted with a high rate of severe and occasionally fatal complications such as infections, granulation tissue formation and dehiscence at the site of the anastomosis. Problems with silk as suture material and the lack of antiseptic therapy were probably the main reasons for the early surgical failures with this method. In the following decades we therefore observe an increasing number of publications dealing with the far less dangerous *partial* resection followed by reconstruction of the airway in several smaller steps.

Most of these surgical attempts to reconstruct the upper airway were developed to overcome stenotic processes due to scar tissue. The 'open trough' technique, creating large defects of the anterior wall of the airway, consequently required the stepwise closure with plastic reconstructive operations. As reconstructive materials in the early literature, skin, bone and nasal septal cartilage were used. The main disadvantages of the open reconstructive procedures were recurrent scar tissue formation, lining the airway with skin instead of mucous epithelium, and the long duration of the therapy. New techniques creating a closed airway by a one-stage operation technique were developed. For both open and closed reconstruction of the upper airway an adequate stabilization of the lumen during the healing process was necessary. Although reports on tracheal tumours are scarce in the early literature, we can find the principles of resection and/or reconstruction of the upper airway being developed by courageous surgeons in the second half of the 19th century and the following decades which are still of great interest and validity for our present therapeutic concepts.

HISTOLOGY AND CLINICAL FINDINGS

As already mentioned, the trachea is rarely involved in malignant processes (Lasson et al 1987). Only one-third of these cases primarily originate from the trachea (Amemiya et al 1990, Inoue & Ishihara 1990). Until 1987 there had been no more than 800 cases published in the international literature (Emami 1987). Among them, the squamous-cell carcinoma presents the predominant histology with about 50% of the cases (Nonoyama et al 1983, Kharchenko et al 1984, Nealon 1986, Li et al 1990) followed by adenoid-cystic carcinoma with 25% (Xu et al 1987, Nomori et al 1988, Li et al 1990). Other malignant tumours described in the literature have to be considered as rare exceptions such as carcinoid tumours Le-Tian et al (1983), plasmocytoma (Taki et al 1987, Dulmet el al 1990), malignant neurolemmoma (Stack & Steckler 1990), fibrous histiocytoma (Sculerati et al 1990), leiomyoma (Koshiishi et al 1988, Douzinas et al 1989, Thedinger et al 1991), adenocarcinomas (Gelder & Hetzel 1990, Li et al 1990), anaplastic carcinoma, large cell carcinoma (Gelder & Hetzel 1990), melanoma (Moulton et al 1990), mucoepidermoid tumours (Said et al 1988), mostly observed in children (Watterson & Wisheart 1990), malignant epitheloid schwannoma (Maurer & Mann 1989), malignant fibrous histiocytoma (Streitz & Shapshay 1991), lymphoepithelial carcinoma (Inizuka 1990), adenoid cystic carcinoma (Randall et al 1990), chondrosarcoma (Neis et al 1989), Kaposi sarcoma (Rajaratnam & Desai 1988) and embryonal rhabdomyosarcoma (Daum et al 1989, Kedar et al 1988, von Ilberg personal observation).

Primary malignant tumours of the trachea have to be distinguished from metastatic manifestation of other lesions like metastases from adenocarcinoma of the lungs (Sakai et al 1986), melanoma (Moulton et al 1990), colon carcinoma (Morency et al 1989), malignant lymphoma (Hessan et al 1988), aesthesioneurofibroma (Franklin et al 1987) and invasive tumours from surrounding regions such as cancer of the thyroid (D'Amico et at 1988, Li et al 1990, Lydiatt et al 1990, Yoshimura & Nakayima 1990) or the mediastinal space (Emami 1987, Petruzzelli et al 1990, Gelder & Hetzel 1990). Altogether Li et al (1990) described in 15 out of 54 patients an association of tracheal carcinoma with other carcinoma of the head and neck region and the lungs.

Emami (1987) pointed out that squamous-cell carcinoma had a predilection for the distal one-third of the trachea, while adenoidcystic carcinoma and adenocarcinoma have a tendency to appear in the upper third of the trachea.

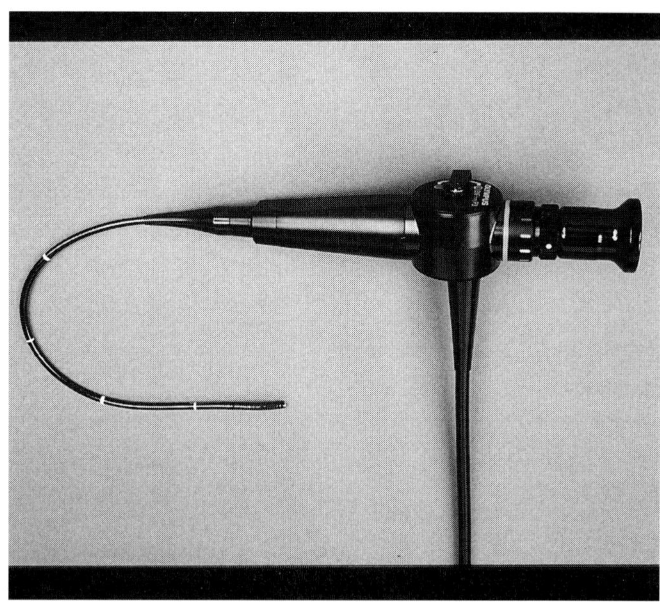

Fig. 15.1 Nasopharyngoscope (Olympus P3).

The first clinical manifestation of tracheal cancer consists of increasing dyspnoea with impending airway obstruction and stridor—sometimes misinterpreted as bronchial asthma or a chronic suppurative bronchitis—brassy cough combined with haemoptysis (Xu et al 1983, Kaiser 1987) or pseudoangina pectoris (Randall et al 1990). In case of infiltration of the recurrent laryngeal nerve, hoarseness as an early symptom of tracheal malignancy may be noticed.

DIAGNOSIS

In the diagnosis of tracheal cancer nowadays, transnasal endoscopy with the flexible fibrescope, with or without local

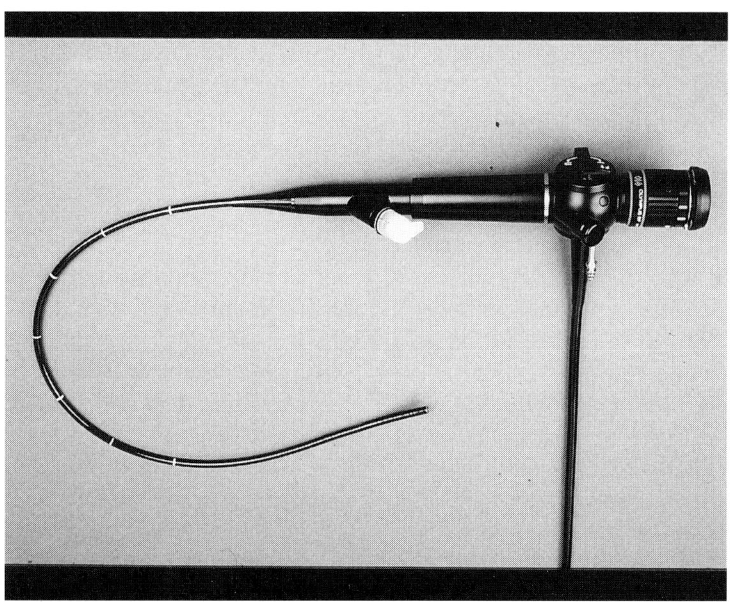

Fig. 15.2 Flexible bronchoscope (Olympus BF type P20D).

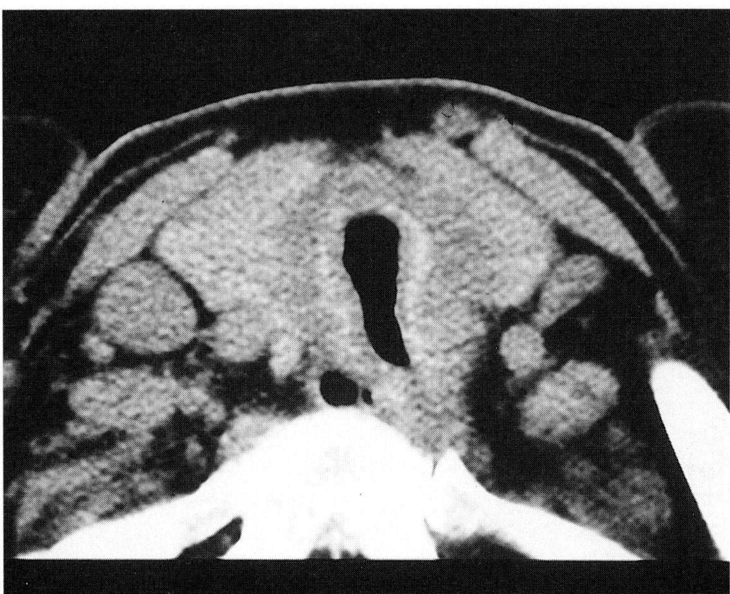

Fig. 15.3 CT scan of a 67-year-old patient with carcinoma of the upper trachea.

anaesthesia, has to be considered as the first method of choice. At our department we use at present the flexible nasopharyngoscope (Fig. 15.1) or the children's bronchoscope (Fig. 15.2) for inspection of the larynx, the upper trachea and the lower trachea—including the bronchial system. For local anaesthesia 10% Xylocain spray is inhaled by the patient for a few minutes prior to the procedure. By this technique we obtain a precise impression of the extent of the airway obstruction without further damage to structures of the larynx and trachea. The tumour mass must not be touched by instruments or the endoscope itself, to avoid bleeding, which can be dangerous. Thus, the procedure

under local anaesthesia is also suitable for emergency cases and can be combined with laser therapy, as we will describe in detail in the following part on tumour excision. Biopsies for histological examination can be taken at the same time. For further determination of the length of the stenotic process and its invasion into the tracheal wall and surrounding tissue, imaging procedures such as ultrasonic examination, xeroradiography, CT scan (Fig. 15.3) and/or MRI are necessary (Gamsu & Webb 1982, Li et al 1990). The documentation of the lesion is performed mainly by rigid-angle optics 0, 30, 70 or 90° (Wolff Instruments) (Fig. 15.4) combined with photocamera (Leica R 5, Olympus

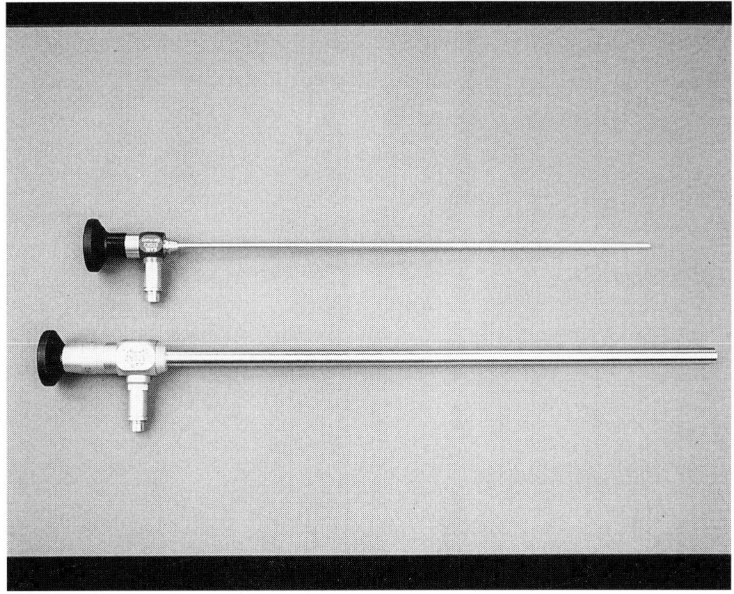

Fig. 15.4 Rigid-angle optics (Storz, Germany) for diagnostic and documentation of the trachea.

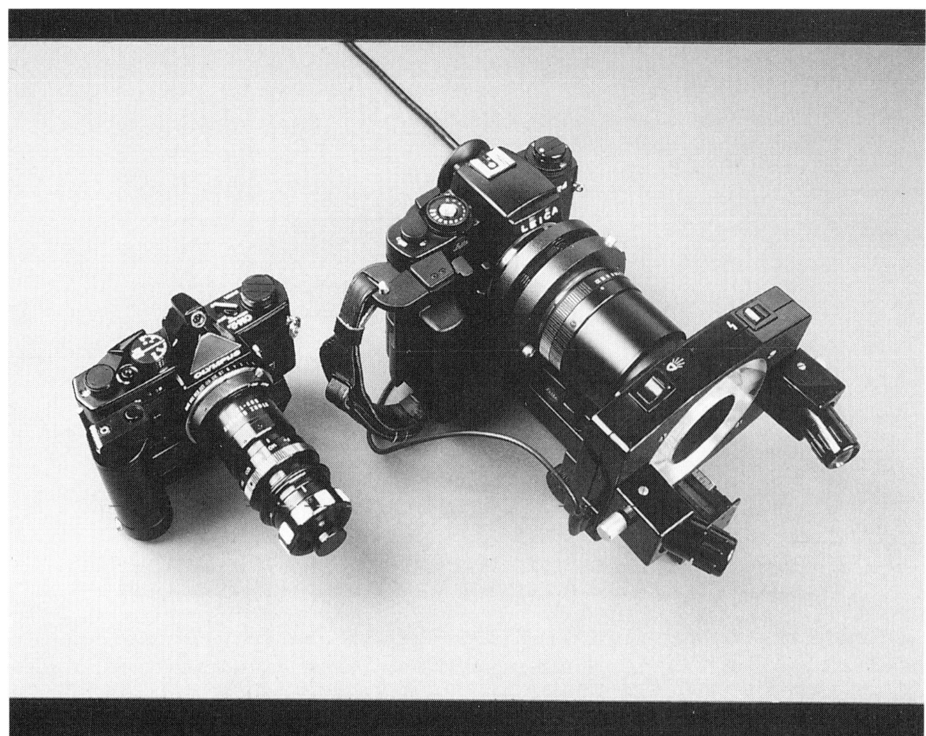

Fig. 15.5   Cameras: Leica R5; Olympus OM2.

OM 2) (Fig. 15.5 and 15.6) or videocamera (Sony DXC 750 P) (Fig. 15.7). During the period between 1977 and 1992 we have seen in our department only five cases with primary malignancies of the trachea among 62 cases with stenotic processes of the same area (Table 15.1).

TUMOUR RESECTION

The surgical approaches in tracheal carcinoma depend largely on the histology, site, and extent of the tumour as well as on the presence or absence of metastases. We therefore

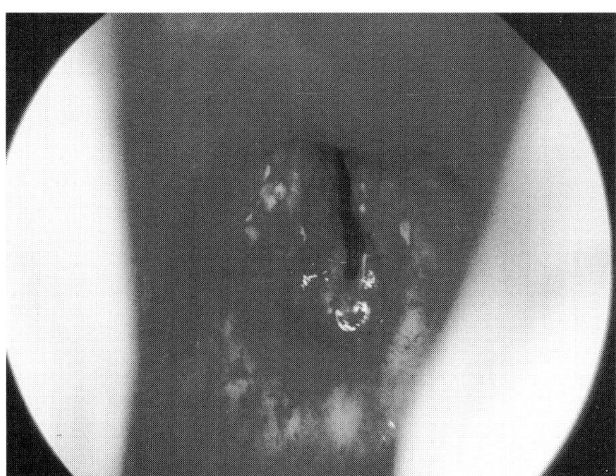

Fig. 15.6   Endoscopic view of a patient with circular growing carcinoma of the upper trachea (0° Optic Storz with Olympus OM2 camera). (See also colour plate section).

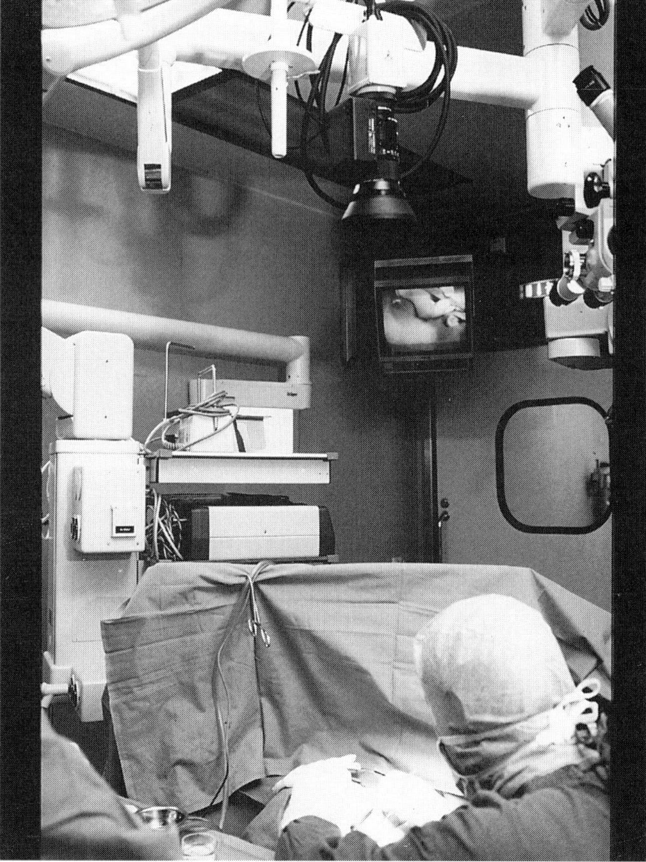

Fig. 15.7   Video camera (Sony DXC 750 P) for micro- and macro documentation.

Table 15.1 Patients with malignancy of the trachea at the ENT Department, University of Frankfurt/Main 1977–1992

B.Z.	12y	F	Rhabdomyosarcoma, upper trachea
R.E.	51y	F	Adenoidcystic carcinoma, uppper trachea and cricoid
F.S.	48y	M	Squamous-cell carcinoma, lower trachea
K.H.B	67y	M	Squamous-cell carcinoma, upper trachea
A.P.	32 y	F	Adenoidcystic carcinoma, upper trachea and cricoid

have to distinguish clearly between curative, palliative and emergency procedures. From the literature it seems to be very difficult to judge the percentage of patients with resectable or non-resectable carcinoma when first seen, because the collection of patients is usually rather limited, and most publications deal with either surgical or palliative (laser, cryotherapy, radiotherapy) treated cases. Inoue & Ishihara (1990) present a statistic of 96 cases with tracheal tumours out of which 79 could be operated. Gelb & Epstein (1987) report 70 patients with tracheal or bronchial carcinoma which have been submitted exclusively to palliative treatment. So we have to decide in each case which therapeutic concept should be applied. It is however, generally accepted that surgical resection—if possible—with primary reconstruction is considered to be the treatment of choice.

To begin with, we would like to present the most common surgical procedures for curative treatment. Smaller lesions of tracheal carcinoma should be treated by resection of the segment involved, followed by immediate end-to-end anastomosis (Fig. 15.8) (Nonoyama et al 1983, 1984, Pearson et al 1984, Kaiser 1985, Grillo & Zannini 1986, Friedman et al 1987, Douzinas et al 1989, Inoue & Ishihara 1990). It is important to point out that sufficiently large margins of the tumour area have to be resected because of the possibility of submucous growth. This is especially the case in adenoidcystic carcinoma (Emami 1987) with its tendency of submucous growth which cannot be recognized by the surgeon.

The technique of sleeve resection with end-to-end re-anastomosis first described by König (1886), Küster (1884) and Foederl at the end of the 19th century was further developed by Grillo (1965), Weerda et al (1974), von Ilberg (1982), von Ilberg & Haas (1985) and Grillo & Zannini (1986). The length of the resected segment should be limited to 6 cm (von Ilberg & Haas 1985, Grillo & Mathisen 1990). In neonates it is obviously possible to increase the segment resection to two-thirds of the trachea (Longaker et al 1990). A preoperatively open tracheostoma can and should be included in the resection (von Ilberg & Haas 1985). An open tracheostoma postoperatively should be restricted to rare exceptions. The restenosis rate at the anastomosis site is about 15% (Weber & von Ilberg 1992); it can be reduced by careful submucous suture technique using re-absorbable stitches (Weerda et al 1974). Any

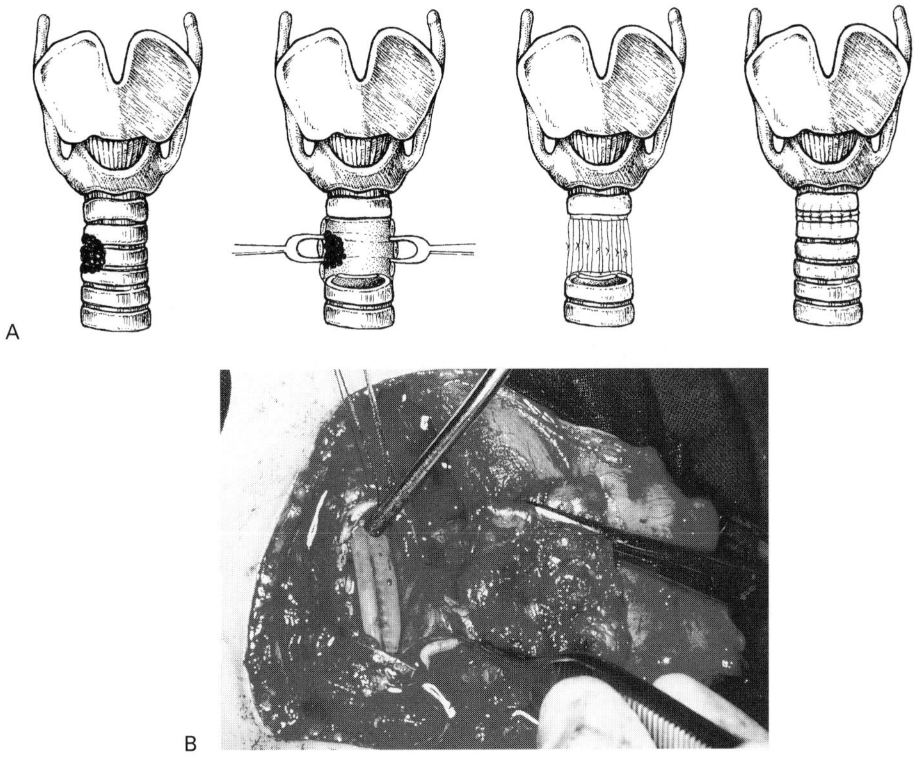

Fig. 15.8 **A.** Surgical technique of tracheal segment resection with end-to-end re-anastomosis. **B.** Tracheal segment resection in a 12-year-old girl with rhabdomyosarcoma of the left upper trachea. (See also colour plate section)

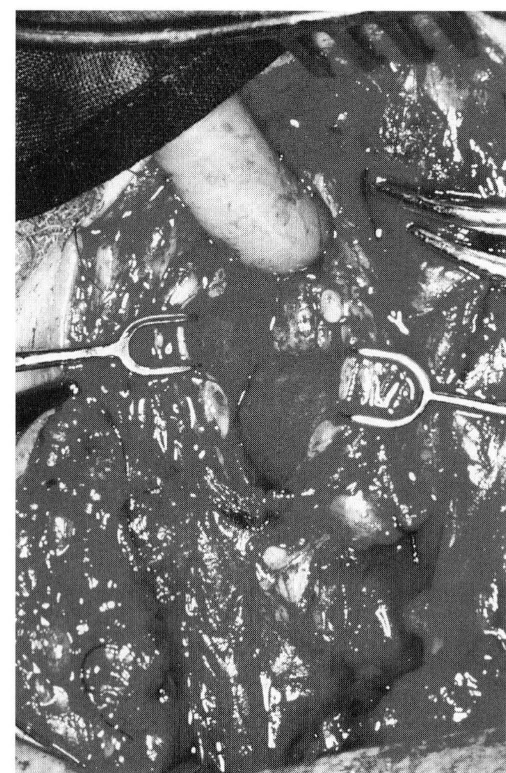

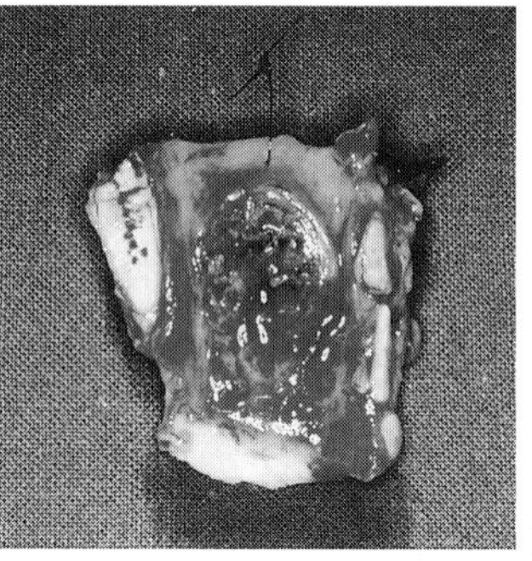

Fig. 15.9 Lateral 'window resection' of the subcricoidal region in a 51-year-old female patient with adenoid cystic carcinoma. (See also colour plate section)

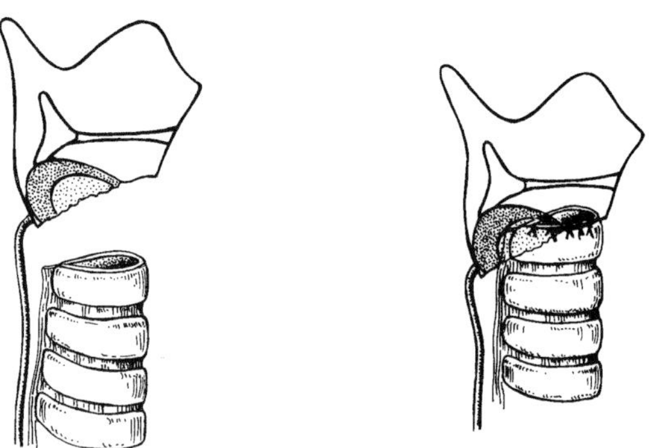

Fig. 15.10 Technique of partial cricoid resection (Pearson 1983).

involves the cricoid ring. In these rare cases, special modifications at the laryngotracheal transition are necessary such as the partial cricoidectomy described by Pearson et al (1984, 1986) (Fig. 15.10), partial cricoid reconstruction with nasal septum (Cotton et al 1989) or with the first intact tracheal ring (von Ilberg & Weber 1991) (Figs. 15.11 and 15.12). If the cricoid plate is infiltrated, in most cases laryngectomy seems to be inevitable.

Primary cancer of the adjacent thyroid gland in advanced stage has a tendency to infiltrate the wall of the upper airway. Shvili et al (1985) described an infiltration of thyroid tumours into the trachea and the larynx in about 5%, Li et al (1990) in 7%. These cases of secondary carcinoma of the trachea most frequently require laryngectomy and partial tracheal resection as a monobloc operation (Shvili et al 1985, Tsumori et al 1985, Grillo et al 1986, Lydiatt et al 1990). In cases with smaller lesions or cases with very poor prognosis partial resection of the trachea without total laryngectomy is recommended (Lipton et al 1987, D'Amico et al 1988, Friedman et al 1986). According to the experience of Lipton et al (1987) and Friedman et al (1988b) debulking or 'shaving' of the thyroid carcinoma from the trachea gave unsatisfactory results. The necessity of an adjuvant chemo- or radiotherapy will not be discussed here.

In other cases, with invasively growing tracheal

postoperative long-term intubation or stenting must be avioded.

In cases with very small restricted primary lesions, a partial lateral (Fig. 15.9) or anterior resection of the trachea may be indicated (Le-Tian et al 1983, Nonoyama et al 1983, Kaiser 1985, Xu et al 1987, Sculerati et al 1990). In these cases, the reconstruction of the tracheal window is necessary (for methods see 'reconstruction').

While most of the sleeve resections of the cervical trachea can be made through a horizontal supraclavicular skin incision, lesions of the lower trachea and the carina require a sternotomy or lateral thoracotomy.

Particular difficulties arise if the carcinomatous lesion

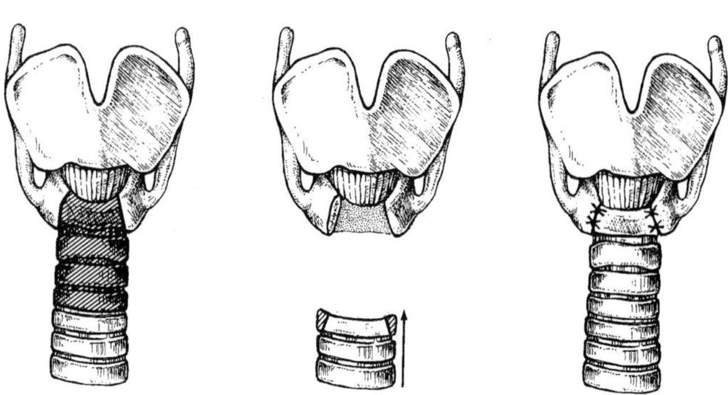

Fig. 15.11 Reconstruction of the anterior cricoid arch with the 'shaped' upper end of the trachea (von Ilberg & Weber 1991).

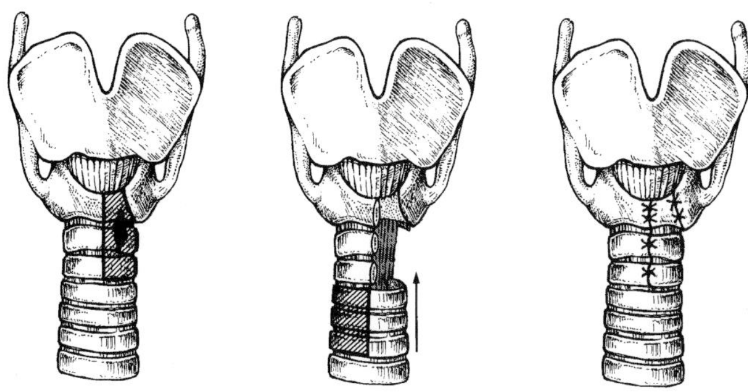

Fig. 15.12 Reconstruction of the lateral cricoid arch with the distal end of the trachea (von Ilberg & Weber 1991).

carcinoma, the infiltration of the dorsal tracheal wall can be occasionally observed. This tumour localization frequently leads to an infiltration of the oesophagus wall and/or uni- or bilateral invasion of the recurrent nerve. The oesophagus involvement has to be verified by CT scan and oeso-phagoscopy. Recurrent nerve paresis or paralysis can easily be recognized by laryngoscopy and electromyography (Fig. 15.13). While smaller lesions of the dorsal trachea can be managed by partial resection and recontruction (Symbas et al 1984, Sakaguchi 1990), deeper infiltration requires more

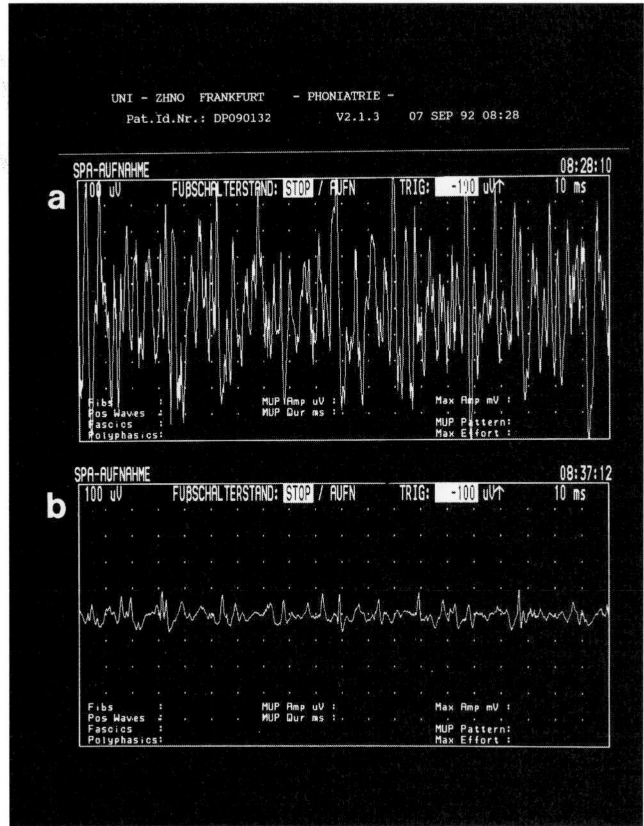

Fig. 15.13 Electromyography of the m. vocalis during phonation: (a) normal side, (b) paralysed side (curve presents single positive spikes).

aggressive surgery. Sleeve resection of the trachea must be combined with horizontal resection of the oesophagus segment involved, followed by reconstruction of the digestive passage using the pulled up stomach, musculocutaneous flaps (Pollard & Harrison 1985, Sakaguchi 1990) or free grafts of colon or jejunum (Fig. 15.14) in a one-stage operation (Grillo et al 1986). Consequently, older reconstructive techniques in two or more steps have become obsolete.

In cases with carcinoma of the upper trachea with involvement of the laryngeal structures this surgical procedure may include laryngectomy (larynx–pharynx–oesophagus–tracheal resection). In these advanced tumours the poor prognosis should be taken into preoperative consideration as we probably reach the border of curative surgery. As soon as the palliative character of the surgery is recognized, in our opinion the improvement of the functional situation of the patient must be given priority over the radical tumour excision.

LYMPH NODES

The exact amount of lymph node involvement in trachea malignancy is difficult to determine. Grillo & Mathisen (1990), among the most experienced authors on this problem, briefly remark that 'squamous cell carcinoma and adenoidcystic carcinoma metastasizes to the regional lymph nodes'; obviously, adenoidcystic carcinoma involves a much smaller number of nodes. As the lymph node involvement will be found especially in squamous-cell carcinoma with advanced tumour stages when the tumour is no longer limited to the tracheal wall, the lymph node resection seems somewhat problematic. To quote Grillo & Mathisen (1990) again: 'Local paratracheal lymph nodes are excised with the specimen when possible'. The problem gets even more evident as a radical systematic mediastinal dissection is impossible for technical reasons. Postoperative radiation therapy therefore seems to be a reasonable procedure in the therapy of these advanced cases, even though its therapeutical value needs further scrutiny.

PALLIATIVE MODALITIES

Approximately one-third of the patients with primary trachea malignancies are not amenable to surgical resection when first seen (Inoue & Ishihara 1990, Grillo & Mathisen 1990). The reasons are local tumour extension, distant metastases, age, or medical condition of the patient. For patients first presenting as emergency cases with a compromised airway, an increasing number of authors recommend endotracheal procedures to open the air passage. This can be carried out by endoscopical electrosurgery (Nakahara 1984, Hooper & Jackson 1985, Frizelli 1986, Gerasin & Shafirovsky 1988), cryosurgery (Homasson et al 1986, Vergnon et al 1987), laser surgery as a general therapeutic technique (Taki et al 1987, Haussinger et al 1988, Hulke &

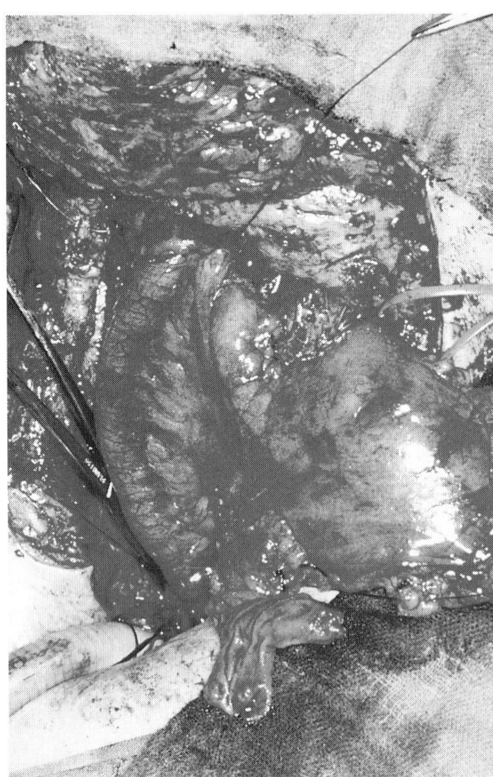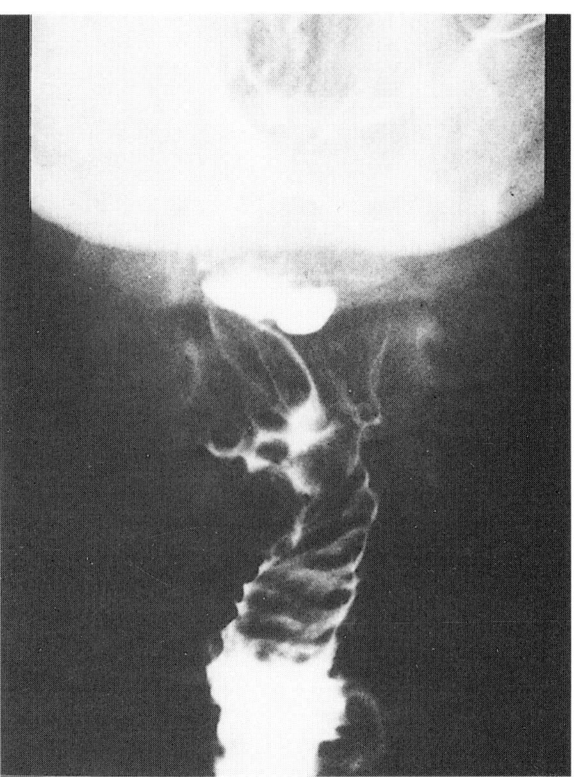

Fig. 15.14 **A.** Reconstruction of the hypopharynx and cervical oesophagus with free jejunum graft. (See also colour plate section) **B.** X-ray control, 3 weeks postoperatively.

Thomson 1988, Kairalla et al 1988), CO_2-laser (McElvein & Zorn 1984, Oswal et al 1988, Shapshay et al 1988, Remacle et al 1989), Neodym-Yag laser (Brutinel et al 1983, Hetzel et al 1983, McElvein & Zorn 1983, Jain et al 1985, Franklin et al 1987, Gelb & Epstein 1987, Kaiser 1987, George et al 1987, Gerasin et al 1987, Gelb et al 1988, Cavaliere et al 1988, Hunt & Pierce 1988, Miro et al 1989, Clarke et al 1989, Castro et al 1990, Sutedja & Stam 1990, Dias-Jiminez et al 1990), argon laser (Hetzel et al 1983), or photodynamic argon laser therapy (McCaughan et al 1988).

Since the early description of von Bruns (1898) it is generally accepted that any kind of endotracheal surgery has a very limited and strictly palliative effect. With improved technology, such as cryo- or laser therapy in selected cases, it may still turn out to be a reasonable emergency procedure prior to resective surgery (Jain et al 1985, Homasson et al 1986, Gerasin et al 1987, Vergnon et al 1987, Kasier 1987, Haussinger et al 1988, Shapshay et al 1988, Sutedja & Stam 1990). To keep a compromised airway open, several endotracheal prostheses are recommended: tracheal T-tubes (Montgomery 1973), plastic or wire nets (Neville 1982, Ehrenberger 1986, Haussinger et al 1988) and balloon-expanded Palmaz-Schantz stents (Johnson & Johnson Interventional Systems) (Fig. 15.15). In most of these cases air moisturizing is mandatory to reduce crust formation at the inner surface of the prothesis.

A segment resection of the trachea in cases of slow-growing tumours such as adenoidcystic carcinoma may afford excellent long-term palliation even when the resection is incomplete. In other cases a deep mediastinal tracheostomy (Wurtz et al 1988) together with intubation may be the ultimate desperate procedure to secure respiration. Other therapeutic non-surgical modalities with pure palliative character—such as radiation and/or chemotherapy—cannot be discussed here.

Of special interest and difficulty are technical details concerning anaesthesia during any manipulation of the trachea. Local anaesthesia may be reasonable in cases where smaller endotracheal procedures such as laser surgery (George et al 1987, Shah & Marg 1989, Sutedja & Stam 1990) or cryosurgery (Vergnon et al 1987) are indicated, or in emergency cases, where a recanalization of the airway by laser or cryosurgery is necessary prior to intubation and surgery. Brutinel et al (1983) advocate Neodym-Yag laser therapy under i.v. anaesthesia. Any other procedures should be carried out exclusively under general anaesthesia. For laser surgery we prefer a modality with alternating intubation through the endoscope and laser application in short intervals with mandatory controlled blood oxygen values. With this technique an optimal visibility is combined with a strongly reduced risk during the application of CO_2 and especially Neodym–Yag laser.

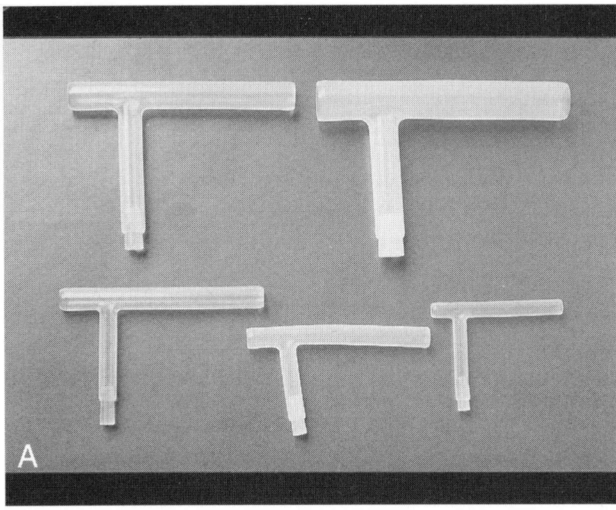

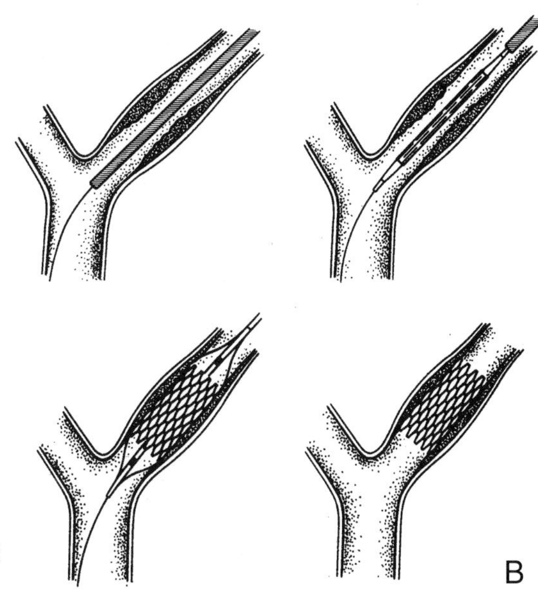

Fig. 15.15 A. Montgomery T-tube. **B.** Palmaz–Schatz stents for immediate and long-term stenting of the trachea.

RECONSTRUCTION

The adequate reconstruction after segment resection of the trachea is the immediate end-to-end reanastomosis, provided that the distal end is carefully freed from surrounding scar tissue at the entrance of the upper mediastinum until it is completely mobilized (Fig. 15.8). An open tracheostoma must be included in the resected segment. This technique is usually possible when the length of the resection does not exceed 6 cm (Weber & von Ilberg 1992). Grillo & Mathisen (1990) point out that, with increasing age, obesity and kyphosis, re-anastomosis becomes more problematic. Any tension at the site of the anastomosis must be avoided. This is achieved by flexing the head anteriorly and sufficient mobilization of the tracheal ends. The suture material and technique seem to be important for a healing process which is free of complications. We use absorbable 2-0 PDS monofil stitches which may comprise cartilage and the mucosal layer. The sutures at the pars membranacea as well as at the anterior circumference have to be knotted exteriorly (Fig. 15.8). Weerda et al (1974) have emphasized that a submucous suture technique may reduce the tendency for local granulation tissue formation. Following segmental resection we found in 15% of our own patients early local restenosis within 50 weeks. After local re-operation, all of these patients could finally be successfully decanulated (Weber & von Ilberg 1992). If parts of the cricoid arch must be included in the tumour specimen—such as in surgery of invasive thyroid carcinoma—the cricoid ring can be reconstructed by shaping the upper end of the distal tracheal stump (Pearson et al 1986, Grillo & Mathisen 1990) or by using the first intact tracheal ring to stabilize the subglottic defect (von Ilberg & Weber 1991) (Fig. 15.10 and 15.11). Smaller defects after lateral or anterior window resection of

the trachea (Fig. 15.9) can be reconstructed with sternohyoid muscle flap (Lange 1976, Weerda 1978, Nonoyama et al 1983, Zalzal et al 1986, Eliachar et al 1989), myoperiostal flap (Friedman et al 1987, 1988a,b), a free perichondral graft from the pinna (Ishikawa & Isshiki 1988), palatal mucoperiostal graft (Yoshimura & Nakajima 1990), sliding flap technique (Gates & Tucker 1989), nasal septum graft (Toohill et al 1976, Zehm 1978, Cotton et al 1981, Duncavage et al 1989) preserved xenograft of tracheal wall (Herberhold et al 1983, Tanimura et al 1989), iliac crest flap (Kambic et al 1986), hyoid-sternohyoid flap (Freeland 1986), rib cartilage (Muntz & Lusk 1990) or hydroxylapatite reinforcement (Hirano et al 1989). Nowadays we personally prefer also the segment resection to any kind of reconstructive surgery in these cases with minor lesions because of its lower stenosis rate.

Defects in the posterior wall of the airway in cases with oesophageal infiltration or tracheo-oesophageal fistula (Symbas et al 1984) may be reconstructed with platysma myocutaneous flap Sakaguchi (1990), skin flaps (Weidenbecher & Thumfart 1979) or by sleeve resection of the involved tracheal and oesophagus segment (von Ilberg personal observation). We feel that most of the cases with partial resections of the trachea in carcinoma surgery would have been better off with a segment resection in terms of radical tumour eradication and postoperative rapid restitution of the airway. Partial resections should therefore in our opinion be restricted to the surgery of benign tumours such as chondroma, leiomyoma and pleomorphic adenoma. In carcinoma with advanced extension—particularly in slow-growing adenoidcystic carcinoma—it may be necessary to remove long segments of the trachea; this makes a primary re-anastomosis impossible. To bridge these large defects, Grillo & Mathisen (1990) advocate a staged reconstruction with muscle flaps stabilized by a Montgomery T-tube. Herberhold et al (1983) suggest the reconstruction of the trachea with preserved tracheal homograft. In rare cases the bridging of large trachea defects with the dacron-prosthesis is reported by Moghissi (1975), Podoshin & Fradis (1976), Weidauer & Vogt-Moykopf (1980) and Neville (1982).

We still have to admit that reconstruction of extremely long trachea defects remains a questionable procedure as neither the oncological nor the functional results have been satisfying so far. The problems with any extra long endotracheal stents or prostheses consist of crust formation at the inner surface or granulation tissue at their upper and lower ends, followed by circular scar tissue formation and airway stenosis as the final consequence. At present, the Montgomery T-tube seems to be the best solution for long-term stenting. The satisfying functional results after reconstruction of long tracheal segments with tracheal homografts reported by Herberhold et al (1983) or fresh human tracheal allograft transplantation reported by Rose & Sesterhenn (1982) require further confirmation.

PROGNOSIS

As we have pointed out earlier, malignancies of the trachea have to be considered as extremely rare diseases. We therefore cannot expect large numbers of patients for valid statistics from single authors. The largest number of cases was published by Grillo & Mathisen (1990) (198 patients), Inoue & Ishihara (1990) (96 patients with primary and secondary carcinoma of the trachea), Nonoyama et al (1983) (53 patients collected from the Japanese literature), Pearson et al (1984) (44 patients with primary tracheal carcinoma), Kharchenko et al (1984) (100 patients with combined radio-surgical treatment, 41 preoperative, 59 postoperative radiation), Emami (1987) (reviews 800 patients from the world literature), Shvili et al (1985) (122 patients with carcinoma of the thyroid out of which he described 7 patients with airway invasion), McElvein & Zorn (1984) (94 patients treated by laser-surgery only), and Li et al (1990) (55 patients with primary carcinoma of the trachea).

It is obvious, therefore, that there is no series of primary tracheal tumours to be found in the literature comparable to Grillo and Mathisen's published in 1990. These 196 cases allow some detailed statements on the prognosis of the disease. Nearly all of Grillo and Mathisen's patients were irradiated after surgery. Twenty out of 41 (49%) survivors after resection of the squamous-cell carcinoma and 39 out of 52 (75%) patients with adenoidcystic carcinoma are living free of disease. Kharchenko et al (1984) found in their patients after combined treatment an overall 5-year survival rate of 57%. Inoue & Ishihara (1990) referred to 11 out of 13 patients with adenoidcystic carcinoma who were alive without recurrence after 2–9 years. In patients with thyroid carcinoma involving the trachea, Inoue & Ishihara observed that 19 out of 29 (65.5%) patients were still alive after 5

years. The effect of the histological differentiation of adenoidcystic carcinoma on the prognosis is pointed out by Nomori et al (1988): while the solid tumour type with low-grade differentiation frequently produces distant metastases, the tubular–cribriform non-solid tumour type has a tendency to infiltrate into the tracheal wall. Tsumori et al (1985) advocate laryngectomy in combination with tracheal resection in patients with thyroid cancer infiltrating the airway, with respect to the poor prognosis.

Positive lymph nodes or invasive disease at resection margins appeared to have an adverse effect on the cure rate Grillo & Mathisen (1990). This effect could not be demonstrated for adenoidcystic carcinoma.

If we compare these results with cases which were exclusively treated by radiotherapy— Fields et al (1989) observed a survival rate of 45% after 1 year, 25% after 5 years and 13% after 10 years,—we may come to the conclusion that radical resection, if possible, combined with postoperative radiation should be the therapy of first choice. This observation corresponds with that of most authors in the earlier literature. Other therapeutic concepts, such as radiotherapy, chemotherapy or lasertherapy alone must be considered as mainly palliative.

PROBLEMS AND COMPLICATIONS

Any planned or emergency surgery at the airway is associated with a high percentage of complications and risks. For tracheobronchial surgery Engelmann et al (1990) described a perioperative mortality of 9.5%. Grillo & Mathisen (1990) observed only 1 death in 82 patients with tracheal resection, but 6 fatal accidents out of 65 patients following reconstruction of the carina. Further early complications after tracheal resection are: granulation tissue formation, dehiscence at the anastomotic site, injury of the recurrent nerve (25%, Weber & von Ilberg 1992), subcutaneous emphysema and heavy bleeding. The main long-term complication is still stricture of the airway by scar tissue (15% Weber & von Ilberg 1992) which sometimes may be hardly distinguishable from recurrent tumour. The variety of further complications is largely dependent on the nature of therapy applied. The high risk of laser therapy is pointed out by McElvein & Zorn (1983) who described in their 43 patients given CO_2 laser therapy four fatal complications: one intraoperative and three in the postoperative phase. About the same results (8 deaths out of 200 patients) are reported by Haussinger et al (1988). It should be pointed out that most of the patients who were submitted to laser therapy were not amenable to surgery because of advanced tumour stage.

Complications, particularly in connection with endotracheal stenting or prosthesis such as secondary strictures, fistulas, dehiscence, subglottic granuloma or granuloma at the distal sutures, are described by Neville et al (1990).

FUTURE DEVELOPMENTS

As many authors have demonstrated that radical resection of tracheal malignancy still produces the best oncological results, future research has to concentrate on new methods for adequate repair and reconstruction of the airway, including parts of the larynx, the trachea and the bronchial system. New alloplastic materials such as hydroxylapatite (Hirano et al 1989), may be used to repair long defects of the airway. Since Connolly and Richards (1951) and Davies et al (1951), a great many authors have tried to introduce tracheal homografts as a substitute in large tracheal defects without convincing results (Flemming & Hommerich 1968, von Ilberg et al 1977). In both alloplastic and homoplastic airway reconstruction the inner epithelial lining remained unsatisfactory. New approaches with cultivated epithelial layers (Kaschke et al 1990) for coating a tracheal prosthesis may indicate a solution to the problem in the future. Herberhold et al (1983) was the first to describe the successful transplantation of methacrylate-preserved tracheal homografts in human surgery. As we pointed out earlier, his positive results could not yet be verified by others.

REFERENCES

Amemiya R, Guang S G, Koshiishi H, Takahashi E, Naitoh J, Oho K 1990 Primary and metastatic tracheal tumours with airway stenosis. Journal of the Japan Broncho-Esophagol Society 41: 374–383

Beck A, Nanko N, Schildge J, Hasse J 1989 Stent implantation as a palliative means of treatment in inoperable bronchial tumours: preliminary experience with an endoscopically implanted stent. Radiologie 29: 399–405

Bergstrom B, Fogh A, Ranudd N E 1985 Late complications after irradiation treatment for cervical adenitis in childhood: a 60-year follow-up study. Acta Oto-Laryngology 100: 151–160

Brutinel W M, McDougall C, Cortese D A 1983 Bronchoscopic therapy with neodymium–yttrium–aluminum–garnet laser during intravenous anesthesia. Effect on arterial blood gas levels, pH, hemoglobin saturation, and production of abnormal hemoglobin. Chest 84: 518–521

Castro D J, Saxton R E, Ward P H, Oddie J W, Layfield L J, Lufkin R B, Calcaterra T C 1990 Flexible Nd-YAG laser palliation of obstructive tracheal metastatic malignancies. Laryngoscope 100: 1208–1214

Cavaliere S, Foccoli P, Farina P L 1988 Nd-YAG laser bronchoscopy. A five-year experience with 1396 applications in 1000 patients (see comments). Chest 94: 15–21

Clarke C P, Jackson K A, Moreland M, Coles J R, Ball D L 1989 Bronchoscopic use of the neodymium–yttrium–aluminium–garnet laser for lesions of the trachea and bronchus. Medical Journal of Australia 150: 260–262

Cohen R C, Filler R M, Konuma K, Bahoric A, Kent G, Smith C, 1985 The successful reconstruction of thoracic tracheal defects with free periosteal grafts. Journal Pediatric Surgery 20: 852–858

Connolly J E, Richards V 1951 The homotransplantation of trachea in dogs. Surgical Forum 1: 47–53

Cotton R T, Richardson M A, Seid A B, 1981 The management of 5 advanced laryngo-tracheal stenoses. Management of combined advanced glottic and subglottic stenosis in infancy and childhood. Laryngoscope 91: 221–225

Cotton R T, Myer C M 3rd, Bratcher G O, Fitton C M 1988 Anterior cricoid split, 1977–1987. Evolution of a technique. Archives of Otolaryngology—Head and Neck Surgery 114: 1300 –1302

Cotton R T, Gray S D, Miller R P 1989 Update of the Cincinnati experience in pediatric laryngotracheal reconstruction. Laryngoscope 99: 1111–1116

D'Amico D, Favia G, Annunziata N 1988 The treatment of tracheal invasion thyroid tumours. Chirurgia 1: 225–228

Daum R, Denecke H J, Roth H 1987 Tumour-induced intraluminal stenoses of the cervical trachea—tumour excision and tracheoplasty. Progress in Pediatric Surgery 21: 50–57

Davies O G, Edmiston J M, McCorkle H J 1951 The repair of experimental tracheal defects with fresh and preserved homologous tracheal grafts. Journal of Thoracic and Cardiovascular Surgery 23: 367–376

Diaz-Jimenez J P, Canela-Cardona M, Maestre-Alcacer J 1990 Nd-YAG laser photoresection of low-grade malignant tumours of the tracheobronchial tree. Chest 97: 920–922

Douzinas M, Sheppard M N, Lennox S C 1989 Leiomyoma of the trachea— an unusual tumour. Thoracic and Cardiovascular Surgeon 37: 285–287

Dulmet E, Verley J M, Levasseur Ph, Jaubert F, Choudat L 1990 Plasmocytome solitaire de la trachée. A propos d'un cas. Solitary plasmacytoma of the trachea. A case report. Annales de Pathologie 10: 275–277

Duncavage J A, Ossoff R H, Toohill R J 1989 Laryngotracheal reconstruction with composite nasal septal cartilage grafts. Annals of Otology, Rhinology and Laryngology 98: 581–585

Ehrenberger K 1986 Expandierende endotracheale Prothesen zur Behandlung von Trachealstenosen. Archives of Otorhinolaryngology suppl, II 154–158

Eliachar I, Tucker H M 1991 Reconstruction of pediatric larynx and upper trachea with the sternohyoid rotary door flap. Archives of Otolaryngology—Head and Neck Surgery 117: 316–320

Eliachar I, Welker K B, Roberts J K, Tucker H M 1989 Advantages of the rotary door flap in laryngotracheal reconstruction: is skeletal support necessary? Annals of Otology, Rhinology and Laryngology 98: 37–40

Emami B 1987 Radiation oncology: tumours of the mediastinum. Principles and practice of radiation oncology. In: Perez C A, Brady L W (eds). Lippincott, Philadelphia, p 684–699

Engelmann C, Liedtke D, Ehlert U 1990 Rekonstruierende Operationen bei tracheobronchialen Tumoren (Reconstructive surgery in tracheobronchial tumours). Zentralblatt für Chirurgie (Leipzig)115: 949–961

Fields J N, Rigaud G, Emami B N 1989 Primary tumours of the trachea. Results of radiation therapy. Cancer 63: 2429–2433

Flemming J, Hommerich K W 1968 Homotransplantation der Trachea im Tierexperiment. Archiv für Klinische und experimentelle Ohren-Nasen-and Kehlkopfheilkunde, Heute: Archives für Oto-Rhino-Laryngology 19: 724–727

Franklin D, Miller R H, Bloom K, Easley J, Stiernberg C M 1987 Esthesioneuroblastoma metastatic to the trachea. Head and Neck Surgery 10: 102–106

Freeland A P 1986 The long-term results of hyoid-sternohyoid grafts in the correction of subglottis stenosis. Journal of Laryngology and Otolaryngology 100: 665–674

Friedman M, Grybauskas V, Toriumi D M, Skolnik E, Chilis T 1987 Sternomastoid myoperiosteal flap for reconstruction of the subglottic larynx. Annals of Otology, Rhinology and Laryngology 96: 163–169

Friedman M, Toriumi D M, Grybauskas V T, Owens R 1988a Experience with the sternocleidomastoid myoperiosteal flap for reconstruction of subglottic and tracheal defects: modification of technique and report of long-term results. Laryngoscope 98: 1003–1011

Friedman M, Toriumi D M, Grybauskas V T 1988b Advances in treatment of thyroid carcinoma invading the aerodigestive tract (meeting abstract). Second International Conference on Head and Neck Cancer. July 31–August 5 1988, Boston MA, American Society for Head and Neck Surgery p 81

Frizelli R 1986 Le Traitement par Electrocoagulation en Pathologie maligne Tracheo-Bronchique. (Treatment by electrocoagulation in malignant tracheobronchial pathology). Revue de Pneumologie Clinique (Paris) 42: 235–237

Gamsu G, Webb W R 1982 Computed tomography of the trachea: normal and abnormal. American Journal of Roentgenology 139: 321–326

Gates G A, Tucker J A 1989 Sliding flap tracheoplasty. Annals of Otology, Rhinology and Laryngology 98: 926–929

Gelb A F, Epstein J D 1987 Neodymium–yttrium–aluminum–garnet laser in lung cancer. Annals of Thoracic Surgery 43: 164–167

Gelb A F, Tashkin D P, Epstein J D, Fairshter R, Zamel N 1988 Diagnosis and Nd-YAG laser treatment of unsuspected malignant tracheal obstruction. Chest 94: 767–771

Gelder C M, Hetzel M R 1990 National survey of primary tracheal tumours. British Thoracic Society Summer Meeting, Birmingham, UK, July 11–13 1990. Thorax 45: 804

George P J M, Garrett C P O, Nixon C, Hetzel M R, Nanson E M, Millard F J C 1987 Laser treament for tracheobronchial tumours: Local or general anesthesia? Thorax 42: 656–660

Gerasin V A, Shafirovsky B B 1988 Endobronchial electrosurgery. Chest 93: 270–274

Gerasin V A, Shafirovsky B B, Berezin Y D, Zhurba V M 1987 Endobronchial surgery of trachea and bronchi. Zeitschrift für Erkrankungen der Atmungsorgane mit Folia bronchologica (Leipzig) 169: 238–241

Grillo H C 1965 Circumferencial resection and reconstruction of the mediastinal and cervical trachea. Annals of Surgery 162: 374–384

Grillo H C, Mathisen D J 1990 Primary tracheal tumours: treatment and results. Annals of Thoracic Surgery 49: 69–77

Grillo H C, Zannini Pl 1986 Resectional management of airway invasion by thyroid carcinoma. Annals of Thoracic Surgery 42: 287–298

Grillo H C, Zannini P, Michelassi F 1986 Complications of tracheal reconstruction. Incidence, treatment, and prevention. Journal of Thoracic and Cardiovascular Surgery 91: 322–328

Haussinger K, Breyer G, Karg O 1988 Die endobronchiale Lasertherapie - eine lebensrettende Sofortmaß-nahme bei stenosierenden Trachealtumoren. Endobronchial laser therapy—a life-saving emergency measure in stenosing tracheal tumours. Praxis und Klinik der Pneumologie 42: 338–339

Herberhold C, R Franz 1971 Deckung offener Rinnen mit cialitkonservierten homologen Tracheateilen. Vortrag 62. Jahrestagung d. Nordwestdeutschen Verein d. HNO-Ärzte, Braunlage

Herberhold C, Westhofen M, Rauchfuss A 1983 Transplantation konservierter homologer Trachealsegmente. Archives of Otorhinolaryngology (suppl) 342

Hessan H, Houck J, Harvey H 1988 Airway obstruction due to lymphoma of the larynx and trachea. Laryngoscope 98: 176–180

Hetzel M R, Millard F J, Ayesh R, Bridges C E, Nanson E M, Swain C P, William I P 1983 Laser treatment for carcinoma of the bronchus. British Medical Journal 286: 12–16

Heymann P, Kronenberger E 1898 In: Handbuch der Laryngologie u. Rhinologie, Hersg. P. Heymann. Wien, p1–53

Hirano M, Yoshida T, Sakaguchi S 1989 Hydroxylapatite for laryngotracheal framework reconstruction. Annals of Otology Rhinology and Laryngology 98: 713–717

Homasson J P, Renault P, Angebault M, Bonniot J P, Bell N J 1986 Bronchoscopic cryotherapy for airway strictures caused by tumours. Chest 90: 159–164

Hooper R G, Jackson F N 1985 Endobronchial electrocautery. Chest 87: 712–714

Hulke B, Thomson N C 1988 Laser treatment of tracheobronchial tumours. Scottish Medical Journal 33: 323–324

Hunt J M, Pierce R J 1988 Tracheal papillomatosis treated with Nd-YAG laser resection. Australian and New Zealand Journal of Medicine 18: 781–784

Inoue H, Ishihara T 1990 Tracheal tumour resection and reconstruction surgery. Japanese Journal of Thoracic Diseases 28: 272–277

Ishikawa K, Isshiki N 1988 Repair of subglotic stenosis with a free perichondrial graft. British Journal of Plastic Surgery 41: 652–656

Jain P R, Dedhia H V, Lapp N L, Thompson A B, Frich J C jr 1985 Nd-YAG laser followed by radiation for treatment of malignant airway lesions. Lasers in Surgery and Medicine 5: 47–53

Kairalla R A, Carvalho C R, Parada A A, Alves V A, Saldiva P H 1988 Solitary plasmacytoma of the trachea treated by loop resection and laser therapy. Thorax 43: 1011–1012

Kaiser D 1985 Operative Maßnahmen bei den sogenannten Bronchusadenomen. Surgical measures in 'broncho-adenomas'. Praxis und Klinik der Pneumologie 39: 844–845

Kaiser L R. 1987 Thoracic emergencies. Tracheobronchial emergencies: use of the neodymium:YAG laser in cancer patients. In: Turnbull A D(ed) Surgery emergencies in the cancer patient. Year Book, Chicago, p137–139

Kambic V, Godina M, Zupevc A 1986 Epithelialized microvascular iliac crest flap for reconstruction of subglottic and upper tracheal stenosis: a preliminary report. American Journal of Otolaryngology 7: 157–162

Kaschke O, Wenzel M, Gerhardt H J, Haake K 1990 Scanning electron microscopic findings after tissue ingrowth into porous (expanded) PTFE implants. A pilot study for the development of an alloplastik tracheal prosthesis. HNO-Praxis 15: 109–115

Kedar A, Cantrel G, Rosen G 1988 Rhabdomyosarcoma of the trachea. Journal of Laryngology Otology 102: 735–736

Kharchenko V P, Chkhikvadze V D, Kuz'Min I V, Pan'Shin G A, Bogdanova L N, Karibov Y U I, Sergeev I E, Sutyushev G M 1984 Combined treatment of tracheal tumours. Meditsinskaia Radiologiia (Moscow) 29: 53–55

Kikuchi K, Ishihara T, Kobayashi K, Suzuki T, Takeshi A, Fukai S 1986 Surgical treatment of tracheal anastomotic stenosis. Journal of the Japanese Association for Thoracic Surgery 34: 1169–1173

Kikuchi K, Kota R, Sakai S, Nishimura Y, Suzuki T, Kaseda S, Kobayashi K, Ishihara T, Nemoto E 1987 Silicone T-tube for the management of 15 patients with laryngeal or tracheal stenosis. Journal of the Japanese Association for Thoracic Surgery 35: 818–823

Killian G 1903 Die Intubationsbehandlung bei laryngealen Stenosen nach Tracheotomie. Verhandlungen des Vereins (Versammlung) Süddeutscher Laryngologen 64–71

Kirstein R 1896 Die Autoskopie des Kehlkopfes und Luftröhre. Berlin

König F 1886 Zur Deckung von Defekten in der vorderen Treachealwand. Berliner Klinische Wochenschrift 33: 1129–1135

Koshiishi Y, Amemiya R, Takizawa N, Okitsu H, Naito J, Tajika E 1988 A case report of tracheal leiomyoma. Journal of the Japanese Association for Thoracic Surgery 36: 1003–1007

Kubota T, Kaku M, Yoshida A, Unno H, Sagawa F, Miyata T 1985 A case of cervical neurofibroma invading into the trachea: a trial of tracheal reconstruction with collagen sheet. Journal of the Japan Broncho-Esophagol Society 36: 317–322

Küster E 1884 Vorstellung eines Patienten, bei welchem der halbe Kehlkopf exstirpiert worden ist. Zentrablatt für Chirurgie (Leipzig)13: 95–97

Lange G 1976 Die narbigen Kehlkopfengen und ihre Behandlung. Zeitschrift für Laryngologie, Rhinologie, Otologie 55: 127–138

Lasson S, Cardillo G, Lepore V 1987 Surgical management of tracheal tumours. Scandinavian Journal of Thoracic and Cardiovascular Surgery 21: 97–103

Le-Tian X, Zhen-Fu S, Ze-Jian L, Hun W L, Zong W Z 1983 Tracheo bronchial tumours: an 18 year series from Capital Hospital. Peking, China. Annals of Thoracic Surgery 35: 590–596

Li W, Ellerbroek N A, Libshitz HI 1990 Primary malignant tumours of the trachea. A radiologic and clinical study. Cancer 66: 894–899

Lipton R J, McCaffrey T V, Von Heerden J A 1987 Surgical treatment of invasion of the upper aerodigestive tract by well-differentiated thyroid carcinoma. American Journal of Surgery 154: 363–367

Little F B, Koufman J A, Kohut R I, Marshall R B 1985 Effect of gastric acid on the pathogensis of subglottic stenosis. Annals of Otology, Rhinology and Laryngology 94: 516–519

Longaker M T, Harrison M R, Adzick N S 1990 Testing the limits of neonatal tracheal resection. Journal of Pediatric Surgery 25: 790–792

Lydiatt D D, Markin R S, Ogren F P 1990 Tracheal invasion by thyroid carcinoma. Ear, Nose and Throat Journal 69: 145–149

Mackenzie M 1880/1884 Manual of diseases of the throat and nose. Verlag August Hirschwald, Berlin

Mackenzie M 1880 Die Krankheiten des Halses und der Nase. Verlag August Hirschwald, Berlin

McCaughan J S jr, Hawley P C, Bethel B H, Walker J 1988 Photodynamic therapy of endobronchial malignancies. Cancer 62: 691–701

McElvein R B, Zorn G 1983 Treatment of malignant disease in trachea and main-stem bronchi by carbon dioxide laser. Journal of Thoracic and Cardiovascular Surgery 86: 858–863

McElvein R B, Zorn G L jr 1984 Indications, results , and complications of bronchoscopic carbon dioxide laser therapy. Annals of Surgery 199: 522–525

Maurer J, Mann W 1989 Maligne Schwannome im HNO-Bereich (malignant schwannoma of the ENT area). Laryngorhinootologie 68: 433–436

Miro A M, Shivaram U, Finch P J 1989 Noncardiogenic pulmonary edema following laser therapy of a tracheal neoplasm. Chest 96: 1430–1431

Moghissi K 1975 Reconstruction of the trachea with marlex mesh and pericardium following circumferential excision. Journal of the Royal College of Surgery of Edinburgh 20: 327–333

Montgomery W W 1973 Surgery of the upper respiratory system. Lea & Febiger, Philadelphia

Morency G, Chalaoui J, Samson L, Sylvestre J 1989 Malignant neoplasms of the trachea. Canadian Association of Radiology Journal 40: 198–200

Moulton M, Wain J, Grillo H C 1990 Primary melanoma of the lower respiratory tract (meeting abstract). World Conference on Lung Health, May 20–24 1990, Boston MA

Muntz H R, Lusk R P 1990 A comparison of the cartilaginous rib graft and Evans-Todd laryngotracheoplasties for subglottic stenosis. Laryngoscope 100: 415–416

Nakahara Y 1984 Endoscopic electrosurgical resection of intra-tracheal tumour: a case. Japanese Journal of Chest Diseases 43: 809–813

Nealon T F jr 1986 Management of the patient with cancer of the lung, the trachea, and the pleura. In Nealon T F (ed) Management of the patient with cancer, 3rd edn. W B Saunders, Philadelphia, p 211–236

Neis P R, McMahon M F, Norris C W 1989 Cartilaginous tumours of the trachea and larynx. Annals of Otology, Rhinology and Laryngology 98: 31–36

Neville W E 1982 Reconstruction of the trachea and stem bronchi with Neville prosthesis. International Surgery 67: 229–234

Neville W E, Bolanowski J P, Kotia G G 1990 Clinical experience with the silicone tracheal prosthesis. Journal of Thoracic and Cardiovascular Surgery 99: 604–612

Nomori H, Kaseda S, Kobayashi K, Ishihara T, Yanai N, Torikata C 1988 Adenoid cystic carcinoma of the trachea and the main stem bronchus, a clinical, histopathologic and immunohistochemical study. Journal of Thoracic and Cardiovascular Surgery 96: 271–277

Nonoyama A, Osaka T, Tanaka K, Ohtomo K, Tatsumi A, Saito Y, Sato T, Kasahara K, Masuda A 1983 Primary tracheal tumours: report of 4 cases with primary cancers of the trachea and of 1 case with benign tumour. Journal of the Japanese Association for Thoracic Surgery 31: 232–239

Nonoyama A, Osaka T, Fukunaka M, Saito Y, Tanaka K, Tatsumi A, Ohmoto K, Umemoto M, Masuda A et al 1984 Primary tumours of the trachea: results of various forms of treatment and review of tracheal reconstruction for primary tracheal reconstruction for primary tracheal tumours in Japan. Journal of the Kansai Medical University (suppl.) 35: 10–15

O'Dwyer J 1885 Intubation of the larynx. New York Medical Journal 7: 145–149

Onizuka M, Doi M, Mitsui K, Ogata T, Hori M 1990 Undifferentiated carcinoma with prominent lymphocytic infiltration (so called lymphoepithelioma) in the trachea. Chest 98: 236–237

Oswal V, Flood L M, Ruckley R W 1988 Use of bronchoscopic CO_2 laser in palliation of obstruction tracheobronchial malignancy. Journal of Laryngology and Otology 102: 159–162

Pearson F G 1983 Advances in tracheal surgery. Advances in Surgery 16: 197–223

Pearson F G, Todd T R, Copper J D 1984 Experience with primary neoplasms of the trachea and carina. Journal of Thoracic and Cardiovascular Surgery 88: 511–518

Pearson F G, Brito-Filomeno L, Cooper J D 1986 Experience with partial cricoid resection and thyrotracheal anastomosis. Annals of Otology, Rhinology and Laryngology 95: 582–585

Petruzzelli G J, De Vries E J, Johnson J, Klein M, Kormos R, Herlich A, Curtin H 1990 Extrinsic tracheal compression from an anterior mediastinal mass in an adult: the multidisciplinary management of the airway emergency. Otolaryngology—Head and Neck Surgery 103: 484–486

Podoshin L M, Fradis 1976 Reconstruction of the anterior wall of the cervical trachea using knitted dacron. Ear Nose and Throat Journal 55: 42–44

Pollard B J, Harrison M J 1985 Subtotal tracheal resection: a case report and review of airway, anaesthetic and post-operative problems. European Journal of Anaesthesiology 2: 387–394

Radleman C D, Unger E R, Mansour K A 1990 Malignant fibrous histiocytoma of the trachea. Annals of Thoracic Surgery 50: 458–459

Rajaratnam K, Desai S 1988 Kaposi's sarcoma of the trachea. Journal of Laryngology and Otology 102: 951–953

Randall D, Parker G S, Savage RW 1990 Adenoid cystic carcinoma of the trachea—a cause of pseudo-angina pectoris. Military Medicine 155: 440–442

Remacle M, Declaye X, Mayne A 1989 Subglottic haemangioma in the infant: contribution by CO_2 laser. Journal of Laryngology and Otology 103: 930–934

Ribet M, Bugnon P, Darras J A, Boucquilon P 1990 Surgery for inflammatory and neoplastic tracheal stenosis. Revue des Maladies Respiratoires (Paris) 7: 349–353

Rose K G, Sesterhenn K 1982 Abschließender Bericht über die erste allogene Transplantation beim Menschen. Archives of Otorhinolaryngology 223: 274–277

Said H, Phang K S, Gibb A G 1988 Mucoepidermoid carcinoma of the trachea (a case report). Journal of Laryngology and Otology 102: 83–86

Sakaguchi M 1990 Reconstruction of posterior wall of trachea in esophogeal cancer by using platysma musculocutaneous flap: report of a case. Otolaryngology—Head and Neck Surgery (Tokyo) 62: 63–67

Sakai T, Ikeda T, Kikuchi K, Maruyama M, Fukayama M, Kaseda S 1986 A case of tracheal metastasis of pulmonary cancer. Journal of the Japanese Association for Thoracic Surgery 34: 1178–1181

Sculerati N, Mittal K R, Greco M A, Ambrosino M M 1990 Fibrous histiocytoma of the trachea: Management of a rare cause of upper airway obstruction. International Journal of Pediatric Otorhinolaryngology 19: 295–301

Shah S, Marg E B 1989 Anesthetic management of thyroid cancer with intratracheal lesions (meeting abstract). Third WAE Cancer Conference, February 19–22 1989, Al Ain, United Arab Emirates, Ministry of Health, p14

Shapshay S M, Bohigian R K, Ruah C B, Beamis J F jr 1988 Obstructing tumours of the subglottic larynx and cervical trachea: airway management and treatment. Annals of Otology, Rhinology and Laryngology 97: 487–492

Shimizu Y 1984 Reconstruction of cervical trachea. Japanese Annals of Thoracic Surgery 4: 669–674

Shvili Y, Zohar Y, Buller N, Laurian N 1985 Conservative surgical management of invasive differentiated thyroid cancer. Journal of Laryngology and Otology 99: 1255–1260

Spizarny D L, Shepard J A, McLoud T C, Grillo H C, Dedrick C G 1986 CT of adenoid cystic carcinoma of the trachea. American Journal of Roentgenology 146: 1129–1132

Stack P S, Steckler R M 1990 Tracheal neurilemmoma: case report and review of the literature. Head and Neck 12: 436–439

Streitz J M jr., Shapshay S M 1991 Malignant fibrous histiocytoma of the trachea (letter). Annals of Thoracic Surgery 51: 695–699

Sutedja G, Stam J 1990 Neodymium–yttrium–aluminum–garnet laser in lung cancer under local anesthesia (meeting abstract). World Conference on Lung Health, May 20–24 1990, Boston MA

Symbas P N, McKeown P P, Hatcher C R jr., Vlasis S E 1984 Tracheoesophageal fistula from carcinoma of the esophagus. Annals of Thoracic Surgery 3: 382–386

Taki T, Ito M, Hitomi S, Shimizu Y, Chiba W, Takashima Y 1987 Extramedullary plasmacytoma of the trachea: surgical cases and review of the literature. Journal of the Japanese Association for Thoracic Surgery 35: 2166–2171

Tanimura S, Banba J et al 1989 A case of thyroid cancer with tracheal invasion treated by means of nasal septum transplant. Japanese Journal of Chest Diseases 48: 746–750

Thedinger B A, Cheney M L, Montgomery W W, Goodman M 1991 Leiomyosarcoma of the trachea. Case report. Annals of Otology, Rhinology and Laryngology 100: 337–340

Toohill R J, Martinelli D L, Janowak M C 1976 Repair of laryngeal stenosis with nasal septal grafts. Annals of Otology, Rhinology and Laryngology 85: 600–608

Tsugawa C, Kimura K, Muraji T, Nishijima E, Matsumoto Y, Murata H 1988 Congenital stenosis involving a long segment of the trachea: further experience in reconstructive surgery. Journal of Pediatric Surgery 23: 471–475

Tsumori T, Nakao K, Miyata M, Izukura M, Monden Y, Sakurai M, Kawashima Y, Nakahara K 1985 Clinicopathologic study of thyroid carcinoma infiltrating the trachea. Cancer 56: 2843–2848

Vergnon J M, Boucheron S, Bonamour D, Fournel P, Emonot A 1987 Destruction endobronchique des lesions tumorales: laser ou cryotherapie? Analyse preliminaire. (Intratracheal destruction of tumour lesions: laser or cryotherapy? A preliminary analysis.) Revue des pneumologie clinique (Paris) 43: 19–25

Von Bruns P 1898 Die Neubildungen der Luftröhre. In: Heyman P (ed) Handbuch der Laryngologie und Rhinologie. A. Hölder Verlag, Vienna

Von Ilberg C 1982 Verletzungen von Kehlkopf und Trachea Hals-, Nasen-Ohrenheilk. In: Berendes J, Link R, Zöllner F (eds) Praxis u. Klinik. G. Thime Verlag, Stuttgart

Von Ilberg C, Haas G 1985 Reconstruction of the upper airway following stenotic processes. Auris Nasus Larynx (suppl.) 12: 75–77

Von Ilberg C, Weber A 1991 Longterm results following tracheal stenosis surgery. The First international Laryngotracheal Reconstruction Symposium Cleveland OH, August 23–27

Von Ilberg C, S Kitano, Schmidt A 1977 Das Cialit-konservierte Trachea-Transplantat. Zeitschrift für Laryngologie, Rhinologie, Otologie 56: 814–823

Von Schroetter A 1876 Beitrag zur Behandlung der Larynxstenosen. Vienna

Watterson K G L, Wisheart J D 1990 Tracheobronchial mucoepidermoid carcinoma in childhood with a ten year follow-up. European Journal of Cardiothoracic Surgery 4: 112–113

Weber A, Von Ilberg C 1992 Tracheaquerresektion— Langzeitergebnisse. Oto-Rhino-Laryngologia NOVA (in press)

Weerda H 1978 Einzeitige Rekonstruktion der Trachea mit einem Insellappen. Archives of Otorhinolaryngology 221: 211–214

Weerda H, Gründjens L, Petersen-Mahrt I 1974 Die Naht am Tracheo-Bronchialbaum. Langenbecks Archiv für Chirurgie 336: 91–102

Weerda H, Zoellner C, Schlenter W 1986 Die Behandlung der Stenosen des laryngo-trachealen Überganges und der zervikalen Trachea. (Treatment of stenoses of the laryngotracheal junction and the cervical trachea.) HNO 34: 156–163

Weidauer H & Vogt-Moykopf I 1980 Der prothetische Tracheaersatz mit Kunststoff. Archives of Otolaryngology 222: 454–456

Weidenbächer M and Thumfart W 1979 Verschluß ösophagotrachealer Fisteln nach Langzeitintubation. HNO (Berlin) 27: 409–412

Wurtz A, Darras J, Sobecki L, Maetz E, Quandalle P 1988 Chirurgie des lesions malignes de la trachée supérieure. A propos de six observations de tracheostomie mediastinale. Surgery for malignant lesions of the upper trachea. Report of a series of six cases of mediastinal tracheostomy. Annals de Chirurgie 42: 209–213

Xu L T, Sun Z F, Li Z J, Wu L H, Wang Z Z 1983 Tracheobronchial tumours: an eighteen year series from Capital Hospital, Peking, China. Annals of Thoracic Surgery 35: 590–596

Xu L T, Sun Z F, Li Z J, Wu L H, Zhang Z Y, Xu X Q 1987 Clinical and pathologic characteristics in patients with tracheobronchial tumour: report of 50 patients. Annals of Thoracic Surgery 43: 276–278

Yoshimura Y, Nakajima T 1990 Tracheoplasty with palatal mucoperiosteal graft. Plastic and Reconstructive Surgery 86: 558–562

Zalzal G H, Cotton R T, McAdams A J 1986 The survival of costal cartilage graft in laryngotracheal reconstruction. Otolaryngology and Head and Neck Surgery 94: 204–211

Zehm S 1978 The use of composite grafts for reconstruction of the trachea and the subglottic airway. Transactions of the American Academy of Ophthalmology and Otolaryngology 84: 934–940

Section 3

16. Ear - the auricle

Hilko Weerda

INTRODUCTION AND HISTORICAL REVIEW

The ear, like the nose and the forehead, is especially exposed to irradiation from the sun because of its prominent position. Approximately 70% of all carcinomas in this region result from actinic damage. A high incidence is seen in certain professional groups, such as farmers, sailors and forestry workers (Chen & Dehner 1978, Müller & Petres 1984).

The auricle is a flexible cartilaginous appendage covered anteriorly and posteriorly by skin. It has an average length of 64 mm, a width of 34 mm and a thickness of 5 mm. The complicated structure form and contours of the auricle present a great challenge to the plastic reconstructive surgeon.

Throughout history, there have been isolated reports of partial reconstructions of the auricle, with very early reports of partial replacement from India, for example. The first detailed account of ear reconstruction was reported by Tagliacozzi in his well-known book *De curtorum chirurgia per insitionem* (1597) where he described partial replacement of the upper and lower auricle. Tagliacozzi initially used pedicle flaps from the hair-bearing areas of the scalp to cover these defects. Zeis (1868) found the operations described by Tagliacozzi difficult to understand and noted that no mention was made of any kind of ear support. It is clear that the portion of the auricle which was reconstructed using a double skin flap was subject to severe shrinkage and was probably not very successful cosmetically. Zeis believed that it was improbable that Tagliacozzi had ever carried out such an operation. Zeis also reported that Velpeau and Dieffenbach also attempted partial reconstructions of the ear. Dieffenbach (1834) sutured his flaps on the freshened wound of the upper ear and left the reverse side of the ear to granulate. Szymanowski (1870) described a case of reconstruction of the upper and lower ear and lobule using reverse rectangular flaps. Dieffenbach (1845) expressed the dominant opinion of the time when he said that 'any attempted replacement of an entire ear is highly questionable endeavour since it will be impossible to give it the needed form. The new ear will remain an unshapely disfigured lump of skin'. Szymanowski (1870) on the other hand felt that reconstruction of the auricle was not beyond the realms of possibility and stated that 'an auricle even without cartilage is still better than no auricle at all'. He termed this 'the fashioning of an artificial ear made of skin' but, judging by the description, we have to assume that Szymanowski himself never carried out the reconstruction of an entire auricle.

Towards the end of the nineteenth century and at the beginning of the twentieth century, partial resections of the ear were increasingly reported (Nelaton & Ombredanne 1907). It was the discovery of cartilage transplantation during this period that led to the concept of using cartilaginous support in partial and total ear reconstruction. In Berlin, Victor Schmieden (1908) probably performed the first rib cartilage transplantation used for reconstruction of an ear. Subsequently, detailed descriptions of auricle reconstruction with rib cartilage were reported by Gillies (1920).

The techniques most commonly used in ear reconstruction today have been developed since the second world war (Converse 1942, 1950, 1963, Mundnich & Terrahe 1962, Weerda 1972, Tanzer 1974, Brent 1976, Davis 1986, Toplak 1986). All of the surgeons mentioned above have made significant contributions to modern ear reconstructive surgery and some of their methods will be described in this chapter.

ANATOMICAL CONSIDERATIONS

The auricle, the auditory canal and the outer surface of the ear drum together form what is commonly known as the external ear. The auricle is composed of elastic cartilage covered with skin on both its anterior surfaces. The skin of the anterior surface has no subcutaneous fat and adheres tightly to the perichondrium. The skin on the posterior aspect however contains an additional layer of fat which makes the skin somewhat thicker, more mobile and less adherent to its underlying supporting structure. The lobule has no cartilaginous support, its fleshy form deriving from the subcutaneous fat.

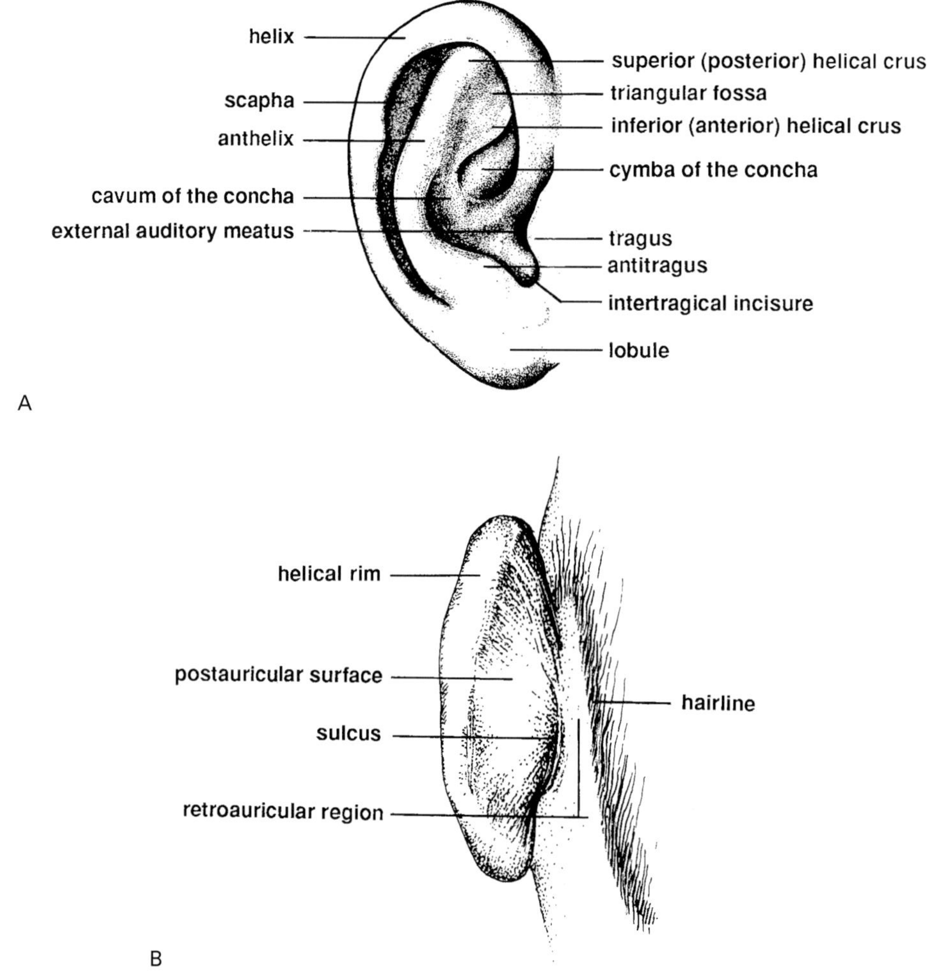

Fig. 16.1 **A.** Anatomy of the anterior surface of the auricle. **B.** Anatomy of the posterior surface of the auricle.

The auricle's characteristic appearance results from its convoluted relief structure (Fig. 16.1). The auricle protrudes from the side of the head at an angle of about 25–30° from the plain of the mastoid and is inclined at an angle of 30° away from the facial profile line. The blood supply is provided by the upper and lower branches of the superficial temporal artery and by perforating branches from the posterior auricular artery. Sensation is supplied by the auricular temporal branch of the mandibular nerve and by the greater auricular nerve from the cervical plexus (Weerda 1985).

PRINCIPLES OF EXCISION

Of all skin tumours, 80–90% occur in the head and neck region, and over 70% of these are so-called light-induced tumours. Precancerous conditions account for about 20–25% of skin lesions in the head and neck and include actinic keratosis, keratoacanthoma, lentigo maligna, Bowen's disease, keratin horns and leukoplakia. In the precancerous stages, all of these tumours have one thing in common: they can all develop into malignant metastatic tumours (Müller & Petres 1984). About two-thirds of all malignant growths of the skin are basal cell carcinomas. Melanoma and other malignant tumours occur at a rate of only 2–3%. Dermatological statistics place the percentage of basal cell carcinomas somewhat higher, but otolaryngologists have often found the percentage of squamous carcinomas to be greater (Pless 1976).

The percentage of tumours occurring in the region of the auricle, including precancerous lesions, is estimated at between 5 and 17%. Müller & Petres (1984) found, in their review of 270 cases of precancerous lesions, that 17% were located in the ear region. Out of 6121 basal-cell carcinomas, 8.6% were located in the ear region, and out of 1796 skin carcinomas, 16.3% were located in the ear region. From their total of 8187 tumours, 865 (10.6%) were to be found in the region of the auricle. Few papers have investigated the distribution of tumours on the ear itself (Table 16.1). Accumulating data from six papers, we have been able to compile statistics on the distribution of 776 tumours which

Table 16.1 Distribution of tumours of the auricle

	Lederman 1965	Bailin et al (1980)	Alvares Cruz et al (1981)	Freedlander & Chung (1983)	Draf (1984)	Niparko et al (1990)	n	%
Helix	60	29	31	95	11	84	310	39.9
Antihelix	23	11	17	15	1	15	82	10.6
Concha	12	4	20	7	10	41	94	12.1
Tragus and antitragus	19	–	4	–	–	3	26	3.4
Lobule	4	1	4	1	1	3	14	1.8
Post-and retro-auricular region and sulcus	46	23	27	29	10	115	250	32.2
Total	164	68	103	147	33	261	776	100.0

show that approximately 70% were located on the anterior surface of the auricle and only 30% on the posterior surface. The rate of metastasis obviously depends on the histology, but on looking at metastatic spread from squamous-cell carcinoma there are widely differing figures in the literature ranging from 3 to 14% (Weerda 1984); Freedlander & Chung (1983) identified metastatic spread in 14% of their cases. In this series, 50% of the tumours however were larger than 3 cm. They also found that the rate of metastasis was higher for squamous-cell carcinomas which had invaded perichondrium and cartilage. Metastasis occurs in the regional lymph nodes of the parotid or in the deep cervical lymph nodes or in both regions regardless of whether the tumour is pre-, post- or retroauricular. It is our practice to perform a lymph node excision, i.e. a parotidectomy, and a neck dissection only when lymph nodes can be detected clinically or by computer tomography and ultrasonic examination. A sonography-guided needle-biopsy of the lymph node assesses its status with a high degree of reliability.

The purpose of all tumour surgery is the radical removal of the lesion, and the surgical method used is determined by the type, size, degree of infiltration and metastasis. With increasing size and malignancy, a greater safety zone around the skin tumour is required.

Microscopically controlled surgical excision (Mohs 1941, 1988, Haas 1982) has proved to be of value. The pathologist is informed as to the exact anatomical position of the tumour by placing a suture for orientation and making an exact diagram. (Fig. 16.2A) The main tumour is cut into serial sections by the pathologist and both of the defined surgical edges and the deep margin of excision are carefully examined to determine whether they are tumour-free. In addition, small sample excisions are removed clockwise from the edges and the base of the wound and sent for separate evaluation (Fig. 16.2B) Should the tumour spread to the cartilage or protrude into the facial nerve, radical surgery will be necessary involving either visualization or resection of the facial nerve. In severe cases, removal of the entire petrous bone may be required (see Ch. 17).

Solid nodular basal-cell carcinomas are excised with a 4–5 mm safety margin. Small squamous-cell carcinomas, sclerosing basal-cell carcinomas and larger tumours are excised with a margin of 10–15 mm. Melanomas and recurrent carcinomas, whose clinical borders cannot be sharply delineated and which exhibit histologically scleroderma-like growth, are resected with a safety margin of 15 mm or more. This also applies to tumours with a history longer than 1 year and tumours larger than 2 cm diameter (Haas 1982). Tumours that extend beyond the auricle, either into the retro- or pre-auricular regions, will require excision beyond the ear to ensure radical tumour clearance (Hauben et al 1982).

When the pathological findings on the edge samples are positive, histologically controlled excisions are continued until the edges are pathohistologically free from disease (Koplin & Zarem 1980). Only then is final wound closure carried out.

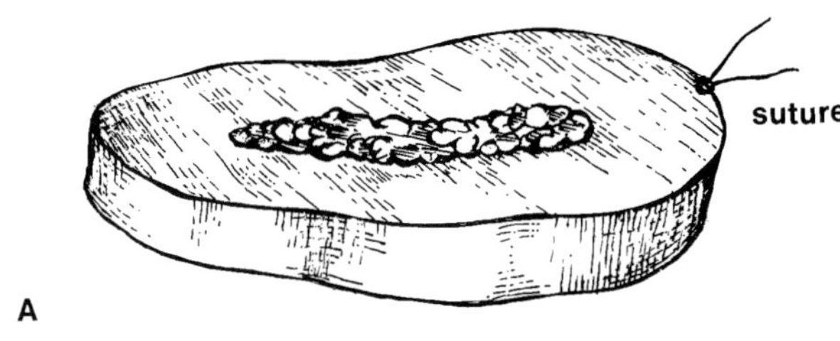

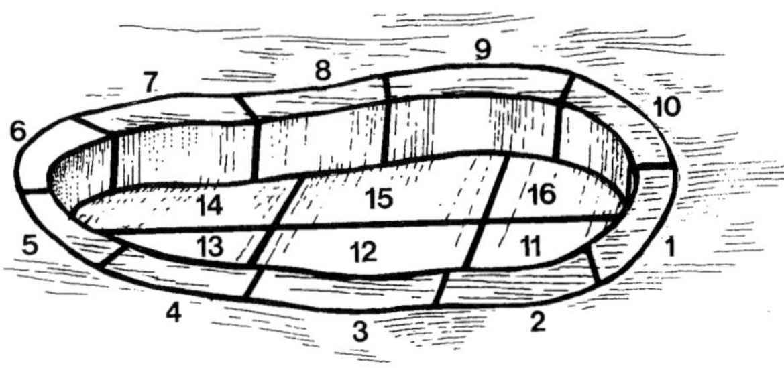

Fig. 16.2 **A.** Microscopically controlled surgery. Specimen of resected tissue marked with suture. **B.** Additional excisions from the margin and base of the wound for histological analysis.

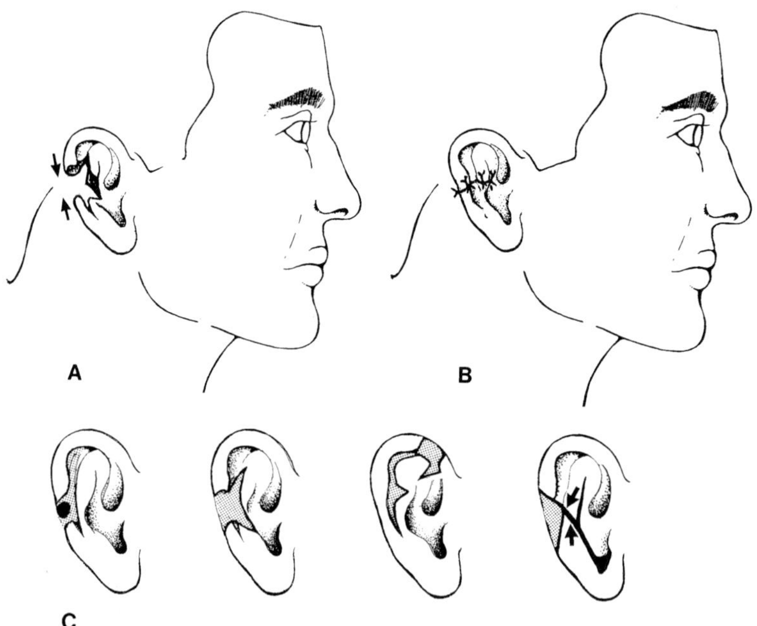

Fig. 16.3 A. Wedge-shaped excision of a helical tumour with removal of Burow's triangles. **B.** Tension-free wound closure, but a smaller ear size. **C.** Variations in surgical technique following removal of marginal helix tumours (after Senechal & Pech 1970).

PRINCIPLES OF RECONSTRUCTION

Primary reconstruction is performed after excision of smaller carcinomas and basal-cell carcinomas of nodular type. Recurrent tumours and all other tumours undergo secondary reconstruction following the histological procedures mentioned previously to ensure that margins are tumour-free.

In order to obtain a proper safety margin around the tumour site, it is often necessary to remove cartilage in the auricle. In optically conspicuous regions, reconstruction with skin from the surrounding area brings the best cosmetic result, whereas in the concha or in the post- and retroauricular regions, postauricular free grafts can be used. If it is expected that shrinkage of a skin flap will lead to a deformity of the auricle, the supporting cartilage must be maintained or a replacement for it must be found. Although there are many methods available for the partial or total reconstruction of the auricle, only a small selection can actually be applied, depending on the nature of the defect.

RECONSTRUCTIVE TECHNIQUES

In reconstruction of the helix, a distinction should be made between those techniques in which materials from the ear itself are used—thus resulting in a slightly smaller ear—and those techniques in which material from other sources, usually from the vicinity of the ear, are used and the size of the ear is maintained.

Reconstruction of the helix with reduction in auricle size

The wedge-shaped excision (Celsus circa 10 AD)

Small tumours in the helical region can be removed with a three-layered wedge-shaped excision. After resection of small Burow's triangles the defect can be closed without tension (Fig. 16.3).

Garsuny-technique (Mündnich & Terrahe 1962, Weerda 1984a, 1988)

Larger defects in the helical region can be closed by two-layered incision in the upper or lower scapha, and also in the crus helicis, and by mobilization of the postauricular skin (Fig. 16.3C). There are countless modifications of this technique which was developed at the beginning of this century for reducing the size of the auricle. Particularly noteworthy are the techniques of Antia & Buch (1967) and Argamaso & Lewin (1968).

Reconstruction of the helix without reduction in auricle size

Maintenance of auricular size is usually achieved by reconstructing with pre-or retroauricular skin flaps. To reconstruct defects along the entire rim of the helix, superiorly or inferiorly pedicled tubed flaps can be prepared and transferred into the defect in the region of the helix. Mulching at

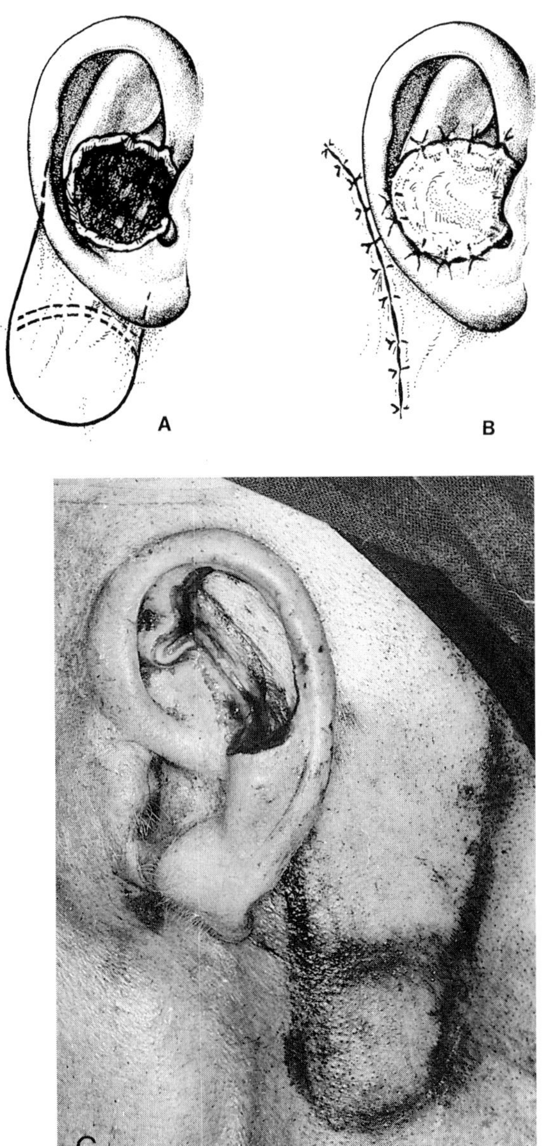

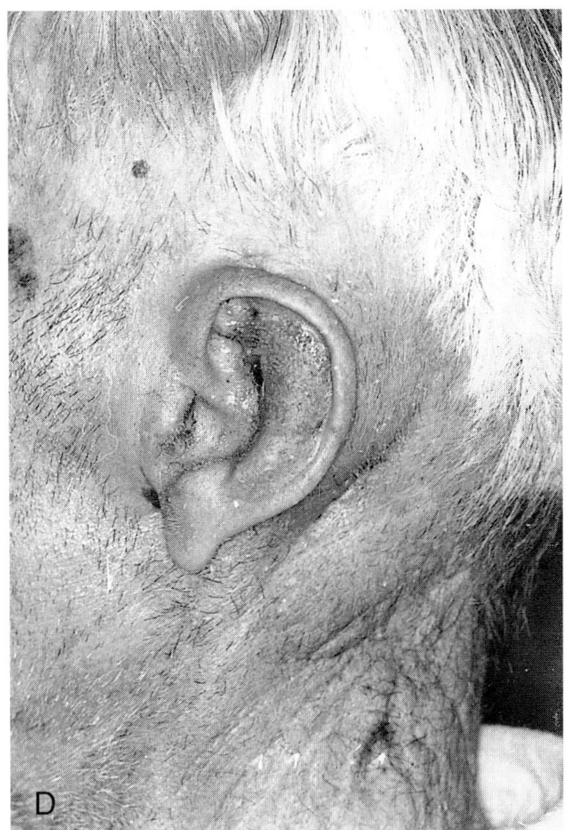

Fig. 16.4 A, B. Superiorly based retro-auricular flap outlined with de-epithelialized bridge segment for primary closure of the defect. **C, D.** Reconstruction of upper concha and antihelix.

the junction of the flap and the residual part of the helix can be minimized by careful slanting of the incisions or using small z-plasties. For long helical defects, Goldstein & Stevenson (1988) recommend the use of a retroauricular bridge flap (bipedicled flap) which can be made very long in the retroauricular hairline region with a middle skin bridge retained to ensure vascularity of the flap.

Reconstruction of the antihelix and concha

For defects in the middle portion of the auricle which are not too large, superiorly or inferiorly pedicled retroauricular flaps can be employed, even for three-layered through-and-through defects. The flap can either be de-epithelialized at the time of primary elevation and insetting or carried out as a two-stage technique (Fig. 16.4). In reconstruction in the area of the antihelix, the helix can be temporarily divided at the time of transfer and insetting the flap. At a second stage, when the flap is separated, the helix can be returned to its original position and repaired. The postauricular defect may occasionally have to be reconstructed with a split-thickness skin graft (Weerda 1984b). Other alternatives include the use of island flaps, pedicled on the posterior auricular artery. Occasionally, free flaps from the retroauricular region or from the sulcus can be sutured into the area of the medial concha.

Reconstruction of the upper part of the auricle

Pocket procedure

If sufficient non-hair-bearing skin is available, an incision is

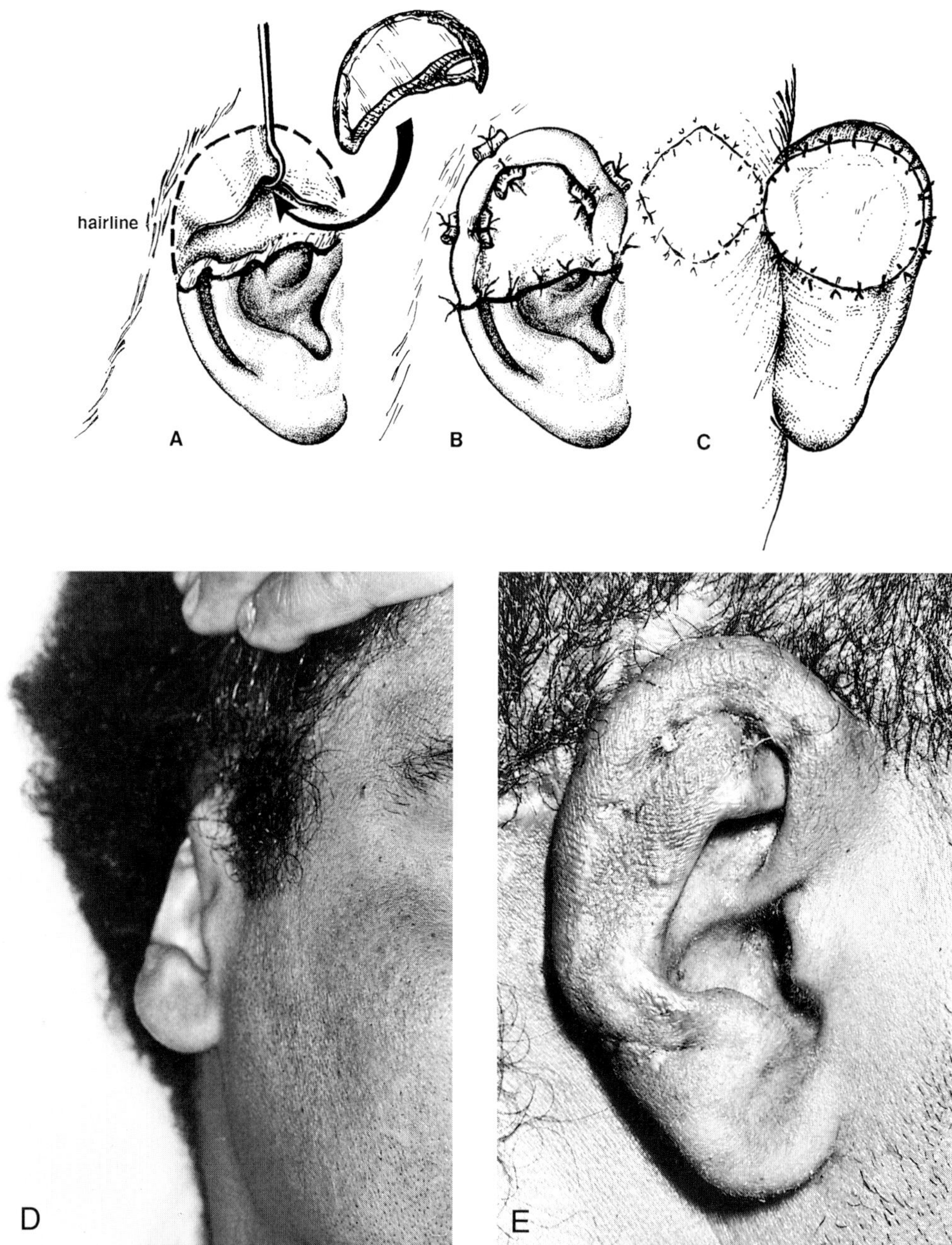

Fig. 16.5 A–C. Pocket technique for reconstruction of the upper part of the auricle. The incision is placed in the retro-auricular region at the level of the auricular stump and the postauricular skin of the stump sutured to the lower margin of the incision. After inserting the rib cartilage the scapha is moulded with mattress sutures. The auricle is released from the side of the head at 6 weeks. **D, E.** Defect in the upper part of the auricle reconstructed using the pocket technique.

made in the retro-auricular region at the level of the auricular stump and a pocket opening upwards is created. The postauricular skin of the ear is sutured to the mastoid at the lower edge of the incision (Fig. 16.5A). A rib cartilage support carved by the surgeon and according to a pattern previously made of the patient's healthy ear, is inserted into the anatomically correct position in the pocket and sutured to the auricular cartilage with 5-0 PDS sutures. The upper edge of the pocket incision is subsequently sutured to the

skin on the front side of the stump. The scapha and helix can then be moulded using a few mattress sutures (Fig. 16.5B).

At a second operation approximately 6 weeks later, the skin along the new helical rim is incised and the postauricular plane is separated (Fig. 16.5C). Care should be taken that tissue with sufficient blood supply remains on the cartilage support. A thick split-thickness skin graft from the buttocks or inguinal region is glued onto the postauricular wound and sutured to the skin of the upper helix with 6-0 PDS. Primary closure of the mastoidal wound is sometimes possible by mobilizing the adjacent tissue. Otherwise a thick split-thickness skin graft is used to cover the defect (Fig.16.5C). If necessary, the contour of the reconstructed auricle can be further improved at a third operation (Weerda 1984a,b, Weerda 1988) (Fig. 16.5, D & E).

Pedicled flaps

For patients with a low hairline we use a superiorly pedicled, retro-auricular flap (Weerda 1980) as suggested by Crikelair (1956). The rib cartilage support is sutured into the correct position as previously described. The flap for reconstruction of the anterior and posterior surface of the auricle is raised and sutured into place and the scapha shaped with mattress

sutures. The resulting defect can be covered by mobilizing skin from the surrounding area or utilizing a split-thickness skin graft. At a second operation in about 6 weeks, the flap is separated and inset both retro- and postauricularly. Further corrections for contour of the auricle can be made in subsequent operations if required.

Reconstruction of the middle part of the auricle

The U-shaped advancement flap

A rib cartilage support, corresponding to a previously prepared pattern from the patient's healthy ear, is carved from the sixth and seventh ribs and sutured to the cartilaginous stump of the auricle (Fig. 16.6, A and B). A wide strip of hair is shaved and a posteriorly based flap which

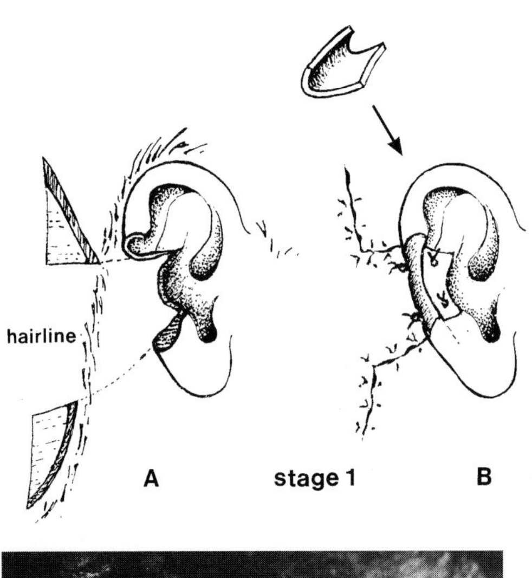

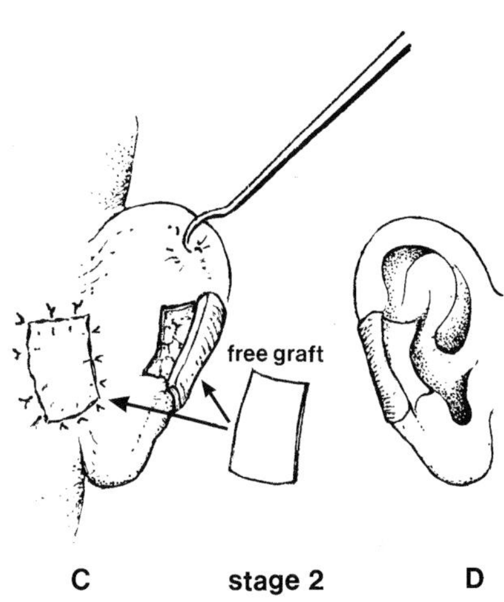

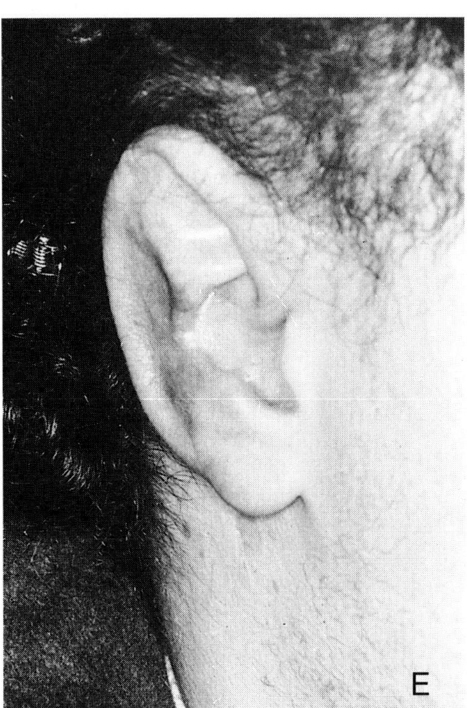

Fig. 16.6 A–D. The U-shaped advancement flap. The defect in the middle part of the auricle is reconstructed using a U-shaped retro-auricular flap with two large Burow's triangles. The second stage is performed at 3 weeks. **E.** Late clinical result. Defect in the middle part of the auricle reconstructed using the U-shaped retro-auricular flap technique.

fits the defect is raised. By mobilizing the entire flap and cutting Burow's triangles, the flap can be advanced and sutured into the defect without tension. The scapha is formed as previously described with through-and-through mattress sutures taking care to ensure the blood supply to the helix. At a second operation in approximately 6 weeks, the flap is divided to form a new outer contour of the helix. As stated previously, care should be taken to ensure that enough soft tissue remains on the newly inserted rib cartilage graft posteriorly so that it can serve as a base for skin grafting. The retro-auricular defect is closed by mobilizing skin from the surrounding area or by covering it with a thick split-thickness skin graft (Berson 1948) (Fig. 16.6, C and D). Numerous variations of this technique have been described in the literature (Senechal & Pech 1970, Mündnich & Terrahe 1962, Converse & Brent 1977, Weerda 1985, 1987, 1988, 1991, Jackson 1985).

Reconstruction of the lower part of the auricle

Reconstruction of the lobule

For reconstructing the lobule, we mainly use the operational procedure described by Gavello in the last century (Weerda 1980, 1984a). An anteriorly based bilobed flap is raised below the resected lobule designed according to a previously prepared pattern from the patient's normal ear. By folding this flap upwards, a cosmetically unobtrusive lobule is created. The secondary defect can be closed directly by mobilizing the adjacent tissue and the scar remains largely invisible, situated behind the ear. It is also possible to employ inferiorly pedicled pre-auricular pedicled flaps or inferiorly based flaps from below the lobule stump.

Pocket procedure

It is possible to reconstruct the lower part of the auricle using retro-auricular skin in a similar way to that described for reconstruction of the upper portion of the auricle. After mobilizing a pocket of skin, a rib cartilage support carved according to a pattern of the patient's normal healthy ear is inserted. The operation is then carried out in a similar fashion to that previously described for reconstruction of the upper part of the auricle.

Large Gavello flaps

A large Gavello flap can be raised and used as a one-stage method of reconstruction for defects of the entire lower portion of the auricle (Fig. 16.7). The secondary defect can be closed by mobilizing the surrounding tissue and closing the wound directly (Brent 1976, Weerda 1988).

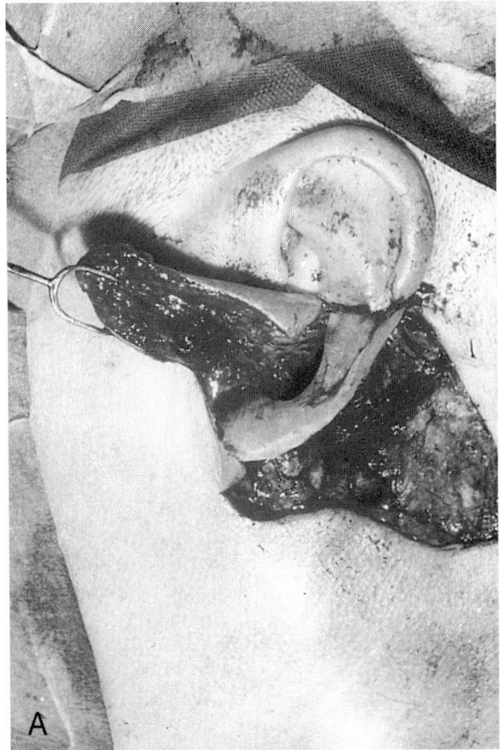
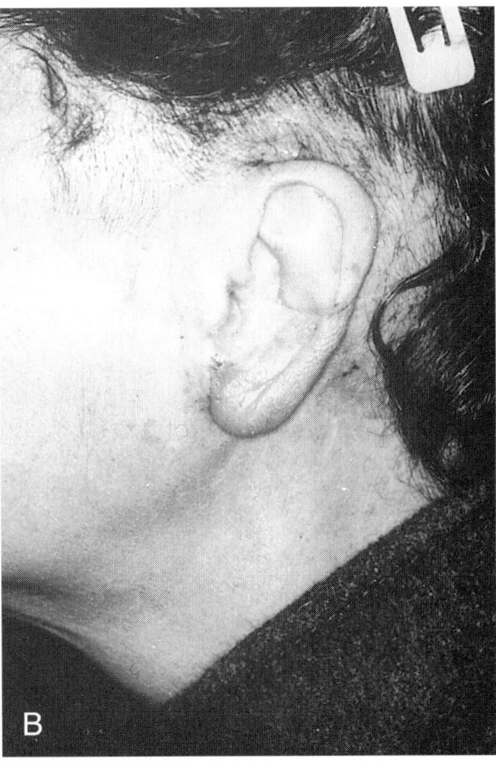

Fig. 16.7 **A.** Reconstruction of the lower portion of the ear using a large anterior superiorly pedicled Gavello flap. A carved rib cartilage support is sutured to the auricular cartilage stump and both the anterior and posterior surfaces covered by the flap. **B.** The secondary defect has been closed directly. The oblique insertion at the helical rim minimizes any notching at the junction with the auricle stump.

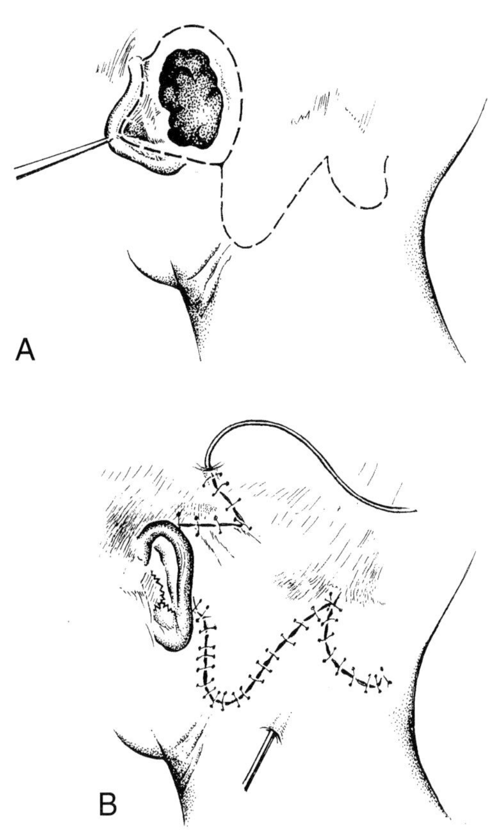

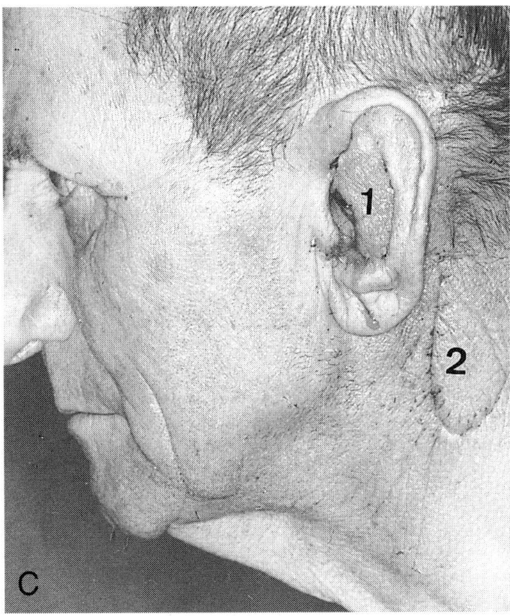

Fig. 16.8   A. Subtotal defect of the auricle with preservation of the helix and lobule. Resection involved part of the mastoid and posterior auditory canal. A bilobed flap is outlined for reconstruction. **B.** The bilobed flap allows reconstruction of the ear and closure of the secondary defect. **C.** The cartilaginous support has been reconstructed with rib cartilage. Flap 1 allows closure of both the anterior and retro-auricular defect and can be performed in one stage with de-epithelialization of part of the flap. Flap 2 is utilized for closing the secondary defect.

Subtotal defects of the antihelix and concha

In cases where large tumours of the retro-auricular side of the ear encroach upon the auricle, large parts of its structure can frequently be preserved by microscopically controlled surgery. Even in partial resection of the mastoid and back of the auditory canal with resection of the concha and a large part of the antihelix, it is possible to preserve the helix and the lobule. Reconstructions with 'bilobed' and large neck flaps have shown good results (Fig. 16.8). Using a rib cartilage support, as previously described, such large flaps, superiorly pedicled, provide sufficient skin to replace both the retro- and postauricular regions as well as the anterior surface of the auricle. The secondary defect is closed utilizing the second flap of the bilobed design (Weerda & Walter 1984, Weerda 1987).

Reconstruction of total and subtotal defects

The pocket procedure

When tumours require extensive excision of the auricle, the author prefers to close the resulting defect by mobilizing the surrounding skin and postponing reconstruction for at least 1 year (Fig. 16.9A). Prior to surgery a pattern of the patient's healthy ear is made using a piece of transparent celluloid. Using this pattern a rib cartilage support can be carved using

cartilage taken from the seventh and eighth ribs. Should the eighth rib be short, the graft can be taken from the sixth and seventh ribs following suggestions by Tanzer (1974) and Converse & Brent (1977). The length of the rib to be used for the helix should be at least 10 cm (Fig. 16.9B). The ear's anatomical position should be marked or determined by measuring the position of the healthy ear.

Via a small incision in the region of the posterior part of the ear canal, all the skin of the mastoid region up to the hairline is generously undermined. The rib cartilage support is then inserted into its correct anatomical position and the auricle formed and contoured using mattress sutures. A suction drain should be placed in situ and remain for at least 7 days to help shape the skin over the rib cartilage support.

As previously described, a second-stage operation follows in approximately 6 weeks, raising the auricle and ensuring soft-tissue coverage throughout the posterior aspect of the cartilage support. The postauricular region and remaining mastoid defect are closed as far as possible and the remaining defect covered by thick split-thickness skin graft obtained from the buttocks. The graft is attached with fibrin glue, and, to achieve good contour for the helix, the free edge is sutured with 6-0 PDS to the edge of the anterior skin of the auricle (Fig. 16.9D). At a third stage, small corrections can be made to obtain a satisfactory end result (Fig. 16.9E)

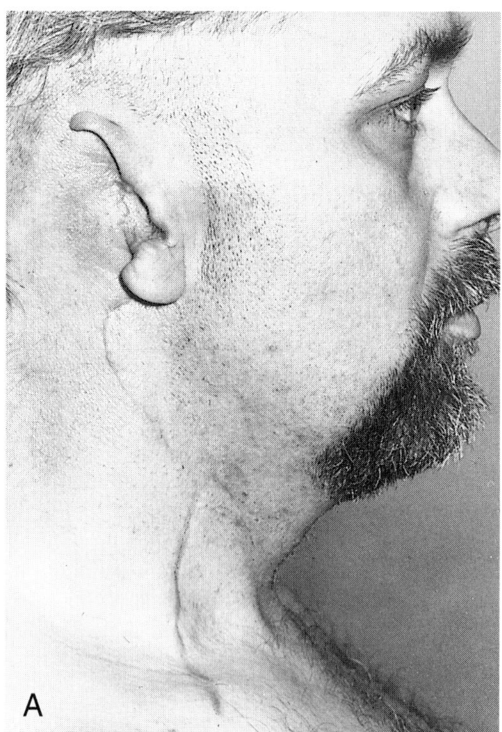

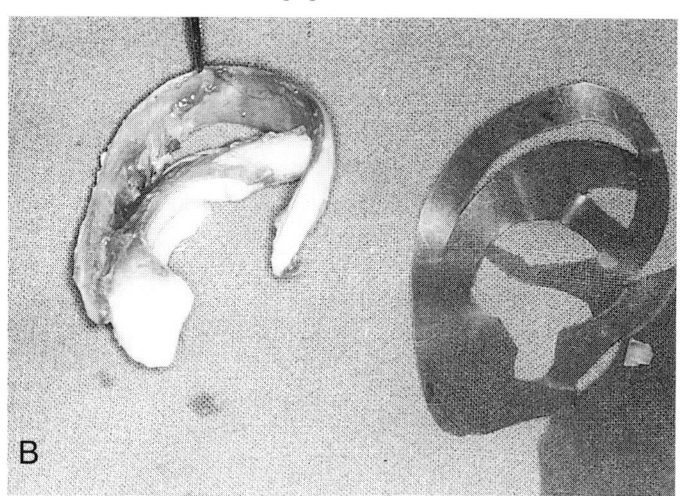

Fig. 16.9 **A.** Defect resulting from an excision of a melanoma of the antihelix. **B.** A rib cartilage support is prepared with the aid of a celluloid pattern. **C.** The cartilage support is inserted into the prepared retro-auricular pocket in the correct anatomical position. The scapha and helix are formed with mattress sutures and suction drainage. **D.** At 6 weeks an incision is made along the helix. The auricle is elevated from the side of the head and the defect closed with a thick split-thickness skin graft. The secondary defect is closed by mobilizing the skin from the surrounding area. **E.** The postoperative result shows good contour and maintenance of the cartilage graft.

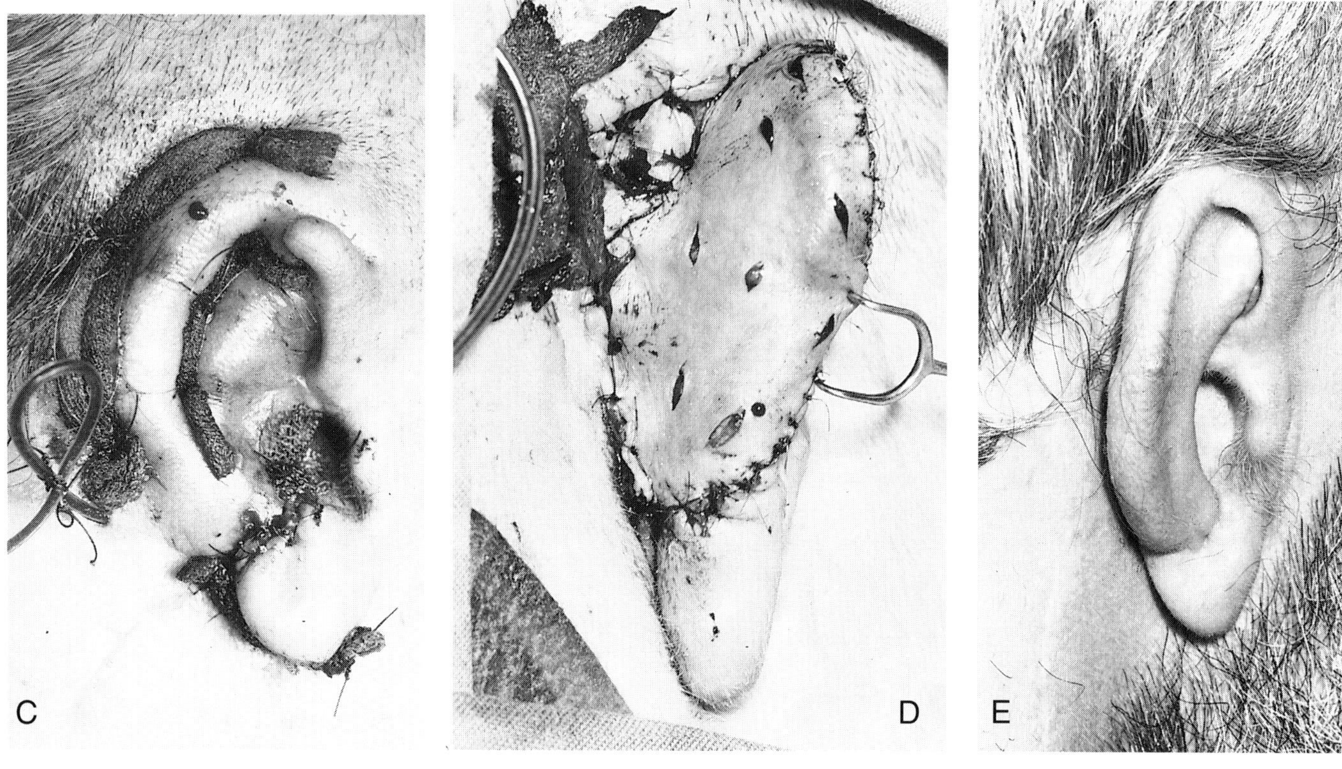

The temporoparietal fascia flap

Tegtmeier & Gooding (1977) and Brent & Byrd (1983) have suggested that if sufficient skin is not available for the reconstruction of the auricle, a temporoparietal fascial flap supplied by the superficial temporal artery may be used. The temporoparietal fascial flap is well vascularized and can cover the rib cartilage support. Using a suction drain, the flap is contoured over the support and a free split-thickness skin graft glued and sutured to the flap. Split-thickness grafts from the buttocks provide a poor colour match, and it is often better to use grafts taken from the postauricular region of the opposite ear or from the supraclavicular area. This technique can provide satisfactory results in auricle reconstruction.

PROBLEMS AND COMPLICATIONS

As in any reconstructive procedure, the established rules of plastic and reconstructive surgery must be observed. It should be remembered that free skin grafts cannot be incorporated onto exposed cartilage without an additional covering of perichondrium. Rib cartilage not covered with skin will become necrotic. After a part or an entire auricle has been raised from the side of the head, the rib cartilage support must be covered with soft tissue that is well supplied with blood in order to allow the incorporation of free skin graft. Poor graft take with areas of necrosis or skin flaps which show partial necrosis may cause exposure of the rib cartilage and subsequent necrosis. Large defects resulting from total ablation of the external ear or extirpation of the petrous temporal bone require different techniques using superiorly or inferiorly pedicled regional flaps or myocutaneous island flaps such as the pectoralis major or latissimus dorsi. In such cases, reconstruction of the external ear is not possible.

FUTURE DEVELOPMENTS

A variety of modalities of treatment for malignant disease of the external ear have been described and these include radiotherapy, cryotherapy and photodynamic laser therapy. The latter particularly is being increasingly utilized in the treatment of smaller auricular tumours, although no long-term results as to its effectiveness have yet been published. The surgical removal of tumours, with reconstruction of the resulting defects, has proved itself to be effective and is still our method of choice in the treatment of auricular tumours. Should metastasis appear in the regional lymph nodes, a parotidectomy and neck dissection must be performed.

In cases where reconstruction is not possible, an auricular prosthesis can be made using coloured silicone fastened to skin loops (Weerda 1972) or via osseo-integrated pressure screws (Tjellström et al 1985) Such external prosthesis—particularly when fixed to the skull — can give very satisfactory results.

REFERENCES

Alvares Cruz N, da Silva Castro D, Luisi A 1981 Carcinomes primitifs de l'oreille externe et de l'oreille moyenne. Annals Oto-Laryngologie (Paris) 98: 613

Antia N, Buch V 1967 Chondrocutaneous advancement flap for the marginal defect of the ear. Plastic and Reconstructive Surgery 39: 472

Argamaso R, Lewin M 1968 Repair of partial ear loss with local composite flap. Plastic and Reconstructive Surgery 42: 437–441

Arons M, Sadin R 1971 Auricular cancer. American Journal of Surgery 122: 770

Bailin P H, Levin H, Wood B, Tucker H 1980 Cutaneous carcinoma of the auricular and periauricular region. Archives of Otolaryngology—Head and Neck Surgery 106: 692

Berson M 1948 Atlas of plastic surgery 10. Grune & Stratton, New York

Brent B 1976 Earlobe construction with an auriculo-mastoid flap. Plastic and Reconstructive Surgery 57: 389

Brent B, Byrd H 1983 Secondary ear reconstruction with cartilage grafts covered by axial, random, and free flaps of temporoparietal fascia. Plastic and Reconstructive Surgery 72: 141

Burow 1853 Cited by Weerda 1991

Celsus Cited by Weerda 1984a

Chen K, Dehner L 1978 Primary tumours of the external and middle ear. Archives of Otolaryngology—Head and Neck Surgery 104: 247

Converse 1942, 1950, 1963 Cited by Converse & Brent 1977, Toplak 1986

Converse J, Brent B 1977 Acquired deformities. In: J M Converse (ed) Reconstructive plastic surgery, 2nd edn. W Saunders, Philadelphia, vol III, p1724

Crikelair G 1956 A method of partial ear reconstruction for avulsion of the upper portion of the ear. Plastic and Reconstructive Surgery 17: 438

Davis 1975 Cited by Davis 1986

Davis J 1986 Aesthetic and reconstructive otoplasty. Springer, New York

Dieffenbach M 1834 Cited by Zeis 1863 and Converse 1977

Dieffenbach M 1845 Cited by Toplak 1986

Draf W 1984 Zur Frage der Rekonstruktion und Lymphknotenausräumung bei Malignomen der Ohrmuschel. In: Müller P, Friedrich H, Petres J (eds) Operative Dermatologie im Kopf-Hals-Bereich. Springer, Berlin-Heidelberg

Freedlander E, Chung F 1983 Squamous cell carcinoma of the pinna. British Journal of Plastic Surgery 36: 171

Gillies H 1920 Cited by Toplak 1986

Goldstein J, Stevenson T H 1988 Reconstruction of ear helix: use of self-tubing pedicle flap. Annals of Plastic Surgery 21: 149

Haas E 1982 Oncological principles of the treatment of malignoma of the facial area (in German). Laryngologie, Rhinologie, Otologie 61: 611

Hauben D, Zirkin H, Mahler D, Sacks M 1982 The biologic behavior of basal cell carcinoma: analysis of recurrence in excised basal cell carcinoma Part II. Plastic and Reconstructive Surgery 69: 110

Jackson I 1985 Local flaps in head and neck reconstruction. Mosby, St Louis

Joseph J 1931 Nasenplastik und sonstige Gesichtsplastik. Curt Kabitzsch, Leipzig

Koplin L, Zarem H 1980 Recurrent basal cell carcinoma. Plastic and Reconstructive Surgery 65: 656

Lederman M 1965 Malignant tumours of the ear. Journal of Laryngology and Otology 71: 85

Mohs F 1941 Chemosurgery, a microscopically controlled method of cancer excision. Archives of Surgery 42: 279

Mohs F 1988 Fixed tissue micrographic surgery for melanoma of the ear. Archives of Otolaryngology—Head and Neck Surgery 114: 625

Müller R, Petres J 1984 Semimaligne und maligne Tumoren der Haut im Kopf-Hals-Bereich (semimalignant and malignant tumours in the head and neck region, in German). In: Müller R, Friedrich H, Petres J (eds) Operative Dermatologie im Kopf-Hals-Bereich. Springer, Heidelberg

Mundnich K, Terrahe K 1962 Plastische Operationen an der Ohrmuschel. In: Sercer A, Mundnich K (eds) Plastische Operation an der Nase und der Ohrmuschel. Thieme, Stuttgart

Nelaton C, Ombredanne L 1907 Les autoplasties: lèvres, joues, oreilles, tronc, membres. Steinheil, Paris

Niparko J, Swanson N, Baker S, Telian St, Sullivan M, Kemink J 1990 Local control of auricular, preauricular, and external canal cutaneous malignancies with Mohs surgery. Laryngoscope 100: 1047

Pless J 1976 Carcinoma of the external ear. Scandinavian Journal of Plastic and Reconstructive Surgery 10: 147

Schmieden V 1908 Cited by Toplak 1986

Senechal G, Pech A 1970 Chirurgie du pavillon de l'oreille. Librairie Arnette, Paris

Tagliacozzi 1597 Cited by Joseph 1931

Tanzer R C 1974 Secondary reconstruction of the auricle. In: Tanzer R C, Edgerton M T (eds) Symposium on reconstruction of the auricle. Mosby, St Louis

Tegtmeier R, Gooding R 1977 The use of fascial flaps in ear reconstruction. Plastic and Reconstructive Surgery 60: 406

Tjellstrom A, Yontchen E, Lindström J, Branemark P-J 1985 Five years experience with bone-anchored auricular prostheses. Otolaryngology 93: 366

Toplak F H 1986 Die Totalrekonstrüktion der Ohrmuschel (The total reconstruction of the auricle, in German). Inaugural Dissertation , Univ-Klinikum Streglitz, Berlin

Von Szymanowski J 1870 Handbuch der Operativen Chirurgie. Vieweg, Braunschweig

Weerda H 1972 Attachments for auricle prostheses (in German). HNO 20: 83

Weerda H 1980 The trauma of the auricle (in German). HNO 28: 209

Weerda H 1984a Kompendium plastisch-rekonstruktiver Eingriffe. Ethicon, Hamburg

Weerda H 1984b Probleme der operativen Therapie der Ohrmuschel-Malignome (Problems of surgery on malignancies of the auricle, in German). In: Müller R, Friedrich H, Petres J (eds) Operative Dermatologie im Kopf-Hals-Bereich. Springer, Berlin

Weerda H 1985 Embryology and structural anatomy of the external ear. Facial Plastic Surgery 2: 85

Weerda H 1987 Plastic surgery of the ear. In: Booth J B (ed) Otology, Scott-Brown's otolaryngology, 5th edn. Butterworths, London vol 3

Weerda H 1988 Reconstructive surgery of the auricle. Facial Plastic Surgery 5: 5

Weerda H, Walter C 1984c Surgery of the pinna and surrounding area. In: Ward P H (ed) Surgery of the head and neck. Mosby, St Louis

Zeis E 1868 Geschichte und Literatur der plastischen Chirurgie, Leipzig. Reprinted by Arnaldo Forini, Bologna (1963)

17. Temporal bone resection for malignant tumours of the middle ear and ear canal

Rammohan Tiwari

INTRODUCTION AND HISTORICAL REVIEW

Malignant tumours of the middle ear and the external ear canal are rare. The first description of the disease was by Politzer in his classic textbook entitled *Lehrbuch der Ohrenheilkunde für Practische Ärzte und Studirende* (Politzer 1883). Politzer described the symptoms of the disease as eczema of the external ear, polyp formation and granulations which may all be associated with the presenting symptoms. He further described facial palsy, meningitis and brain abscess as complications and talked about amputation of the ear. Secondary involvement of the external auditory canal as a result of invasion from a primary malignant process of the parotid gland was mentioned, and a reference to American literature was quoted. The next milestone was a review by Zeroni in the *Archeives Ohrenheilkunde* in the German language (Zeroni 1899). The first review on the subject in the American literature appeared in the early part of this century (Newhart 1917). Newhart reported 34 cases which he collected as a result of a survey.

Broders' study on the subject of epitheliomas of the ear included the middle ear, external auditory meatus and the auricle (Broders 1921). This was the first pathological account of a sizable number of cases. Since the advent of radiotherapy in 1922 its use in the treatment of cancer of the middle ear and external ear canal was attempted, but the results were disappointing (Schall 1934). In modern times radiotherapy alone as a modality for treating these cancers has been reported only from the Christie hospital in Manchester, England (Holmes 1965, Birzgalis et al 1992). Boland & Patterson (1955) and Wang (1975) advised against radiotherapy for cancer of the external ear canal, middle ear and mastoid. Other radiotherapy centres in Britain also reported poor results with radiotherapy alone (Lederman 1965). In recent years attempts have been made to use brachytherapy for carcinoma of the external ear canal (Martinez et al 1991). The futility of salvage surgery after initial radiotherapy was reported by Stell & Miles (1986). On the other hand, encouraging results were reported by Lederman using postoperative radiotherapy after initial radical mastoidectomy for middle ear carcinomas (Lederman 1965). A surgical procedure to extirpate the tumour in an oncological sense was first described in the United States by Ward et al (1951). This was subsequently modified by Parson & Lewis (1954). Lewis subsequently reported his experience on the largest number of surgically treated cases (Lewis 1975). It would appear that few selection criteria were employed for radiotherapy or surgery. Lederman subjected all cases to radiotherapy, and Lewis operated on all his cases (Stell 1984). In recent years improved results have been reported using systematic ablation of the tumour followed by postoperative radiotherapy (Kinney & Wood 1987, Tiwari et al 1992).

SURGICAL PATHOLOGY

In the majority of cases it is not possible to assess the exact site of origin of these tumours. Tumours of the ear canal may grow into the middle ear, and middle ear tumours may extend into the external auditory meatus. These tumours are therefore best considered as a single entity. The mastoid is often secondarily involved in cases of middle ear carcinoma. Histopathological confirmation is essential as a prelude to the precise planning of therapy. These tumours may be:

1. Primary, i.e. those originating in the middle ear or the external ear canal
2. Secondary—as a result of invasion from neighbouring structures, e.g. the parotid gland, the infratemporal fossa, temporomandibular joint, or nasopharynx (in the case of the middle ear)
3. Metastatic—as a result of a haematogenous spread from kidney, breast, prostate, bones and uterus (Lewis 1979, Sahin et al 1991).

Radiation-induced carcinoma of the mastoid has been reported (Beal et al 1965). Recently, bilateral carcinoma of the external auditory meatus has also been reported (Munk-Nielsen & Hansen 1991).

The primary malignant tumours may be epithelial or mesenchymal in origin. The epithelial tumours are squamous-cell carcinomas in about 86%, and basal-cell carcinoma in approximately 8% of cases. Adenocarcinomas, ceruminomas, adenoid cystic carcinomas, adenoid epitheliomas (Brooks tumour), malignant melanomas and sarcomas are rare and comprise the rest (6%). At the Free University Hospital, Amsterdam, in a period of 12 years between 1979 and 1990, a total of 56 140 new cases with pathologies of the ear, nose and throat were seen. Of these, 3966 were histologically proven cases of malignant tumours of the head and neck region. Only 21 cases of primary malignant tumours of the external auditory meatus and middle ear were seen during the same period, making it 0.037% of all ENT pathologies and 0.5% of all malignancies of the head and neck. Of the 21 malignant tumours, 18 were squamous-cell carcinoma, two basal-cell carcinoma and one adenoid cystic carcinoma.

Carcinoid tumours which are adenomas exhibiting neuro-endocrine characteristics have been described in the middle ear (Manni et al 1984). They are very rare and are locally malignant requiring repeated local excisions. Malignant mesenchymal tumours or sarcomas of the temporal bone are rare. Except for rhabdomyosarcomas all other types of sarcoma are rarely encountered. The average age in our patients was 55 years. The youngest patient seen was a female aged 27 years, and the oldest patient was 72 years of age. The male-to-female ratio was 1.3:1.

According to the only epidemiological report on middle ear cleft carcinoma in the literature, the disease is predominant in males with a rising incidence until the 75th year. If the reported association with chronic otitis media is correct then, with the changing trends in treatment, one would expect a proportionate decline in the incidence of the disease (Morton et al 1984).

SURGICAL ANATOMY AND MODE OF SPREAD

The external ear canal is cartilagenous in its outer third and is continuous with the concha of the pinna of the ear. This part of the canal is rich in ceruminous glands and ceruminomas are therefore localized in the outer third of the ear canal. The cartilage is discontinuous in places, and tumours spread easily through direct extension. Besides, this area is rich in lymphatics. The bony part of the ear canal comprises of the medial two-thirds. Its anterior, inferior and part of the posterior walls are formed by the tympanic plate of the temporal bone and is slightly concave anteriorly. Posterosuperiorly it is completed by the mastoid part of the temporal bone and the tympanomastoid suture marks this junction. The average length of the external ear canal is 2.4 cm in an adult, but because of the obliquity of the tympanic membrane the anterior and inferior walls are slightly longer (Fig. 17.1). The skin over the bony meatus is thin and closely adherent to the bone. The bony ear canal is often involved in a carcinomatous process extending from the

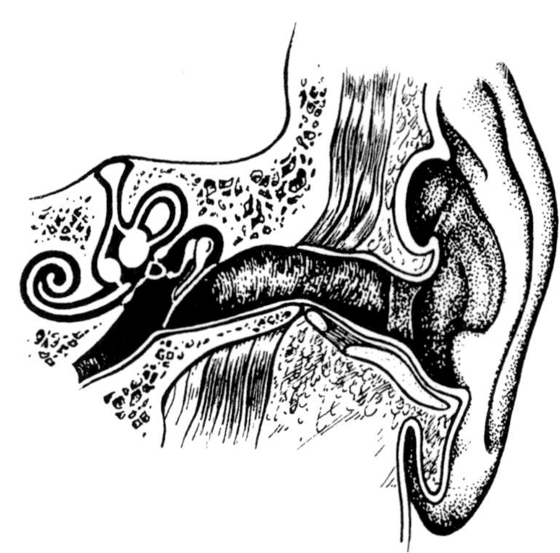

Fig. 17.1   Anatomy of the left external ear canal and middle ear and their immediate relationship.

middle ear. Tumours arising in the bony canal itself spread easily towards the cartilagenous meatus.

The tympanic membrane is attached to the tympanic ring. The middle ear is lined with cuboidal mucosa which may be ciliated or non-ciliated and is normally filled with air. The anterior wall has the opening of the tensor tympani canal in its upper part and the Eustachian tube in its middle part. The lowest part of the anterior wall separates it from the carotid canal. Posteriorly, the middle ear cleft communicates with the mastoid antrum through the aditus which provides easy access to the spread of cancer to the mastoid air cells. The canal for the facial nerve runs on the posterior wall of the middle ear. It may be dehiscent from birth, thus providing easy access for the spread of cancer. The sigmoid sinus is posterior to the mastoid process.

The middle ear cleft is narrowest at its centre. Its average height is 15 mm. The jugular bulb is the immediate inferior relation to the middle ear cleft with the IX, X and XI nerves lateral to the bulb and the inferior petrosal sinus in its medial part. The medial wall of the middle ear separates it from the labyrinth and lodges the oval and round windows. It is uncommon for the disease process to involve the labyrinth by direct extension. The superior wall of the middle ear cleft or the tegmen is a thin bone often pierced by a tiny vein or two and is the most commonly eroded wall in a malignant process causing immediate threat of extension to the meninges. The dura incidentally offers a potent barrier to the spread of the disease. The superior petrosal sinus runs along the superior border of the petrous temporal. The anterior surface of the petrous temporal is marked superiorly by a bulge, the arcuate eminence produced by the superior semicircular canal. This bulge forms the medial limit of the excision in temporal bone resection. The styloid process holds a topographically important position in relation to the jugular bulb and the carotid canal (Anson & Donaldson

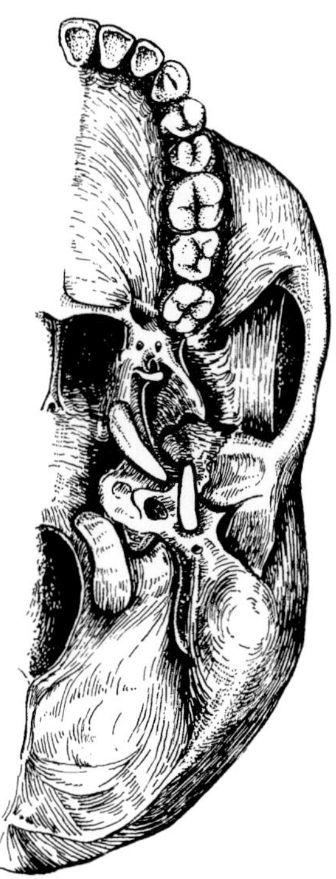

Fig. 17.2 Skull base left. Note that the entrance to the carotid canal is medial to the styloid process, while the stylomastoid foramen is posterolateral to it. The infratemporal space and the glenoid cavity are its anterior relations.

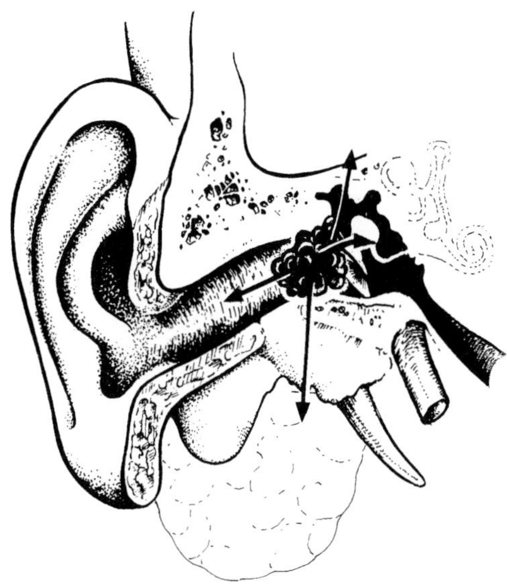

Fig. 17.3 Directions of spread of carcinoma of the middle ear and external ear canal. Tumour spreads superiorly to the middle cranial fossa through the roof and may involve the dura. Spread inferiorly is into the parotid gland and the infratemporal space. Medially, the tumour seldom involves the labyrinth, but commonly spreads through the Eustachian tube. Lateral spread into the cartilagenous ear canal occurs frequently.

1973). It is lateral to the jugular bulb and posterolateral to the carotid canal (Fig. 17.2). In addition, it is just anterior to the stylomastoid foramen which marks the exit of the facial nerve. The process is absent in about a third of patients. When present it is enclosed in a sheath. Its length varies from 1 to 9 mm, but ossification of the stylomandibular ligament may give the impression of a long styloid process and the process may assume a maximum length of 4.2 cm. It is an important landmark in temporal bone resections as the inferior plane of excision traverses between it and the carotid canal.

The numerous fissures, foramina and tiny communicating veins offer an easy pathway for the spread of cancer from the ear canal and middle ear cleft. Tumours may spread by direct extension or through perivascular and perineural pathways in addition to the spread through lymphatic channels.

Direct spread may also occur to the infratemporal fossa, external ear canal and the middle cranial fossa (Fig. 17.3). Lymphatics drain into the pre- or postauricular lymph nodes and via the node of Rouviere to the subdigastric nodes. The incidence of lymph node metastases varies from 10 to 21% in various series reported (Jesse et al 1967). In the author's own series, 3 of the 21 cases (14.3%) presented with lymph node metastases. Another patient developed lymph node metastases 6 months following treatment of the primary tumour and lived 4 years subsequently following a comprehensive neck dissection.

STAGING

Neither the UICC nor the AJC offer a staging system for carcinoma of the external ear canal and middle ear.

Stell & McCormick (1985) suggested a system of staging based essentially on the principles of the UICC. Their classification is as follows:

T1   Tumour limited to the site of origin, i.e. no facial nerve paralysis and no bone destruction

T2   Tumours extending beyond the site of origin indicated by facial paralysis or radiological evidence of bone destruction, but no extension beyond the organ of origin

T3   Clinical or radiological evidence of extension to surrounding structures (dura, base of skull, parotid gland, temporomandibular joint, etc.)

Tx   Patients with insufficient data for classification, including patients previously seen and treated elsewhere.

Stell claimed that the above staging system significantly predicts survival in carcinoma of the ear.

The N and M classifications are the same as in the UICC or AJC classifications. According to Stell & McCormick, stage-for-stage there is no significant difference in survival between tumours of the external ear canal and middle ear. However, some other authors reported progressively poorer prognosis in more medially localized tumours (Goodwin & Jesse 1980). In the majority of cases, however, a clear-cut differentiation between middle ear and external ear canal tumour is difficult. Histology, lymph node metastases, dural invasion and patients' general condition are significant predictors of prognosis.

PRINCIPLES OF TREATMENT

An en bloc resection of the tumour and, when necessary, clearance of the regional lymphatics is ideal. Modern imaging techniques make an accurate assessment possible. Selection of cases is important. Increasing awareness on the part of the general practitioners and specialists has increased the number of operable cases to several centres. Early localized lesions, especially of the ear canal, would therefore sometimes permit excision with free margin. Such cases are, however, rare. Of 24 cases seen so far by the author, only one was found suitable for partial excision. The proximity of the parotid gland to the meatus requires a parotidectomy so that the inframeatal lymphatics are not violated and the parotid nodes can be removed en bloc with the tumour. Postoperative radiotherapy is an integral part of treatment of all cancers of the external ear canal and middle ear. Modern megavoltage radiotherapy with linear accelerators has made a significant difference. In all medially located lesions a subtotal temporal bone resection described by Lewis is preferred. Reconstruction after temporal bone resection needs careful thought and planning. Modern techniques permit early rehabilitation, so that radiotherapy can be started as soon as possible and, in any case, within 6 weeks of surgery. Its value in preventing locoregional recurrence is well documented (Vikram et al 1984). In the 1960s, Lewis reported a 40% recurrence rate when no postoperative radiotherapy was administered (Lewis 1965).

PRE-OPERATIVE PLANNING

Pre-operative evaluation includes documentation of the Karnofsky index, audiometric evaluation of patients' hearing, CT scan of the temporal bones and, if necessary, MRI (magnetic resonance imaging) of the infratemporal region. If the neck nodes are palpable, a fine-needle aspiration cytology of the suspected nodes is carried out. Temporal bone resection is a major surgical undertaking. Before embarking on actual operation, it is important to evaluate the local and regional extent of the tumour and to assess whether a partial or total excision of the temporal bone is called for. Careful history taking and local, general and neurological examination must precede. The oft-mentioned association of squamous carcinoma with chronic otitis media is not frequently seen. This author concurs with Lewis that these findings are more likely to be coincidental. More than half the patients seen at the Free University Hospital did not have chronic otitis media. Documentation of the hearing through an audiogram is important. The affected ear may be the better ear for the patient as regards his hearing, and appropriate steps such as fitting of a hearing aid to the opposite ear may have to be taken. Excisions for basal-cell carcinoma may be limited and, when excised completely, do not need postoperative radiotherapy. Except for rhabdomyosarcoma, which responds well to chemoradiotherapy, all other sarcomas—as well as adenoid cystic carcinoma—are treated in a similar way to squamous-cell carcinomas. Bony erosion is not necessarily a contraindication for surgery (Fig. 17.4). The tegment tympani is the most commonly involved bone. Localized dural involvement can be salvaged, but the prognosis is poor. Several patients with destruction of the tegmen in the author's series are alive and well more than 5 years after surgery and radiation.

EXCISION TECHNIQUES

Excision of the ear canal

Excision of the auditory canal is indicated in those rare circumstances when the pathology is limited and leaves a clear margin between it and the tympanic membrane or the medial wall of the middle ear and there is no bony erosion. Lewis advocated a U-shaped incision with the base above. A flap consisting of the skin, superficial fascia, temporalis muscle and the superficial lobe of the parotid gland is raised from below upwards. The external auditory canal is transected at the level of the external meatus, and the flap is raised superiorly for a distance of 4 cm. A cortical mastoidectomy is performed and the facial canal is exposed. The facial nerve is preserved. The external auditory canal is excised in close proximity to the temporomandibular joint antero-inferiorly to the level of the tympanic membrane. Lewis recommends using a 0.4 cm thick (0.16 inch) split-skin graft and suturing it to the edge of the incision to recreate a 'new' lined external

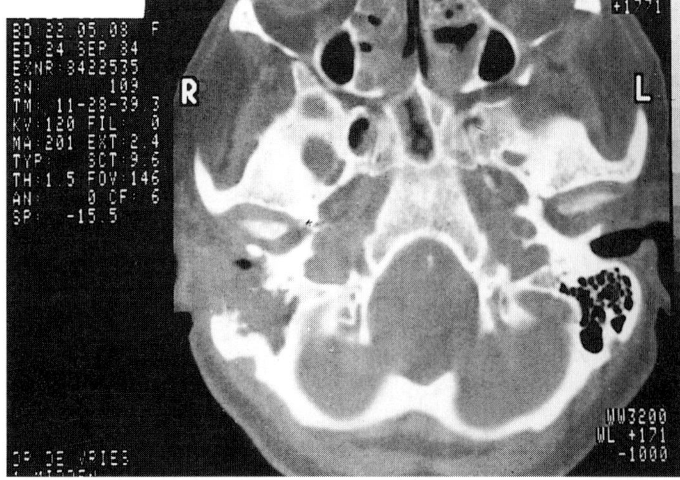

Fig. 17.4 CT scan showing gross destruction of bone in all but the medial direction in a female with squamous-cell cancer. The dura was not involved. Following temporal bone resection followed by radiotherapy, the patient is alive and well 12 years after treatment.

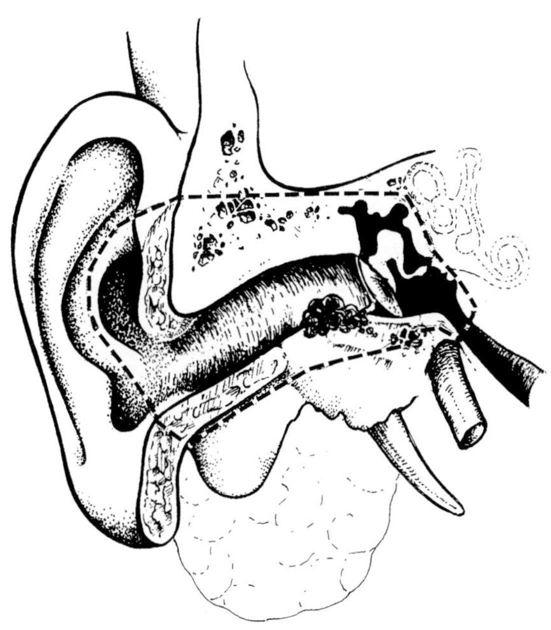

Fig. 17.5 Partial temporal bone resection.

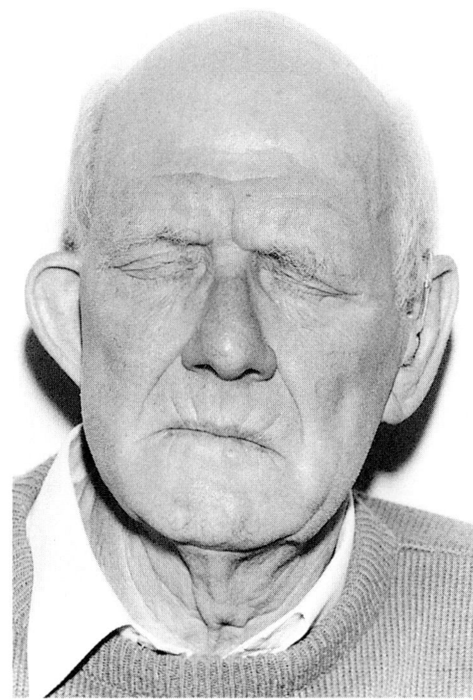

Fig. 17.6 Clinical photograph after partial temporal bone resection and re-routing of the facial nerve. Note completely normal facial expression.

auditory meatus. The graft is held in place by vaseline gauze immersed in bacitracin and left for 4 to 6 weeks.

Another approach to 'limited' cancers with radical mastoidectomy and irradiation was described by Tabb and his collegues (Tabb et al 1964).

Partial temporal bone resection

This approach is indicated when tumour involving the external auditory canal impinges on to the tympanic membrane, but does not actually involve it (Lewis 1981). Carcinoma of the external ear canal is seldom so small as to permit a sleeve resection and to indulge in a conservative resection is risking safe margins. Lewis advocated mobilization and preservation of the facial nerve, excision of the posterior canal wall, malleus and incus and the temporomandibular joint with the anterior canal wall. He advocated the use of a U-shaped incision and a split skin graft. For partial resections, this author uses a single vertical postauricular incision. The auricle is retracted forwards. A complete excision of the ear canal with the tympanic membrane, incus and malleus with the temporomandibular joint and superficial parotidectomy is performed. The facial nerve is re-routed and preserved (Fisch 1978). The cavity is filled with a free non-vascularized fat graft from the abdomen or thigh and the meatus is stitched. In case of a squamous-cell carcinoma or an adenocystic carcinoma a full course of radiotherapy is administered postoperatively (Figs. 17.5, 17.6). Having accepted the fact that the anatomical localization of these cancers demands a combined treatment in the form of radical surgery followed by radiotherapy, the

concept of skin grafting and packing for 4 to 6 weeks is contrary to the aim and may even defeat the very purpose. Not only is the chance of taking a free skin graft in this kind of cavity technically uncertain but, more importantly, it delays radiotherapy. The residual hearing is practically of no use to the patient who is left with a cavity which needs regular care. When a single vertical incision is used there is no cavity and recovery is quicker.

In all partial procedures, oncologically safe margins must be the goal, and partial procedures must not compromise a complete excision. At the end of the day the patient is not going to be left with a normal functional ear. We should therefore endeavour to provide him with a disease-free ear.

Subtotal resection of temporal bone

The procedure is carried out as a team with the otologist and the head and neck surgeon working together. The incision begins on the temple about 2 cm cranial and a little in front of the superior attachment of the helix. It follows the pre-auricular crease of skin and is extended onto the concha through the incisura terminalis. The concha is incised as close to the entrance of the ear canal as possible, depending upon the lateral extent of the tumour. The incision is now extended through the incisura intertragica back to the pre-auricular skin crease and then under the lobule of the ear to the tip of the mastoid. It curves round and is extended

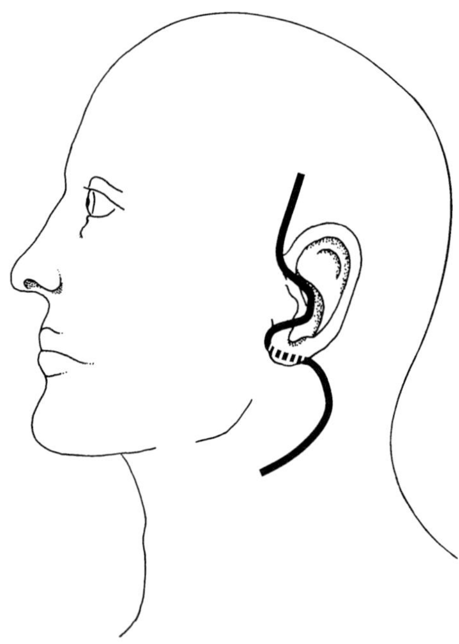

Fig. 17.7 Incision, developed and used by the author. It provides adequate access, avoids three-point junction, and can be adapted to incorporate a neck dissection should this be found necessary. (Reproduced with permission from the American Journal of Surgery.)

downwards and forwards to the level of the greater cornu of the hyoid bone (Fig. 17.7). If a neck dissection is contemplated, this extension is placed a little lower and no additional incisions are necessary. Alternatively, another supraclavicular transverse incision may be added. If a neck dissection is not needed and a sternomastoid myocutaneous flap—used by the author—is contemplated, then the integrity of the skin over the clavicle is preserved. The use of a single incision described above permits adequate exposure of the middle cranial fossa, parotid gland, sigmoid sinus and the neck and avoids a three-point junction (Tiwari 1985). The skin flaps are raised. The pinna of the ear is retracted posteriorly and superiorly and held by means of a self-retaining retractor. The marginal branch of the facial nerve is identified and is followed cranially in a retrograde fashion through the parotid gland. The cervicomandibular division is identified and followed cranially until the main trunk and its orbitotemporal division is identified. The orbital branch is exposed and the main trunk of the nerve is divided a few millimetres cranial to the bifurcation. Further dissection of the nerve is avoided. A superficial parotidectomy is done and the parotid gland is left attached to the under and anterior surface of the external auditory meatus.

The internal jugular vein, and the external and internal carotid arteries are exposed from the level of the posterior belly of the digastric to the level of the styloid process and the jugular foramen. The IX, X, XI and XII nerves are dissected and fully exposed (Fig. 17.8). Soft rubber catheters are used to put around the vessels for identification and eventual control. This exposure permits full control of the major

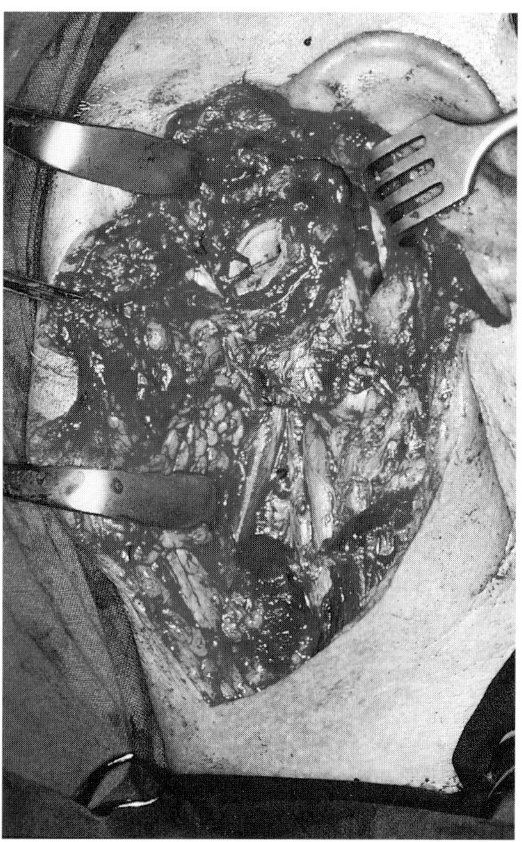

Fig. 17.8 Exposure of the infratemporal region. The ear canal has been transected. The facial nerve is dissected in a retrograde fashion from its marginal branch and divided. The parotid gland can be seen attached to the antero-inferior aspect of the ear canal. The carotid vessels, internal jugular vein and the X, XI and XII nerves have been dissected. (See also colour plate section.)

vessels and allows palpation and eventually the opportunity to obtain a frozen section of the subdigastric lymph node. The sigmoid sinus is exposed, and the sinodural angle is reached.

The anaesthesist is informed and a mannitol drip is commenced. Carbon dioxide concentration is lowered to 25–30 vol%. A spinal tap is usually not needed. This manoeuvre relaxes the dura. The temporalis muscle and the pericranium are raised in one layer and left attached anteriorly. The squama is removed to provide adequate exposure of the dura and the petrous bone. At its anterior end the incision on the squama joins the vertical incision through the zygoma (Fig. 17.9). The neck of the mandible is cut with an electric saw. The dura is now carefully lifted off the superior surface of the petrous temporal. Should the dura be involved over the roof of the middle ear, the dissection is carried through the tumour until the medial end of the tumour and the healthy dura is reached. Proper pre-operative evaluation usually helps to prevent such a situation. The involved part of the dura is excised separately. The dura is retracted gently until the petrous apex is visualized. Care is taken to protect

Fig. 17.9 **Fig. 17.10**

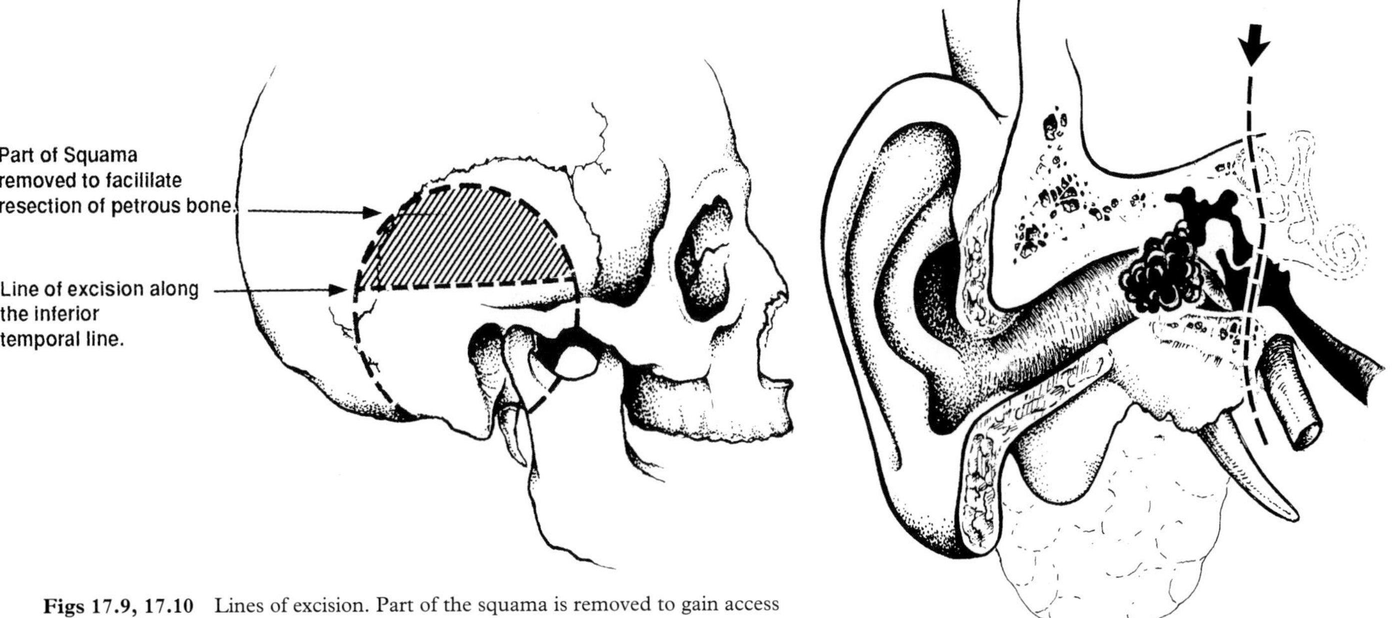

Figs 17.9, 17.10 Lines of excision. Part of the squama is removed to gain access to the superior surface of the petrous temporal.

the dura with patties, and continuous traction is avoided. The superior petrosal sinus is coagulated and cut. The arcuate eminence is identified and the incision over the petrous temporal is marked with a burr just medial to the arcuate eminence. This is extended anteriorly over the floor of the middle cranial fossa up to the incision over the squama at the level of the cut on the zygoma. Posteriorly, the incision is marked with the burr until just in front of the sigmoid sinus. With a small electric saw the cut is deepened. An osteotome completes this bony excision. At this point the internal carotid artery is protected by one of the surgeons keeping the index finger between the styloid process and the internal carotid artery. The bony excision traverses just lateral to the artery which is protected (Figs 17.10, 17.11). If a neck dissection is planned it is carried out first and left attached to the mastoid process so that, with this last bony

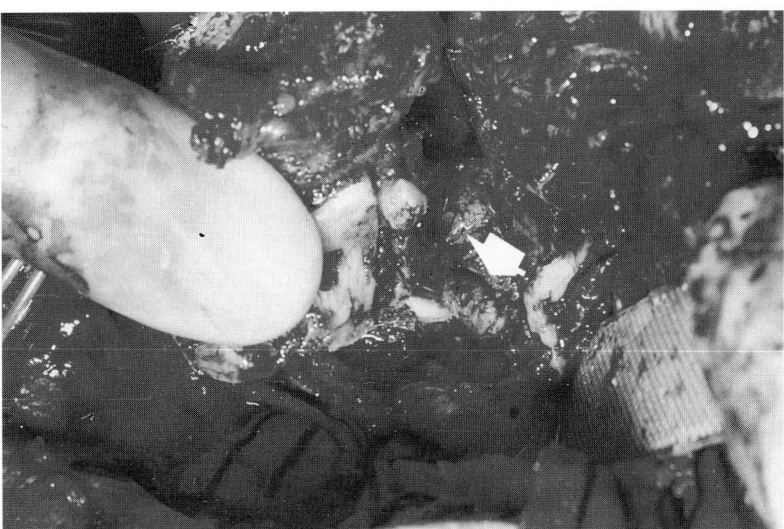

Fig. 17.11 Intra-operative photograph of left temporal bone resection. The specimen is being detached from the petrous apex. The dura is being retracted medially. The internal carotid artery is visible in the carotid canal (arrow). (See also colour plate section.)

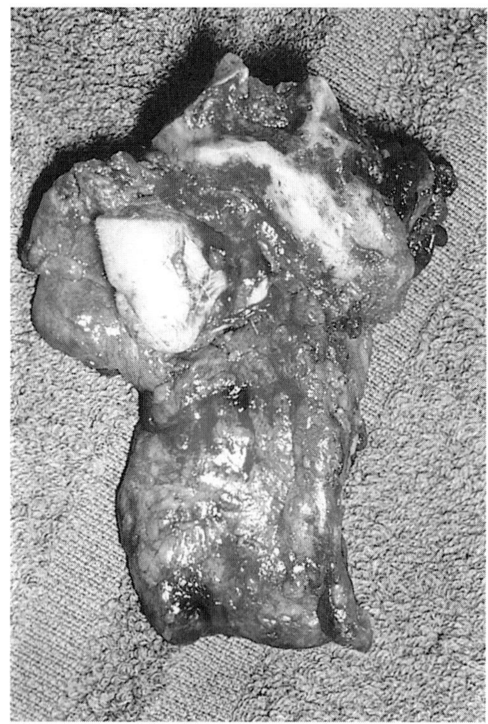

Fig. 17.12

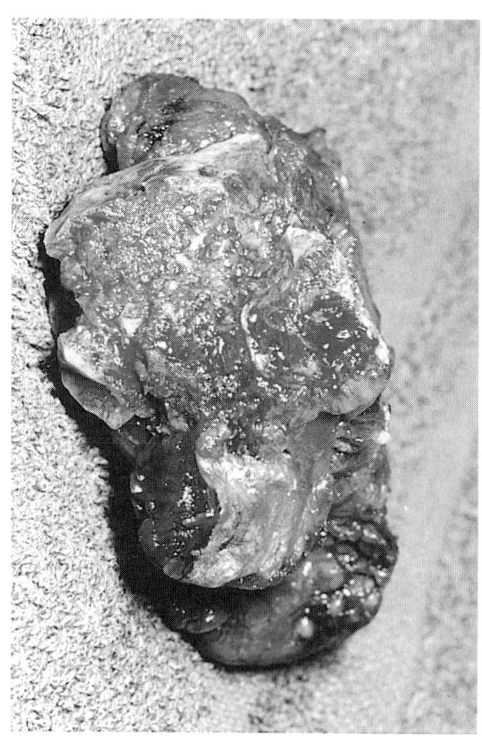

Fig. 17.13

Figs 17.12, 17.13 Medial and lateral views of the specimen. Note the tragus attached to the specimen laterally. Medially, the thick intact bone provides safe margin from tumour tissue in the middle ear. Impression of the bony superior semicircular canal is visible superiorly.

cut, the specimen can be removed en bloc (Figs 17.12–17.14). Bleeding from the inferior petrosal sinus is controlled by packing with surgicel. The dura is carefully inspected for any cerebrospinal fluid leak, and any tear is closed with 5'0' ethylon. If a part of the dura is removed the defect is covered by lyodura. The operating field is thoroughly irrigated with saline.

RECONSTRUCTION

The hypoglossus nerve is dissected and cut close to the lateral border of the mylohyoid. The nerve is mobilized and anastomosed under the operating microscope to the main trunk of the facial nerve with four to six sutures of 9'0' ethylon. Mobilization of the hypoglossus should be enough to have a tension-free anastomoses (Figs 17.15, 17.16). Several options are available for closure of the defect, and the operator must assess the defect and decide upon the

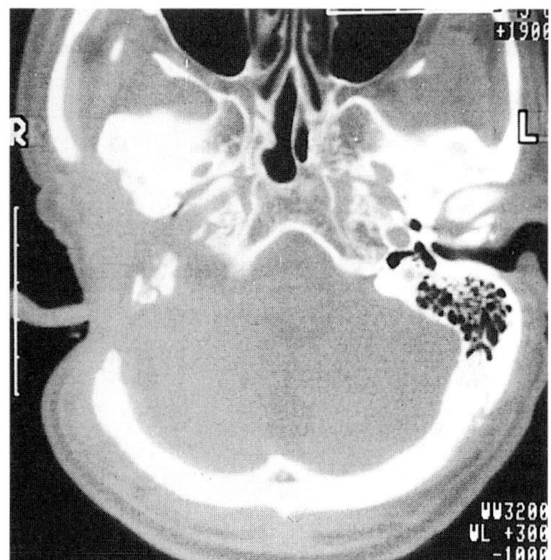

Fig. 17.14 Postoperative CT scan after right temporal bone resection.

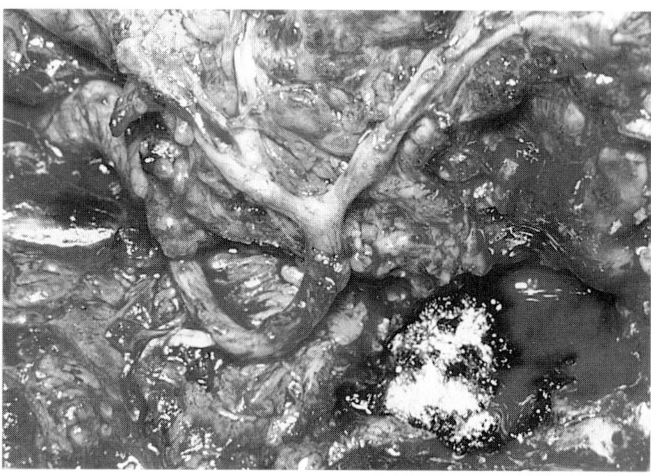

Fig. 17.15 Faciohypoglossal anastomoses.

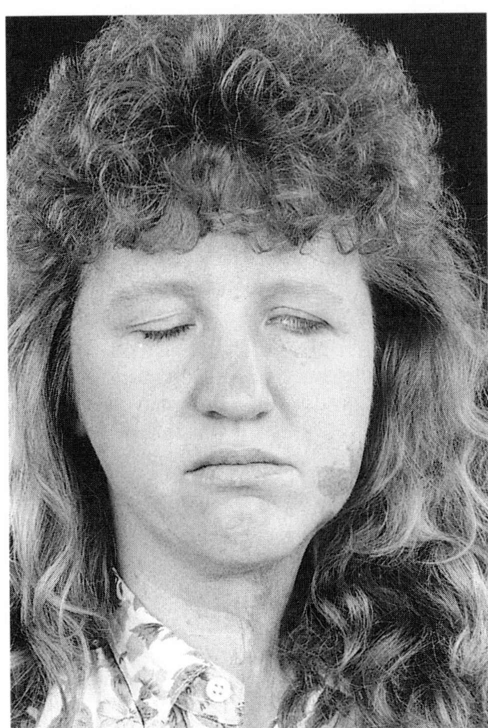

Fig. 17.16   Clinical photograph of a patient 9 months after treatment. Note minimal facial deformity and reasonably good closure of the eye.

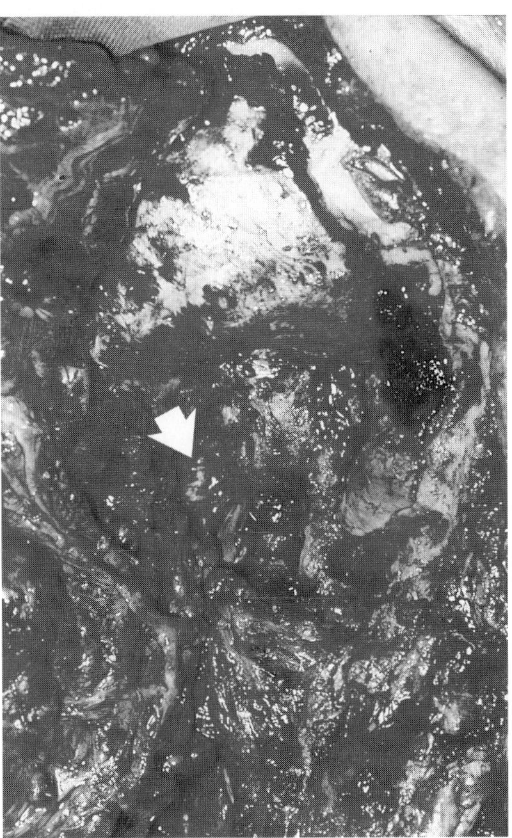

Fig. 17.17   Intraoperative photograph. The specimen has been removed. The sigmoid sinus is visible posteriorly and the jugular bulb slightly anterior to it. The dura is seen superiorly, and the sectioned main stem of the facial nerve with the main trunks is clearly seen on the left. The internal carotid artery is seen medially and slightly superior to the jugular bulb (arrow). (See also colour plate section.)

most suitable technique for reconstruction in each individual case. The use of the temporalis muscle has been mentioned in the literature, but this muscle alone is insufficient to obliterate such a defect. Regional flaps of skin can be used, but they lack thickness and bulk. Mobilization of skin flaps is fraught with danger of breakdown. The use of a skin flap from the nape of the neck was suggested by Conley & Schuller (1977). When neck dissection is not carried out, this author prefers to use a superiorly based sternomastoid muscle or myocutaneous flap (Figs 17.17, 17.18). The muscle is approximated to the temporalis. This muscle mass fills the defect and protects the dura, the nerves and the vessels. The technique is easy to execute and saves time. It is seldom necessary to sacrifice the accessory nerve. The morbidity is minimal (Tiwari 1990). When a sternomastoid myocutaneous flap is needed, the donor area may need skin grafting. Subcutaneous fat from the thigh or abdominal wall is a useful alternative. Strict aseptic precautions are necessary. Where the loss of overlying soft tissue is extensive, both pedicled and free vascularized myocutaneous flaps either from the pectoralis major or latissimus dorsi offer an alternative.

PROBLEMS AND COMPLICATIONS

An accurate preoperative assessment will go a long way in avoiding surprises at the time of surgery. Most problems can

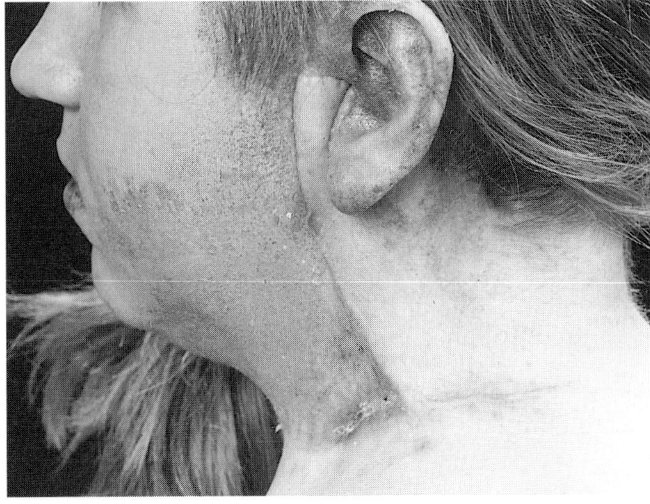

Fig. 17.18   Closure of the defect with sternomastoid myocutaneous flap. No skin grafting of the donor site was needed in this patient. (Reproduced with permission from the American Journal of Surgery.)

be attributed to two factors, namely: selection of cases and inadequate planning. It is a mistake to plan these procedures purely as an otological operation. Unless the operator has experience with neuro-otological, head and neck and reconstructive techniques, it is better to plan a team approach. Proper surgical techniques, avoiding dural injury and blood loss, are essential steps. Any dural tear must be repaired immediately. Protection of the eye against corneal injury in the first few weeks after surgery is essential. Use of methylcellulose drops and the wearing of an eye shield are advisable. Dizziness is transient and usually lasts from 2 to 3 days but may be present for 2 to 3 weeks. It is never severe enough to prevent early ambulation. The period of acclimatization is longer in older individuals. Provided the opposite ear has adequate hearing, or is well compensated by means of a hearing aid, most patients have no problem adjusting to the unilateral loss of hearing. Dysphagia is a rare complication and can arise if the glossopharyngeal nerve is traumatized. The use of muscle flaps can lead to seroma formation and it is better to keep the drains a little longer.

With the techniques described above the morbidity is minimal, and in the 21 cases operated so far there was no mortality attached to the procedure. The quality of life is, to a great extent, preserved.

Radiotherapy is well tolerated by patients. All patients with squamous-cell and adenoid cystic carcinoma received a total of 65 Gy in 35 sittings in 7 weeks. Piecemeal surgery should be avoided. Ultraradical procedures reported in the literature with sacrifice of the internal carotid artery and several cranial nerves leave the patient with a quality of life that can hardly justify such procedures (Graham et al 1984, Sataloff et al 1987). What is important is that the tumour be excised in one piece with good margins whenever possible, that the defect be reconstructed well in the shortest time, and that the patients be left in a fit state for radiotherapy. In all results reported so far this problem has seldom been addressed. Following this strategy a 3–11-year overall survival of 42% for all cancers and 38.8% for squamous-cell carcinomas was achieved, in spite of the fact that the earlier cases were treated with conventional techniques mentioned in the literature—with their added problem of delayed healing (Tiwari et al 1992).

FUTURE DEVELOPMENTS

One of the features of malignant tumours of the external ear canal and the middle ear is their infrequency. Treatment should therefore be centralized in centres of head and neck surgery. Brachytherapy for external ear canal cancer sounds promising. Temporal bone resections with postoperative radiotherapy remain the most suitable form of therapy for middle-ear tumours. With increasing successful control of nasopharyngeal and middle-ear infections, it would be expected that the incidence of this disease would decline. Further improvements in the already sophisticated methods of imaging techniques such as three-dimensional views, are going to prove increasingly helpful in the accurate preoperative assessment of the disease process.

REFERENCES

Anson B J, Donaldson J A 1973 Surgical anatomy of the temporal bone and ear. In: Anson B J, Donaldson J A (eds) W B Saunders, Philadelphia, pp 10–362

Beal D D, Lindsay J R, Ward P H 1965 Radiation induced carcinoma of the mastoid. Archives of Otolaryngology 81: 9–16

Birzgalis A R, Keith A O, Farrington W T 1992 Radiotherapy in the treatment of middle ear and mastoid. Carcinoma 17: 113–116

Boland J, Patterson R 1955 Cancer of the middle and external auditory meatus. Journal of Laryngology and Otology 69: 468–478

Broders A C 1921 Epithelioma of the ear. A study of 63 cases. Surgical Clinics of North America 1: 1401–1410

Conley J J, Schuller D E 1977 Reconstruction following temporal bone resections. Archives of Otolaryngology 103: 34–37

Fisch U 1978 Infratemporal fossa approach to tumours of the temporal bone and base of skull. Journal of Laryngology and Otology 92: 949–967

Fisch U 1982 Subtotal petrosectomy with permanent anterior dislocation of the facial nerve and obliteration of the cavity. In: Naumann H H (ed) Head and neck surgery. Thieme, Stuttgart, vol III, pp 544–551

Goodwin W J, Jesse R H 1980 Malignant neoplasms of external auditory canal and temporal bone. Archives of Otolaryngology 100: 45–49

Graham M D, Sataloff R T, Kemink J L, Wolf G T, McGuillicuddy J E 1984 Total en bloc resection of the temporal bone and carotid artery for malignant tumours of the ear and temporal bone. Laryngoscope 94: 528–533

Holmes K S 1965 Carcinoma of the middle ear. Clinical Radiology 16: 400–404

Jesse R H, Healey J E, Wiley D B 1967 External auditory canal, middle ear and mastoid. In: Mcomb W S, Fletcher G H (eds) Williams & Wilkins, Baltimore, pp 412–417

Kinney S E, Wood B G 1987 Malignancies of the external ear canal and temporal bone. Surgical techniques and results. Laryngoscope 97: 158–163

Lederman M 1965 Malignant tumours of the ear. Journal of Laryngology and Otology 79: 85–119

Lewis J 1965 Radical surgery for malignant tumours of the ear. Archives of Otolaryngology 83: 56–61

Lewis J S 1975 Temporal bone resection review of 100 cases. Archives of Otolaryngology 101: 23–25

Lewis J S 1979 Tumours of the middle ear cleft and temporal bone. In: Ballantyne J, Groves J (eds) Scott's Brown diseases of the ear, nose and throat, 4th edn. Butterworth, London, pp 385–404

Lewis J S 1981 Cancer of the external auditory canal, middle ear and mastoid. In: Suen J, Myers E (eds) Cancer of the head and neck. Churchill Livingstone, New York, pp 557–575

Manni J J, Haelst U J G M, Kubat K, Marres E H M A 1984 Primäres Karzinoid des Mittelohres. HNO 32: 419–423

Martinez A, Edmundson G, Borrego C, Brown D, Kader F, Clarke D 1991 High dose rate treatment of ear canal carcinoma. Activity—Selectron Brachytherapy Journal 5: 2–6

Morton R P, Stell P M, Derrick P P O 1984 Epidemiology of cancer of the middle ear cleft. Cancer 53: 1612–1617

Munk-Nielsen L, Hansen H S 1991 Bilateral carcinoma of the external auditory meatus. Journal of Laryngology and Otology 105: 112–114

Newhart H 1917 Primary carcinoma of the middle ear. Laryngoscope 27: 543–555

Parson H, Lewis J H 1954 Subtotal resection of the temporal bone for cancer of the ear. Cancer 7: 995–1001

Politzer A 1883 Epitheliom der Ohrmuschel und des ausseren Gehörorganes. In: Politzer A (ed) Lehrbuch des Ohrenheilkunde. Verlag von Ferdinande Enke, Stuttgart, pp 421–423

Sahin A A, Ro J Y, Ordonez N G, Luna M A, Weber R S, Ayala A G 1991 Temporal bone involvement by prostatic adenocarcinoma. Head and Neck 13: 349–354

Sataloff R T, Myers D L, Lowry L D, Spiegel J R 1987 Total temporal bone resection for squamous cell carcinoma. Otolaryngology Head and Neck Surgery 96: 4–14

Schall L A 1934 Neoplasma involving the middle ear. Archives of Otolaryngology 32: 548–553

Stell P M 1984 Carcinoma of the external auditory meatus and middle ear. Clinical Otolaryngology 9: 281–299

Stell P M, McCormick 1985 Carcinoma of the external auditory meatus and middle ear. Prognostic factors and a suggested staging system. Journal of Laryngology and Otology 99: 847–850

Stell P M, Miles J B 1986 The place of salvage petrosectomy. Journal of Laryngology and Otology 100: 145–147

Tabb H G, Komet H, McLaurin J W 1964 Cancer of the external auditory canal. Treatment with radical mastoidectomy and irradiation. Laryngoscope 74: 634–643

Tiwari R M 1985 Reconstruction after subtotal temporal bone resections. Journal of Laryngology and Otology 99: 143–146

Tiwari R M 1990 Experiences with the sternocleidomastoid myocutaneous flaps. Journal of Laryngology and Otology 104: 315–321

Tiwari R M, Feenstra L, Karim A B F M 1992 Temporal bone resections for carcinoma of the middle ear and external ear canal. American Journal of Surgery 164: 648–650

Vikram B, Strong E W, Shah J P, Spiro R 1984 Failure in the neck following multimodality treatment for advanced head and neck cancer. Head and Neck Surgery 6: 724–729

Wang C C 1975 Radiation therapy in the management of carcinoma of the external auditory canal, middle ear or mastoid. Radiology 116: 713–715

Ward G E, Loch W E, Lawrence W 1951 Radical operation for carcinoma of the external auditory canal and middle ear. American Journal of Surgery 82: 169–178

Zeroni 1899 Über das Carcinom des Gehörorganes. Archieve Ohrenheilkunde 8: 141–190

18. The nose

Louis C. Argenta

ANATOMICAL CONSIDERATIONS

Because it is one of the central focal points of the face, any surgery of the nose must be performed with skill and attention to detail. Contours of the nose vary from convex to concave, and both subtle and sharp contrast occurs within aesthetic subunits of the nose. The eye quickly focuses on asymmetry or subtle differences in colour and texture. Gonzalez-Ulloa et al (1954) considered the entire nose to be one subunit of the face. Subsequently, others have divided the nose into subunits (Burget & Menick 1985), taking into account various light reflections on the nose, colour and skin texture. Ideally, suture lines are placed to lie between subunits (Fig. 18.1). Occasionally, adjacent uninvolved tissue in a subunit is resected so that reconstruction can be performed as a single unit to avoid conspicuous suture lines.

The skin varies significantly in colour, texture, and sebaceous quality in different areas of the nose. In the glabella, the skin is thick, pale, and readily movable. The skin covering the nasal bones and upper lateral cartilages is thin,

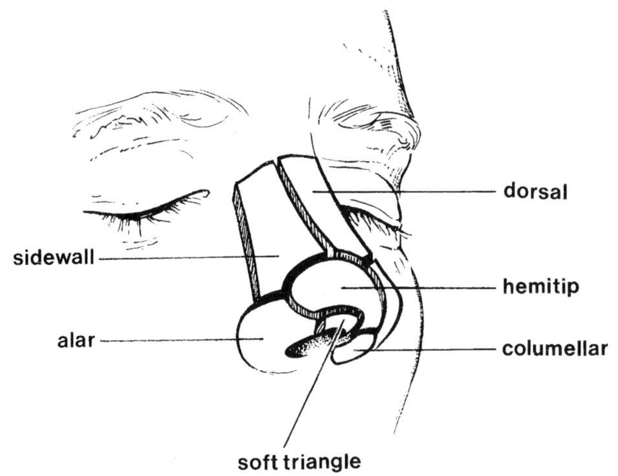

Fig. 18.1 The aesthetic subunits of the nose as described by Burget and Menick (1985). When possible, suture lines should rest in the lines between the subunits to avoid being conspicuous. Occasionally, the entire subunit is resurfaced to minimize colour and texture contrasts.

pale, and begins a transition to acquire more sebaceous glands. In the nasal tip, the skin is usually quite thick, oily and more pigmented. As the patient ages the subtle differences in nasal skin become less obvious and less important, relative to reconstructive procedures. None the less, the surgeon should spare no effort to arrive at a normal post-operative appearance.

PATHOLOGY CONSIDERATIONS

Any of the neoplasms which occur in skin, subcutaneous tissue, bone or cartilage in the human body can occur in the nose. The vast majority of neoplasms occurring in the nose, however, are basal-cell carcinomas, followed by squamous-cell carcinomas in the ratio of 10 : 1. A pathological diagnosis should always be established by excisional biopsy, if possible, or by incisional marginal biopsy if the lesion is large.

Basal-cell carcinoma usually occurs in the elderly but may occasionally occur in a young individual. Sebaceous nevi, irradiation, or excessive sun exposure frequently precede these neoplasms. Although these tumours are usually slow-growing, they can infiltrate widely and deeply. Metastases are extremely rare with only 200 cases reported prior to 1984 (von Domarus & Stevens 1984). Metastases occur most frequently in very large long-standing neglected tumours. Basal-cell tumours must be histologically distinguished from adnexal tumours and adenoid cystic carcinoma, which have a significant potential for metastasis (Hamm et al 1987).

The margins of resection of basal-cell carcinoma can frequently be determined by clinical examination. A cystic basal-cell carcinoma usually has very clear margins which can be delineated from adjacent uninvolved tissue. Ulcerated basal-cell carcinomas, however, have extremely indistinct margins, and the surrounding tissue can be indurated and erythematous, but still not involved with tumour. The margins of morphea and sclerosing basal-cell carcinomas are also extremely difficult to determine clinically in all planes and must be treated with considerable respect. Lesions which occur in previously irradiated tissue, or recurrences of basal-cell carcinoma in the site of previous excision, are difficult in that involved margins may be impossible to ascertain without careful histological confirmation. The surgical margins around previously untouched lesions should be 3–5 mm. Ulcerated or large lesions frequently require margins of 8–10 mm, but these should always be confirmed histologically.

Of equal importance to the lateral margins, it is critical to assess the depth of the lesion prior to any reconstructive procedure. In the upper two-thirds of the nose, where there is mobility of the skin over the nasal bones and upper lateral cartilages, invasion of the deeper structures is unusual. In the lower third of the nose, however, there is intimate attachment of the skin and lower lateral cartilages such that invasion of the cartilage occurs relatively soon in the course of the disease. While the clinical appearance of the periosteum and perichondrium can give some indication as to involvement, biopsy of at least the periosteum or perichondrium should be obtained. If this is positive, the underlying bone and cartilage should be resected with adequate lateral margins to the underlying mucosa. Since frozen section cannot be obtained on bone and cartilage, the question then arises as to whether mucosa should be sacrificed. If the mucosa strips easily and bloodlessly from the overlying cartilage, the odds of involvement are relatively low. In areas of question, however, a small biopsy of the underlying mucosa can be taken and examined under frozen section. If the frozen section is not available, permanent sections are used, leaving the wound open in the interim. The time lost in guaranteeing total excision is well worth the avoidance of late complications.

In the United States, frozen section control to ensure total removal of tumour is used much more frequently than in Europe. A significant incentive may be litigious concerns. The use of frozen section with Mohs' technique has been particularly useful in sparing as much normal tissue as possible. With those experienced in the technique, a control rate of greater than 95% can be obtained (Mohs 1978). In the United States, dermatologists trained in this technique frequently work closely with surgical colleagues. The presence of any tumour cells in the margins after excision is an indication for a secondary resection. In one study a recurrence rate of 33% of basal-cell carcinomas of the face was noted where tumour cells were found on the margin (Gooding & Yatsuhashill 1965). While occasionally a re-excision of a lesion with positive margins reveals no histological tumour, Koplin & Zrem (1980) found residual tumour in 50% of cases where positive margins had been found at the initial sample. It is particularly important to assure resection of all the tumour if flaps are to be used for reconstruction. When there is any question of residual tumour, the wound should be left open—closure being delayed until permanent sections are available. Another alternative is the placement of a thin split-thickness skin graft through which the excised area can be observed for an indefinite period of time.

Cosmetic considerations for compromising margins of resection of the nose are at this time untenable. Adequate techniques exist for reconstruction of almost any defect of the nose with very pleasing aesthetic results. The tumour, therefore, should be resected until all margins are free of residual histological tumour.

Recurrent basal-cell carcinoma

Recurrent basal-cell carcinoma is a warning that the surgeon is dealing with an aggressive lesion. Histologically controlled margins of resection in all planes are necessary for successful treatment. Failure rate after treatment of recurrent basal-cell carcinoma approach 20% (Hayes 1962), but may be as low as 5% with Mohs' technique (Mohs 1978). While some of these 'recurrences' may be the result of multiple or multicentric lesions, most are local failures of original treatment. When basal-cell carcinoma recurs in scar, flap or graft, the entire scar, flap or graft should be excised as these tumours tend to move in previously dissected planes.

Squamous-cell carcinoma

Most surgeons feel that squamous-cell carcinoma is a more aggressive tumour than basal-cell lesions and that it should be treated more aggressively. While very small lesions are adequately treated with resections of 3–5 mm margins, larger deeper lesions require significantly larger resections. Some surgeons believe that squamous-cell carcinoma arising in actinically damaged skin are usually more benign lesions and require less aggressive resection. Large, recurrent, or ulcerated lesions in actinically damaged skin, however, may be extremely aggressive. An increasing depth of penetration of squamous-cell invasion correlates well with metastases and local recurrence.

Treatment of squamous-cell lesions of the nose always includes evaluation of the neck nodes—particularly in the submental area. Fine-needle aspiration may be helpful in delineating tumour-involved nodes from inflammatory lesions. Positive needle aspirates of neck nodes found with squamous-cell lesions of the nose require careful and thorough evaluation of the entire aerodigestive tract in search of a second primary. Most squamous-cell lesions of the nasopharynx and mouth have a higher predilection for metastasis than does squamous-cell carcinoma of the nose.

As with basal cell carcinoma, the limits of resection are ultimately dictated by the histological margins of involvement. Positive margins indicate the need for a second or third resection until margins are clear. Unfortunately, the diagnosis of adjacent 'dysplastic' changes frequently makes histological determination of the margins worrisome. Careful follow-up of all lesions after squamous-cell carcinoma resection for several years is indicated.

SURGICAL TECHNIQUES: direct wound closure

Many small defects can be closed with direct wound approximation. Some undermining in the subdermal plane is particularly helpful to achieve primary closure. Direct closure is most applicable to lesions on the upper two-thirds of the nose, where there is pre-existing mobility of skin and the possibility of distortion asymmetry is minimal. More soft tissue can be mobilized by closing the lesion in a vertical direction. If necessary, the length of wound should be extended to avoid 'standing cones' at the wound end. In the lower third of the nose, direct closure becomes more difficult because of the significant fixation of skin to the underlying cartilages and the tendency to develop asymmetry. In the elderly drooping nose, a transverse closure may often be achieved, lifting the tip of the nose as an added bonus. Wounds should be closed with deep absorbable sutures and fine monofilament skin sutures.

Scars from direct closure are usually minimal, particularly in the elderly population in whom tumours usually occur. If the scar is significantly depressed 6 to 8 months following surgery, it should be excised and the edges re-approximated. In unsightly non-depressed scars, dermabrasion 8 to 12 months postoperatively may be of help.

Healing by secondary intention

Defects in the area of the medial canthus, the alar crease, and the nasal dorsum heal relatively well by secondary intention (Goldwyn & Rueckert 1977). Defects of the lower third of the nose, however, tend to develop distortion and prominent scars. The time loss and inconvenience incurred in allowing wounds to heal by secondary intention is ill spent since most of these wounds can be closed relatively easily by a skilled physician. In rare, selected patients, however, this technique may be permissible.

Split-thickness skin grafting

Split-thickness grafts are usually used in the very debilitated or very elderly patient with a large defect. The aesthetic results from split-thickness skin grafting are usually compromised since they result in a pale shining irregular surface and secondary contracture and distortion. There must be a continuous sheet of periosteum and perichondrium present or the graft will fail. If the defect is significantly large, the possibility of covering the entire aesthetic unit of the nose with a split-thickness skin graft should be entertained since the contrast to the adjacent tissue, both in colour and contour, will be minimized. Thicker grafts of the order of 18–20 thousandths of an inch (0.45–0.5 mm) are better than thin grafts. The skin graft is held in place with a tie-over dressing for at least 5 days and then protected from sun for 8 to 12 months.

Split-thickness skin grafts are also useful in patients where there is significant risk or previous history of recurrence or when biological activity of an unusual neoplasm is in question. Cases in which previous surgery have consumed enough local tissue so that local flaps are impossible or compromised, also can be grafted. Skin grafts are left in place for 12 to 18 months, since most recurrences will occur in this interval (Pascal et al 1968). Secondary excision of the graft and reconstruction with more aesthetic flaps can then be performed.

Another situation in which a split-thickness skin graft may be useful is in the pale, thin-skinned, young patient who develops a neoplasm at the tip of the nose which cannot be closed primarily. A split-thickness skin graft can be applied to the residual area, with the thought of resecting it 1 to 2 months later to achieve primary closure.

Full-thickness grafts

Full-thickness grafts produce a cosmetically better result than split-thickness grafts because of a better colour and texture match. A small amount of fat can be left on the underside of the graft to increase bulk, realizing that excess fat can result in flap death. Potential donor sites should be carefully examined under natural light to discern the best colour match to the remaining nose. The postauricular skin is usually ruberous and thinner than nasal skin. The pre-auricular skin usually has a better colour and texture match to the nose, but is significantly limited in size, particularly in males where the facial hair intervenes. The supraclavicular area can provide sufficient skin to reconstruct very large areas of the nose. Again in these cases, consideration should be given to excising an entire subunit of the nose and covering it with a single full-thickness graft. In younger patients, the supraclavicular area can be expanded and a full-thickness graft of any size harvested. Preparation of the donor site is even more critical in full-thickness grafts than in split-thickness ones. The slightest amount of haematoma will result in loss of the graft. Haemostasis should therefore be meticulous and the graft held securely in place for 7 days with a tie-over dressing. Final determination as to colour match cannot be made for 6 to 12 months during which time the sun should be avoided to avoid hyperpigmentation (Fig. 18.2).

Composite grafts

Small deep excisions, and lesions along the alar margin, are well treated with composite chondrocutaneous grafts harvested from the ear (Avelar et al 1984). Such grafts have been used successfully for the past century for defects of up to 2 cm. The root of the helix is an ideal donor site for small defects (Argomoso 1975). The donor site can be closed by advancing and raising the pre-auricular skin. Such grafts can be used to reconstruct the alar margin and the lining on both

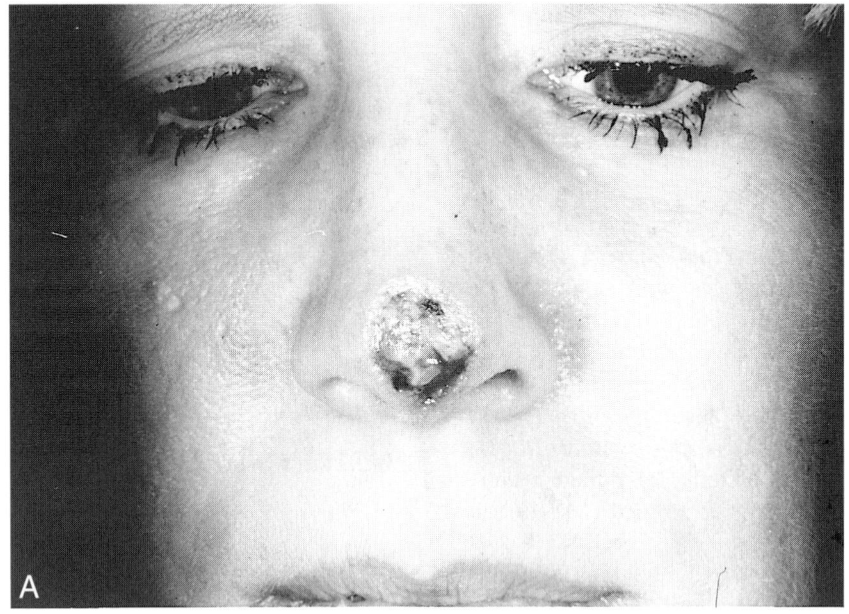

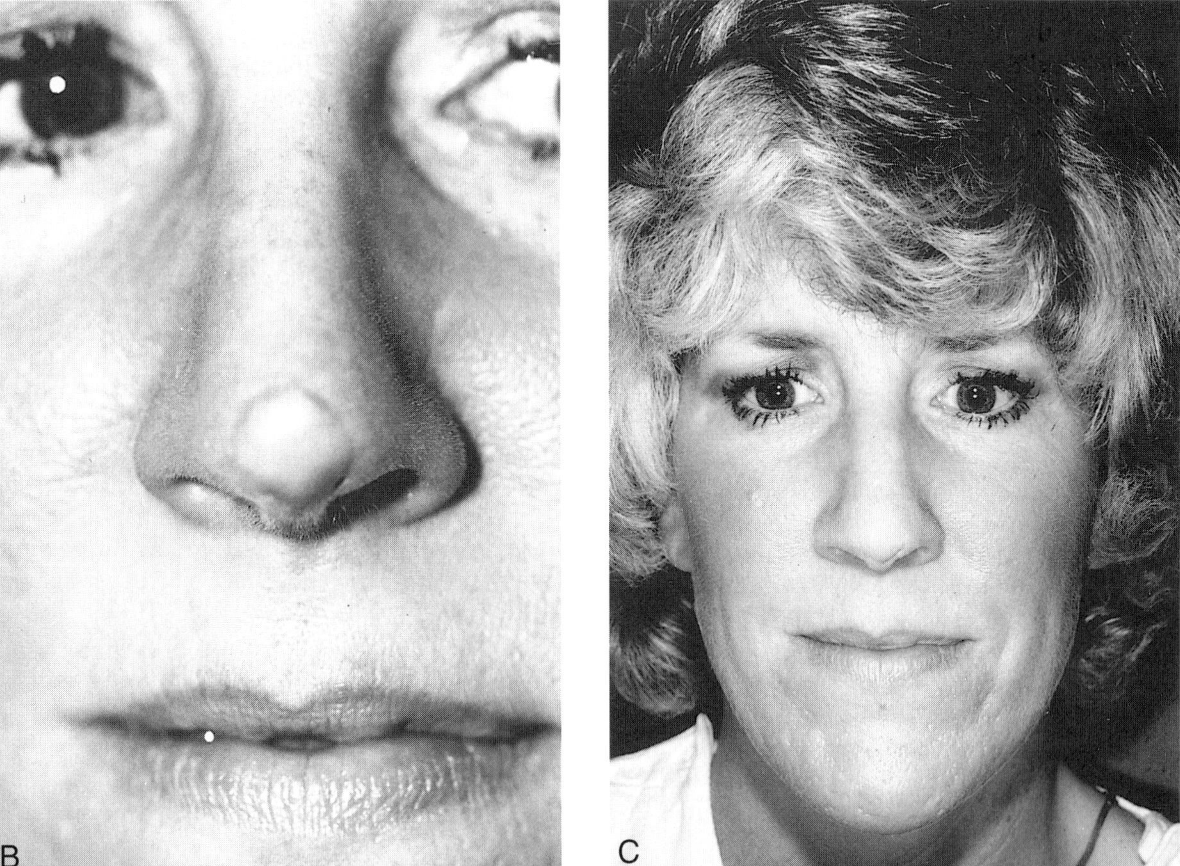

Fig. 18.2 Full-thickness skin graft. **A.** A young female with a deep excision of the nasal tip. Flaps are particularly obvious in a young patient and are best avoided. **B.** A full-thickness graft harvested from the pre-auricular area 1 month after surgery. **C.** Four months after surgery. The graft has blended well with the colour match. The distortion along the alar rim will require secondary revision or dermabrasion.

surfaces (Fig. 18.3). Grafts can also be harvested from the helical rim and the concha, depending on which contour is needed. Composite grafts have the benefit of being relatively simple procedures, which can provide excellent results and minimum compromise if they do fail. Areas which have been previously irradiated or are scarred after excision of multiple previous lesions are less favourable for receiving composite grafts. In these cases, flaps with an intact blood supply are safer.

Revascularization of the composite graft occurs primarily from the edges of the remaining bed. Techniques of varying efficacy to increase the survival of grafts have been attempted. These include cooling of the recipient site (Medawar 1942), avoiding epinephrine (adrenalin) solutions in the graft and recipient bed, and various pharmacological manipulates. Allowing the recipient site to granulate for 3 days increases the size and probability of composite graft take (McCollum & Grabb 1977). Suturing the graft to the margins of the defect should be done as atraumatically and as exactly as possible to encourage neovascularization of the graft. Using a step-type of excision of skin adjacent to the defect to increase the surface area of skin in contact with the recipient site, is helpful to increase revascularization. Postoperatively, the composite graft should not be traumatized. The skin of the graft frequently becomes dark, and often the superficial layer of epidermis will slough. Debridement of the graft should be delayed for as long as possible and allowed to proceed spontaneously if possible. The composite graft is usually more hyperpigmented for the first several months, but then gradually fades, and a relatively good colour match can be achieved. The occurrence of a notch on either side of the graft along the alar margin is the rule rather than the exception. Correction of these notches should be delayed for approximately 6 months and then corrected under local anaesthesia.

Skin flaps

The history of plastic surgery can be traced in the various types of flaps which have been devised to reconstruct the nose. Flaps were used in India in 3000 BC, in Roman and Greek times, and later by the Brancas, and Tagliacozzi of Italy in the Middle Ages (Tagliacozzi 1597). A better understanding of anatomy and microcirculation has allowed a very large number of safe flaps to be described in the past 100 years. Sophisticated flaps have progressed to the point that, at this time, the use of local flaps for reconstructing the nose is the most common and reliable technique for almost all defects. Most local flap procedures take advantage of the laxity of skin in the upper two-thirds of the nose

for advancement or rotation into a horizontal or inferior position. Wide undermining of the skin allows the mobilization of a significant amount of tissue. The extensive blood supply of the nose almost guarantees the survival of most local flaps, if properly designed and executed. The skin of the upper nose is usually of sufficient thickness so that many defects of bone or cartilage can be ignored. In the lower third of the nose, however, reconstruction of the cartilaginous support may be necessary with cartilage grafts prior to rotation of flap to avoid deformation or airway collapse with deep inspiration.

Transposition flaps

A large number of small flaps which mobilize the lax dorsal nasal skin have proven very efficacious. The Banner flap, Limberg flap and finger flap are all simple and reliable (Elliott 1969). These flaps all geometrically transpose skin flaps up to 2 cm in diameter into the defect and allow primary closure of the donor defect. Wide undermining both in the donor and recipient margins are very useful to minimize late distortion. Resulting contour defects should be allowed to remain for 4–6 months before any surgical attempt at revision is carried out. Most of these defects will resolve spontaneously with minimal tape pressure or the injection of local steroids (Kenalog-10). These flaps all do better in the upper three-quarters of the nose where distortion of the lower lateral cartilages is minimized.

The finger flap is an inferiorly based midline transposition flap in the upper two-thirds of the nose. The flap is transposed to the lateral surfaces of the nose or medial canthus and the donor site closed primarily. Problems with this flap are related to its relative thickness which may accentuate a pre-existing bony nasal hump. Scars are usually minimal (Fig.18.4).

The Banner flap (Masson & Mendelson 1977) is a small modified finger flap described for the lower half of the nose. Because of the paucity of available skin as the tip is approached, this flap has limited use. The design of the flap is accomplished by extending the medial edge of the defect superiorly to create a vertical inferiorly based flap. The flap is transposed horizontally and the donor defect closed primarily. The major difficulty with this flap is the tendency to form standing cones and pin cushioning (Fig. 18.4).

The Limberg flap (Limberg & Gibson 1972) is essentially a rhomboid flap and is useful for small defects. The donor rhomboid is positioned in one of the vertical limbs after the defect has been made into a rhomboid. Such flaps tend to have less secondary problems than Banner flaps, particularly if there is wide undermining of adjacent skin (Fig. 18.5).

Fig. 18.3 Composite graft. **A.** A full-thickness defect of the alar rim, including skin, mucosa and cartilage. **B.** A full-thickness graft is harvested from the helix encompassing skin, cartilage and posterior surface skin. **C.** The graft sutured in place to the margins of the defect. Note the discoloration which will persist for 5 to 7 days. **D.** Patient 1 year after surgery with good colour and texture match and an inconspicuous reconstruction of the alar margin.

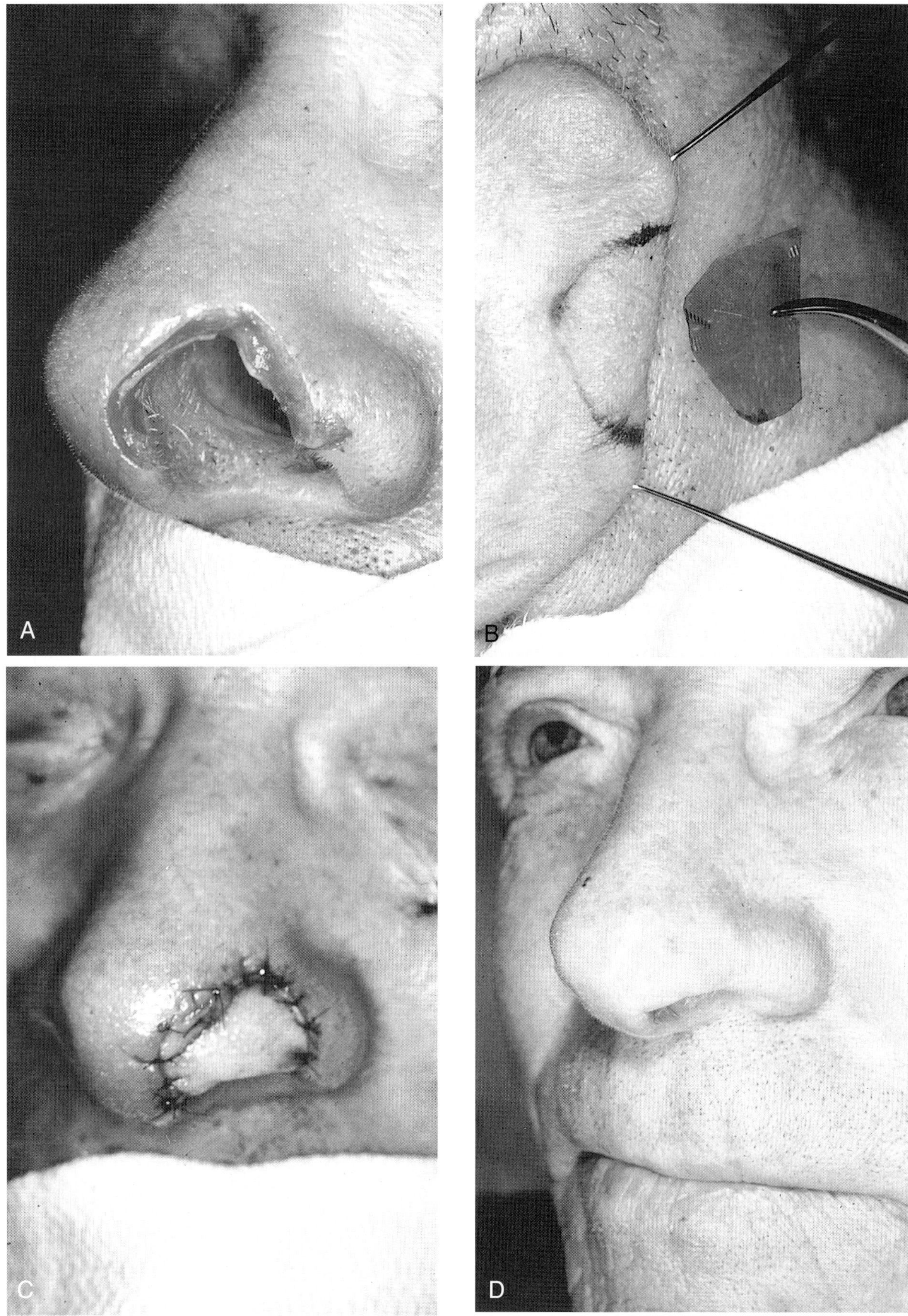

Fig. 18.3

Finger Flap

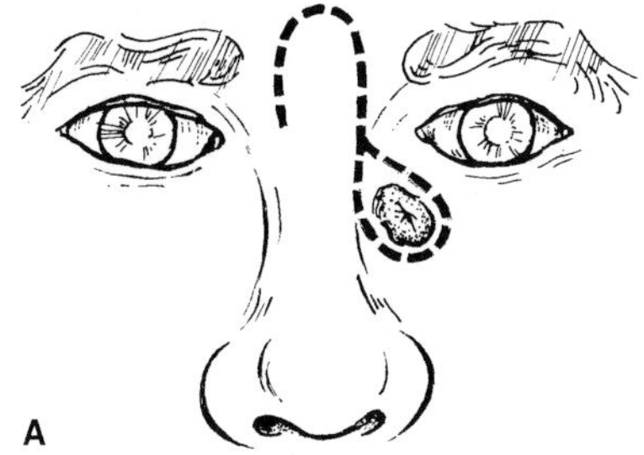

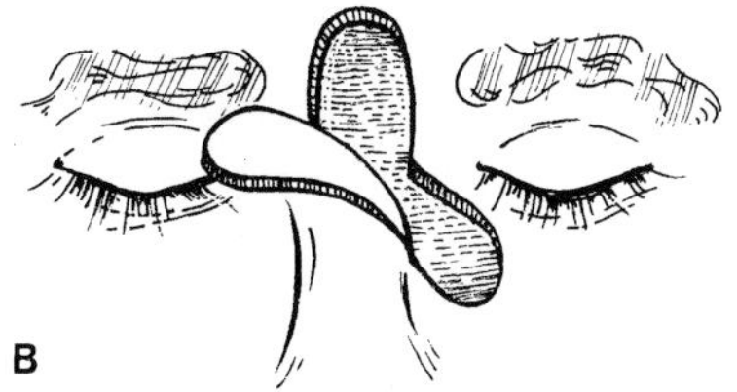

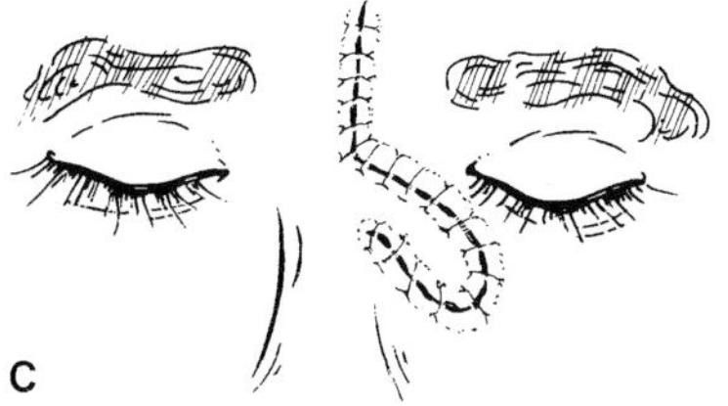

Banner Flap

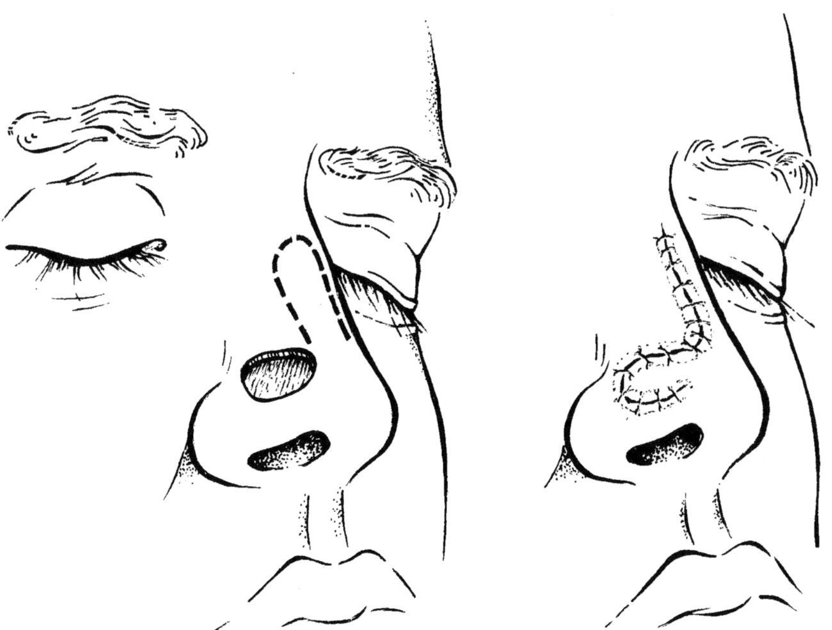

Fig. 18.4 The Finger flap and Banner flap are essentially the same flap. **A–C.** The Finger flap is usually described for the upper nose, taking the flap from the glabellar skin or upper third of the nose. The flap is undermined and transposed transversely. **D.** The Banner flap is used primarily in the lower half of the nose. **E.** Tissue taken from the midline is transposed transversely for defects of this area.

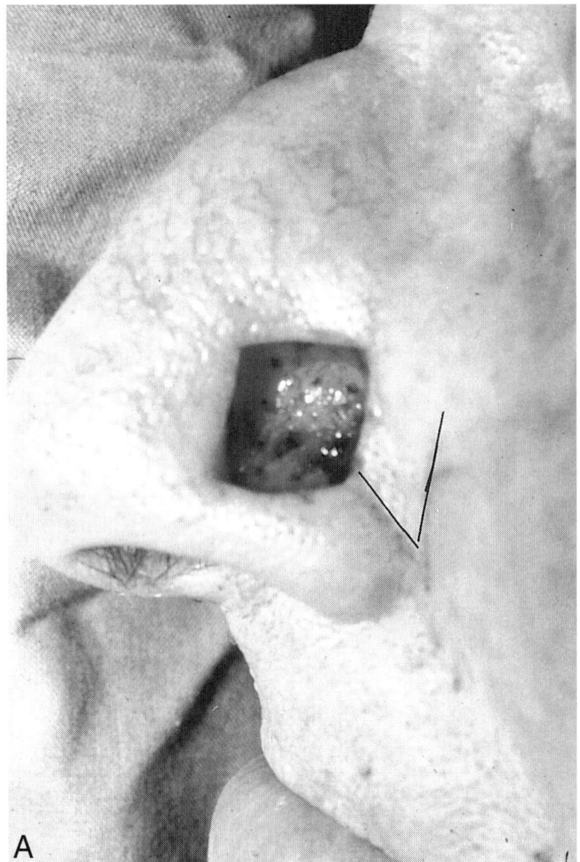

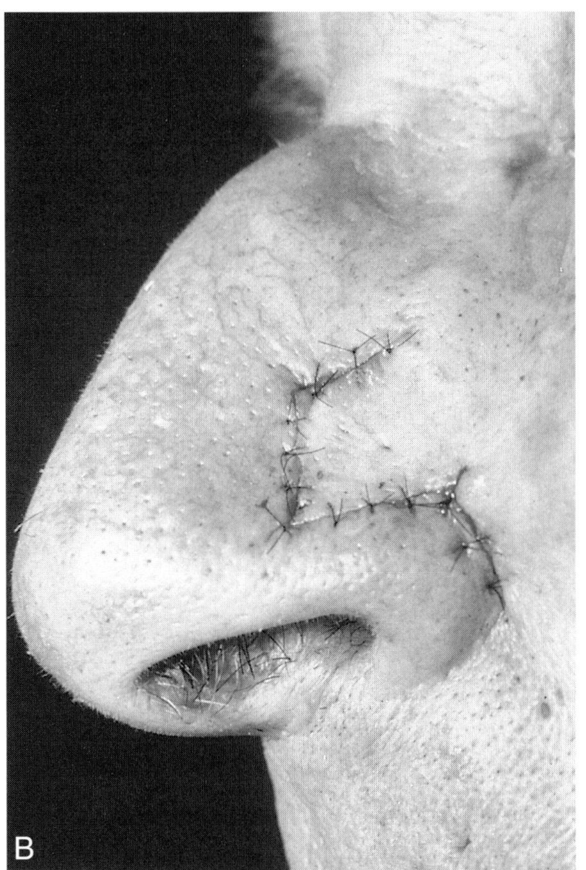

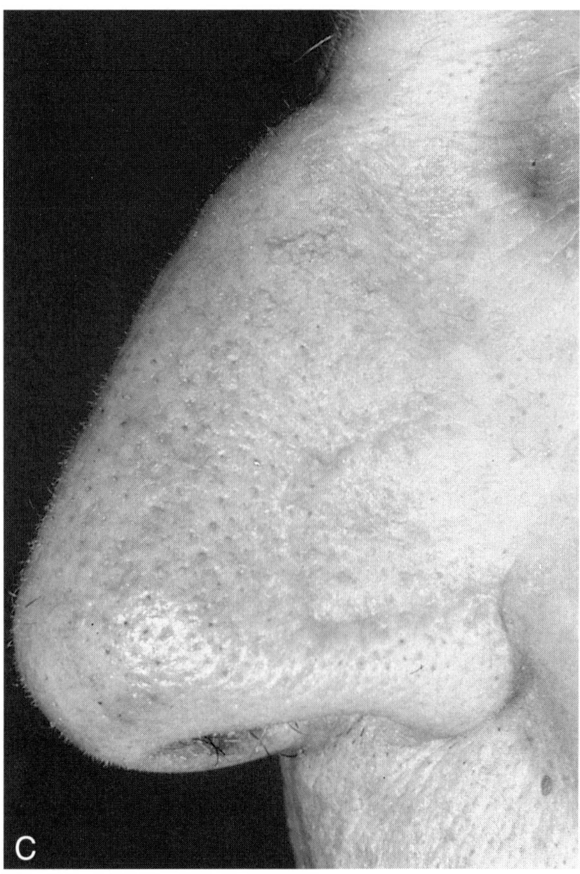

Fig. 18.5 A rhomboid flap. **A.** The defect has been outlined as a rhomboid and the donor flap designed. **B.** After undermining of the recipient bed margins and transposition of the flap. **C.** One year later, with almost inconspicuous margins and no distortion of the alar margin. Such flaps are usually less distorting than Banner flaps for defects of the lower half of the nose.

Bilobed flap

The bilobed flap (Esser 1918, Tardy et al 1972) allows the mobilization of a larger amount of tissue on the nose by creating two commonly based transposition flaps. The flaps are designed with the first flap having a mid-axis 45° to the defect. A second smaller flap with a common base to the first is designed 45° to the first flap and 90° to the axis of the defect (Fig. 18.6). By developing a second flap approximately one-half the size of the first flap, a larger defect can be closed while still achieving closure of the donor site. In general, results are better if the second flap is rotated from the vertical axis of the nose, so that it can be closed where there is maximum laxity of the adjacent tissues. In lesions of the upper half of the nose, the second flap is ideally positioned in the glabellar tissue. This technique allows the redistribution of tension in different directions over a larger area and minimizes postoperative distortion, even though a longer total incision is created. Bilobed flaps require more experience and more careful planning than a simple transposition flap. The most common problem with this flap is

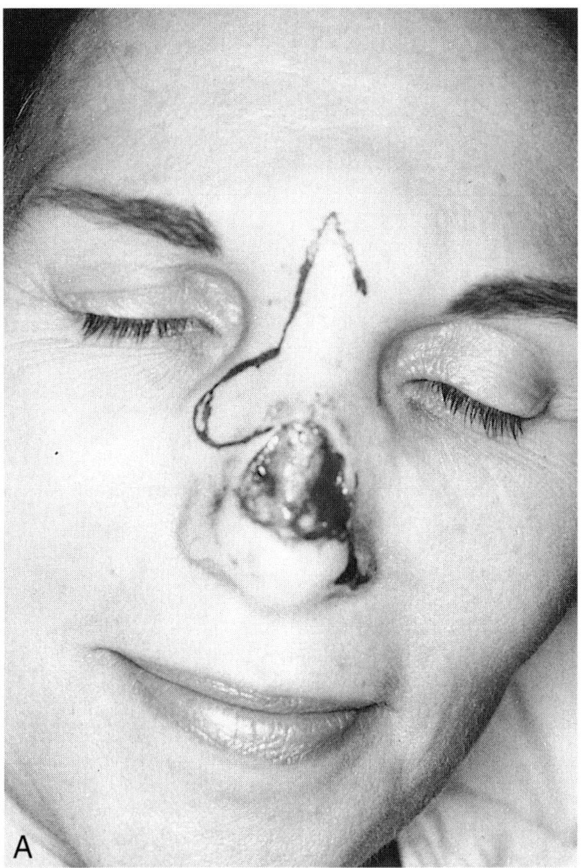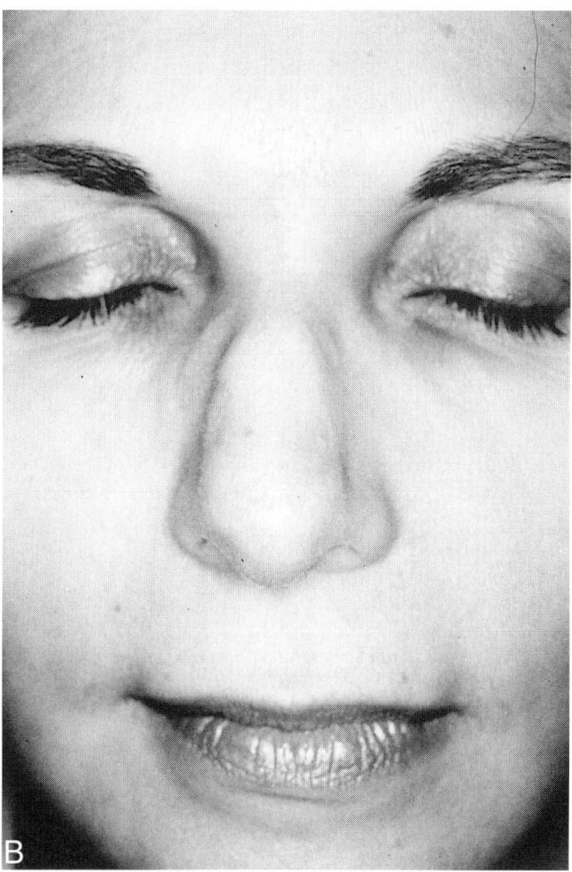

Fig. 18.6 Bilobed flap for a defect in the central third of the nose. **A.** The first flap is designed 45° from the defect, with a second flap designed at 90° from the defect in the glabellar area. **B.** One year after transposition of the flaps, the edges of the flap are barely visible. A slight nasal hump is present at the base of rotation of the flap. This can be minimized by rasping the nasal bones prior to insetting the flap.

poor planning and flaps that are too small. These result in inadequate rotation and distortion.

Glabellar flap

This flap was first described by McGregor (1962), refined by Rieger (1967), and again refined by Marchac & Toth (1990) and de Fontaine et al (1993). This is a safe, useful, large rotation advancement flap which can be used over the entire nasal dorsum to cover a wide variety of defects. The procedure takes advantage of the abundant loose tissue in the inner canthal area, and provides a good colour and texture match for the upper two-thirds of the nose. A cutaneous arterial branch which diverges from the angular artery at the medial canthus will safely supply a very large flap. The entire flap can be mobilized in an inferior direction to reach the lower third of the nose safely (Fig. 18.7). Attempts to reach the alar margin with this flap, however, may result in some distortion of the nose that requires secondary revision.

The margins of the flap should be planned so that the transposed flap suture lines come to lie at the margins of an aesthetic unit. In some cases, superior results can be obtained by sacrificing tissue around the defect and using a large flap to resurface a larger aesthetic unit. The superior margin of the inverted 'V' flap takes advantage of excess tissue between glabellar frown lines, avoiding the eyebrows. The flap is then ideally designed down the opposite side of the nose, at least one-half of the width of the lateral wall of the nose. The plane beneath the flap dissects easily and the vascular pedicle can be well visualized. The flap should be sutured in place in two layers using an absorbable deep suture and a fine monofilament skin suture.

Problems with this flap are largely related to its thickness. If the patient has a prominent bony nasal hump, this can be exaggerated, and therefore the hump should be rasped down prior to inset of the flap.

Subcutaneously based island flaps

The paranasal area of the nose includes well vascularized muscles supplied by the angular artery with direct perpendicular supply to the overlying skin (Herbert & DeGieus 1975). Subcutaneously based V–Y flaps are therefore easily created in the lateral nose and nasolabial fold and advanced

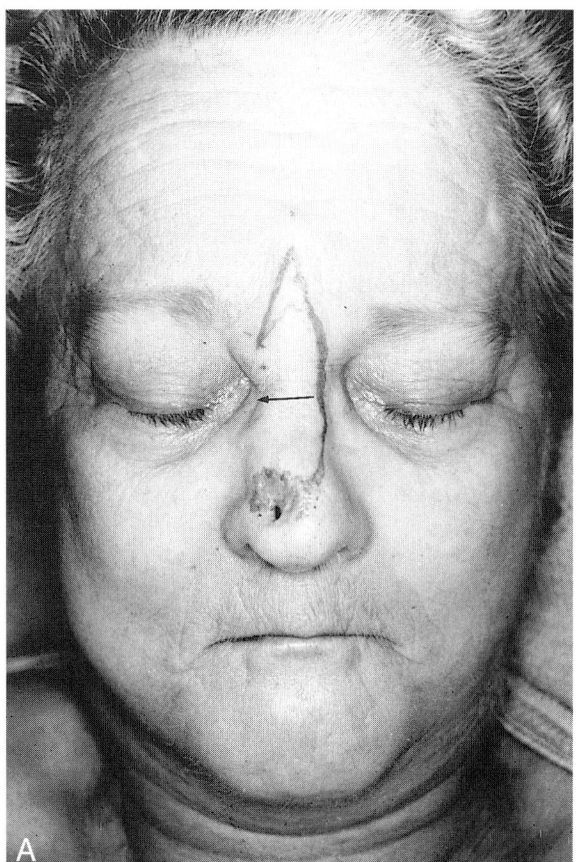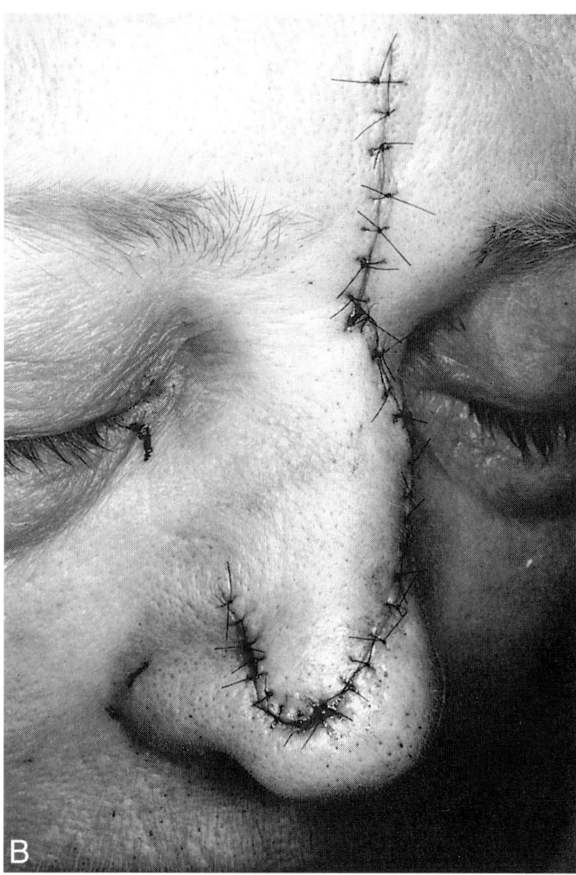

Fig. 18.7 A. The glabellar flap for a full-thickness defect of the lower third of the nose. The indurated area above the full-thickness loss was also removed. The flap is outlined to allow rotation on a branch of the angular artery at the medial canthus (arrow). **B.** The flap inset after undermining the edges of the recipient bed.

toward the middle of the nose (Barron & Emmett 1965, Rybka 1983). Such flaps cover defects of up to 2 cm in diameter and can advance up to 2 cm in the elderly. The excess bulk transposed with the underlying muscle usually resolves spontaneously (Fig. 18.8). In contradistinction, however, subcutaneously based flaps in the lower third of the nose, and particularly in the alar margin, are not recommended. The subcutaneous leash is much shorter and densely adherent to the underlying alar cartilages. Such flaps are usually forced into the defect of the alar rim where there is little to hold them in place. Over time, they tend to retract, resulting in notching of the alar margins (Eisenbaum 1991).

A second subcutaneously based flap employs the galea frontalis to transpose an island of skin from the frontal area onto the nose. Although popular several years ago, such flaps are technically difficult and have a significant rate of failure.

The aim of such flaps was to transpose forehead skin onto the nose without the vertical skin scar and to make this a one-stage procedure so that the pedicle supplying the forehead tissue did not need division and inset. The amount of dissection to supply a safe pedicle and an adequate arc of rotation make this operation more difficult than the standard forehead flap. The safest way to develop such a flap is to perform a transcoronal Misterschmitt incision in the hair-bearing scalp, dissected down to the periosteum of the skull. The flap is then dissected from the back side of the turned down forehead flap, and rotated on a leash of galea frontalis muscle onto the dorsum of the nose. An adequate tunnel must be developed to minimize risk of later compromise. Few of these flaps are used today because of the significant loss rate.

MAJOR RECONSTRUCTION

Before undertaking a major nasal reconstruction it must be pointed out that some patients may not need a reconstruction and may be better off with a prosthesis. Very debilitated, very elderly or non-motivated patients may have silicone nasal prostheses custom-fabricated. These prostheses can be worn when the patient desires by adhering them to adjacent tissue with an adhesive (Fig. 18.9).

When all or a substantial part of the nose has been lost,

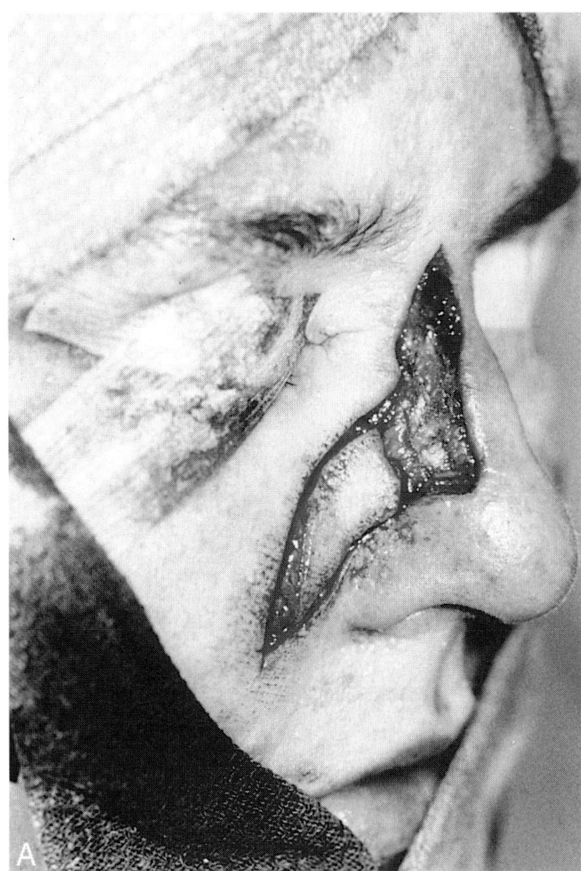

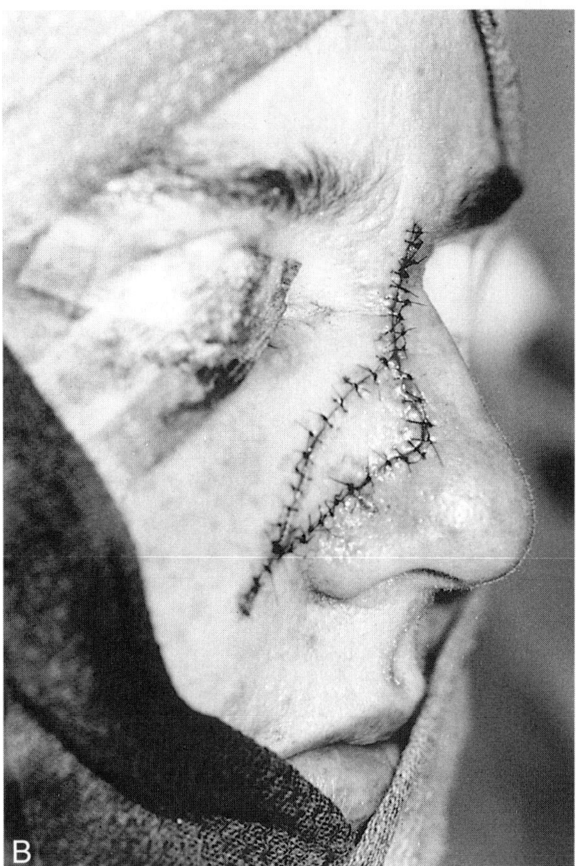

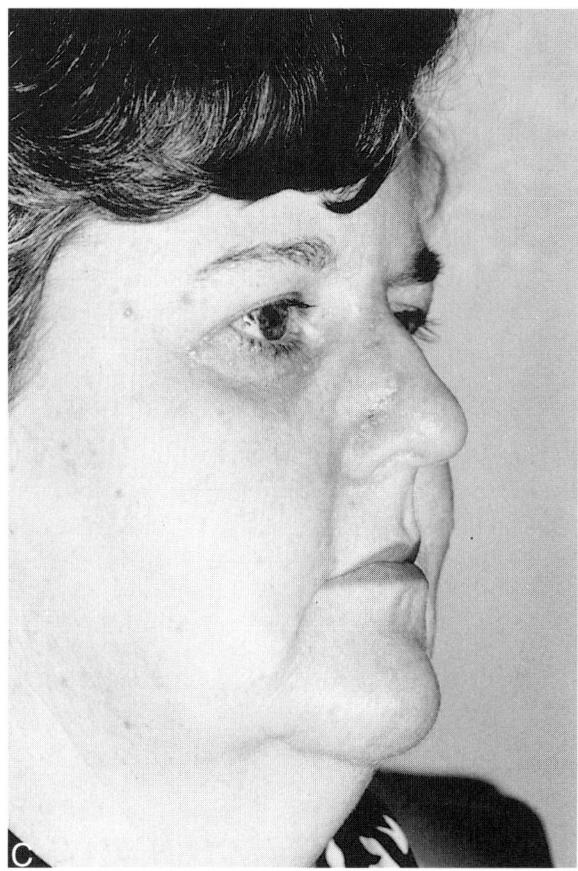

Fig. 18.8 Subcutaneously based V–Y advancement flap. **A.** The flap is based on perforating vessels overlying the muscles of the lateral nose. **B.** The flap is then advanced in a V–Y fashion to the defect with a portion of the defect closed primarily. **C.** The flap 3 months later. Note that there is some thickening of the flap which subsides spontaneously over time.

the use of tissue from elsewhere is required for reconstruction. Historically, a large number of flaps have been devised, many of which have gone into disuse because of the high incidence of complications or poor results. Tube flaps, delayed and taken from the neck or supraclavicular area (Song 1956, Maccomber & Berkeley 1967) frequently necrosed in the course of passage to the required destination.

The Tagliacozzi flap from the upper arm is used only rarely today because of the need for extended immobilization and the poor final results. The Schmid flap (Schmid 1961, 1964) is a delayed transverse forehead flap and designed immediately above the eyebrow to harvest a paddle on lateral to the brow. This is a non-anatomical procedure which does not follow the vascular supply of the forehead and, even worse, may compromise the later use of the forehead. The Washio flap (Washio 1969, 1972) attempted to reconstruct the nose with postauricular skin carried on a flap, based on the temporal artery. The flap depends on the retrograde flow between the temporal artery and the postauricular vessels to supply the postauricular skin. While

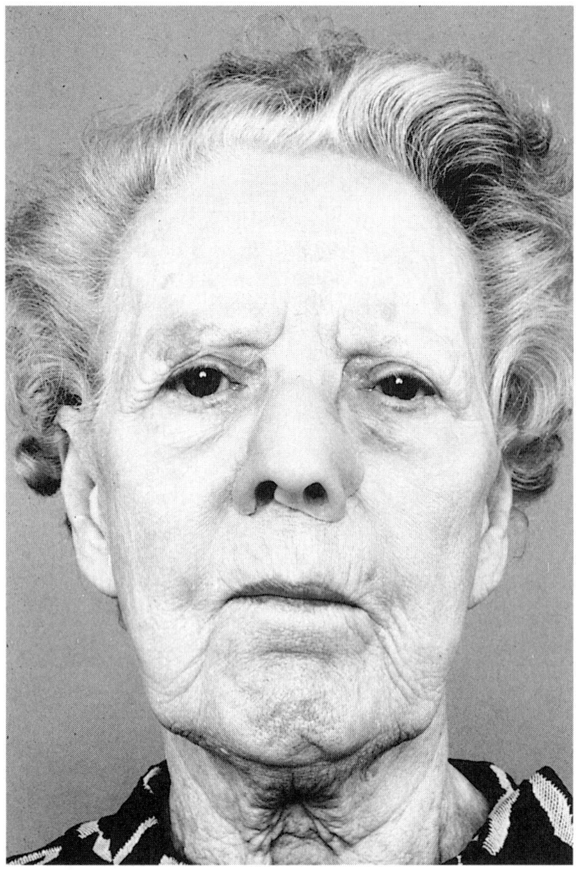

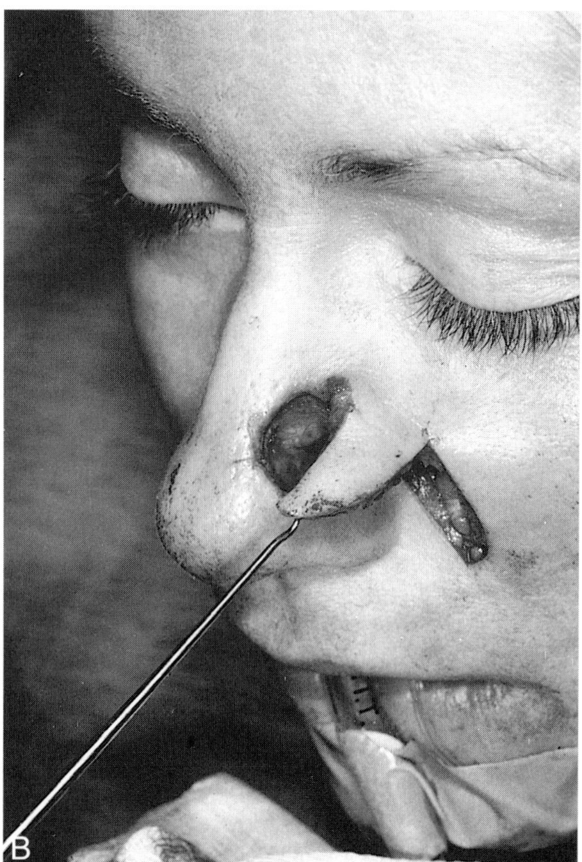

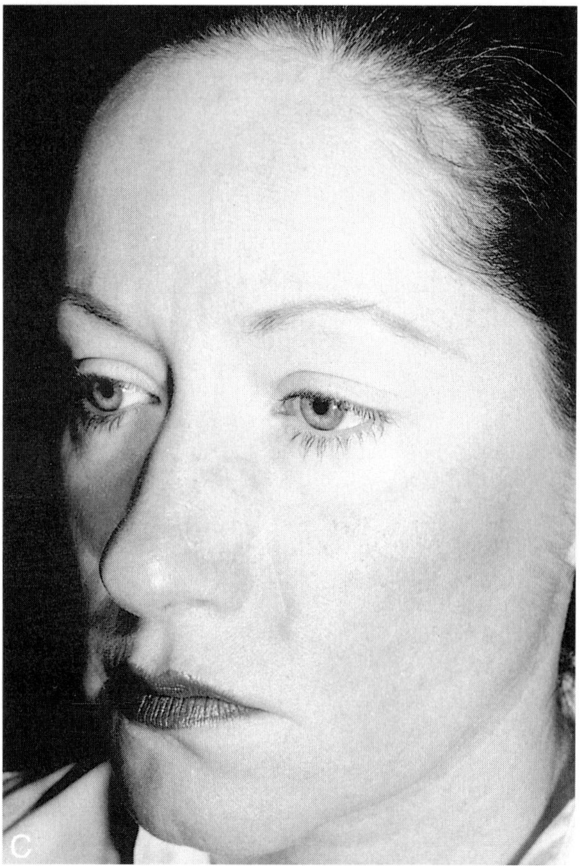

Fig. 18.9 The prosthetic nose fabricated of silicone elastomer and held in place with a skin adhesive. Such prostheses may be helpful in patients unwilling or unfit to undergo reconstruction or as a temporizing procedure to observe for recurrence.

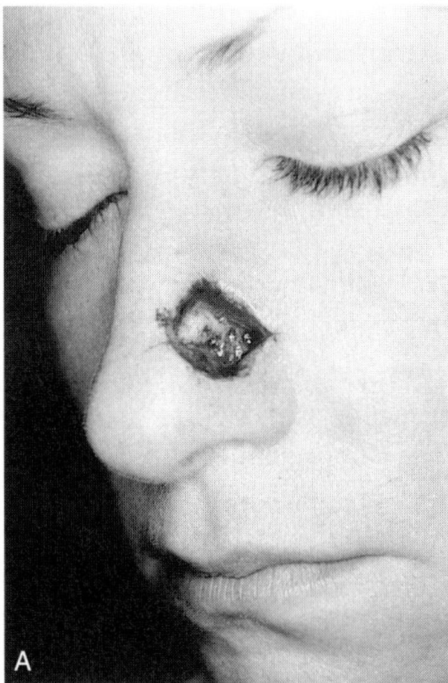

Fig. 18.10 **A.** A young female with a large defect of the lateral nose. **B.** The flap is outlined in the nasolabial fold, sparing the junction of the nose with the face. The flap is swung into place when the donor defect is closed primarily. **C.** One year postoperatively. The flap has contoured well after two injections of local steroids (Kenalog 10).

helpful in some reconstructions in children (Maillard & Montandon 1982), the procedure frequently results in inadequate amounts of skin being delivered to the nose at high risk. This flap is infrequently used today. Free flaps taken from the dorsalis pedis, forearm and scapular areas have been described (Shaw 1981). Because extensive prolonged surgery with below average results are usually produced, these flaps are infrequently employed. In cases of extensive neoplasm invading the deeper face and forehead, they may, however, be life-saving.

The two ideally situated donor sites that offer aesthetic and safe reconstructive possibilities are the medial cheek in the nasolabial fold and the forehead.

The nasolabial flap

Approximately 2–3 cm of skin can be mobilized from the nasolabial fold for reconstruction of the nose, particularly in the older patient. The nasolabial flap can be based either inferiorly or superiorly (Dieffenbach 1845). The superior pedicle technique is thought to be safer and to provide a better reconstruction (Hagerty & Smith 1958). The flap is usually raised and transferred at a single stage based on subcutaneous random blood supply from the angular artery. In the male, careful attention to the facial hair pattern is necessary so as not to transpose hair. If larger flaps are necessary, a delay to extend the length of the flap may be necessary. When a superiorly based flap is used, every attempt should be made to leave the lateral nasal crease intact so as to provide better definition later (Fig. 18.10). Although this may require a two-step procedure in which the flap is first transferred and 6 weeks later divided, the results are superior. Inferiorly based nasolabial flaps may be necessary in some cases, but these flaps tend to 'pin-cushion' more and to remain more oedematous for a longer period of time.

The rotation point in the nasolabial fold is frequently distorted and requires secondary revision. Monthly injections of Kenalog-10 are very useful in minimizing this oedema and achieving final contour. When the nasolabial flap is used to reconstruct the alar margin, underlying cartilage may be necessary if this has been previously sacrificed (Guerrero-Santos & Dicksheet 1981). The flap can also be folded upon itself to recreate both the nasal lining

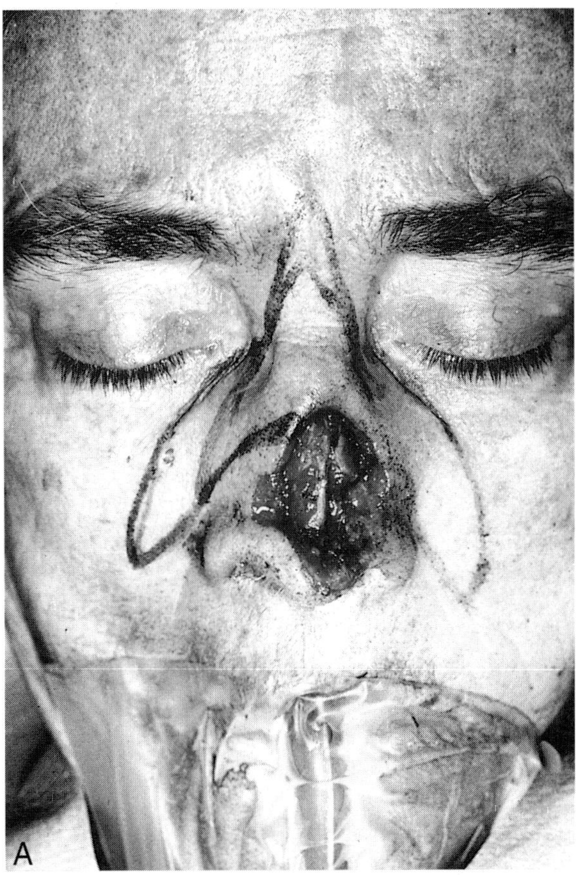
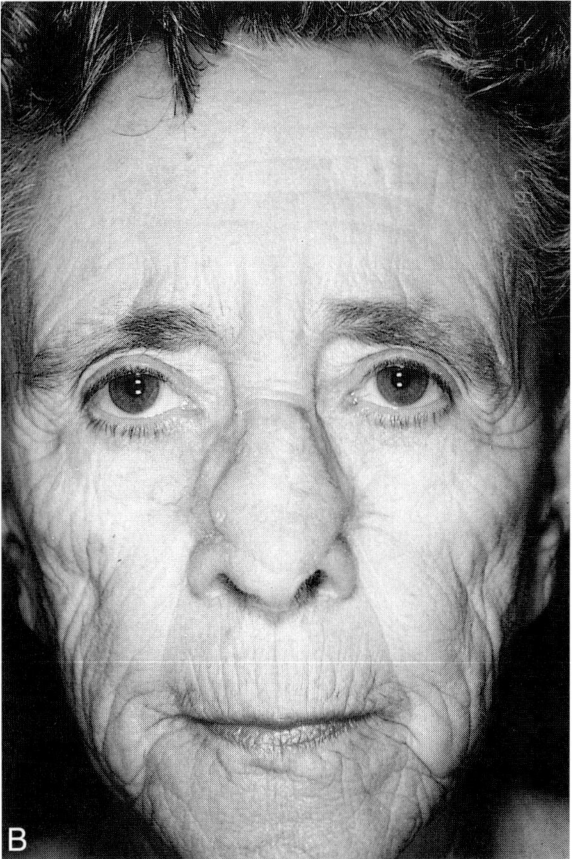

Fig. 18.11 **A.** A large through-and-through defect of the nose resurfaced with bilateral nasolabial flaps. This procedure may be useful in the elderly with large amounts of excess skin, particularly when the forehead has been compromised with previous neoplasms and scars. **B.** The patient 6 months later with some residual oedema in the flaps. This usually resolves over time with pressure or injected steroids.

and the overlying skin, but these are usually bulky. Bilateral superiorly based nasolabial flaps can be used to reconstruct very large defects of the nose safely (Fig. 18.11). These flaps are useful if the forehead tissue is compromised; they remain oedematous for a significant period of time, but, with pressure, injected steroids, and occasional defatting, reasonable results can be achieved, particularly in the elderly individual with large nasolabial folds.

In general, the more experienced the surgeon, the less nasolabial flaps are used. Long-term aesthetic results are frequently suboptimal. The colour and texture match of the flap to the nose are usually only fair. Pin-cushioning and oedema of the flap are common, and late distortion when these flaps are used in the lower third of the nose is common. Harvesting the flap too far superiorly can result in ectropion when the donor defect is closed.

Forehead flap

A very large amount of skin can be harvested from the forehead for reconstruction of large defects of the nose (Kazanjian 1946, Escoffier 1958) (Fig. 18.12). The axial blood supply of the forehead originates from the supra-orbital and supratrochlear vessels and allows the reconstruction of long flaps that can be rotated inferiorly to the pyriform area. Probably owing to its common embryological origin in the frontonasal process, the skin of the forehead is remarkably similar in colour, texture and sebaceous quality to the nose. Reconstructions of the nose using forehead tissue are aesthetically quite good. The forehead donor defect can usually be closed primarily, but, with larger flaps, skin grafts or secondary intention healing may be necessary. Because of the potential for disfigurement of the forehead, some surgeons refuse to use this area as a donor site. This fear is unfounded.

Large defects for the hemi-nose can be reconstructed by a vertical or oblique forehead flap based on the supra-orbital or supratrochlear vessels (Millard 1967). The author prefers general anaesthesia for this procedure, and no local anaesthesia or vasoactive drugs are used. The flap is usually planned in reverse with a three-dimensional folded thin wax template from the defect transposed into two dimensions on the forehead and pivoted over a dopplered vessel. Only by planning for a three-dimensional reconstruction can the proper quantity of tissue needed be estimated. A slightly larger flap than is required is usually taken with a base of

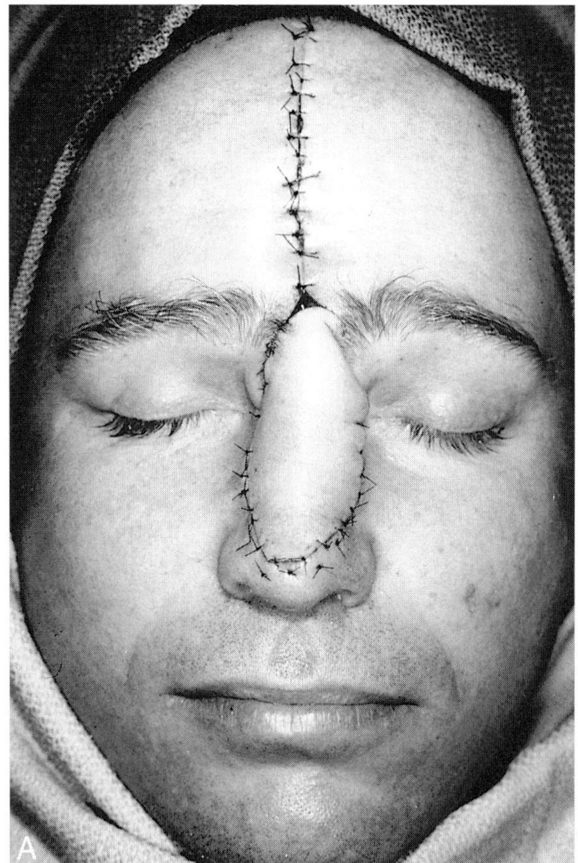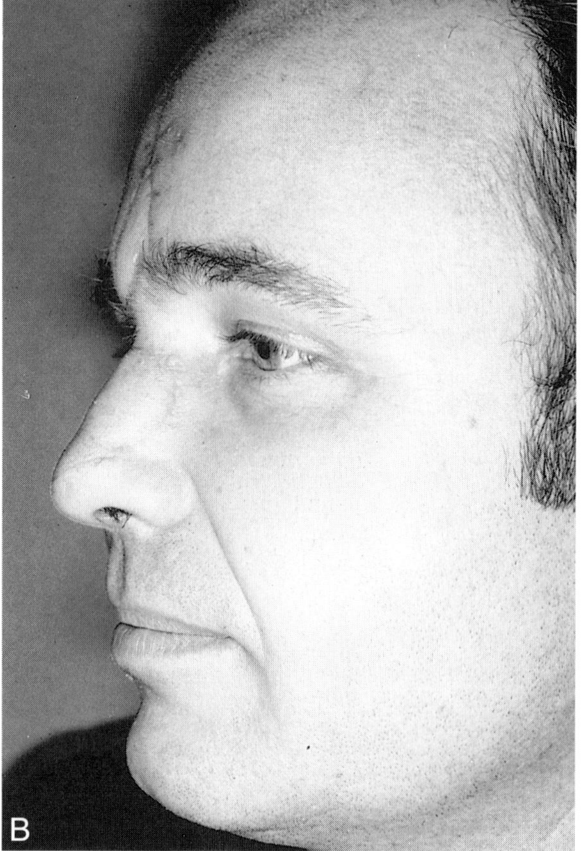

Fig. 18.12 **A.** The forehead flap based in the supratrochlear artery used to cover a full-thickness loss of the entire dorsum of the nose. The flap is outlined in reverse and transposed to the margin of the defect as described in the text. **B.** Five months later: colour, texture and contour match quite well. The forehead scar visible in this patient is avoided with techniques described in the text.

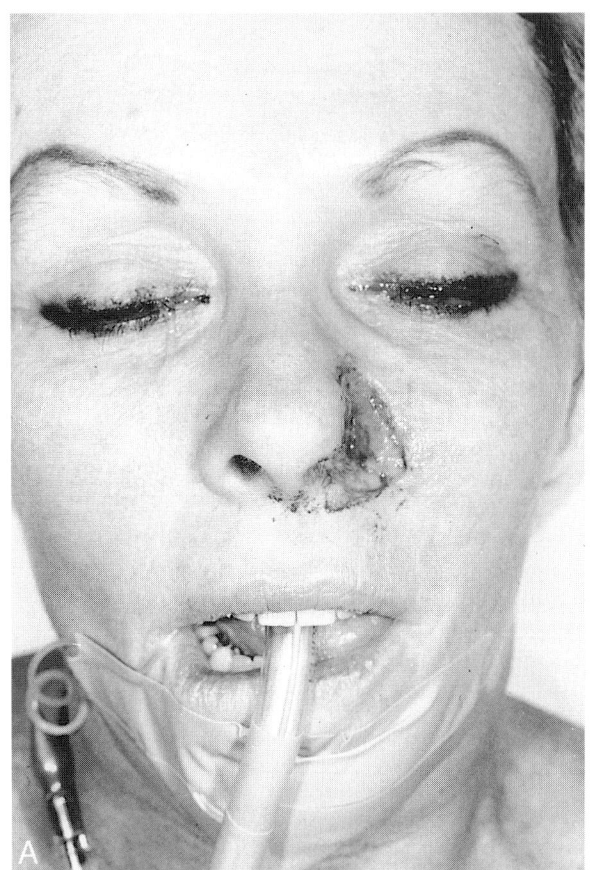

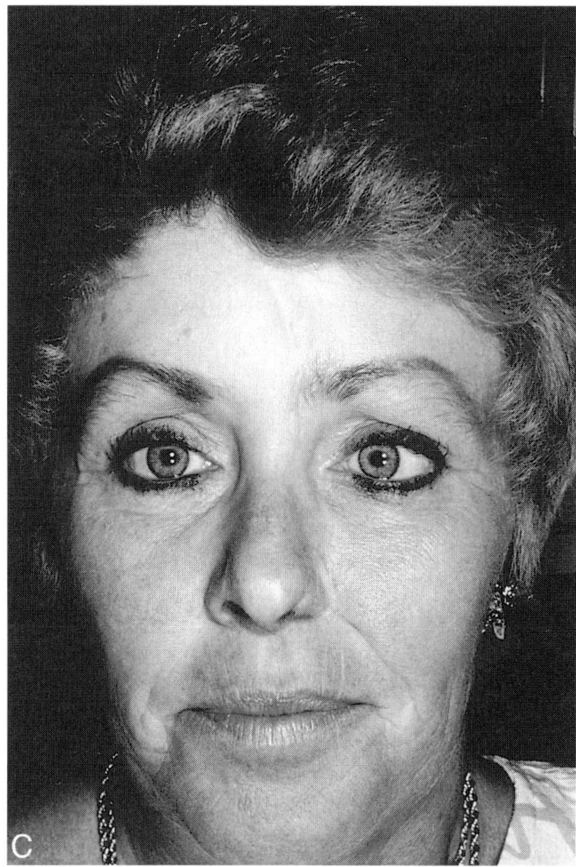

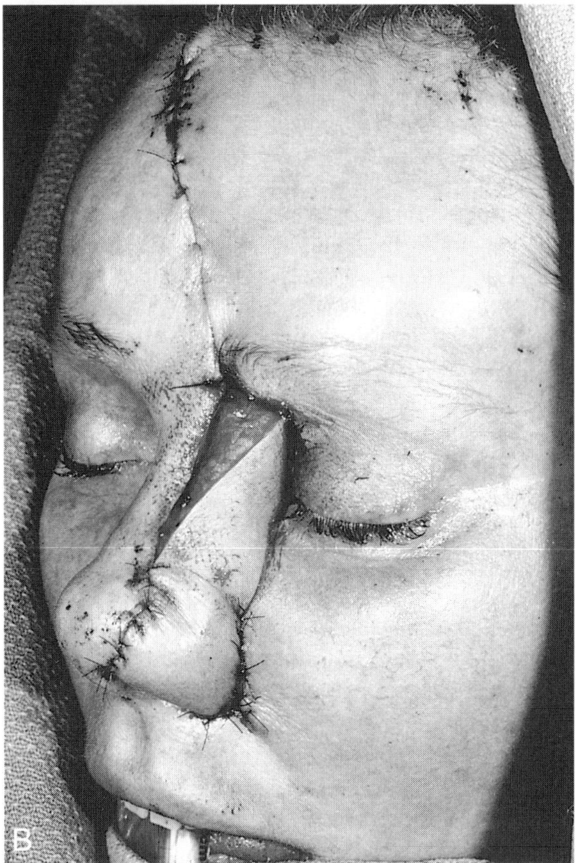

Fig. 18.13 **A.** A large defect of the ala and lateral nose in a 35-year-old woman. **B.** An oblique forehead flap to increase the length of reach is used to reconstruct both the inner lining and external surface. An interposed cartilage graft was placed to reconstruct the missing cartilage. Note arc of rotation taken at the medial canthus by the technique described in the text. **C.** The patient 6 months after rotation of the flap. Note the defect on the forehead, as described in Fig. 18.12, is minimized by discarding some of the forehead flap, rather than repositioning it. The small notch along the alar margin requires secondary revision.

2–2.5 cm. If the patient has a short forehead or a longer flap is required, the flap can be made obliquely, with little risk of significant compromise, or extended into hair-bearing scalp (Fig. 18.13). The hair follicles are removed from the back side of the flap when the flap is transposed. The flap is cut through the galeal frontalis muscle which contains the vessels near the brow, and the distal end is then thinned to the dermis to match the contour of the remaining nose. This can be safely done in the distal part of the flap because the axial vessels become more superficial and are within dermis near the hairline. Optimal rotation and use of all of the flap can be safely achieved by dissecting down to about 2 cm above the supra-orbital rim, leaving the periosteum of the skull intact. At this point, the periosteum is incised and the dissection carried inferiorly into the orbit to the level of the medial canthus in the subperiosteal plane. This safeguards the supra-orbital and supratrochlear vessels and allows the flap to be rotated from a much lower position in the orbit without tension. The flap is sutured in place for 2 to 3 weeks. The pedicle is allowed to tube spontaneously without sutures. The donor defect is closed primarily. If a wide flap is taken, the forehead is undermined extensively on each side and closed under significant tension. Occasionally scars of the forehead may require revision but the scar usually subsides remarkably. The forehead can be decreased 20% in width by advancing the scalp and still be barely perceptible to the viewer.

At a second procedure 3 weeks later, the flap is divided and inset. The remaining flap is returned to the forehead only to the level of the eyebrow. Excess pedicle is discarded rather than making an obvious flap in the forehead.

If the mucosa has been sacrificed during the tumour ablation, the nasal cavity must be recreated with some form of lining, because unlined flaps shrink and become distorted. The standard procedures for accomplishing this are turn-over flaps based on the medial scar of the defect. In the upper nose, full-thickness flaps of skin are rolled medially, based on scar. The lower nasal cavity lining is usually reconstructed by employing a nasolabial flap turned into the nasal cavity. The forehead flap is then used to cover this defect. Unfortunately, these lining flaps frequently result in a rather bulbous nose and airway compromise with significant secondary distortion as flaps subside. Split-thickness and full-thickness grafts used to line the nasal cavity usually suffer the same fate, but much more rapidly. The author's preferred technique for lining will be described later under expanded forehead flap.

Total nose reconstruction

Loss of the full-thickness nose—skin, bone, cartilage and mucosa presents an enormous reconstructive problem. Historically, many operations are usually necessary to achieve an acceptable result (Millard 1966, Mazzola & Marcus 1983, Rybka 1983). When the total nose has been lost, a very large amount of skin is needed of the external surface. The usual dictum is 3 x 3 inches (7.5 x 7.5 cm) of forehead must be used to replace the nose. Our planimetric measurements on 50 individuals indicate that approximately 35% of the forehead skin is needed to reconstruct the external nasal skin in a male and 45% of the forehead in the female. If the forehead flap is to be doubled upon itself in the Converse fashion to form lining as well as the external nose, 60% of the average male forehead is required and 70% of the average female forehead. The loss of such a significant area of forehead requires the use of a split-thickness skin graft that occasionally is more unsightly than the nose reconstruction (Fig. 18.14). To avoid a graft, many times the surgeon compromises in the amount of skin harvested. This results in a small nose with an inadequate airway.

Because of the quantity of skin required, modifications have been described to create a multiple flap gull-wing pattern to recreate the components of the distal nose (Millard

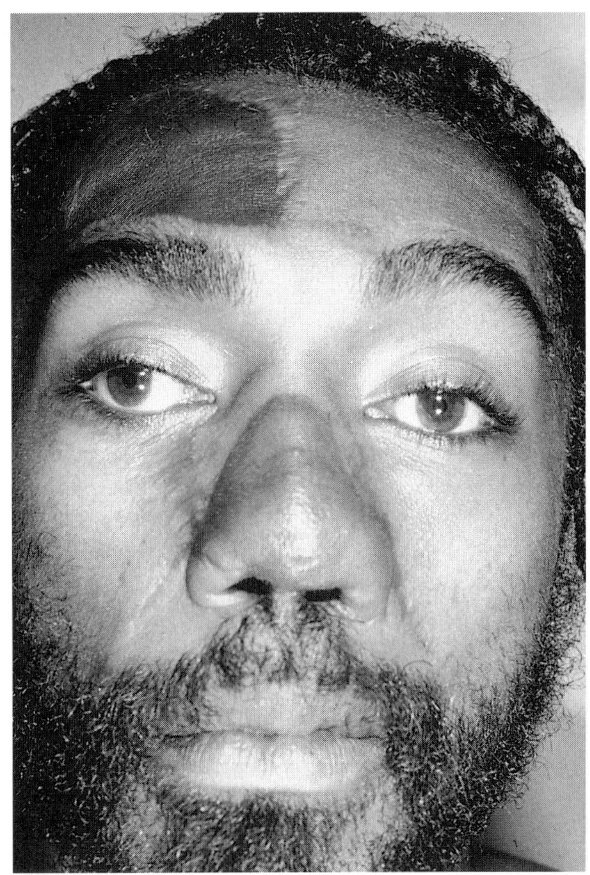

Fig. 18.14 A black male with a total nose reconstruction using the Converse technique. While the nasal reconstruction is acceptable, the hyperpigmented donor site in the forehead attracts attention.

1966). Two other flaps are designed to deliver one-half of the forehead to the pyriform area. The Converse scalping flap bases the forehead tissue on the opposite temporal vessel and mobilizes the anterior scalp as a pedicle (Converse 1942) (Fig. 18.15). The sickle flap (New 1945) is based on the opposite brow and incorporates the supraorbital, supratrochlear or temporal vessels and extends into the scalp. From here, the flap is directed in a downward direction. In this flap, one side of the forehead is used as the pedicle for the opposite side. A very large flap can be generated with either of these flaps to cover all of the nose with frequently pleasing results. Cartilage grafts or chondrocutaneous grafts can be placed in a preplanned position prior to transfer of the flap to create a more contoured natural nasal tip. Cartilage grafts placed prior to transfer of the flap seem to survive better than grafts placed later. Unfortunately, it is difficult to plan where these prefabricated noses will end up after transfer of the flap (Fig. 18.16). Both flaps can be brought down into the nasal area usually with minimal or no tension. It is sutured in place for 2 to 3 weeks after which time the pedicle is divided.

Historically, rib or iliac crest bone grafts have been placed

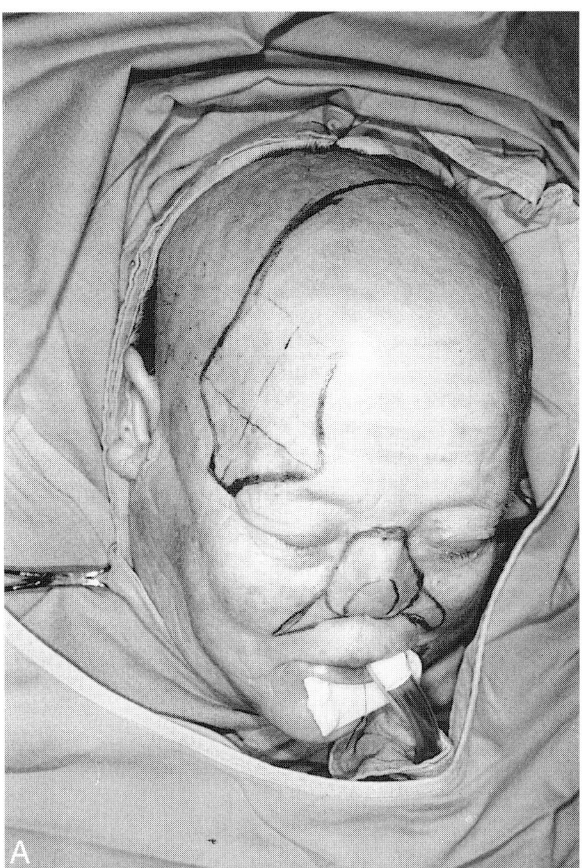 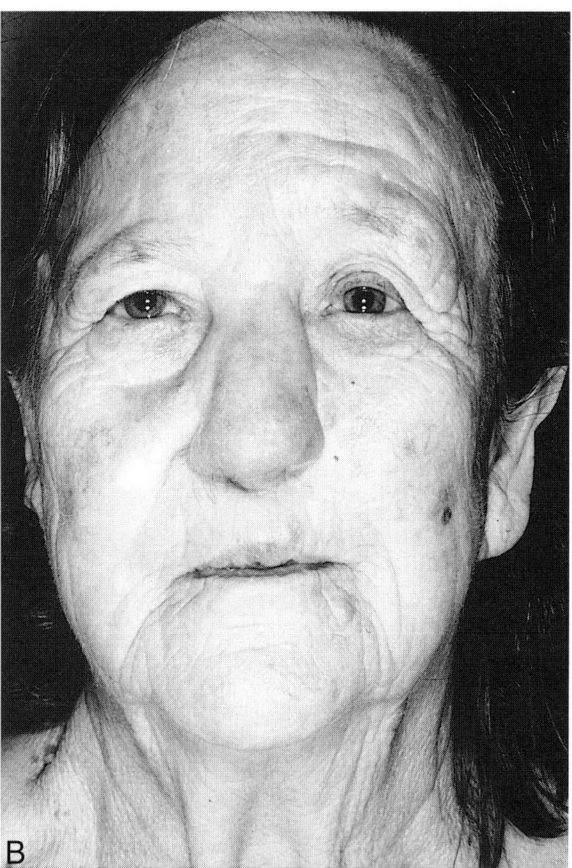

Fig. 18.15 **A.** The Converse scalping flap is useful for major defects of the nose. Full-thickness excision of the nose was required in this patient and the lining reconstructed with the outlined nasolabial flaps. **B.** After transposition and insetting of the flaps and division of the pedicle. Although this patient has an acceptable result, the slight smallness of the nose, the skin graft on the right forehead, and the brow ptosis, should be noted. These are all common secondary complications with this procedure.

to support the nasal dorsum 3 to 6 weeks after the flap has been divided. Cranial bone grafts are today usually placed at the same time as the flap is rotated into position. All total nose reconstructions require that lining of the nasal cavity be replaced (Burget & Menick 1989). Failure to replace the lining as described in the previous sections results in very poor results and frequently obliteration of the airway. Many of these reconstructed noses are bulky and become distorted with time with scar formation. Revisions, defatting, and secondary placement of support bone grafts frequently occur, and skin grafts on the forehead are unsightly. Despite these tribulations, frequently an aesthetically pleasing nose can be created.

Total nose reconstructed with expanded tissue

Tissue expansion allows the surgeon to overcome many of the problems inherent in total nose reconstruction (Fig. 18.17). The increase in vascularity of the expanded flap makes possible very large tissue transfers pedicled on a small base. This vascularity safeguards cartilage and bone grafts placed during the reconstruction. Expansion thins the tissue dramatically, allowing a more refined, detailed, non-bulky nose. A large amount of tissue can be generated so that the thinned forehead tissue can be doubled upon itself to form lining, as well as the exterior surface. The adequately expanded forehead can be closed primarily without the need for skin grafts. A functional, normal-sized nose can be created with this technique.

At the first procedure, a transverse incision is made in the hair-bearing scalp and a large tissue-expander encompassing the entire forehead and adjacent scalp is placed in the subgaleal space. Expanders (400–600 cm^3) are utilized and over-inflated to 600–800 cm^3. Over a course of 4 to 6 weeks, the expander is filled, resulting in a very significant increase in the amount of skin available in the forehead, not only for reconstruction of the nose but for primary closure of the donor defect as well.

At the second procedure, under general anaesthesia, a very large flap is based on the supra-orbital or supratrochlear

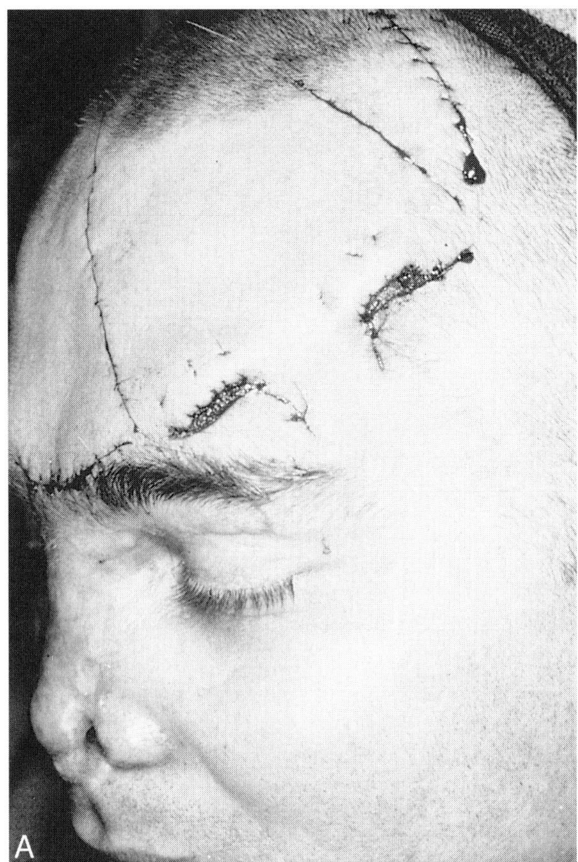

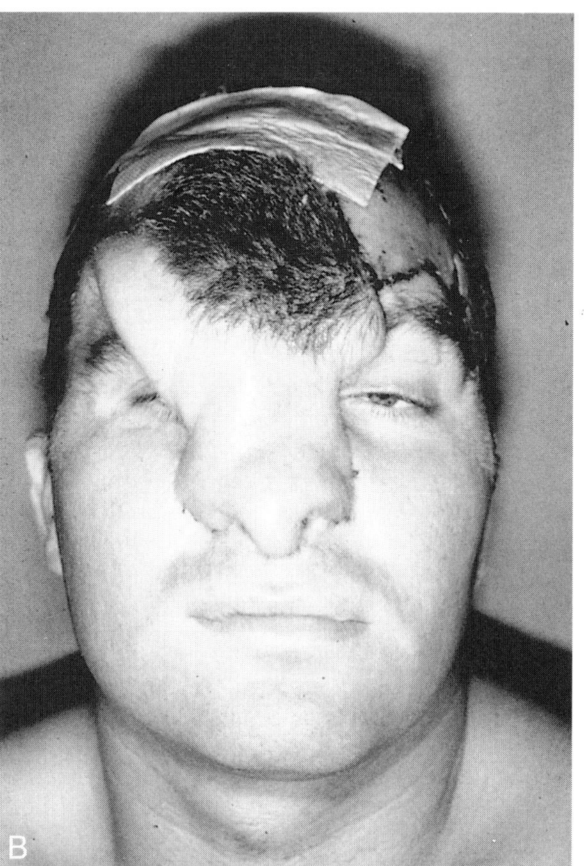

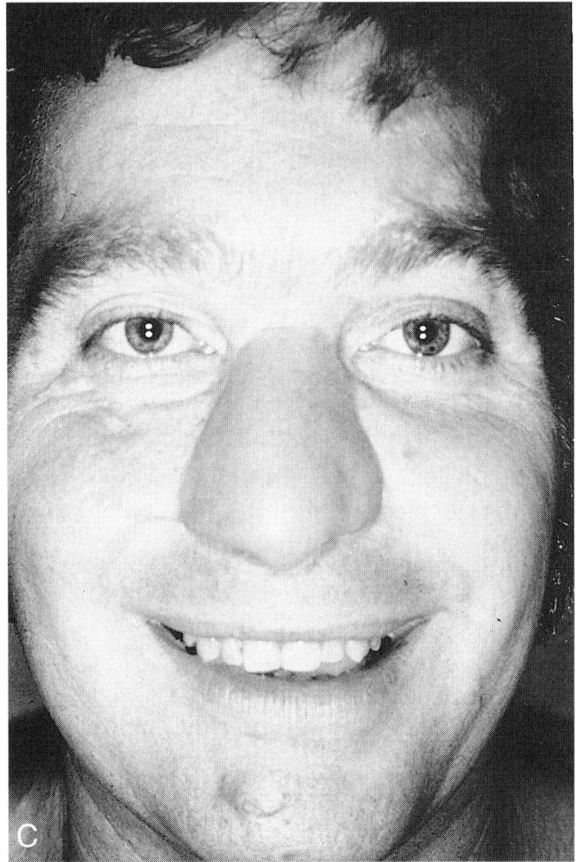

Fig. 18.16 Total nose reconstruction with the Converse scalping technique. **A.** In this patient, cartilage grafts were placed beneath the delayed forehead flap in an attempt to achieve better contour of the nasal tip. **B.** Three weeks later the flap is transferred on a large scalp pedicle. **C.** The final result reveals an acceptable, but large nose with significant loss of detail. When local flaps are rotated to reconstruct lining, such bulbousness is frequently noted.

vessels. The nose is devised retrograde using soft wax or a cloth to outline a nose both of adequate size and position. The template is folded upon itself to create a three-dimensional model—not only the external surface of the nose but the lining as well (Converse 1942). This template is then transposed to the expanded forehead in two dimensions. A pedicle of 2 cm is designed. The outlined flap is then cut while the expander prosthesis is still in place. The capsule of the expander is incised and incorporated into the flap. The dissection continues inferiorly, leaving the periosteum of the skull and the posterior capsule intact until approximately 2 cm above the supra-orbital rim. At this point, the periosteum is incised transversely and the dissection carried down inferiorly toward the medial canthus in a subperiosteal plane. This technique allows the forehead flap to be safely rotated from a much lower point and in a manner that will not obstruct vision. If the supra-orbital or supratrochlear vessels are found encased in bony foramen, the foramen is released with an osteotome to mobilize the flap maximally. Prior to reconstructing the external nose, an adequate framework is mandatory. Many of the early nasal reconstructions

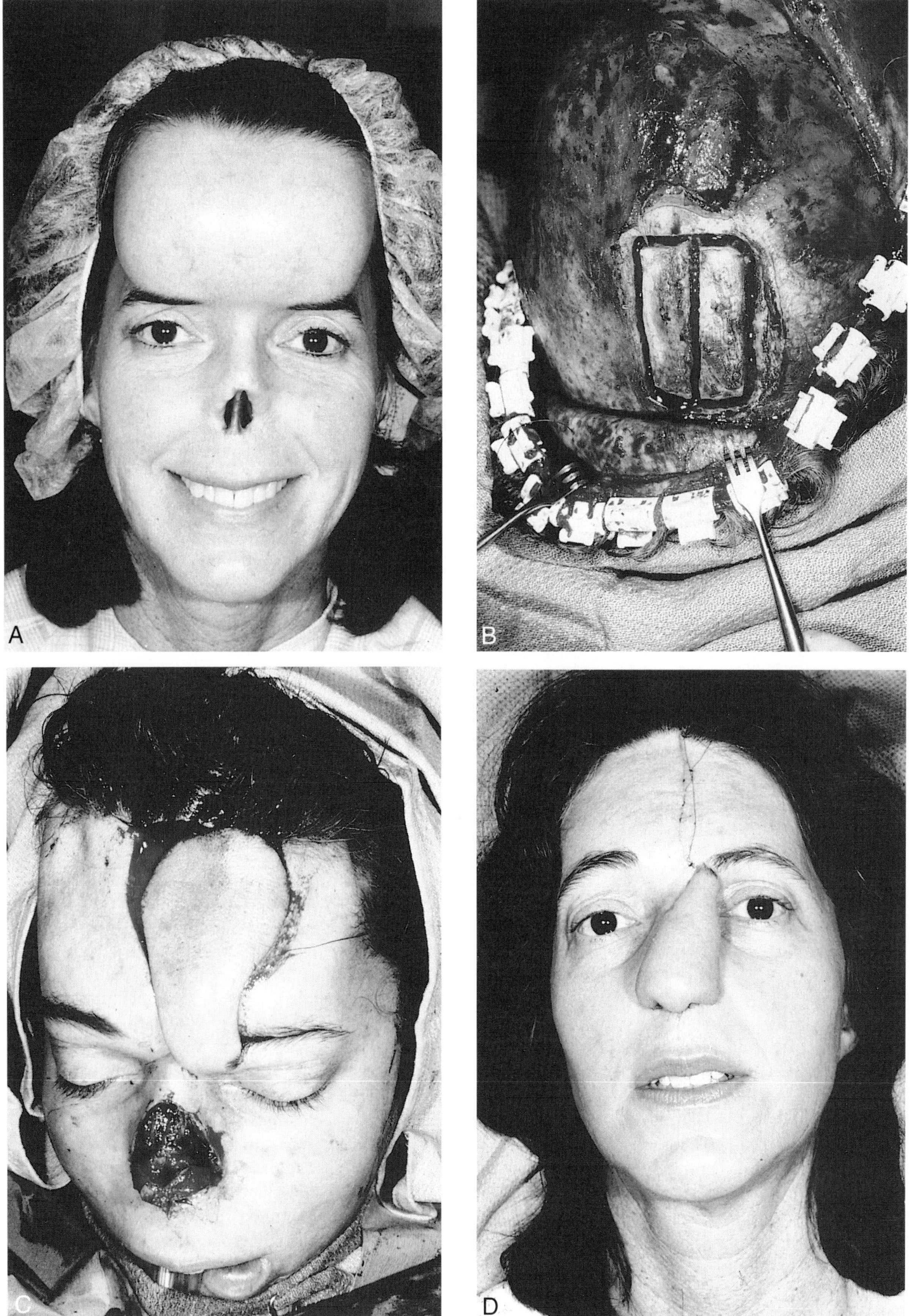

Fig. 18.17

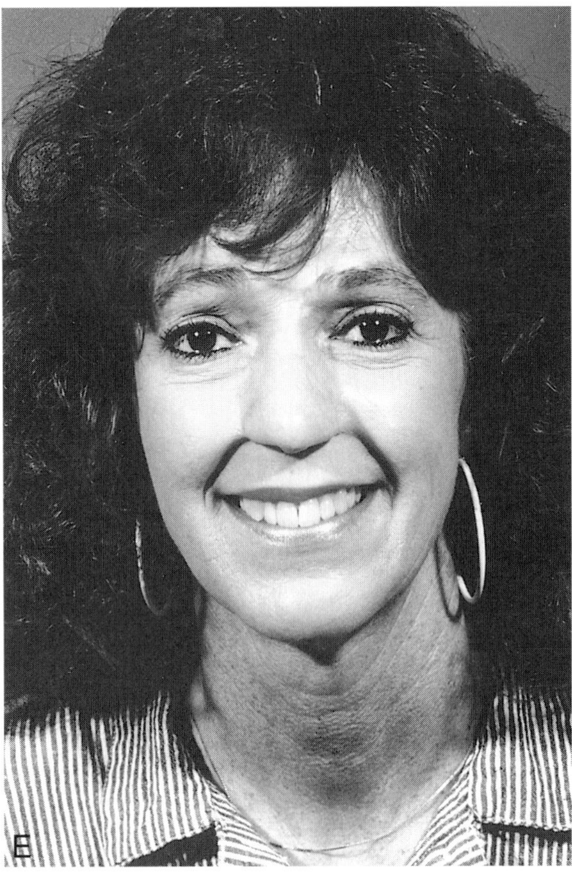 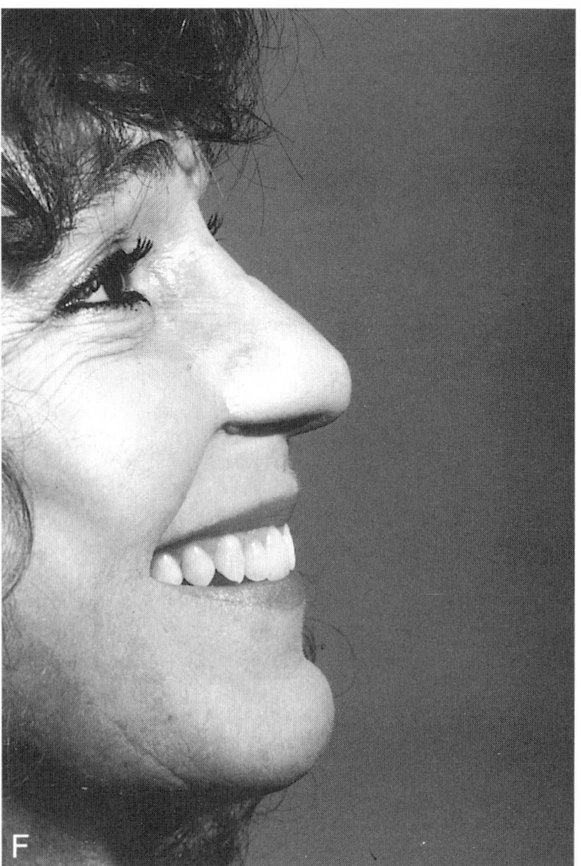

Fig. 18.17 Total reconstruction of the nose with expanded tissue. **A.** A 36-year-old female with loss of the entire nose secondary to a resection of a melanoma 6 years prior to presentation. A tissue expander, placed in the forehead through a separate incision in the scalp is expanded over 8 weeks to create sufficient tissue for reconstruction of the nose as well as to allow primary closure of the defect. **B.** The cranial bone grafts are harvested from below the hair-bearing scalp to reconstruct the dorsum of the nose. These grafts are contoured to an exact size since resorption is minimal. **C.** The infrastructure of the nose has been recreated with cartilage grafts harvested from both conchal bowls. The cranial bone graft has been wired into position to reconstruct the dorsum. The forehead flap is ready for rotation. **D.** After the first procedure, note that the flap is rotated from a point within the orbit to maximize distal reach of the flap. The forehead is closed with buried absorbable sutures and a subcuticular monofilament closure. **E, F.** The patient, 5 years after total reconstruction. There has been no secondary distortion of the nose. The patient has patent airways bilaterally. The nose is of adequate size, colour and contour. The forehead has been closed primarily.

with the expanded tissue resulted in contracted and deformed noses because of inadequate support structure. When a significant part of the bony dorsum has been lost, a cantilever cranial bone graft is placed to reconstruct this segment (Jackson et al 1983). While previous authors have used bulky rib (Millard 1966) or iliac crest bone, today's standards favour the cranial bone graft. Cranial grafts are much less prone to resorption, and a perfect size can be cut and secured in place without the need for over-correction. The graft is harvested through the superior edge of the nasal flap donor site to one side of the midline and within hair-bearing scalp. If a bony prominence is present on the remaining nasal bones it is rasped down with a burr. The cranial bone graft is then inset and wired or screwed to the remaining bony skeleton.

The lower cartilaginous portion of the nose must be reconstructed with cartilage grafts from the conchal bowl, harvested from both ears. A significant piece of cartilage is necessary to reconstruct the alar cartilages medially. Cartilages are trimmed to the exact size needed and sutured to each other and to the cantilevered bone graft medially. This graft is then secured laterally to the periosteum of the pyriform aperture. Suturing the graft laterally to subcutaneous tissue is inadequate and may result in collapse of the airway during deep inspiration. If the tip of the nose needs to be enlarged, additional cartilage grafts from the conchal bowl or septum are onlayed.

The expanded flap is then turned down and the portion to become the alar rim marked with indelible ink. The flap distal to this is radically thinned, removing both the capsule and as much subcutaneous tissue as is necessary to create a thin, yet well vascularized dermal flap which can be rotated upon itself to reconstruct both the lining and the columella (Converse 1942). The new 'lining' is sutured to what remains of the nasal mucosa and preferably to what remains of the nasal bones with absorbable suture. The external surface is then sutured to the lateral margins of the remaining nose or medial cheek. Several large monofilament sutures are used to secure the flap inferiorly as all of these flaps tend to retract superiorly. If possible, the entire aesthetic unit of the nose is reconstructed, even if some normal tissue must be discarded.

The pedicle is allowed to tube spontaneously and the small portion of exposed skull is left covered with a Vaseline gauze. The forehead is closed primarily using towel clips to approximate the edges while the nose is being fabricated. If more mobilization is needed, the lateral capsule is incised. Deep absorbable and smaller subcuticular monofilament sutures are used on the skin.

Two to three weeks later the pedicle is divided and the nose inset. Rather than returning the entire remaining pedicle to the forehead, only enough tissue to reconstruct to the level of the eyebrow and exposed frontal bone is returned. The tissue above the eyebrow is discarded so that above the eyebrow there is only one suture line. We feel that avoidance of the two parallel suture lines of the pedicle returned to the forehead makes the donor site much less obvious. Secondary contouring and defatting can be carried out after 1 month. Usually, however, the injection of small amounts of Kenalog-10 into the bulky areas of the nasal reconstruction at monthly intervals produces enough atrophy to make secondary debulking unnecessary.

REFERENCES

Argomoso R V 1975 An ideal site for the auricular composite graft. British Journal of Plastic Surgery 28: 219–221

Avelar J M, Psillakis J M, Viterbo F 1984 Use of large composite grafts in the reconstruction of deformities of the nose and ear. British Journal of Plastic Surgery 37: 55–60

Barron J N, Emmett A J J 1965 Subcutaneous island flaps. British Journal of Plastic Surgery 18: 51–78

Burget G C, Menick F J 1985 The subunit principle in nasal reconstruction. Plastic and Reconstructive Surgery 76: 239–247

Burget G C, Menick F J 1989 Nasal support and lining: the marriage of beauty and blood supply. Plastic and Reconstructive Surgery 84: 189–203

Converse J M 1942 New forehead flap for nasal reconstruction. Proceedings of the Royal Society of Medicine 35: 811–812

de Fontaine S, Klassen M, Soutar D S 1993 Refinements in the axial frontonasal flap. British Journal of Plastic Surgery 46: 371–374

Dieffenbach J F 1845 Dienasen behandlung. Operatie Chirurgie. F A Brockhaus, Leipzig

Eisenbaum S 1991 VY Reconstruction for nostril defects. Annals of Plastic Surgery 26: 488–492

Elliott R A 1969 Rotation flaps of the nose. Plastic and Reconstructive Surgery 44: 147–154

Escoffier J B 1958 The forehead flap in nasal repair. Plastic and Reconstructive Surgery 21: 94–111

Esser J F S 1918 Gestielte lokale nasanplastik mit zweizipfligem lappen, deckung des sekundaren defektes vom ersten zipfel durch den sweiten. Deutsch Zeitung für Chirurgie 143: 385–390

Goldwyn R M, Rueckert F 1977 The value of healing by secondary intention for sizeable defects of the face. Archives of Surgery 112: 285–292

Gonzales-Ulloa M et al 1954 Preliminary study of the total restoration of the facial skin. Plastic and Reconstructive Surgery 13: 151–166

Gooding C A, Yatsuhashill 1965 Significance of marginal extension in excised basal cell carcinoma. New England Journal of Medicine 273: 923–925

Guerrero-Santos J, Dicksheet S 1981 Nasolabial flap with simultaneous cartilage graft in nasal alar reconstruction. Clinics in Plastic Surgery 8: 599–602

Hagerty R F, Smith W 1958 The nasolabial cheek flap. Annals of Surgery 24: 506–510

Hamm J C, Argenta L C, Swanson N 1987 Microcystic adnexal carcinoma: an unpredictable aggressive neoplasm. Annals of Plastic Surgery 19: 173–180

Hayes H 1962 Basal cell carcinoma: the East Grinstead experience. Plastic and Reconstructive Surgery 30: 273–280

Herbert D C, DeGieus J 1975 Nasolabial subcutaneous pedicled flaps II: Clinical experience. British Journal of Plastic Surgery 28: 90–96

Jackson I T, Smith J, Mixter R C 1983 Nasal bone grafting using split skull grafts. Annals of Plastic Surgery 11: 533–540

Kazanjian V H 1946 The repair of nasal defects with the median forehead flap: primary closure of the forehead wound. Surgery, Gynecology and Obstetrics 83: 37–49

Koplin L, Zrem H A 1980 Recurrent basal cell carcinoma. Plastic and Reconstructive Surgery 65: 656–664

Limberg G D, Gibson T 1972 Closure of rhomboid skin defects. British Journal of Plastic Surgery 25: 300–314

McCollum M S & Grabb W C 1977 Increasing the incidence and size of successful experimental composite ear grafts by advance preparation of the recipient bed. Plastic and Reconstructive Surgery 60: 759–762

Maccomber W B, Berkeley W T 1967 Use of neck-tubed pedicles in reconstruction of defects of the face. Plastic and Reconstructive Surgery 2: 585–596

McGregor I 1962 Fundamental techniques of plastic surgery. Livingstone, Edinburgh

Maillard G F, Montandon D 1982 The Washio tempororetroauricular flap: its use in twenty patients. Plastic and Reconstructive Surgery 70: 550–559

Marchac D, Toth B 1990 The axial frontonasal flaps revisited. Plastic and Reconstructive Surgery 76: 686–695

Masson J K, Mendelson B C 1977 The Banner flap. American Journal of Surgery 134: 419–423

Mazzola R, Marcus S 1983 History of total nasal reconstruction with particular emphasis on the folded forehead flap technique. Plastic and Reconstructive Surgery 72: 408–414

Medawar P D 1942 Notes on problems of skin homografts. Bulletin of War Medicine 4: 1–4

Millard D R 1966 Total reconstructive rhinoplasty and a missing link. Plastic and Reconstructive Surgery 37: 167–183

Millard D R 1967 Hemirhinoplasty. Plastic and Reconstructive Surgery 40: 440–445

Mohs F E 1978 Chemosurgery: microscopically controlled surgery for skin cancer—past, present and future. Journal of Dermatologic Surgery and Oncology 4: 41–54

New G B 1945 Sickle flap for nasal reconstruction. Surgery, Gynecology and Obstetrics 80: 497–499

Pascal R R, Hobby L W, Lattes R, Crikelair G F 1968 Prognosis of 'incompletely excised' versus 'completely excised' basal cell carcinoma. Plastic and Reconstructive Surgery 41: 328–332

Rieger R A 1967 A local flap for repair of the nasal tip. Plastic and Reconstructive Surgery 40: 147–152

Rybka F J 1983 Reconstruction of nasal tip using nasalis myocutaneous sliding flaps. Plastic and Reconstructive Surgery 71: 40–44

Schmid E 1961 Partielle und totale nasenplastik. Fortschritt für kiefer und Geischtschirurgie 7: 80–88

Schmid E 1964 Nasal reconstruction. In: Gibson T (ed) Modern trends in plastic surgery. Butterworth, London, pp 145–172

Shaw W W 1981 Microvascular reconstruction of the nose. Clinics in Plastic Surgery 8: 471–480

Song R Y 1956 Total nose reconstruction: an infraclavicular tube method. Chinese Journal of Medicine 74: 223–233

Tagliacozzi G 1597 De curtorum chirurgia per insitionem. Gasper-Bindoni, Venice

Tardy M, Tental L, Azem K 1972 The bilobed flap in nasal repair. Archives of Otolaryngology 95: 1–5

von Domarus H, Stevens P J 1984 Metastatic basal cell carcinoma. Report of five cases and review of 170 cases in the literature. Journal of American Academy of Dermatology 10: 1043–1060

Washio H 1969 Retroauricular temporal flap. Plastic and Reconstructive Surgery 43: 162–166

Washio H 1972 Further experience with the retroauricular temporal flap. Plastic and Reconstructive Surgery 50: 160–162

19. Malignant tumours of the paranasal sinuses

Rammohan Tiwari   David S. Soutar

INTRODUCTION AND HISTORICAL REVIEW

Malignant tumours of the paranasal sinuses are rare in western countries, with a reported incidence of less than 1% of all cancers of the body and around 3% of all malignancies of the head and neck region. Squamous-cell carcinoma is the most common tumour and comprises approximately 2% of all squamous-cell carcinomas of the head and neck (Ali et al 1986). In some other parts of the world, particularly Japan, Indonesia and Uganda, the incidence is reported to be higher (Roush 1979, Rifki 1985, Fukuda et al 1987).

This group of malignant tumours is most frequently seen in later years of life, and most commonly in the sixth and seventh decades in the west, but younger age groups can be affected—particularly in other countries such as Japan. An association with chronic sinusitis has been reported by some authors but this remains to be confirmed. Risk factors associated with occupation have been identified with the association of adenocarcinoma of the maxillary sinus first reported in workers in the furniture industry in England (Hadfield 1970). Other occupations involving nickel, chromium, boot and shoe manufacturing, petroleum and chemical industries, polyaromatic hydrocarbons, formaldehyde and peat dust have all been said to be associated with a high incidence of malignant tumours (Roush 1979, Hernberg et al 1983, Herity 1984).

The maxillary antrum is the most commonly affected of all the paranasal sinuses, with nasal cavity, ethmoid, sphenoid and frontal sinuses following in that order (Roush 1979).

Surgery with or without radiotherapy has been the mainstay of treatment. It is difficult to be certain who first described surgery to the maxilla and paranasal sinuses. According to Fergusson, operations for tumours of the upper jaw were performed as early as the seventeenth century. White of Manchester and later Lizars of Scotland performed maxillectomy in 1826 (Fergusson 1842). In France Dupuytren claimed to be the first to propose and execute the operation and, about the same time, Gensoul also performed this procedure (Fergusson 1842, Curtin 1957). Fergusson's name is closely linked with maxillectomy and he introduced the lip-splitting incision with paranasal extension which bears his name. This incision was described in his book entitled *A System of Practical Surgery* published by John Churchill of London in 1842. History was made when President Grover Cleveland of the United States in 1833 successfully underwent maxillectomy for carcinoma (Brook 1982).

The introduction of radiotherapy to the treatment of laryngeal cancer in 1919 by Coutard attracted attention, and for a while radiotherapy became the primary mode of therapy for the treatment of malignant tumours of the paranasal sinuses (Coutard 1932). In Sweden, Ohngren and Berven introduced electrocoagulation followed by radiotherapy, and a report of 187 cases of malignant tumours of the maxilla and ethmoid treated in this way was reported by Ohngren (1933). Ohngren observed that tumours located inferior and anterior to an imaginary line drawn from the medial canthus of the eye to the angle of the mandible did well when compared to those tumours located superior and posterior to this imaginary plane. This later became known as the Ohngren line and was subsequently to form the basis for the TNM classification of maxillary tumours.

Failures in treatment under radiotherapy continued to outnumber successes to such an extent that there was a revival of surgical treatment in the 1940s. This was marked by a concurrent development in anaesthesia. Combination therapy with radiation followed by surgery was introduced but the complication rates were higher than desired. As radiotherapeutic techniques and primary surgical techniques improved, the pendulum swung towards primary surgery followed by postoperative radiotherapy and this trend continues to the present day. The results of ethmoidal cancer, however, continue to elude the therapist, because of the proximity to the base of the skull. Smith and his colleagues first attempted a transcranial and transfacial resection of a paranasal sinus tumour (Smith et al 1954). Subsequently Ketcham et al (1963) developed the craniofacial approach to ethmoidal cancer which is still in use at the present time. These techniques have now been expanded and developed so that massive craniofacial resections are now possible (see Chs 21 and 26).

Chemotherapy was suggested and used extensively (Clifford 1976) with the object of improving results. More than two decades of its use, however, has not changed the long-term survival of patients (Stell 1990).

In Japan, faced with a larger number of carcinomas of the paranasal sinuses, Sato et al (1970) introduced an unconventional regime of radiotherapy, limited surgery and topical use of chemotherapeutic agents. The regime was repeated several times and appeared to show improved results with certain types of epithelial tumour, especially adenocarcinomas (Sato et al 1970, Knegt et al 1985).

There continue to be significant problems when assessing the results of various treatment modalities in paranasal sinus tumours. There are widely differing pathologies to be taken into account and a wide variation in site. Palatal tumours, for example, sooner or later involve the floor of the maxillary antrum and partial resection of the maxilla is often performed as treatment for these tumours. In many series, such palatal tumours are included together with tumours of the maxilla. It would appear, however, that, as with other head and neck tumours, long-term results with malignant tumours of the paranasal sinuses have reached a plateau, and efforts continue to be made to improve results as well as the quality of life of these patients.

SURGICAL ANATOMY

The surgical anatomy of the paranasal sinuses which comprise the maxillary, ethmoidal, sphenoidal, and frontal air sinuses is complex (Fig. 19.1) but the advent of modern imaging techniques has made both visualization and teaching somewhat easier.

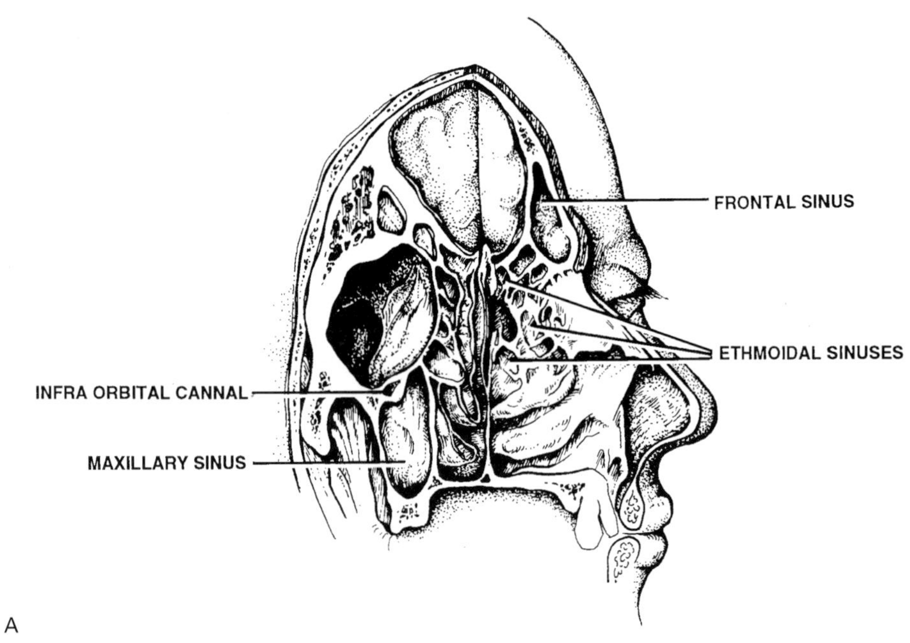

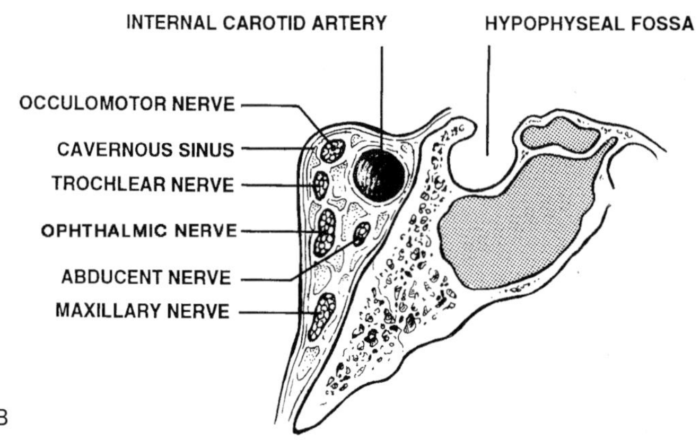

Fig. 19.1 Surgical anatomy of the paranasal sinuses.

Maxilla

The two maxillae together form the upper jaw, which is horseshoe-shaped. In a dentate patient, the roots of the canine teeth, the premolars and the molars are close to the floor and the anterior wall of the maxillary sinuses. Tumours of the paranasal sinuses may present with dentogenic symptoms, and the superior alveolus has to be sacrificed in the vast majority of cancers originating in this area. The infraorbital nerve emerging under the infraorbital margin is an important landmark. It serves as a ready pathway for the spread of cancer intracranially, and its involvement or sacrifice leads to numbness of the cheek and paranasal area.

Not all the walls of the maxilla are of the same thickness. The anterior and posterior walls of the maxillary antrum are especially thin and are relatively easily eroded by tumour. Equally, they can easily be damaged during surgery. The orbital floor is a thin bone formed by the maxilla, the zygoma and the sphenoid. It is often incomplete due to the presence of the infra-orbital canal which runs through it. Inferiorly it is lined by the mucoperiosteum of the maxillary sinus. Superiorly the periosteum of the orbital floor provides a crucial layer in the preservation of the eye and the orbital contents. It forms a strong barrier to the spread of cancer, and the inferior oblique muscle of the eye is attached to it. Laterally, the maxilla fuses with the zygoma which forms the lateral boundary of the infratemporal fossa. The posterior inferior extent of the maxilla is marked by a buttress of bone known as the maxillary tuberosity which lies against the pterygoid process of the sphenoid. The pterygoid muscles are attached to the pterygoid process.

The space between the posterior wall of the antrum and the anterior surface of the body of the sphenoid is the pterygopalatine fossa, also called the pterygomaxillary fossa. The maxillary artery enters here through a triangular space, the pterygomaxillary fissure, just above the articulation of the maxillary tuberosity and the pterygoid plates. The greater wing of the sphenoid forms the superior relation of this aperture, and extension of malignant disease into the pterygomaxillary space therefore opens the possibility of intracranial extension of disease which is often surgically not resectable. Spread of tumour from the maxillary sinus can occur by extension through the ostium or by erosion of the lateral nasal wall.

Ohngren's observation that tumours originating anterior and inferior to an imaginary line between the medial canthus of the eye and the angle of the mandible had a better prognosis is still significant and valid. Present staging for carcinoma of the maxillary antrum takes this into account (Table 19.1). Both UICC and AJC classifications are, in this respect, similar, and are based on the initial attempts at staging of the paranasal sinuses by Sisson et al (1963).

Ethmoid

The ethmoid labyrinth is located between the two orbits and

Table 19.1   Staging of carcinoma of the maxillary sinus TNM classification

T	Primary tumour
TX	Primary tumour cannot be assessed
T0	No evidence of primary tumour
Tis	Carcinoma in situ
T1	Tumour limited to the antral mucosa with no erosion or destruction of bone
T2	Tumour with erosion or destruction of the infrastructure (see anatomical division above) including the hard palate and/or the middle nasal meatus
T3	Tumour invades any of the following: skin of cheek, posterior wall of the maxillary sinus, floor or medial wall of orbit, anterior ethmoid sinus
T4	Tumour invades the orbital contents and/or any of the following: cribriform plate, posterior ethmoid or sphenoid sinuses, nasopharynx, soft palate, pterygomaxillary or temporal fossae, base of skull

just above the level of the maxillary antra. The ethmoid labyrinth is like a honeycomb with cells varying in size. The posterior ethmoid cell is the largest, and the optic foramen is its immediate posterolateral relation. The sphenoid sinus is posteromedial to it. The anterior and posterior ethmoidal foramina indicate the superior limit of the lamina papyracea and are located 2.4 and 3.6 cm from the anterior lacrimal crest. The optic foramen is said to be 4.2 cm from the anterior lacrimal crest (Rontal et al 1979). These measurements, however, were made on skulls imported from India (Harrison 1971), and racial variations are to be expected. The cribriform plate is reputed to be approximately at the level of the pupils, but in the experience of the authors it is frequently located at a slightly higher level. According to Harrison its measurements are 20 mm in length, 5 mm in breadth and 2 mm in thickness (Harrison 1972). The ethmoid labyrinth in an adult is 3–4 cm in length and 1.5 cm in width posteriorly, and 0.5–1 cm anteriorly (Mosher 1929). The perpendicular plate forms the midline partition between the two sides and continues antero-inferiorly to articulate with the vomer and the septal cartilage.

Sphenoid

The sphenoid sinuses are often asymmetrical and may expand laterally into the greater wings. The optic chiasma lies immediately posterosuperior and the cavernous sinus and internal carotid artery are closely situated laterally. The optic foramen is superolateral and anterior to these sinuses. Where a large sinus is present, these structures may be very close to the mucosa and pulsation of the artery should be looked for in such cases. The ostia of the sinuses are located superiorly on the anterior wall but very occasionally the sphenoid may not be aerated. Occasionally the sinus cavity contains another septum. The lateral attachment of this septum marks the location of the internal carotid artery.

Frontal

The frontal sinuses are very variable in size, extending superiorly into the frontal bone and laterally into the superior wall of the orbit. They may not develop at all and this is found in approximately 4% of normal individuals (Schaeffer 1920).

PATHOLOGY

Malignant tumours of the paranasal sinuses and maxilla may be osseous, connective tissue epithelial or stem cell in origin (Table 19.2). As stated previously, squamous-cell carcinoma is the most common tumour of the paranasal sinuses. The maxillary antrum is the most commonly affected of all the sinuses followed by the nasal cavity, ethmoid, sphenoid and frontal sinus in that order. Lymph node metastasis in paranasal sinus tumours, except the maxillary antrum, is rare. Tumours of the maxillary sinus have a tendency to develop lymph node metastasis when the oral mucosa, particularly the buccal surface of the alveolus and the anterolateral wall, is involved by tumour. The overall incidence at the time of first presentation is around 10% (St Pierre & Baker 1983, Sisson et al 1989). The Glasgow experience is similar, with only 6 out of 62 patients with squamous-cell carcinoma of the maxillary antrum having lymph node metastasis at the time of presentation (Robertson et al 1992).

Malignancy in the sphenoid and frontal sinuses is very rare and accounts for only 1% of all malignancies in the region. In a period of 15 years only three cases of malignant tumour of the frontal sinus and three cases of malignancy of the sphenoid sinuses were encountered by the first author at the Free University Hospital, Amsterdam. There are no known lymphatics in these two cavities, and lymph node metastasis is unknown. The behaviour of these tumours, however, is usually very aggressive.

Table 19.2 Primary malignant tumours of the paranasal sinuses

Osseous	Osteogenic sarcoma Ewing's sarcoma
Connective tissue	Chondrosarcoma Fibrosarcoma Rhabdomyosarcoma Myxosarcoma Haemangio-endotheliosarcoma Malignant fibrous histiocytoma
Epithelial	Squamous-cell carcinoma Adenocarcinoma Adenoidcystic carcinoma Muco-epidermoid carcinoma Malignant melanoma Olfactory neuroblastoma Neuro-endocrine carcinoma Malignant Schwannomas Malignant pleomorphic tumours
Other	Non-Hodgkin's lymphoma Plasmacytoma

INVESTIGATION OF PARANASAL SINUS TUMOURS

In the past, the clinical presentation and radiological appearance provided the basis for decision making. While clinical signs and symptoms remain an important step in diagnosis, the evolution of modern imaging techniques over the last two decades has revolutionized the evaluation of patients with malignant tumours. Computerized tomography in axial and coronal planes, together with magnetic resonance imaging when necessary, offers a three-dimensional look into the depths of the anatomy of this area and can provide the clinician with a reasonably accurate assessment of the extent of the tumour (Fig. 19.2).

Assessment of tumours of the paranasal sinuses begins with an accurate analysis of the nature of the malignant tumour since the therapeutic guidelines are entirely dependent on this information. The age and general condition of the patient is assessed together with the extent of the tumour

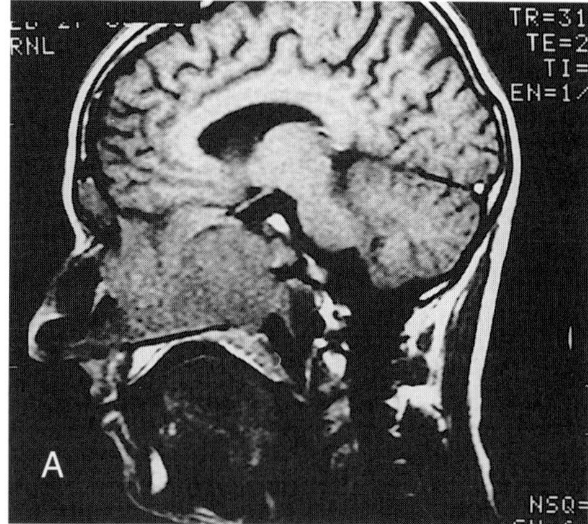
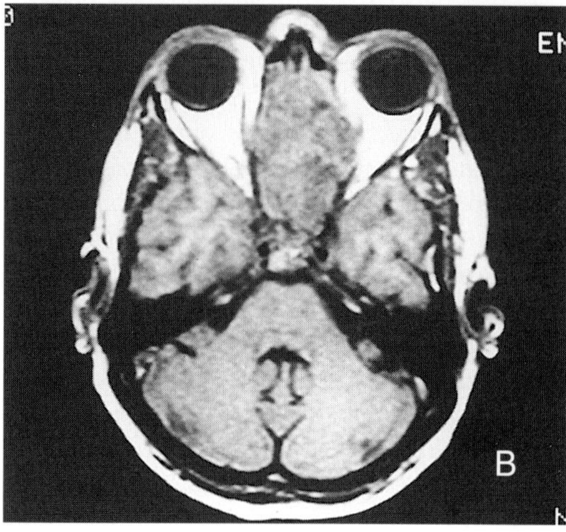

Fig. 19.2 An extensive adenocarcinoma of the ethmoid in a young male. MRI clearly shows invasion of the cranium by tumour and this necessitated a craniofacial resection (**A**). The tumour extends into the orbit (**B**) but could be dissected off the orbital periosteum on both sides.

and the presence or otherwise of palpable regional lymph nodes. Signs and symptoms should be considered as oral, nasal, ocular, facial and neurological. Clinically, the presence of trismus, displacement of the eyeball, perpetual headache and/or pain, trigeminal neuralgia and the presence of metastatic cervical lymph nodes are poor prognostic signs. Clinical assessment can be substantiated in certain cases by endoscopic examination, and where lymph nodes are palpable aspiration cytology can be performed. Where doubt exists with regard to cervical lymph node metastasis, an ultrasound-guided aspiration cytology can be performed and may be supplemented by MRI. These investigations have been shown to have a high degree of precision (van den Brekel et al 1992). Examination under anaesthetic can also provide useful information, and a biopsy for histological diagnosis is an essential prerequisite to determining treatment. CT scans in both axial and coronal planes provide

information on the extent of the tumour. Coronal scans are particularly valuable in assessing the spread of tumour in a vertical direction, e.g. extension of a maxillary antral tumour into the orbit or an ethmoidal tumour (Fig. 19.3) into the cribriform plate or intracranially. Magnetic resonance imaging (MRI) is useful in visualizing the extent of soft-tissue involvement (Fig. 19.4), particularly in the sagittal plane. While MRI delineates soft-tissue extension better, CT scan is more accurate for the assessment of bony involvement. This accuracy approaches 80% (Tiwari et al 1986). With modern software such computerized investigations can build up a three-dimensional picture of the true extent of the tumour.

PRINCIPLES OF MANAGEMENT

The principles governing treatment of malignant tumours of the palate, maxilla and paranasal sinuses relate to the patient and to the tumour itself. Patient factors such as age, general health, nutritional status, systemic illness, presence or absence of distant metastasis are similar to considerations in other branches of head and neck surgery. The significant tumour factors are the histopathology and the stage of disease. Not all malignant tumours of paranasal sinuses should be treated by surgery. Malignant lymphoma, for example, responds well to chemotherapy and/or radiotherapy, and sarcomas are often best treated with systemic chemotherapy in the first instance. With these two exceptions, most other mesenchymal tumours and epithelial tumours are treated by surgery or radiotherapy, either as single modality treatments or in combination. Many surgeons still practice pre-operative radiotherapy followed by surgery. Although radiotherapy administered before surgery shrinks the tumour, it has not proved to be very effective in disease that involves bone, and the majority of paranasal

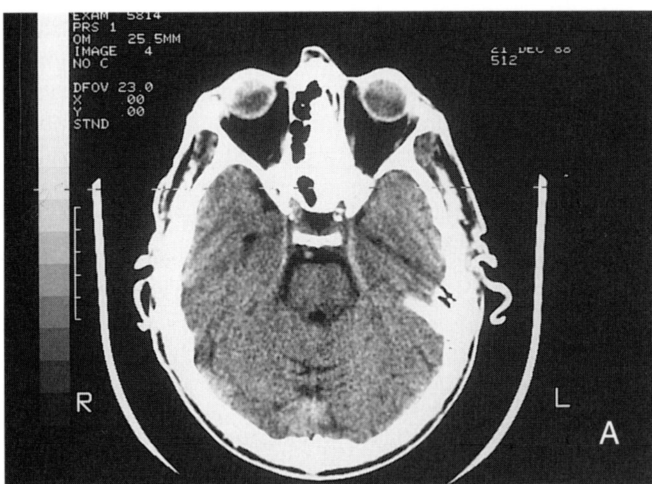

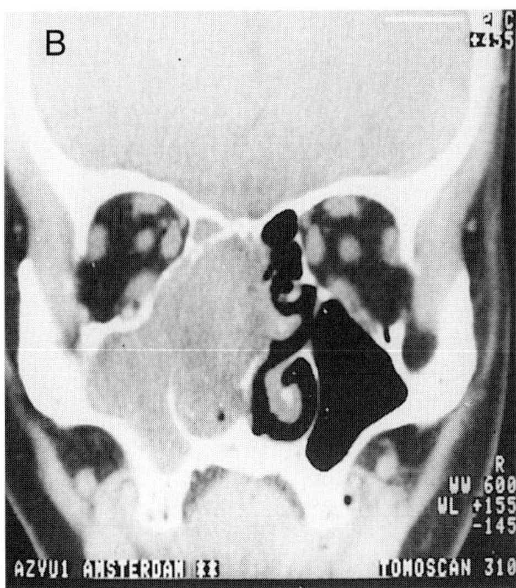

Fig. 19.3 CT scan of the paranasal sinuses in a patient with adenocarcinoma of the ethmoid. **A.** Axial view. **B.** Coronal view. Differentiation between tumour tissue and secretions is not clear.

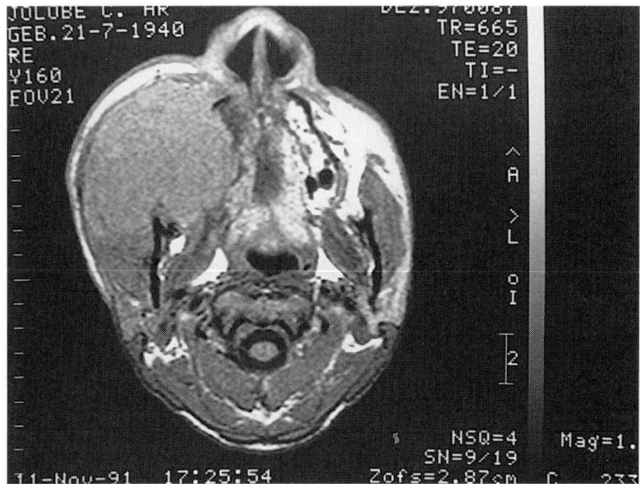

Fig. 19.4 MRI of a arge squamous-cell carcinoma (T4) in a young man. Invasion of the pterygomaxillary space and the soft tissues of the cheek is clearly delineated and proved helpful in planning surgery.

sinus tumours—particularly in the maxillary antrum—present at an advanced stage. Both the authors prefer to perform surgery as the primary treatment combined with early radical postoperative radiotherapy. Surgery allows a very accurate assessment of the extent of the disease and can significantly help in the planning of the radiotherapy postoperatively. It also provides the ideal opportunity to place accurately tubes for subsequent brachytherapy if this is indicated. Postsurgery, the tumour volume to be irradiated is much smaller and, furthermore, the complications of operating on an irradiated patient are avoided. The most important advantage, however, is that the surgeon can direct the radiotherapist precisely to the areas of concern. Areas of doubtful excision can be marked using metal clips which can subsequently be identified on the CT planning films for radiotherapy. The authors do not use chemotherapy as an integral part of management either in the form of adjuvant or induction chemotherapy. Chemotherapy is still used occasionally as intra-arterial infusion prior to other forms of treatment in cases where the general state of the patient or the advanced stage of the disease does not permit surgical intervention and the treatment is regarded as palliative.

Maxilla

Relatively small tumours (T1) are infrequent in western countries. Frequently, signs and symptoms do not occur until the tumour has breached the maxillary sinus and the majority present with advanced disease. The exception is tumours of the palate which can present early, and these can readily be treated by primary surgery or radiotherapy. This particularly applies to lesions extending onto the soft palate where excisional surgery can have debilitating effects with regard to speech and oral competence. Elsewhere, both authors prefer primary surgery with wide surgical excision to achieve clear margins. Primary radiotherapy is reserved for cases where recovery is likely to be prolonged or problems in reconstruction are anticipated. Slightly larger lesions, such as T2 tumours located anteriorly and inferiorly and not extending into the pterygopalatine space, can also be treated by radiotherapy. The problems are in accurately defining the extent of the disease—particularly when there is tumour invasion of bone. For this reason, the authors prefer primary surgery since, at this level, there is a reasonable chance of obtaining clear surgical margins, and reconstruction can be simply affected using dental obturation (Fig. 19.5). Whenever surgery is contemplated for maxillary lesions, the maxillofacial prosthodontist is always consulted beforehand and the necessary impressions taken to prepare a temporary plate or obturator. Combined planning by the surgeon and prosthodontist can have significant benefits in subsequent rehabilitation of the patient (see Ch. 8). All other maxillary lesions, i.e. T3 with extension to the pterygopalatine space or T4 involving the adjacent structures, are treated surgically followed by a full course of radiotherapy in the form of 60–65 Gy over 6 weeks using external megavoltage radiation.

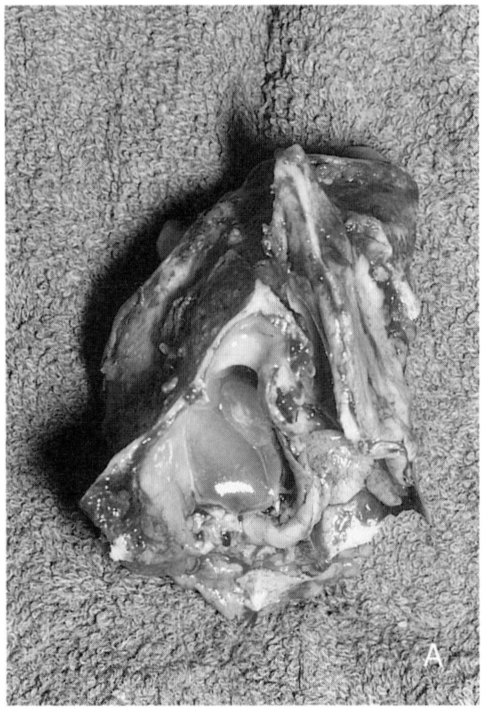
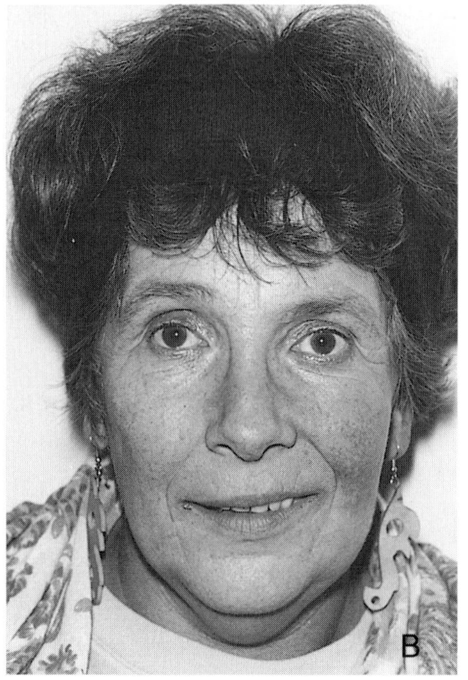

Fig. 19.5 A large osteosarcoma of the upper jaw removed transorally with histopathological confirmation of complete tumour removal **(A)**. Patient 3 years postoperatively. Note absence of external facial scars. **(B)**.

If the orbital floor or medial wall of the orbit is eroded the orbital periosteum is carefully elevated and examined. If uninvolved, the position of the globe of the eye will be maintained. If the tumour invades the orbital periosteum minimally, without extension to the ocular surface, local excision of the periosteum may be considered. The eye will need to be supported in such cases and a prosthesis will not suffice, and some form of formal reconstruction will be required. Where there is more extensive involvement of the orbital periosteum or gross invasion into the extra-ocular fat, the eye is sacrificed and orbital exenteration is carried out. Ketcham et al (1963), in a series of 86 patients, reported that whenever excision was compromised by preserving the eye it was at the cost of long-term survival. The authors agree that every attempt should be made to preserve the eye in a patient where long-term control of the disease is possible, but preservation of the eye should not be at the cost of diminishing the chance of cure. In selected patients, preservation of the eye does not appear to jeopardize survival (Bridger et al 1991).

Loss of the eye is certainly one of the most emotive factors for the patient to deal with. Sometimes it is the function of the eye, i.e. eyesight, that is most important to the patient, but most commonly it is the cosmetic deformity following exenteration which worries the patient most. In preserving the eye, therefore, the surgeon must consider both function and cosmesis. It should be remembered that in such cases postoperative radiotherapy will frequently be required and, depending on the extent of the tumour, it is often not possible to shield the retina and optic nerve satisfactorily so that a number of patients may eventually lose visual function following radiotherapy. In such cases, the only advantage of preserving the eye lies in cosmesis and, to preserve this, accurate reconstruction at the time of surgery may be required.

Whenever the periosteum is breached, there will be herniation of the extra-ocular fat and subsequent displacement of the globe unless Tenon's capsule is preserved intact. This will result in a degree of enophthalmus and globe displacement and postoperative diplopia. It is essential therefore in reconstruction to maintain the position of the globe and the volume of the orbital contents. Extension to the pterygopalatine fossa is frequent in T3–T4 tumours. In these cases, following removal of the maxilla, the pterygoid processes and pterygoid muscles are resected along with the tumour up to the sphenoid.

Extension of maxillary antral tumours to ethmoids, base of the skull and cribriform plate can usually be determined pre-operatively with the aid of CT and MRI scans. In such situations, the surgeon should consider a combined craniofacial approach. Much depends on the training and experience of the operator but in the absence of proper neurosurgical training it is advisable to carry out this surgery in combination with a neurosurgeon. Although excision of lesions involving the cribriform plate through a rhinological approach has been described (Suarez Nieto et al 1988), both authors prefer an intracranial approach. This allows identification of the intracranial extent of the tumour and the feasibility of resection. Limited involvement of the dura is not a contraindication to surgery. The dura can be radically excised and substituted with lyophilized dura or fascia most readily obtained overlying the temporalis muscle. In experienced hands, craniofacial tumour resection has proved worthwhile in selected cases (see Ch. 21).

We do not advocate elective lymph node dissections since lymph node metastasis is, on the whole, rare in paranasal sinus tumours. Whenever cervical lymph node metastasis is present (N+) a formal neck dissection is performed. In the presence of positive nodes, postoperative radiotherapy is extended to incorporate the cervical area. Lymph node involvement especially occurs when tumours spread to the soft palate, buccal mucosa or the outer surface of the alveolus and is associated with a poor prognosis.

Following excision of large lesions, a tracheostomy is advisable to ensure a safe airway. In lower maxillectomies, however, this is not generally required. In extensive surgery, it is also advisable to carry out a middle ear drainage with placement of a grommet on the side of surgery to prevent secretory otitis. In excisions for T1 and T2 tumours, a temporary obturator can usually be wired in situ using circumzygomatic wires. This allows immediate oral competence and function and such patients can commence an oral diet. For more extensive resections, nasogastric feeding may be required for a period of 7 to 10 days. Temporary obturators are usually removed under general anaesthetic at 2 to 3 weeks, at which time further impression can be taken for dental prosthesis. Postoperative radiotherapy commences between 4 and 6 weeks following surgery and, wherever possible, the patient is fitted with a temporary dental prosthesis.

Ethmoid

Malignant tumours of the ethmoid, without involvement of the cribriform plate, but with extension to the nose or maxillary sinus, are treated by surgery followed by full-course radiotherapy. Macroscopic removal of the tumour is performed through a lateral rhinotomy. The frontal, ethmoid, sphenoid and maxillary sinuses on the side of the lesion and, if necessary, on the other side, and the nasal cavity on the side of the lesion, are converted into one cavity (Fig. 19.6).

The maxillary antrum on the involved side is entered through the anterior wall with an electric drill. The opening is enlarged to encompass the anterior wall almost completely while preserving the inferior orbital vessels and nerve. The mucosa and/or tumour is systematically removed and marked appropriately for the pathologist. The periosteum of the lateral wall of the nose is separated from the bony anterior nasal aperture and this dissection is pursued posteriorly. The frontal process of the maxilla and

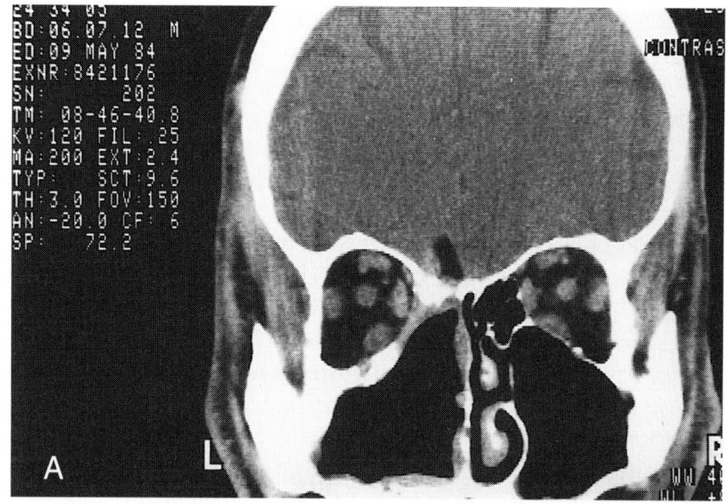

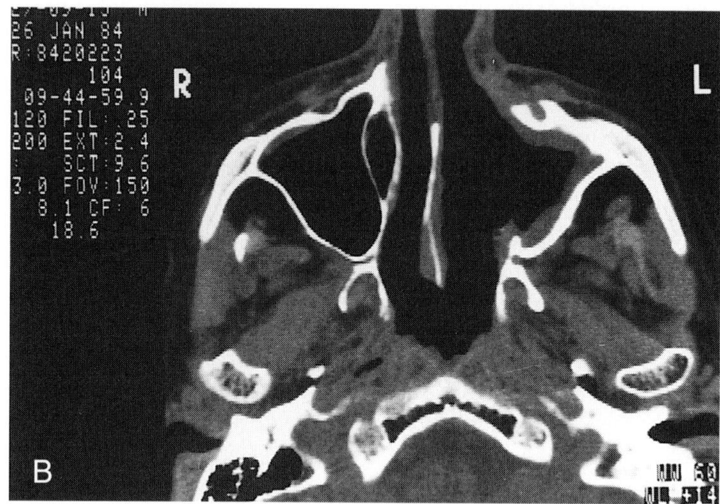

Fig. 19.6 Postoperative coronal (**A**) and axial (**B**) CT scans following macroscopic tumour removal through a left lateral rhinotomy.

part of the nasal bone is removed while preserving the margin of the orbit. The membranous lateral wall of the nose is entered just caudal to the bony anterior nasal aperture and the nasal cavity is examined. The bony defect created as a result of the removal of the frontal process and part of the nasal bone provides entrance into the anterior ethmoid. The periosteum of the orbit is elevated from the lamina papyracea and the anterior and posterior ethmoidal arteries are coagulated. The nasolacrimal duct is divided.

The posterior ethmoidal cell is medial and posterior to the posterior ethmoidal artery and also serves as a guide to the sphenoid sinus. The optic canal is just lateral to the posterior ethmoid cell. With this in mind, the entire ethmoid complex can be removed.

To enter the ethmoid on the opposite side, the perpendicular plate is removed and the cells on the opposite side dissected out. Specimens obtained from the ethmoid and sphenoid sinuses and the nasal cavity are sent separately for histological examination. The cavity is irrigated and the rough bony edges smoothed. The information obtained on histological examination from the differing specimens provides the radiotherapist with essential information regarding site or sites where treatment should be focused.

The palate and the orbit, except in exceptional cases, remain intact. A fine silicone tube is inserted into the nasolacrimal duct after initial dilatation to prevent obstruction. The tube is kept in place for 3 months following completion of postoperative radiotherapy (Fig. 19.7). A temporary vaseline pack is kept for 48 to 72 hours following surgery, and radiotherapy is instituted as soon as possible, preferably within 6 weeks of surgery. This can be followed by brachytherapy to the site of the primary tumour, i.e. the ethmoid region (Karim et al 1990). The advantage of this regime is that the cavity can be regularly inspected and kept clean.

More extensive ethmoid tumours require a craniofacial approach. A bicoronal incision gives the best cosmetic result but it sometimes interferes with access during a combined

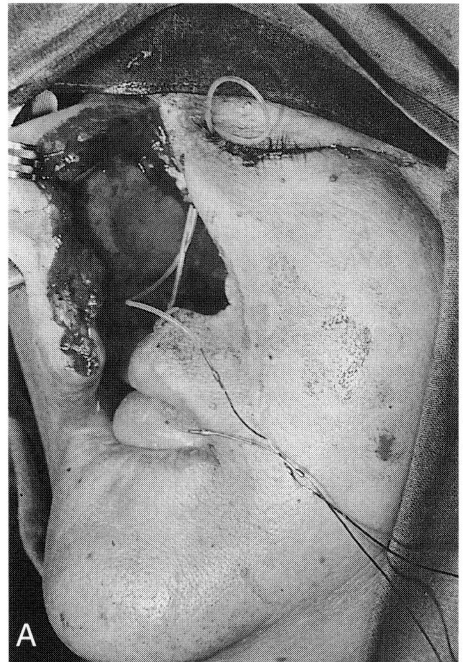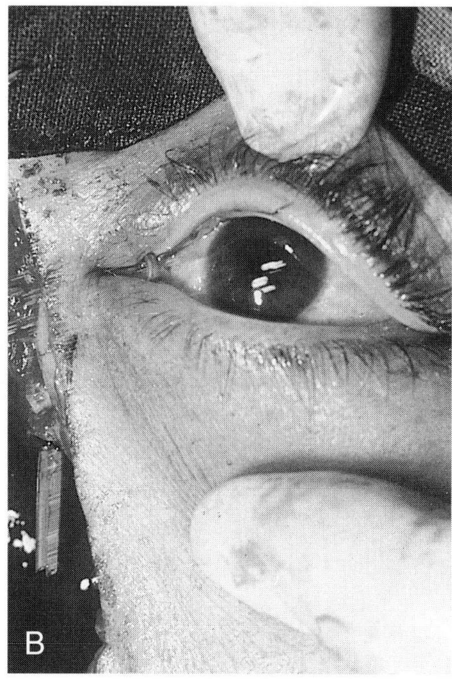

Fig. 19.7 Canalization of the nasolacrimal duct in a patient following total maxillectomy (**A**). The silicone tube is maintained in position in the nasolacrimal duct (**B**).

nasal and transcranial approach, particularly towards the end of the procedure. The vertical extension of the lateral rhinotomy incision provides easier access and satisfactory cosmetic results. Before embarking on this incision, it is useful to get an idea of the dimensions of a pericranial flap that might be needed to replace bone. A one-to-one lateral X-ray of the skull provides accurate assessment of the distance between the glabella and the hypophyseal fossa. A length 2 cm longer than this distance will cover the defect satisfactorily. No bony replacement of the ethmoid is required. A segment of frontal bone is removed in a block either as a trefine or in the form of a pentagon or shield (Fig. 19.8). The ethmoid is explored by careful elevation of the dura which is coagulated with a bipolar diathermy at points where the branches of the olfactory nerves enter the nasal cavity. Bony excision includes the posterior wall of the frontal sinuses, the jugum sphenoidale and part of the orbital plates of the frontal bone on both sides. The incision is marked with a fine burr and completed using a thin osteotome. If the superior orbital wall requires to be included in the excision then these incisions are altered accordingly. At the end of the operation, the pericranial flap is lined on the nasal side using a split-thickness skin graft (Fig. 19.8).

Frontal sinuses

Malignant tumours of the frontal sinuses are exceptionally rare but the authors favour primary surgery followed by radical radiotherapy. A craniofacial approach is ideal.

Sphenoid sinuses

Tumours of the sphenoid sinuses are seldom seen. Radiotherapy is the mainstay of treatment. The sphenoid sinus, however, usually requires a transnasal–trans-septal approach for the purpose of a biopsy to determine the histological diagnosis. Most commonly at this time a debulking procedure of the tumour is carried out prior to irradiation (Fig. 19.9). Intracranial extension of these tumours requires close co-operation with a neurosurgical team, trained in skull-base surgery.

SURGICAL APPROACHES

Access to malignant tumours of the paranasal sinuses may be through the following approaches which may be used either singly or in combination.

Transoral

This is a suitable route for smaller lesions of the palate and the superior alveolus. However, even larger tumours may be successfully and totally removed through this approach using a wide sublabial incision and raising a cheek flap in a degloving manoeuvre. Large tumours involving half of the

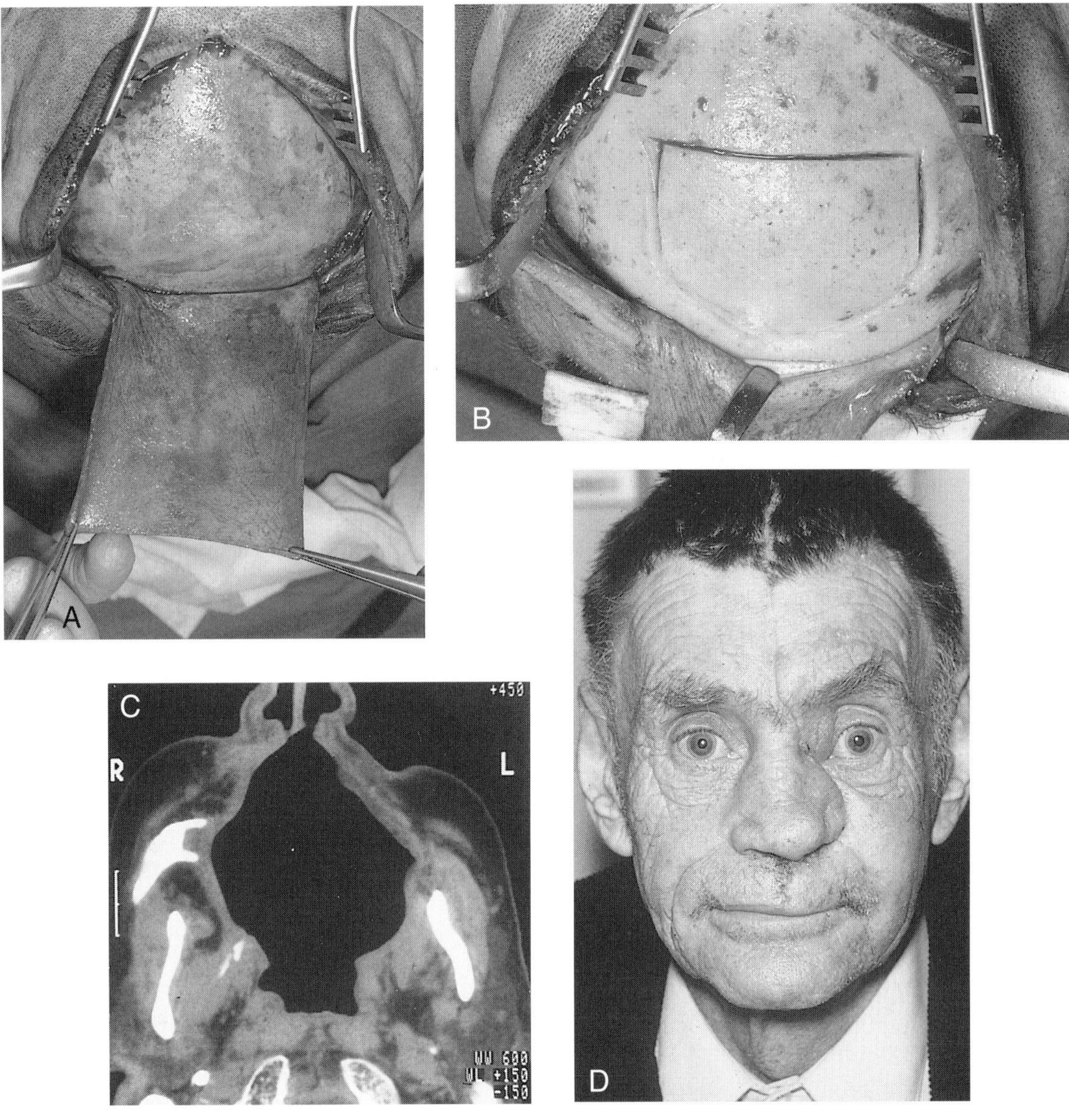

Fig. 19.8 Craniofacial resection for squamous-cell carcinoma of the ethmoid in a patient who had previously undergone a left maxillectomy. A pericranial flap is raised via a midline vertical forehead approach (**A**). A shield-shaped portion of frontal bone is removed. (**B**). A single cavity defect is created (**C**). A satisfactory recovery and cosmetic result is achieved 4 weeks following surgery (**D**).

upper jaw have been removed and total maxillectomy performed (Fig. 19.10). Selection of cases and experience of the operators are crucial factors. The technique has the advantage of preserving the integrity of the patient's face but it should not be used at the cost of incomplete tumour removal. Gross tumour extension into the soft tissues of the cheek can make this approach difficult but suitable retractors (Brunnings) can be helpful.

Lateral rhinotomy

This approach is used especially for tumours of the ethmoid and nasal cavities when the tumour does not involve the cribriform plate.

Paranasal lip-splitting incision

This has greatly simplified the procedure of maxillectomy and was originally described by Fergusson (1842). It can be extended laterally infra-orbitally as a Weber or Dieffenbach extension or superiorly over the forehead as a Lynch extension. The paranasal incision is in most cases adequate even to visualize the periosteum on the infraorbital rim and explore the orbit. Only when the anterior extent of the

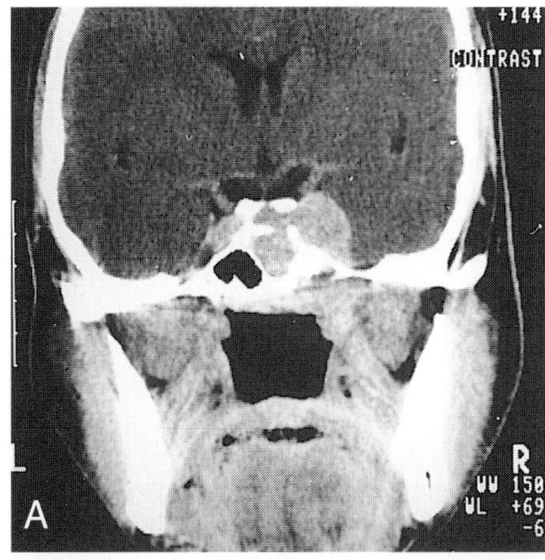

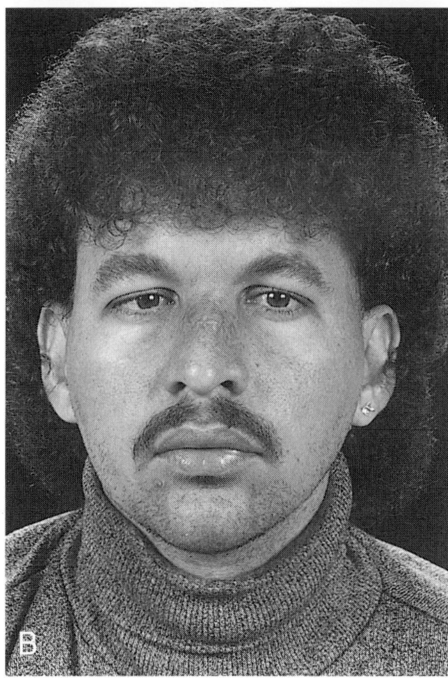

Fig. 19.9 CT scan showing presence of an adenoidcystic carcinoma of the sphenoid with intracranial extension. This young man presented with a history of headaches. **A**. Debulking of the tumour was performed via a transnasal osteoplastic flap approach. There is an acceptable cosmetic result. Note the abducent paresis on the right **(B)**.

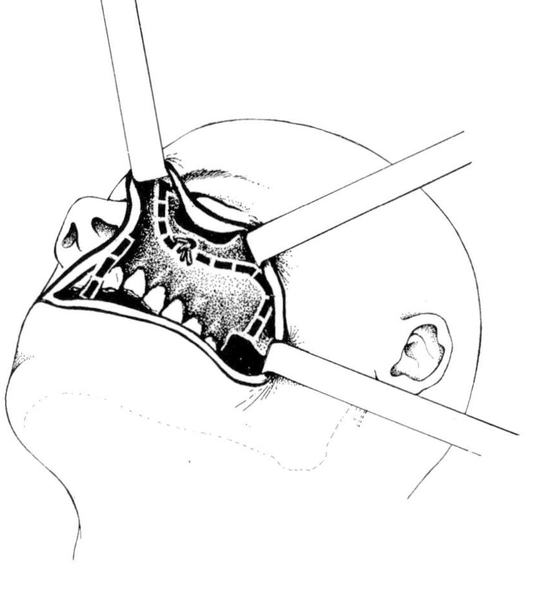

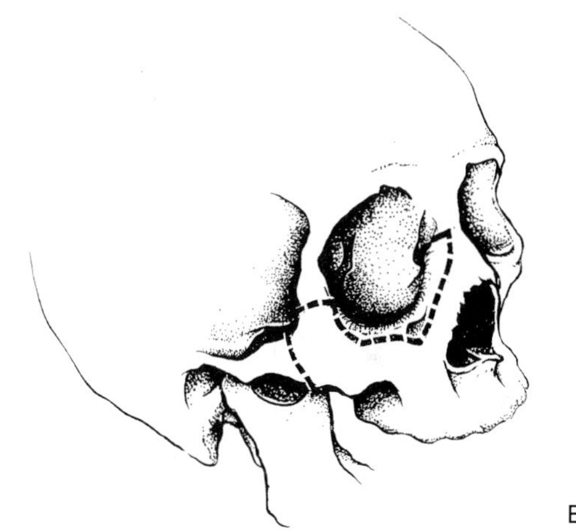

Fig. 19.10 Transoral partial maxillectomy showing the extent of exposure **(A)** for access to the bony incisions **(B)**.

tumour in the soft tissues of the cheek is large or orbital exenteration is contemplated, do the authors use the infraorbital extension. Suturing the subcutaneous lid tissues to the periosteum can help minimize postoperative ectropion. In recent years, modifications and improvements of this approach have been described and these are said to improve the end results (Osborne et al 1987).

Craniofacial approach

This has now become a standard approach for tumours involving the cribriform plate and the anterior base of the skull. A bicoronal incision is particularly useful in gaining access and craniofacial approaches have proved to be safe and effective and are used even in children (Supance & Seid 1981). In recent years, modifications have been described where the head and neck surgeon and the neurosurgeon approach the tumour through the same incision instead of separate incisions (Panje et al 1989).

Transmandibular

Barbosa described a transmandibular approach for extensive tumours of the paranasal sinuses (Barbosa 1961). This certainly provides good exposure of the pterygopalatine fossa and also gives access to the skull base.

Trans-septal

The trans-septal approach to sphenoid sinuses, commonly

used in hypophysectomy, can also be useful for debulking tumours in this area.

Transfacial approach

The transfacial approach described by Hernandez Altimer (1986) provides a facial split which gives excellent access to the postnasal space and retromaxillary structures and base of skull. Essentially, the maxilla and zygoma are osteotomized to allow it to be swung laterally with the bone still attached to the cheek tissues. The sites of the osteotomies can be varied depending on the proposed tumour extension making this a very versatile osteoplastic technique (Brown et al 1991).

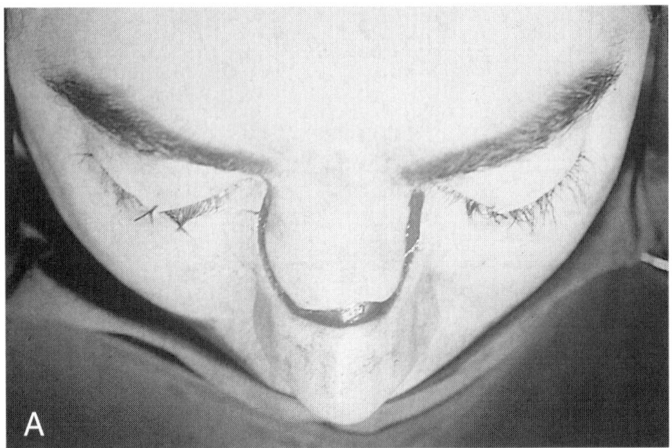

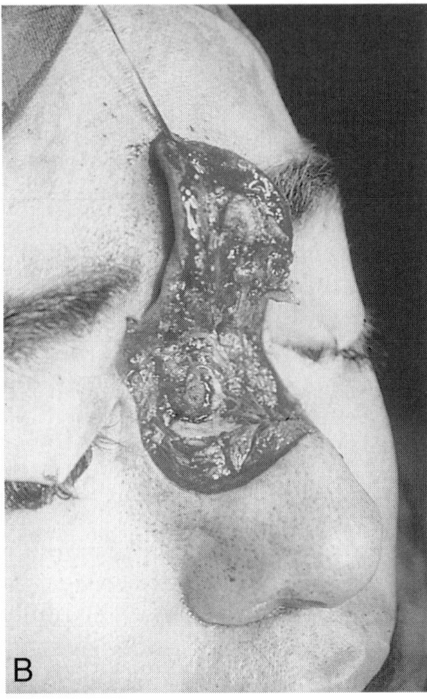

Fig. 19.11 The incision for a transnasal osteoplastic approach to the ethmoid and sphenoid sinuses (**A**). The skin flap is raised, including the nasal bones, to give direct access to the sinuses (**B**).

Transnasal osteoplastic flap

This is an alternative approach used by the first author. It consists of a U-shaped incision from the medial end of one eyebrow to the other. The nasal bones along with the attached skin are lifted cranially as an osteoplastic flap. This provides direct access to the ethmoid and sphenoid sinuses (Fig. 19.11).

RECONSTRUCTION

Radical surgery can result in large defects of the palate, maxilla and orbit, including orbital exenteration, but these can often satisfactorily be obturated and the patient rehabilitated. The advent of osseo-integrated Branemark implants for both dental rehabilitation and for external facial prosthesis has placed increasing demands on the reconstructive elements of surgery. Here again, the expertise of the maxillofacial prosthodontist is essential in designing appropriate reconstruction. This applies particularly to reconstruction of the facial skeleton at key points which allow for osseo-integration of implants to permit a satisfactory facial prosthesis to be worn postoperatively. In such extensive excisions, reconstruction must be planned beforehand and the alternatives discussed with the patient.

There remains a debate as to whether to obturate so that a cavity can be regularly inspected for tumour recurrence or whether the defect should be reconstructed, perhaps obliterating the defect and hiding any evidence of tumour recurrence. Obturation of defects which allows regular inspection is acceptable only if there are other treatment modalities available should the tumour recur. All too often, however, the tumour recurs in a site which is not amenable to further surgery or any treatment other than palliation. Such patients often die in misery with fungating, ulcerating and bleeding tumours extruding from an open defect. On the other hand, immediate reconstruction of the defect is sometimes mandatory, for example, to preserve the position of the eye following removal of the periosteum or to pack off and protect the brain from ascending infection in extensive resections involving the skull base. It is now the authors' practice to obturate dentally all patients where there is no danger of collapse of the cheek and where the zygoma and orbital margins have been preserved intact. This applies essentially to smaller resectable lesions. In more extensive lesions, where the meninges and/or orbital contents are exposed, primary reconstruction is performed and this policy has allowed for more radical excision of the tumour with confidence that the reconstruction can prevent ascending infection to the brain and maintain satisfactory cosmesis.

Unfortunately, there are very few local flaps available for reconstruction of such extensive defects. Flaps such as the pericranial flap (Schramm et al 1979), the galeofrontalis flap, the temporogaleal flap, and the temporalis muscle flap (Arden et al 1987), although useful in protecting the brain

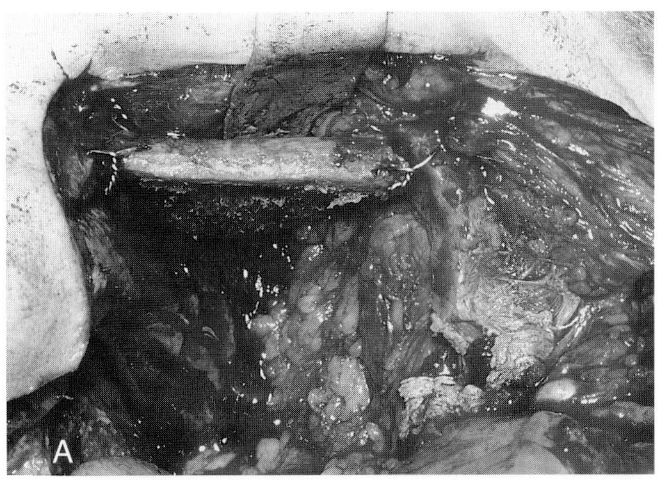
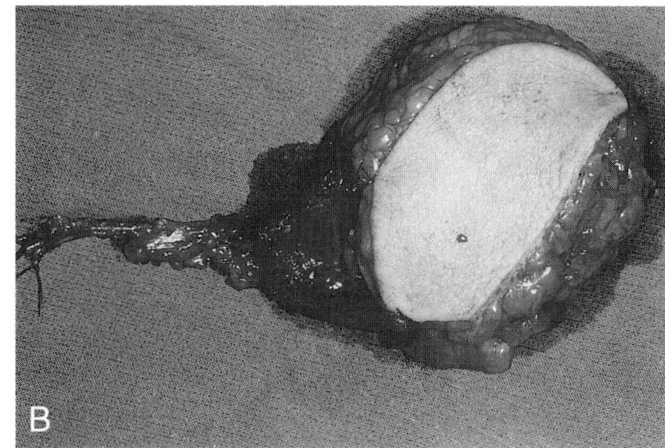
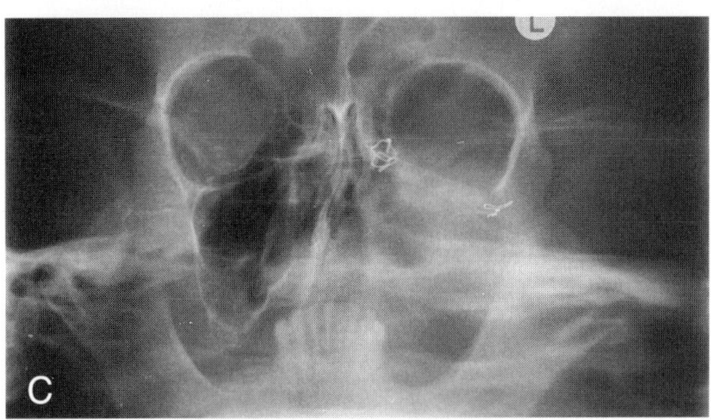
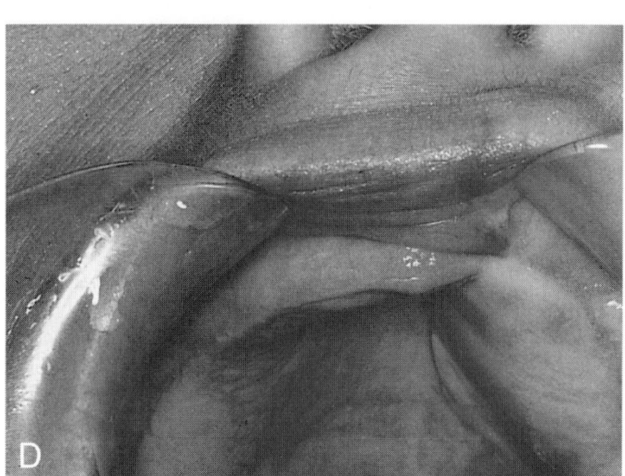
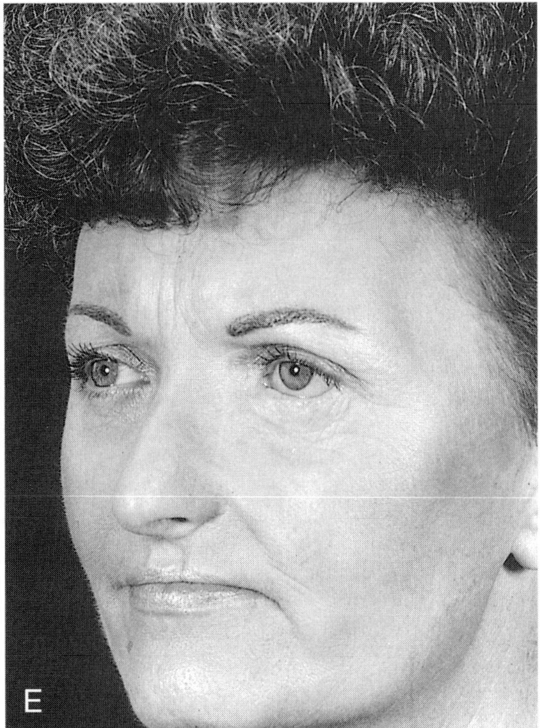

Fig. 19.12 Total maxillectomy including the orbital floor and adjacent periosteum. An iliac crest free bone graft is wired in place to reconstruct the orbital floor and support the globe of the eye (**A**). The oronasal defect is closed using a rectus abdominus myocutaneous free flap (**B**). The patient underwent postoperative radiotherapy and the appearance of the bone graft at 1 year is shown (**C**). The patient remains disease-free at 5 years. The skin of the rectus abdominus flap lines the oral cavity (**D**). The eye has been preserved, and there has been no loss of vision at 5 years (**E**).

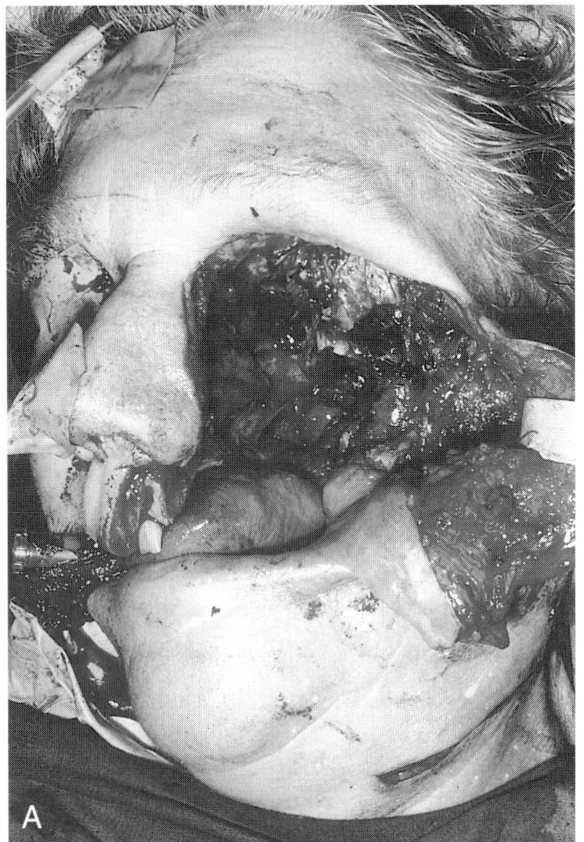
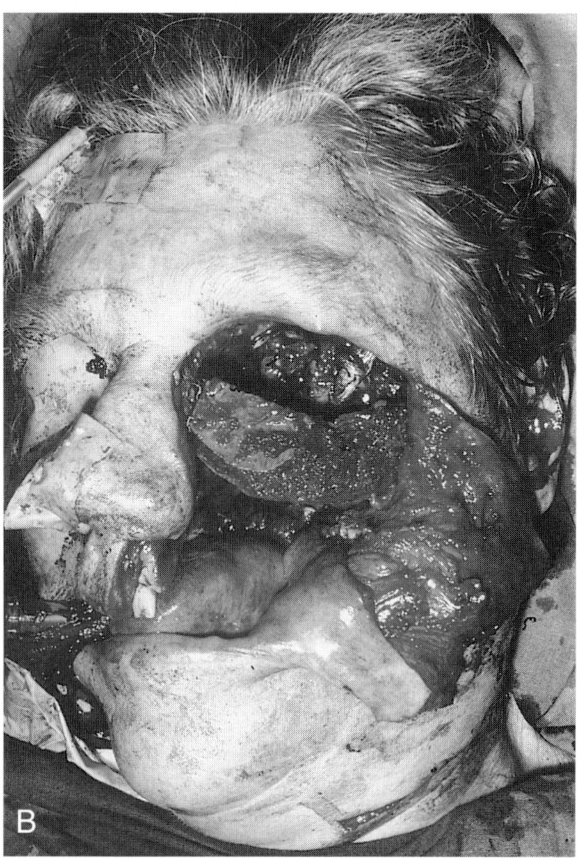
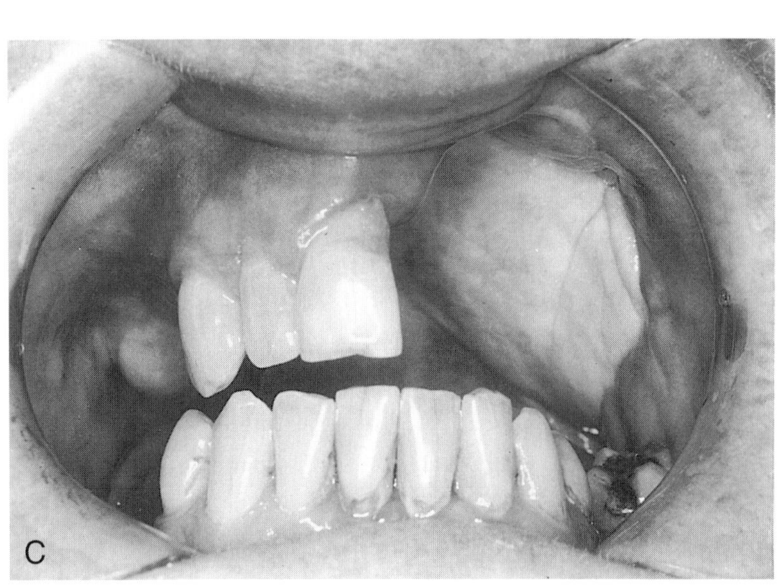
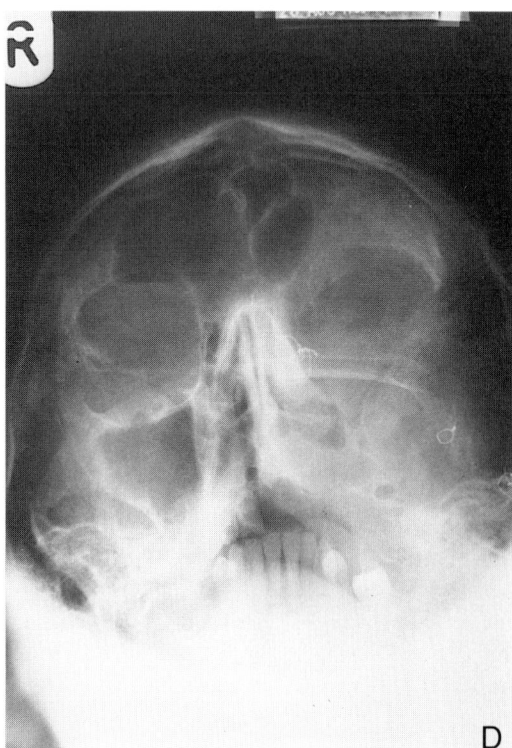

Fig. 19.13

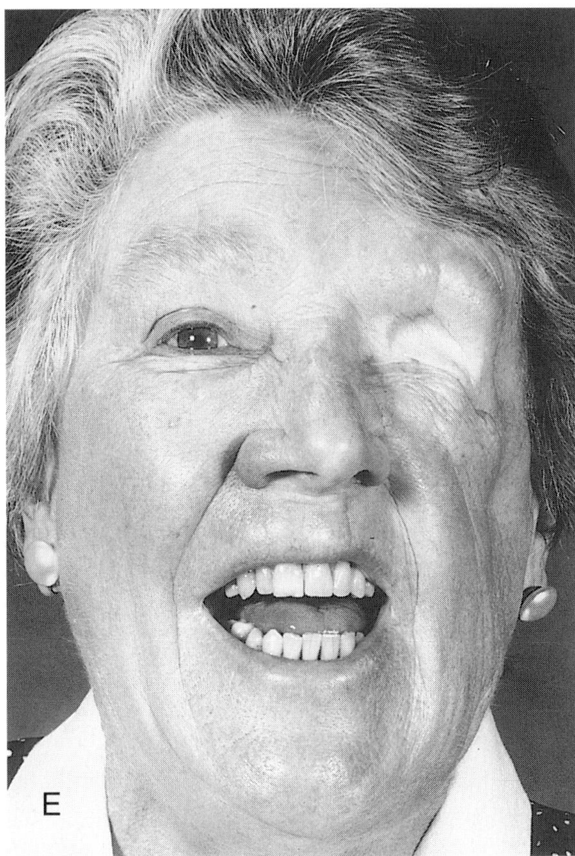

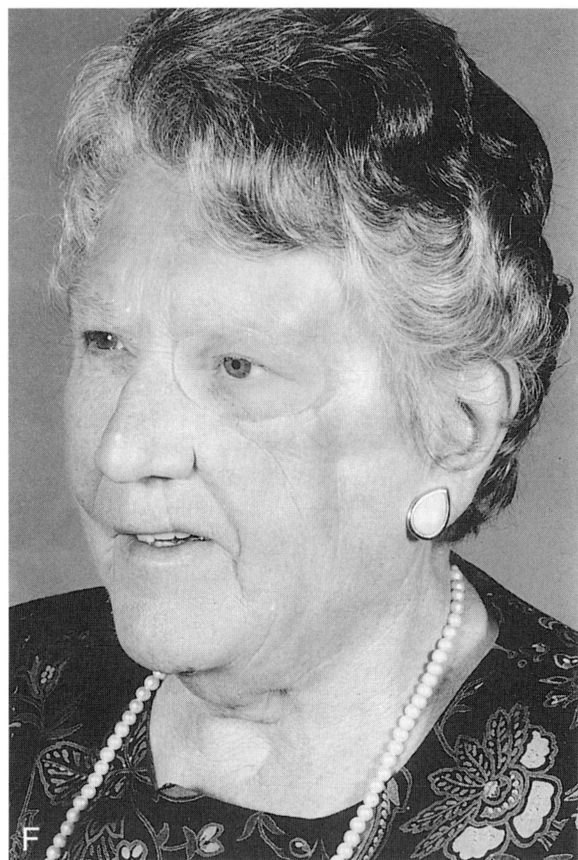

Fig. 19.13 A radical maxillectomy for squamous-cell carcinoma, including exenteration and removal of the orbit (**A**). A free non-vascularized iliac crest bone graft is wired in place to reconstruct the zygoma and anterior maxilla (**B**). A rectus abdominus myocutaneous free flap was used to close the defect and vascularize the bone graft, the skin replacing the oral mucosa (**C**). The patient underwent postoperative radiotherapy. The position of the bone graft at 18 months is shown (**D**). With the cavity closed satisfactorily, dental obturation has been achieved (**E**). Reconstruction of the bone to prevent facial collapse allows a small orbital prosthesis to be worn (**F**).

from ascending infection, do not provide sufficient bulk to reconstruct the defects adequately. There is often a need to reconstruct part of the facial skeleton to prevent facial collapse and simplify the requirements for an external facial prosthesis.

Increasingly, the second author has tended towards the use of free flaps revascularized with microvascular anastomosis. Although at first site it would appear appealing to consider composite flaps that include vascularized bone as well as soft tissue, these have proved difficult to contour satisfactorily into the various shapes that are required in the upper part of the facial skeleton. For this reason, the author has tended towards the use of non-vascularized bone which can be shaped and moulded to replace the facial skeleton and act as a traditional bone graft. A soft-tissue free flap is then wrapped around the bone grafts to ensure their adequate vascularity and survival. There are two techniques which the author has found particularly useful and reliable and which have proved able to withstand early postoperative radical radiotherapy without ill effect.

Rectus abdominus free flap with iliac crest

The rectus abdominus is probably the first choice for maxillary reconstruction. This donor site permits simultaneous operating without the necessity of changing the position of the patient on the operating table. The rectus abdominus provides well-vascularized muscle with the potential of an isolated skin paddle which can be used for mucosal or skin closure. Via the same incision, access can be gained to the iliac crest for a traditional non-vascularized iliac crest bone graft (Fig. 19.12). Such bone grafts can be contoured to reconstruct part of the facial skeleton and the viability ensured by wrapping the bone in vascularized rectus abdominus muscle (Fig. 19.13).

Latissimus dorsi flap with rib

Initially, the author used this technique as a vascularized transfer, taking rib on the serratus anterior as well as latissimus dorsi. Orientation of the bone, however, proved

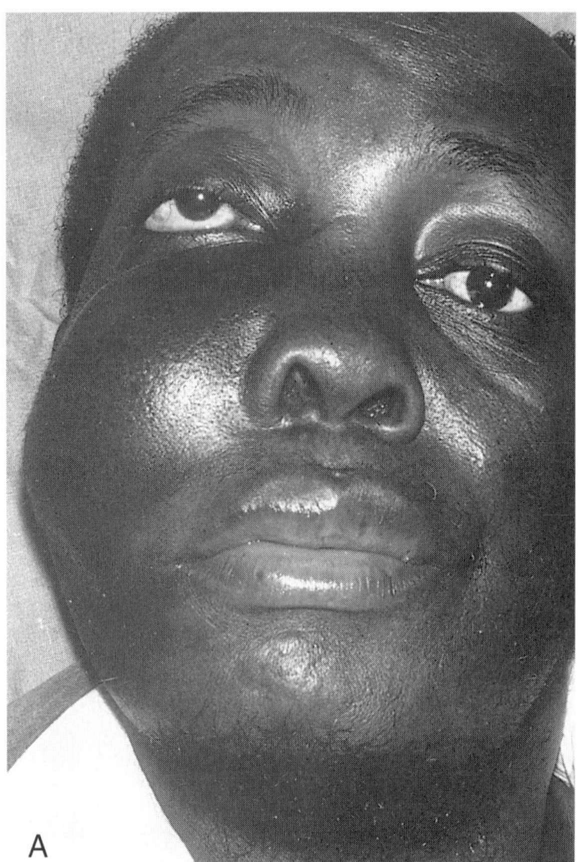

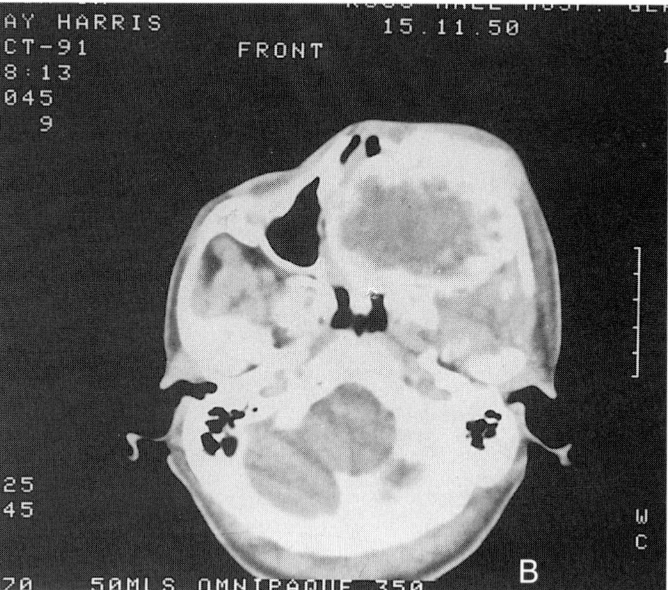

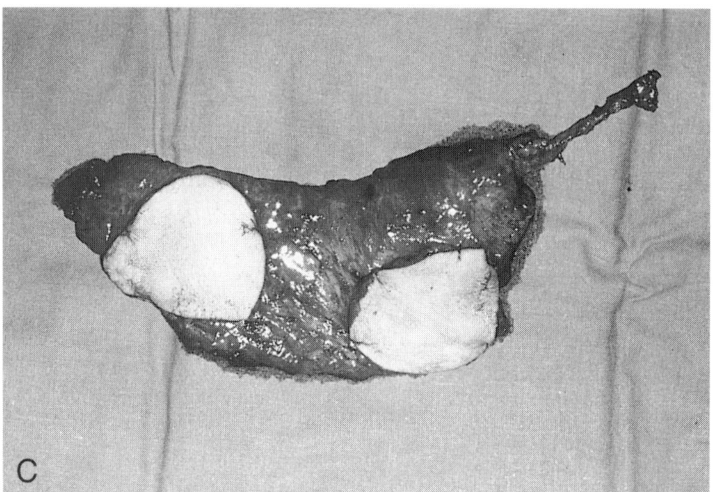

Fig. 19.14 This extensive sarcoma failed to respond to radiotherapy and chemotherapy (**A**). CT scan shows the extent of the tumour and involvement of the overlying skin (**B**). A latissimus dorsi flap incorporating two skin paddles is shown in this photograph of a different patient (**C**). A free non-vascularized rib graft was used for reconstructing the zygoma and anterior maxilla and the latissimus dorsi muscle wrapped round this bone graft to aid vascularization (**D**). Early postoperative X-rays showing placement of rib graft (**E**). One skin paddle was used to reconstruct the oral cavity (**F**) while the other replaced the skin loss of the cheek (**G**).

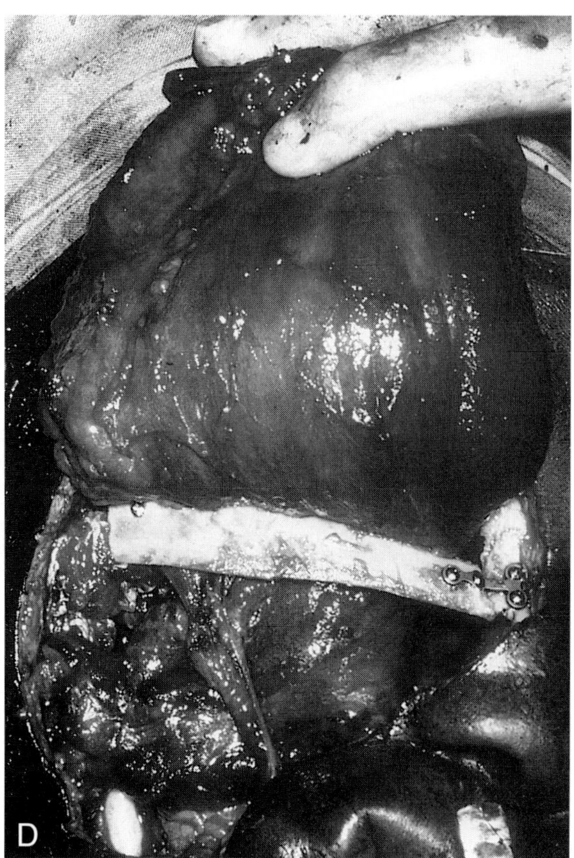

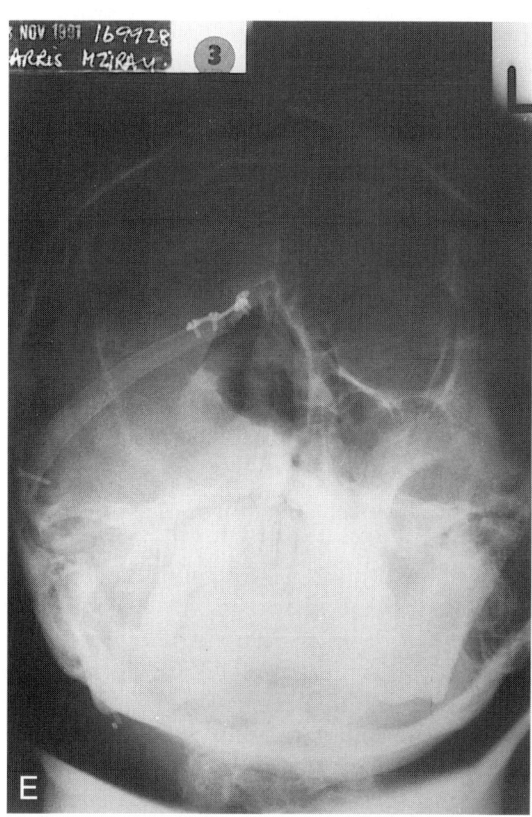

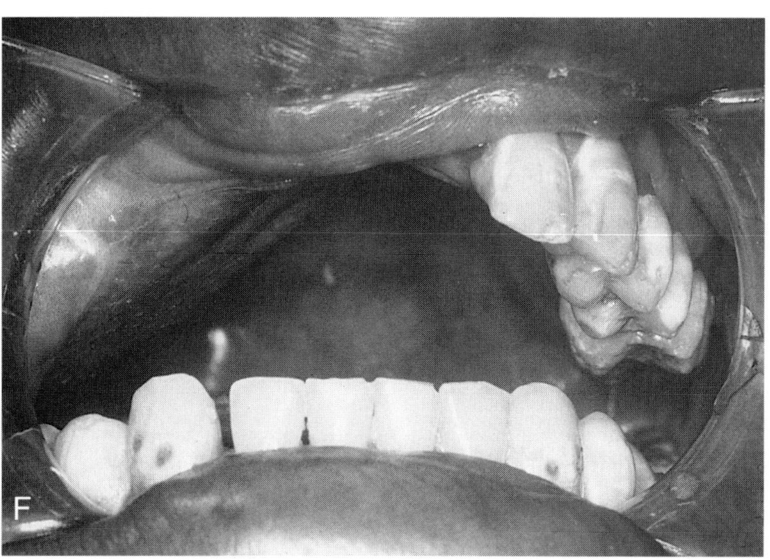

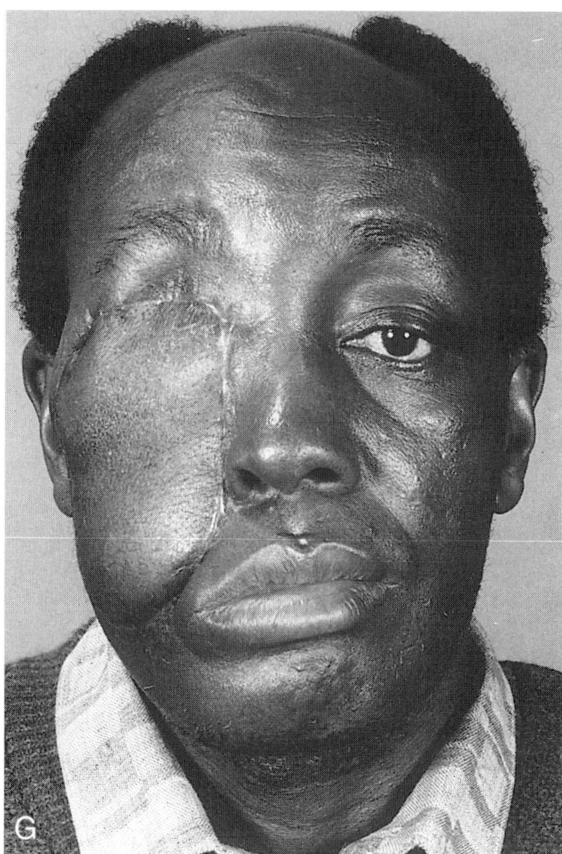

Fig. 19.14

exceptionally difficult and the technique has now been modified to use non-vascularized traditional rib grafts which can be moulded into the particular shape of the facial skeleton. The latissimus dorsi muscle provides excellent vascularity for these bone grafts to ensure their survival. A skin paddle can be taken when there is a necessity to provide skin and/or mucosal lining (Fig. 19.14). The vascularity of free flaps, particularly muscle, provides a barrier against ascending infection and can help close off the brain in composite resections. In over 20 composite resections in which the dura has been exposed, the author has yet to see a case of meningitis or ascending infection.

COMPLICATIONS AND RESULTS

Proper pre-operative evaluation can prevent many problems and complications. The surgeon should be alerted to possible difficulties, particularly when tumours extend intracranially or extend posteriorly into the pterygopalatine fossa. Significant bleeding can be encountered in the pterygopalatine fossa, and the maxillary artery should be ligated before its entry into this space. In a personal series of 80 patients (R.T.) it was never found necessary to ligate the maxillary artery before embarking on a maxillectomy. If the artery is identified during surgery and its location is anticipated, it can be ligated at that time so that blood loss is kept to a minimum.

During craniofacial resections a conscious effort should be made to avoid excessive retraction on the brain and prevent cerebral oedema. Dura should be sealed—whether it is the result of tears or excision of the dura—and here the use of the pericranial flap (Schramm et al 1979) can prove useful. Techniques of using non-vascularized lyophilized dura or fascial grafts should also be considered, but these techniques require ancilliary procedures (see Ch. 21) to provide vascular tissue and ensure graft survival and primary wound healing and prevent ascending infection. When the cranial cavity is breached, particular neurosurgical complications should be actively sought, including infection, oedema, diplopia, diabetes insipidis and subdural haematoma.

Trismus following maxillectomy is encountered particularly after postoperative radiotherapy. The authors routinely excise the coronoid process and the anterior part of the ascending ramus of the mandible, detaching the musculature in this region in an attempt to prevent this complication. Wound breakdown is occasionally encountered—particularly in cases who have undergone radiotherapy. These anterocutaneous fistulae require careful reconstruction and this should be attempted only after the reaction around the wound has settled (Fig. 19.15).

As mentioned previously, assessing the results in terms of control of disease in paranasal sinus tumours has proved difficult because of the wide diversity of sites and tumour types. The results of treatment by surgery and radiotherapy in some of the reported literature are shown in Table 19.3.

An analysis of 62 patients with squamous-cell carcinoma of the maxillary antrum treated in Glasgow showed that early squamous-cell carcinoma (T2N0) was adequately controlled by radical radiotherapy alone with a 5-year survival of 69.1%. More advanced tumours (T3N0 and T4N0) showed a fall in 5-year survival to 19% using radical radiotherapy alone. Combined modality treatment comprising radical surgery followed by postoperative radiotherapy improved 5-year survival in advanced squamous-cell carcinoma to 61% (Robertson et al 1992). Radical surgery

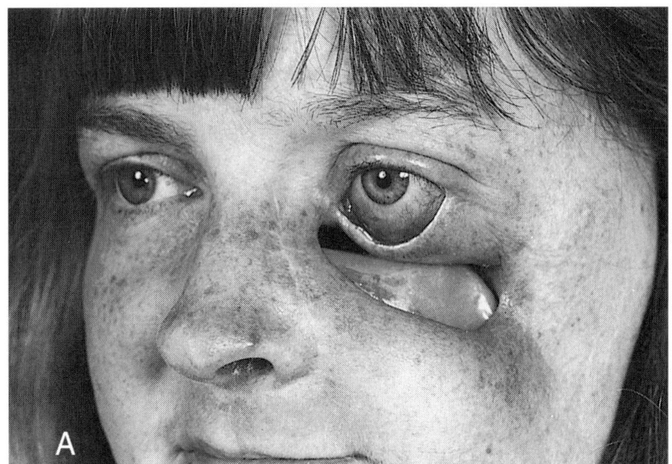

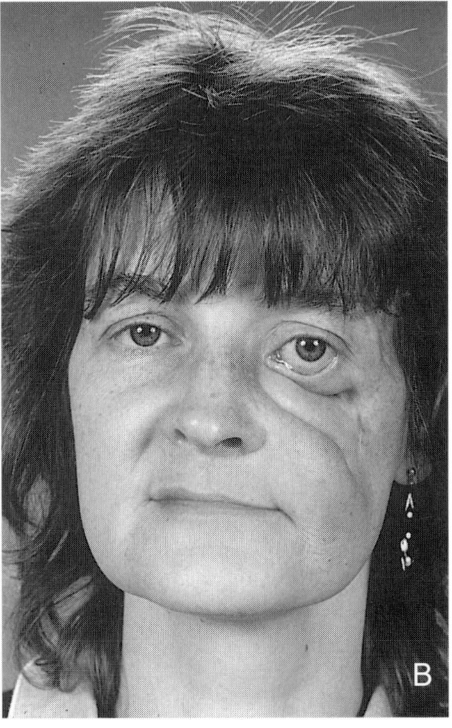

Fig. 19.15 Infraorbital wound breakdown following total maxillectomy and postoperative radiotherapy (**A**). The defect was reconstructed using a temporal flap. The patient remains well and disease-free 7 years postoperatively (**B**).

Table 19.3 Results in paranasal sinus tumours treated by surgery and radiotherapy

Author	Year reported	Number of cases	Site	Results (5-year overall survival)
Jesse et al	1975	146	Antro-ethmoid	40%
Harrison	1972		Antro-ethmoid	30%
Simon et al	1980		Antro-ethmoid	40%
Ahmad et al	1981	59	Maxillary sinus (T3 and T4)	39.3%
St Pierre & Baker	1983	66	Maxillary sinus (T3 and T4)	58%
Ketcham & van Buren	1985	89	Maxillo-ethmoid	43.8%
Cheesman et al	1986	60	Maxillo-ethmoid	48%
Sisson et al	1989	60	Maxillary sinus Ethmoid	48% 68%
Spiro et al	1989	105	Maxillary sinus Ethmoid	38% 13%
Karim et al	1990	45	Ethmoid	68%
Sakai et al	1983	134	Antro-ethmoid	54%
Sato et al	1978			70%
Knegt et al	1985	92	Antrum Ethmoid	52% 100%

Reproduced with permission from Cancer.

followed by postoperative radiotherapy is now our treatment of choice in advanced squamous carcinomas of the maxillary antrum.

The technique of Sato for the treatment of malignant tumours of the paranasal sinuses used in Japan consists of 2 Gy of megavoltage external radiotherapy followed by debulking of the tumour through a Caldwell Luc approach and local application of cytotoxic agents, such as 5FU cream, followed by 2 Gy of radiotherapy, followed by removal of necrotic tissue and re-application of the 5FU cream. This regime is followed for a period of months (Sato et al 1970). Knegt et al (1983) have also shown good results with this method in the treatment of adenocarcinoma but less satisfactory results with squamous-cell carcinoma. Sakai et al (1983) reported a 54% 5-year survival in 134 cases using cobalt-60 gamma ray irradiation of 50 Gy in 5 weeks, continuous arterial infusion of 5FU in a total dose of 2000 mg, and a reduction of tumour mass mainly by cryosurgery. This was further supplemented by immunotherapy with maxillectomy reserved for cases of recurrence. Mukarami (1992) has reported 78–87% 5-year survival in carcinoma of the maxillary antrum and ethmoid in Japan.

Three different policies of combinations and permutions of surgery, radiotherapy and chemotherapy with minor differences are presently in vogue in Japan. The policy yielding the longest survival (87%) is advocated by Takahashi and consists of 800 CGy radiotherapy in 1 to 4 days followed by transantral debulking. Between the sixth and tenth days another 800 CGy are administered followed by transantral daily cleaning. This is followed by partial maxillectomy. It is claimed that no radical surgery is required. The protagonists of this approach believe that microscopic residual tumour can disappear as a result of the patient's own immune system assisted by small amounts of combined therapy. Such small doses of radiotherapy cannot eliminate tumour if used alone but may act as an immune activator. Macroscopic residual tumour must be eliminated by transantral surgery for this procedure to be successful.

No satisfactory improvement in local control rates using this trimodal combination therapy however has been reported by Shibuya et al (1982). These approaches, of course, require frequent visits and treatment over a fairly long period of time.

Few studies address themselves to advanced disease. Choi et al (1991) reported 58% 4-year survival in tumours which were at least T4 treated using split-course hyperfractionated radiation (120 CGy fractions) and concomitant cisplatinum infusion (5–7 g/m^2 per 24 h). Another modality of treatment, namely, intra-operative radiotherapy, has been used for recurrent cancers in which a 2-year survival has been reported as 54.9% (Rate et al 1991).

Interpretation of these results is difficult, but there is little doubt that advanced disease remains a major problem in therapeutic management. However, advances in both excisional and reconstructive surgical techniques have recently opened up new pathways for additional combined modality treatments following radical debulking of disease previously considered inoperable. It is to be hoped that such radical approaches will, in the future, show an improvement in survival. Even if this is not the case, improved reconstructive techniques can do much to reduce the morbidity in this group of patients.

The association of various aetiological factors and the development of cancer in the paranasal sinuses is now well known (Hadfield 1970, Roush 1979, Muir & Nectoux 1980, Hernberg et al 1983, Becker et al 1985, Brinton et al 1985, Olsen & Asnaes 1986). The increasing awareness of society and cancer prevention organizations are likely to mobilize opinion so that appropriate measures can be taken to protect industrial workers from exposure and the risk of developing paranasal sinus cancer. The successes of trimodality treatment reported by the Japanese will no doubt stimulate other centres throughout the world to look again at the differing modalities of treatment, and it is likely that we will see over the next decade a wide variety of schedules using the traditional combinations of surgery, radiotherapy and chemotherapy.

REFERENCES

Ahmad K, Cordoba R B, Fayos J V 1981 Squamous cell carcinoma of the maxillary sinus. Archives of Otolaryngology 107: 48–51

Ali S, Tiwari R M, van der Waal I, Snow G B 1986 Incidence of squamous cell carcinoma of the head and neck. Journal of Laryngology and Otology 100: 315–327

Arden R L, Mathog R H, Thomas L M 1987 Temporalis muscle—galea flap in craniofacial reconstruction 97: 1336–1342

Barbosa J F 1961 Surgery of extensive cancer of paranasal sinuses. Archives of Otolaryngology 73: 129–138

Becker N, Claude J, Frentzel-Beyme R 1985 Cancer risk of arc welders exposed to fumes containing chromium and nickel. Scandinavian Journal of Work Environment and Health 11: 75–82

Bridger G P, Mendelsohn M S, Baldwin M et al 1991 Paranasal sinus cancer. Australia and New Zealand Journal of Surgery 61: 290–294

Brinton L A, Blot W J, Fraumeni J F 1985 Nasal cancer in textile and clothing industries. British Journal of Industrial Medicine 42: 469–474

Brook S J 1982 President Cleveland's curative surgery for oral carcinoma. Contemporary Surgery 20: 49–64

Brown A M S, Lavery K M, Millar B G 1991 The transfacial approach to the postnasal space and retromaxillary structures. British Journal of Oral and Maxillofacial Surgery 29: 230–236

Cheesman A D, Lund V J, Howard 1986 Craniofacial resection for tumours of the nasal cavity and paranasal sinuses. Head and Neck Surgery 8: 429–435

Choi K N, Rotman M, Aziz H et al 1991 Locally advanced paranasal sinus and nasopharynx tumours treated with hyperfractionated radiation and concomitant infusion cisplatin. Cancer 67: 2748–2752

Clifford P 1976 Prospectives in head and neck oncology. Journal of Laryngology and Otology 90: 221–250

Coutard H 1932 Roentgen therapy of epitheliomas of the tonsillar region, hypopharynx and larynx from 1920 to 1926. American Journal of Roentgenology 28: 269–313

Curtin J M 1957 Malignant diseases of the ethmoid and maxillary antrum. Irish Journal of Medical Sciences 6: 488–500

Fergusson W 1842 A system of practical surgery. John Churchill, London, p 449

Fergusson W 1857 Plastic operations on the face. British Medical Journal 5: 81

Fukuda K, Shibata A, Harada K 1987 Squamous cell carcinoma of the maxillary sinus in Hokkaido, Japan. A case control study. British Journal of Industrial Medicine 44: 263–266

Hadfield E H 1970 A study of adenocarcinoma of the paranasal sinuses in woodworkers in the furniture industry. Annals of the Royal College of Surgeons in England 46: 301–319

Harrison D F N 1971 Surgical anatomy of maxillary and ethmoidal sinuses. A reappraisal. Laryngoscope 81: 1658–1661

Harrison D F N 1972 The ENT surgeon looks at the orbit. Journal of Laryngology and Otology 82: 1–43

Herity B 1984 Carcinoma of the paranasal sinus. A possible new aetiology. British Journal of Cancer 49: 371–373

Hernandez Altimer F 1986 Transfacial access to the retromaxillary area. Journal of Maxillofacial Surgery 14: 165–170

Hernberg S, Westerholm P, Schultz-Larsen K et al 1983 Nasal and sinonasal cancer. Connection with occupational exposures in Denmark, Finland and Sweden. Scandinavian Journal of Work Environment and Health 9: 315–326

Jesse R H, Goepfert H, Lindberg R D 1975 Carcinoma of the sinuses. A review of treatment. Cancer of the Head and Neck. Amsterdam, Excerpta Medica, pp 153–159

Karim A B M F, Kralendonk J H, Njo K H et al 1990 Ethmoid and upper nasal cavity carcinoma: treatment results and complications. Radiotherapy and Oncology 19: 109–120

Ketcham A S, van Buren J M 1985 Tumours of the paranasal sinuses: a therapeutic challenge. American Journal of Surgery 150: 406–413

Ketcham A S, Wilkins R H, van Buren J M, Smith R R 1963 A combined intracranial facial approach to the paranasal sinuses. American Journal of Surgery 106: 698–703

Knegt P P, De Jong P C, Van Andel J G et al 1985 Carcinoma of the paranasal sinuses. Results of a prospective pilot study. Cancer 56: 57–62

Mosher H P 1929 The surgical anatomy of the ethmoid labyrinth. Transactions of the American Academy of Ophthalmology and Otolaryngology, p 409

Muir C S, Nectoux J 1980 Descriptive epidemiology of the malignant neoplasms of nose, nasal cavities, middle ear and accessory sinuses. Clinical Otolaryngology 5: 195–211

Mukarami Y Y 1992 Cancer of the paranasal sinuses. In: Helmuth Goepfert (programme chairman) Third International Conference on Head and Neck Cancer, p 37

Ohngren L G 1933 Malignant tumours of the maxillo-ethmoid region. Acta Otolaryngologica Supplement 19: 1

Olsen J H, Asnaes S 1986 Formaldehyde and the risk of squamous cell carcinoma of the sinonasal cavities. British Journal of Industrial Medicine 43: 769–774

Osborne J E, Clayton M, Fenwick J D 1987 The Leeds modified Weber Fergusson incision. Journal of Laryngology and Otology 101: 465–466

Panje W R, Dohrmann G J, Pitock J K et al 1989 The transfacial approach for combined anterior craniofacial tumour ablation. Archives of Otolaryngology Head and Neck Surgery 115: 301–307

Rate W R, Garrett P, Hamaker R et al 1991 Intraoperative radiation therapy for recurrent head and neck cancer. Cancer 67: 2738–2740

Rifki N 1985 Problems of paranasal sinuses malignancy in Indonesia. O R L Indonesia 16: 175–180

Robertson A G, Rao G S, Al-Sammarie A, Soutar D S 1992 The management of tumours arising in the maxillary antrum. Clinical Oncology 4: 240

Rontal E, Rontal M, Guilford F T 1979 Surgical anatomy of the orbit. Annals of Otology, Rhinology and Laryngology 88: 382

Roush G C 1979 Epidemiology of cancer of the nose and paranasal sinuses. Current concepts. Head and Neck Surgery 2: 3–11

St Pierre S, Baker S R 1983 Squamous cell carcinoma of the maxillary sinus. Analysis of 66 cases. Head and Neck Surgery 5: 508–513

Sakai S, Hohki A, Fuchihata H, Tanaka Y 1983 Multidisciplinary treatment of maxillary sinus carcinoma. Cancer 52: 1360–1364

Sato Y, Morita M, Takahashi H et al 1970 Combined surgery, radiotherapy and regional chemotherapy in carcinoma of the paranasal sinuses. Cancer 25: 571–579

Sato Y, Inouye K, Yamamoto E, Takahashi H 1978 Combined immunotherapy for head and neck cancer. Japanese Journal of Cancer Clinics 24: 561–567

Schaeffer J P 1920 The embryology development and anatomy of the nose, paranasal sinuses, nasolacrimal passages and olfactory organ in man. P. Blakistons Son, Philadelphia

Schramm V L, Myers E N, Maroon J C 1979 Anterior skull base surgery for benign and malignant disease. Laryngoscope 59: 1077–1091

Shibuya H, Suzuki S, Horuchi J I et al 1982 Reappraisal of trimodal combination therapy for maxillary sinus carcinoma. Cancer 50: 2790–2794

Simon C L, Barthelme A, Chobaut J C, Wayoff M 1980 La paralateronasale technique chirurgicale et résultats à propos de 55 cas cancers ethmoido-maxillaires. Journal Français Otorhinolaryngology 29: 121–127

Sisson G A, Johnson N E, Amire C S 1963 Cancer of the maxillary sinus. Clinical classification and management. Annals of Otology Rhinology and Laryngology 72: 1050–1059

Sisson G A Sr, Toriumi D M, Atiyah A R 1989 Paranasal sinus malignancy. A comprehensive update. Laryngoscope 99: 143–150

Smith R E, Klopp C T, Williams J M 1954 Surgical treatment of cancer of the frontal sinus and adjacent areas. Cancer 7: 991–994

Spiro J D, Soo K C, Spiro R H 1989 Squamous carcinoma of the nasal cavity and paranasal sinuses. American Journal of Surgery 158: 328–332

Stell P M 1990 Adjuvant chemotherapy in head and neck cancer. Clinical Otolaryngology 15: 193–195

Suarez Nieto S C, Gomis J E, Llorente Pedas J L 1988 A rhinological approach for the craniofacial resection of the ethmoid. Rhinology 26: 273–279

Supance J S, Seid A B 1981 Craniofacial resection for ethmoid carcinoma in children. International Journal of Paediatric Otorhinolaryngology 3: 185–194

Tiwari R M, Gerritsen G J, Balm A J M, Snow G B 1986 Critical evaluation of the role of CT scanning in ethmoidal cancer. Journal of Laryngology and Otology 100: 421–428

van den Brekel M W M, Castelijns J A, Stel H V et al 1992 Computed tomography, magnetic resonance ultrasound and ultrasound guided aspiration cytology for the assessment of the neck. A comparative study. Thesis, Free University of Amsterdam, pp 102–117

20. The orbit and mid-face

Shan R. Baker

INTRODUCTION

The history of the treatment of head and neck cancer has been one of continual applications of new techniques in the hope of improving cure rates and functional rehabilitation after tumour ablation. In the 1930s, orthovoltage radiation therapy dominated the management of head and neck cancer, following the Coutard fractionation method, which cured perhaps 25% of oral, pharyngeal and laryngeal cancers (Moore 1980). In the 1940s, Martin improved the survival statistics by developing new techniques of radical surgery that combined wide resection of the primary tumour in continuity with neck dissection for regional metastases. The philosophy of 'one operation fits all' prevailed, and functional and cosmetic disability was a common trade-off for improved survival rates. In the 1950s, improvement in radiation therapy equipment enabled MacComb and Fletcher to introduce the concept of combined therapy, consisting of radiotherapy and surgery. Treatment results again improved while the surgeon's ability to reconstruct the head and neck lagged behind. It was not until the 1960s that new surgical concepts such as immediate repair of large defects of the head and neck using regional skin flap repair began to expand the clinician's options for reconstruction of head and neck defects following tumour ablation.

Conservative laryngeal surgery emerged as another surgical advancement. In the 1970s, the concept of adjuvant chemotherapy was developed and continues to be investigated. The staging of disease was standardized (Moore 1980). Modifications of radical surgery became popular, and new concepts of reconstructive surgery were introduced, including the use of musculocutaneous regional flaps (Ariyan & Krizek 1977) and revascularized free flaps (Panje et al 1977).

The 1980s have seen refinements in surgical techniques, particularly in the area of microvascular surgery. These improved surgical techniques have enabled the surgeon to perform major resections of neoplasms of the head and neck without the degree of concern for restoration of form and function experienced by clinicians in the past decade.

This chapter attempts to place into perspective the numerous alternatives now available for excision of orbital and mid-facial neoplasms and reconstruction of the resulting surgical defect. Remarks concerning orbital surgery will be confined to surgical techniques used in orbital exenteration and subsequent reconstruction. A discussion of resection and reconstruction of the eyelids is beyond the scope of this chapter. The chapter will help to clarify which surgical approaches are preferable for resection of tumour, and which reconstructive option is best for a given condition. It is not the purpose to offer a detailed discussion of surgical techniques as much as it is to offer the author's indications and perceptions as to the advantages and disadvantages of a particular ablative and reconstructive technique, based not only on the criteria of form and function, but also on cost effectiveness. This latter criterion is included because of its increasing importance in our society as it strives to contain the rising cost of medical care.

EXCISION TECHNIQUES

Excision of cancer of the nasal and mid-facial skin

Most defects of the mid-face result from the need to excise skin cancers. Skin cancer is the most common form of malignancy in man, and basal-cell carcinoma is the predominant histological type. Fortunately, the mortality rate from basal-cell carcinoma is negligible, but its morbidity can be significant when such tumours are not treated early and properly. Most frequently, basal-cell carcinoma, like actinic keratosis and squamous-cell carcinoma, is found in sun-exposed areas. Thus, 97% of these tumours present in the area of the head and neck. There are several histologically identifiable patterns of basal-cell carcinoma and these include nodulo-ulcerative (most common), superficial, cystic, adenoid, morpheic and basisquamous carcinoma. Tumour histology is correlated with frequency of recurrence; however, the site of the tumour appears to be a far more important factor in predicting treatment failure. The mid-face is the location of the highest risk of recurrence. In general, recurrence rates for the entire face range from 0.05 to 14%, with an average recurrence in the United States of 7%. Highest recurrence rates are seen when basal-cell carcinoma is managed by curettage and electrodesiccation, and the lowest recurrence rate is observed with surgical excision with complete histological controlled margins (Mohs' surgery).

The question often arises as to why certain basal-cell carcinomas are more invasive and difficult to treat than others. Such tumours send out silent contiguous subclinical extensions which have affinity for certain structures such as dermis, fascial planes, periosteum, perichondrium, nerve sheaths and blood vessels. The spread of basal-cell carcinoma along these structures is related to mechanical factors, that is, tumour tends to follow the path of least resistance. Tumour often approaches certain anatomical structures and spreads along them before invading. Specific examples of this phenomena in the mid-face are: tumour spread along periosteum of nasal bones, perichondrium of alar cartilages and the tarsal plate of the eyelid. Basal-cell carcinoma spreads along nerve sheaths and blood vessels by invasion along the perineural sheath and adventitia of arteries.

Another mode of spread of basal-cell carcinoma is along embryonic fusion planes. Tumours arising in areas of fusion planes may invade to an unexpected depth because embryonic fusion planes extend in a direction perpendicular to the surface of the skin. Important sites where this occurs in the mid-face are along the columella of the nose and at the junction of the nasal ala with the nasolabial fold.

Curettage and electrodesiccation is an ideal method for removing small basal-cell carcinomas less that 0.5 cm in diameter. However, the technique is not as effective for larger tumours, and other therapeutic modalities should be used. Ring curettes are used to scrape out the tumour from the surrounding normal tissue. This is followed by electrodesiccation of the wound base margins. A biopsy should be obtained to confirm the presence of malignancy prior to performing this technique. The advantage of curettage and electrodesiccation is that it is easily and rapidly performed and is highly reliable for small basal-cell carcinomas; however, it leaves a rather unsatisfactory scar compared with excision and primary closure or cryosurgery. Recurrent and morpheic basal-cell carcinomas should not be managed with curettage and electrodesiccation because the tactile difference between tumour and surrounding normal tissue is lost, making tumour removal difficult.

Cryosurgery is also an acceptable method of managing small basal-cell carcinomas less than 0.5 cm in diameter. A localized spray of liquid nitrogen (–197°C) is applied to the lesion and surrounding tissue. The advantage of cryosurgery is that it is easily employed with little discomfort to the patient and does not require surgical equipment. The degree of subsequent scarring is minimal. Similar to curettage and electrodesiccation, cryosurgery should be reserved for small basal-cell carcinomas less than 0.5 cm in diameter and

areas where there is not a propensity for recurrence of neoplasm.

Radiotherapy offers a high cure rate for basal-cell carcinoma and compares favourably with that resulting from surgical excision. Medium-sized tumours, from 0.5 cm to 2.0 cm in diameter, can be readily managed by this approach. Utilizing the electron beam, superficial irradiation can be applied over a relatively short time period to maximize expediency and minimize the effects on normal tissue deep to the tumour. Radiotherapy is a relatively non-invasive method of treating basal-cell carcinoma and is therefore particularly amenable to the very elderly or ill patient.

Disadvantages of radiotherapy include the problem with determining the correct port size for a tumour that may run for a considerable distance under the skin surface and may not be clinically visible. Late sequelae may result from radiotherapy—including atrophy of the skin, pigmentary abnormalities, telangectases and the development of cutaneous carcinomas in the irradiated site. Because of these disadvantages, radiotherapy should be avoided in younger patients and in patients with neoplasms larger than 2 cm in diameter.

As in the case with radiotherapy, surgical excision is a particularly useful method of treating small and medium-sized basal-cell carcinomas of less than 2.0 cm in diameter. A 0.5 cm margin of normal tissue surrounding the neoplasm should be removed with excision of the tumour. Surgical excision is particularly advantageous in instances where local flaps and grafts are required for closure. The advantage of surgical excision is that the specimen as well as the margins may be histologically examined; however, complete histological examination of the entire margin, providing total microscopic control, is quite difficult by conventional methods of surgical excision. More extensive tumours treated with surgery should make use of an extended follow-up period of 6 to 12 months before reconstructive procedures are initiated.

The most contemporary method of managing basal-cell carcinoma is by microscopically controlled excision (Mohs' surgery). The cornerstone of this surgical method is total microscopic control of excision. Using local anaesthesia, the tumour mass is excised and then a thin layer of tissue is removed, maintaining orientation of the specimen in relationship to the patient. The specimen is diagrammed, divided into sections of appropriate size for frozen sectioning, and the edges marked with coloured dye corresponding to a diagrammed map. Horizontal frozen sections, 5–7 μm thick, are then taken from the undersurface of each specimen and examined under the microscope. Persistent microscopic tumour can then be pin-pointed. In this way, the entire undersurface as well as the epidermal edges of the excised specimen can be examined. Additional layers of tissue are then removed and carefully handled in the same manner only in areas where tumour is persistent. This layer-by-layer removal continues until total tumour extirpation has been achieved. The indications for the use of Mohs' surgery for the treatment of facial basal-cell carcinoma are governed by tumour size, histology and location. In addition, all recurrent basal-cell carcinomas should be managed with the Mohs' technique.

The algorithm of Table 20.1 summarizes the author's approach to the management of basal-cell carcinoma of the mid-face (Baker & Swanson 1983). The majority of primary tumours may be treated with conventional methods discussed. Primarily basal-cell carcinoma occurring in high-risk locations, specifically the nasolabial crease, nasal columella and the region of the medial canthus should be resected by Mohs' surgery. Likewise, tumours having morpheic or basisquamous histology, greater than 2 cm in size, having an aggressive growth pattern or multicentric in origin, should be treated initially using Mohs' surgery. Additionally, inadequately excised basal-cell carcinomas and recurrent tumours should be treated by Mohs' surgery whenever the expertise is available in the medical community.

Excision of cancer of the orbit

The orbit can be defined as a bony cavity in which are housed those tissues and organs contributing to the function of the eye. The orbit conforms to the shape of a pear, with the optic canal its stock. There are a number of tumours that may arise within the orbit, and most are benign. These include haemangioma, choristoma, pseudotumor, meningioma, glioma, and tumours of the lacrimal gland. Primary malignant tumours occur within the orbit such as lymphoma, lymphosarcoma and rhabdomyosarcoma; however, more commonly the orbit is involved with malignant disease by secondary involvement. This occurs from skin cancer around the eye, directly extending into the orbit, or by paranasal sinus cancer extending to the orbit.

A general principle when dealing with cancer of the orbit should be that the diagnosis must be established before treatment can be planned. Biopsy of primary orbital tumours suspected of being cancerous can be accomplished through a simple canthotomy or, if necessary, a Kronlein operation which offers the surgeon an opportunity to explore the orbit and appraise the tumour. This procedure is accomplished by performing a wide canthotomy and severing the lateral canthal ligament. This permits the entrance of the surgeon's finger into the orbit for the purpose of palpation, and provides access for the biopsy of most tumours within the orbit. Tumours from adjacent structures extending into the orbit are best biopsied at the primary source of the tumour. An example would be a transnasal biopsy to confirm a malignancy of the ethmoid or maxillary sinus involving the orbit. Although biopsy prior to resecting orbital tumours is generally preferred, some well-circumscribed or encapsulated primary orbital tumours which are accessible may be removed transorbitally without a preliminary biopsy. Likewise, in some instances, the diagnosis may be clear without the need for a biopsy.

Malignant tumours of the eyelid and periorbital facial skin with secondary involvement of the orbit may be resected by incisions placed in the lids. Very small malignant tumours of the lacrimal gland may also be removed in this manner, or through a Kronlein operation which involves removing the bony lateral wall of the orbit entirely back to the thick cancellous bone where the lateral orbital wall meets the lateral cranial wall. A Stryker saw is used to perform the bony osteotomy creating an osteoplastic bone flap hinged on the zygomatic sphenoid suture. The peri-orbita is incised as far posteriorly as possible. All dissections should be

Table 20.1 Management of mid-facial basal-cell carcinoma

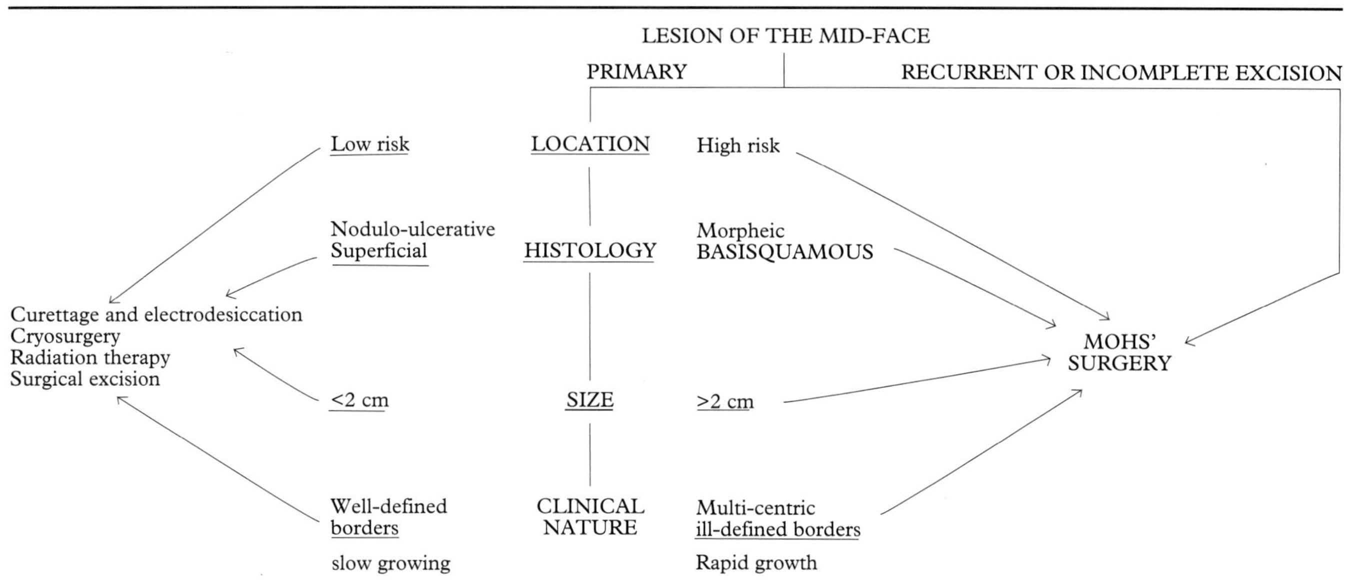

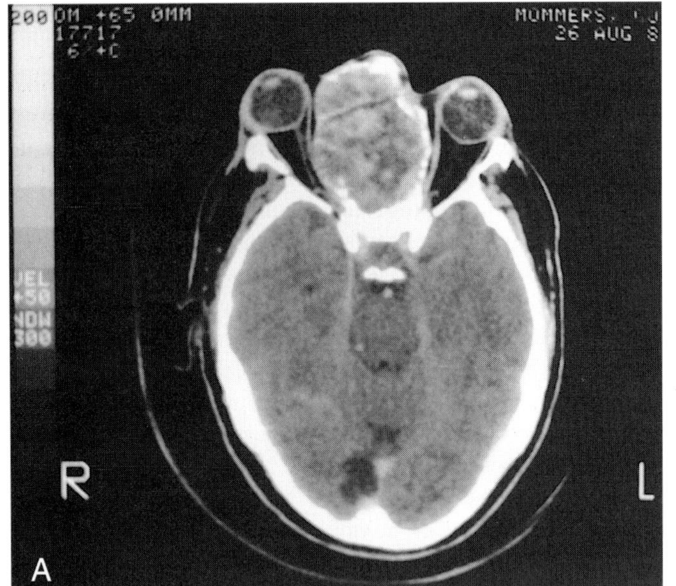
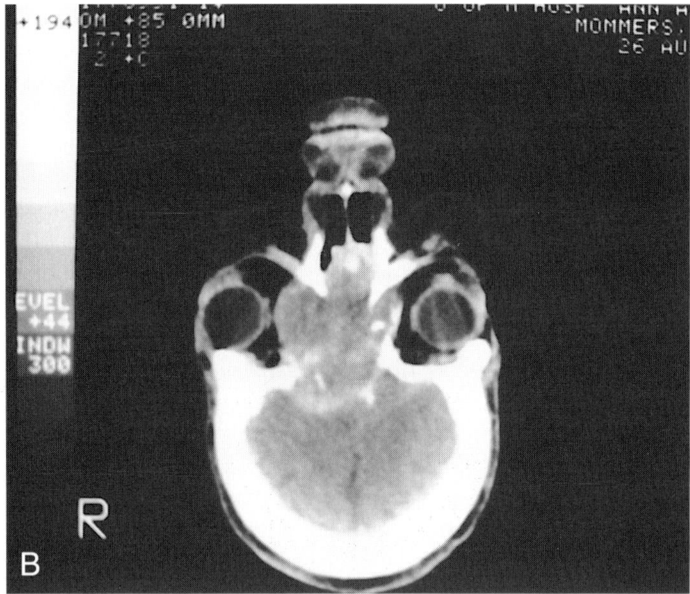
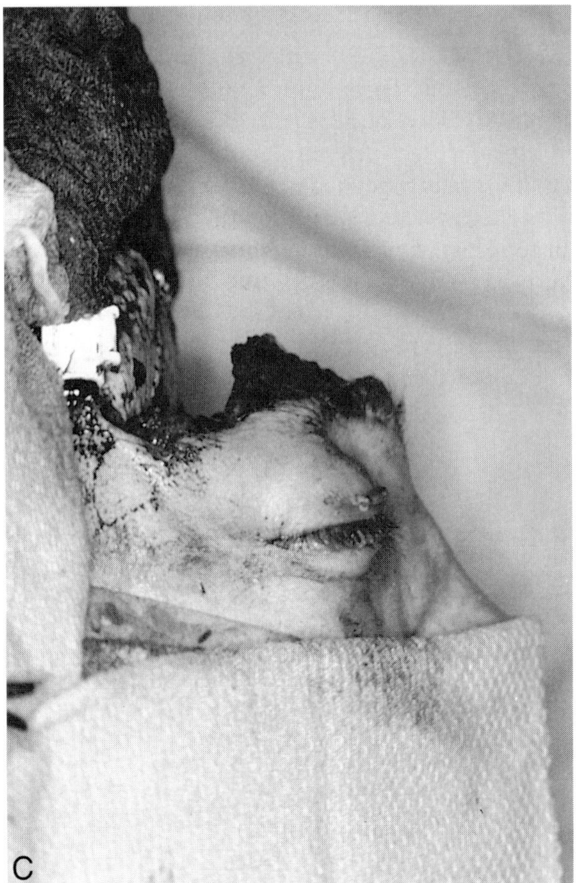
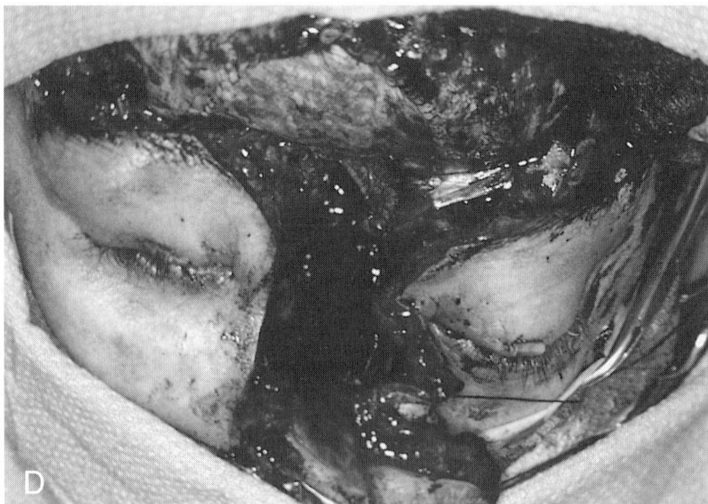

Fig. 20.1   Upper left **(A)** and upper right **(B)** views of axial and coronal CT scan of an extensive chondrosarcoma of the frontal sinus. Lower left **(C)** and lower right **(D).** An anterior craniotomy (left) combined with a lateral rhinotomy (right) enabled en bloc removal of tumour.

accomplished by blunt dissection once the bone has been immobilized.

The transcranial approach provides excellent visualization for tumours that have spread to include both the orbit and the intracranial cavity such as sphenoid ridge meningiomas, optic nerve gliomas, and ophthalmic neurilemmomas. The approach may also be used for en bloc resection of malignancies of the orbit or paranasal sinuses that require resection of the roof of the orbit. A craniotomy flap allows anterior and lateral exposure of the anterior cranial fossa. This is a particularly good approach for removing tumour arising from the ethmoid or frontal sinus with extension to both orbits (Fig. 20.1).

Subtotal exenteration, in which part of the eyelids and peri-orbita are saved, may be possible with indolent malignancies of the eyelids and malignant tumours of the paranasal sinuses that have destroyed portions of the bony orbit but have not invaded through the protective peri-orbita (Baker & Swanson 1983, Baker & Swanson 1984a). In such instances, portions of the peri-orbita may be resected along with an adequate bony margin around the tumour while sparing the globe and extra-ocular muscles. A split-thickness skin graft may be applied directly over the peri-orbital fat to provide external covering of the eye. Unfortunately in some cases of subtotal exenteration, even though the eye may be salvaged, the usefulness may be diminished because of enophthalmos, diplopia, or an unaesthetic appearance as a result of surgery.

A group of patients particularly amenable to subtotal exenteration are those with cancer of the skin of the nose, forehead, cheek or temple which has encroached upon the orbit. The most common scenario is a chronically recurring basal-cell carcinoma located adjacent to the region of the inner canthus. These cancers are often treated with irradiation or electrodesiccation and curettage without marginal control. Recurrences may be deceptive and subclinical, frequently tracking along the periosteum of the medial orbit and penetrating into the lacrimal sac and adjacent ethmoid sinus. When treatment is initiated at an early stage of invasion of the orbit by basal-cell carcinoma, the globe can often be preserved, although some appendages and supportive structures may require resection.

Conservative approaches to surgical resection of portions of the orbit may also be practised in treating some paranasal sinus cancers with limited orbital extension. An example would be the removal of the medial and inferior peri-orbita and even portions of the peri-orbital fat concurrent with a radical ethmoidectomy and maxillectomy (Baker & Swanson 1984a). This could include all bony support laterally from the inferior orbital fissure to the frontal ethmoid suture line medially (Fig. 20.2). The orbital contents are supported by a skin graft and antral packing. Sufficient fibrosis occurs during healing usually to support the soft tissue of the orbit without causing undue difficulties with enophthalmos, inferior displacement of the globe or peripheral diplopia.

Once the cancer has invaded the muscles and fat of the eye, exenteration is necessary in an attempt to cure the patient. This frequently occurs with malignant tumours of the paranasal sinuses, pterygopalatine fossa, and temporal fossa that spread to the orbit through the superior or infraorbital fissure or by direct extension from orbital bone erosion. The need for orbital exenteration for the treatment of cancer of the paranasal sinuses ranges from 20 to 45%, depending upon the method of management at different institutions. The sinuses involved with the primary tumour are resected en bloc with the orbital contents. Sufficient bony orbit is removed to ensure adequate margins around the tumour. Maxillectomy is commonly combined with orbital exenteration in cases of carcinoma of the maxillary sinus displaying tumour extension into the orbit. Ethmoidal cancer involving the orbit often also invades the cribriform plate and fovea ethmoidalis, necessitating a cranial facial resection with concomitant orbital exenteration.

RECONSTRUCTIVE TECHNIQUES

A hard and fast 'cook book' approach to reconstruction of mid-facial defects is not feasible because of the many variables that influence methodology. Age, sex, social habits and associated health problems are but a few of the patient variables that the surgeon must consider. Size and location of orbital or mid-facial defects along with a concomitant partial or total loss of adjacent nervous, vascular, muscular and skeletal tissues are a few of the anatomical variables that must also be considered. Each of these variables is added to a formula called clinical judgement in the mind of the surgeon so that a plan can be synthesized which will provide a reliable method of reconstruction that maximizes the rehabilitation and cosmesis and minimizes acute and delayed morbidity. Ultimately the two factors governing the method of repair of defects of the orbit or mid-face are the deficits in form and function that will be left after finalizing all reconstructive efforts. Both factors are to some degree related and to some degree exclusive of each other, and both play an important role in formulating a final plan of reconstruction.

An example of this is a large skin defect of the medial cheek that is closed primarily to the detriment of form (cosmesis), but not function, contrasted to a small defect of the nasal ala closed primarily to the detriment of function (i.e. airway) with minimal impairment of cosmesis.

Reconstruction of mid-facial skin defects

The algorithm in Table 20.2 (Baker 1989) is an attempt to integrate form and function into a logical approach for formulating a method of repairing general surface defects of the mid-face. The first consideration of the clinician is a choice of repair by primary closure of the wound or use of a skin graft. Occasionally, primary closure may not be feasible

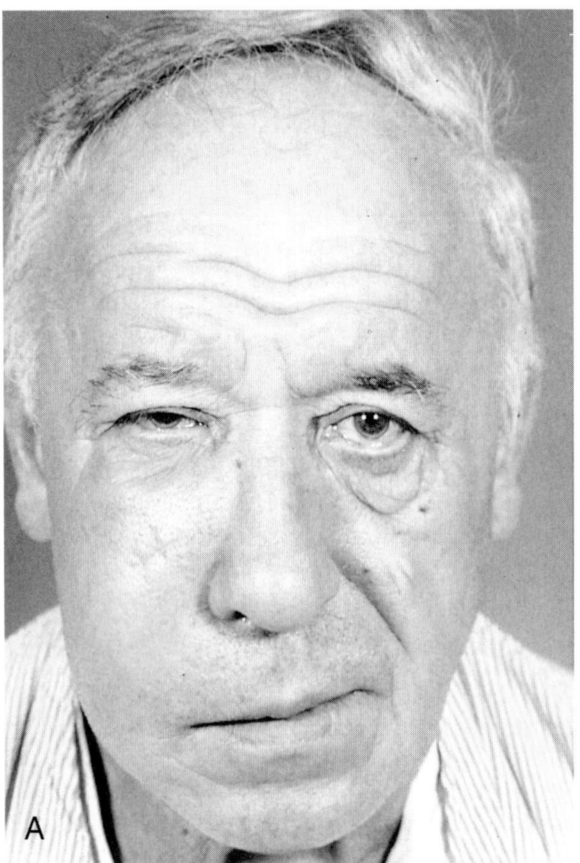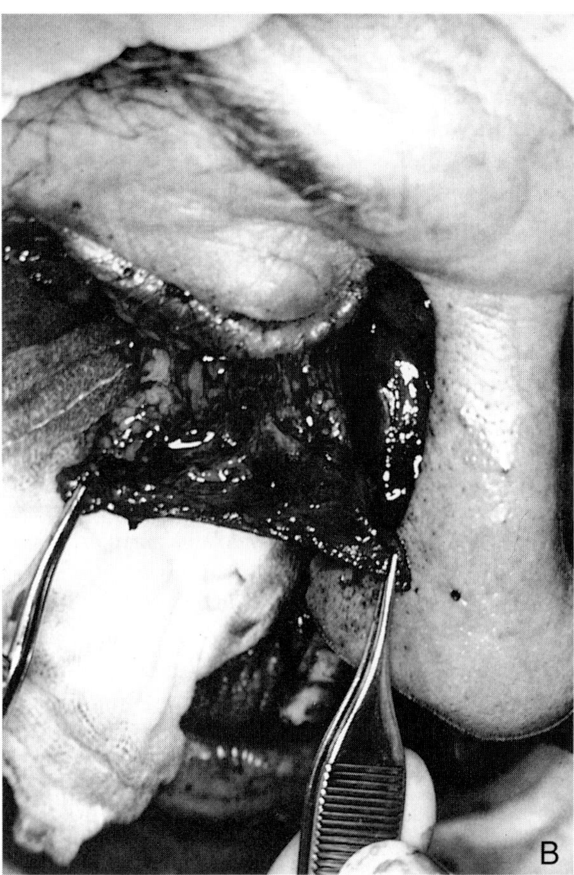

Fig. 20.2 A. Extensive squamous-cell carcinoma of the right maxillary sinus with encroachment of the peri-orbita. **B.** Dissection of peri-orbita at the time of maxillectomy. This method allowed removal of portions of the peri-orbita and the inferior rectus muscle while preserving the globe and optic nerve for useful vision. (From Head and Neck Surgery 6: 918 (1984) with permission of the publisher, John Wiley.)

and a skin graft can be used without unduly affecting form and function. Larger defects of necessity may frequently require alternative methods of reconstruction. The next echelon in the order of thinking is consideration of use of local flaps. Similar to primary closure or the use of skin grafts, the detriment of form and function resulting from the use of local flaps must be considered, and, if the detriment is excessive, consideration must be given to the use of regional flaps. This natural progression from simple to more complex methods of reconstruction provides a systematic approach for evaluating any combination of defects of the orbit or mid-face. Each step in the algorithm is governed by the experience and clinical judgement of the person responsible for reconstruction.

Skin grafts

In general, primary closure is preferred when it does not compromise cosmesis or function. When selecting a skin graft for closure, the split-thickness (0.02 inches—0.5 mm —or greater) or full-thickness grafts are preferred to thinner split-thickness skin grafts because the thicker grafts provide

a better colour and texture match with adjacent skin, and they contract less severely.

The advantages of a skin graft for resurfacing defects of the mid-face include ease of repair, single-stage procedure, and no additional incisions or scars are necessary in the area of the defect. Skin grafts also provide coverage of large defects which cannot be repaired with local flaps. The disadvantages of skin grafts preclude their general use and include poor colour and texture match with surrounding skin, scar contracture at the recipient site, and an unsightly donor scar.

Local flaps

Defects in the skin of the mid-face that cannot be closed primarily without significant compromise of form or function can be resurfaced with a skin graft; however, local flaps are preferred.

The author defines local flaps as those adjacent to or in the immediate vicinity of the defect. Advantages of local flaps for resurfacing defects of the mid-face include excellent colour and texture match with surrounding skin, repair

Table 20.2 Options for reconstruction of surface defects of the mid-face

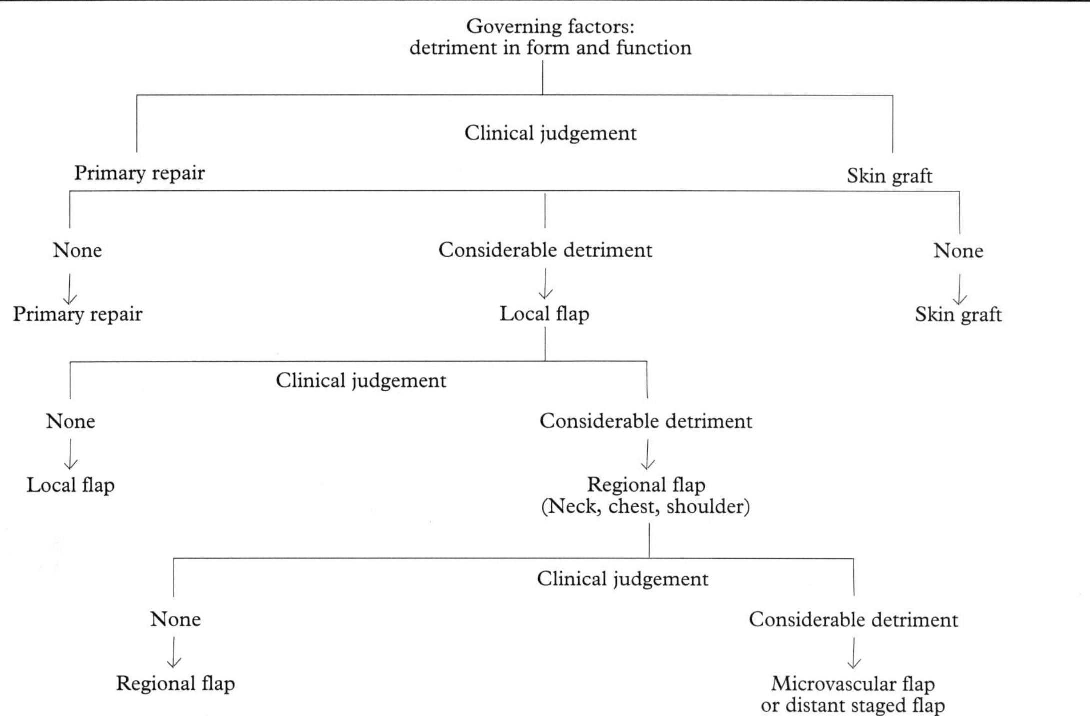

of the defect with like tissues, and a one-stage surgical procedure. Disadvantages are few, and they relate to the need for additional scars in the area and a more extensive surgical procedure compared to primary closure.

Regional flaps

Defects of the mid-face that are large may be difficult to resurface with local flaps without considerable impairment in form or function (Table 20.2) (Baker 1989). When this is the case, consideration must be given to the use of a regional flap. The author defines a regional flap as one located near a defect but not in the immediate proximity.

The selection of a specific regional flap is dependent upon the location and size of the defect and the intrinsic properties of the regional flap. Single pedicle peninsular or island axial pattern flaps are usually selected because of their superior blood supply compared to random flaps. For most skin defects of the mid-face, a medially based deltopectoral or Bakamjian flap (Bakamjian 1965) is preferable to regional musculocutaneous flaps because it is less bulky, more supple and produces less functional deficits at the donor site. When mid-facial skin defects are accompanied by underlying soft tissue or bone deficits, compound flaps are selected because they provide greater tissue bulk for restoring contour, thus providing better overall restoration of form and function (Baker 1991).

The advantages of regional flaps for resurfacing skin defects of the mid-face include the following: (i) large

surface areas of skin are available with concomitant soft-tissue bulk if needed; (ii) flaps can be transferred in a one-stage surgical procedure; (iii) donor site functional morbidity is usually limited; (iv) the donor site can usually be covered by appropriate clothing. Disadvantages include poor colour and texture match of the flap compared to the skin of the face, excessive bulkiness of the flap, particularly when using compound flaps, and donor site deformity.

Revascularized flaps

Massive defects of the skin of the mid-face may on occasion be difficult or impossible to reconstruct with regional flaps. In such instances, microvascular or revascularized flaps are appropriate. Even when such defects can be reconstructed with regional flaps, microvascular flaps may be preferred if the flap ultimately provides better restoration of overall form and function.

Revascularized flaps provide the capability of transferring almost an unlimited quantity of skin to reconstruct massive surface defects of the face. Defects involving only skin of the mid-face are best covered by revascularized cutaneous or musculocutaneous flaps harvested from the shoulder (scapular flap), groin (inguinal flap) or axilla because of the large axial vessels located in these regions (Baker 1981). Skin defects accompanied by loss of underlying muscle and/or bone are restored by transferring revascularized compound flaps containing like tissue, if possible, to that lost, i.e. skin plus muscle and/or bone (Fig. 20.3) (Baker 1984b).

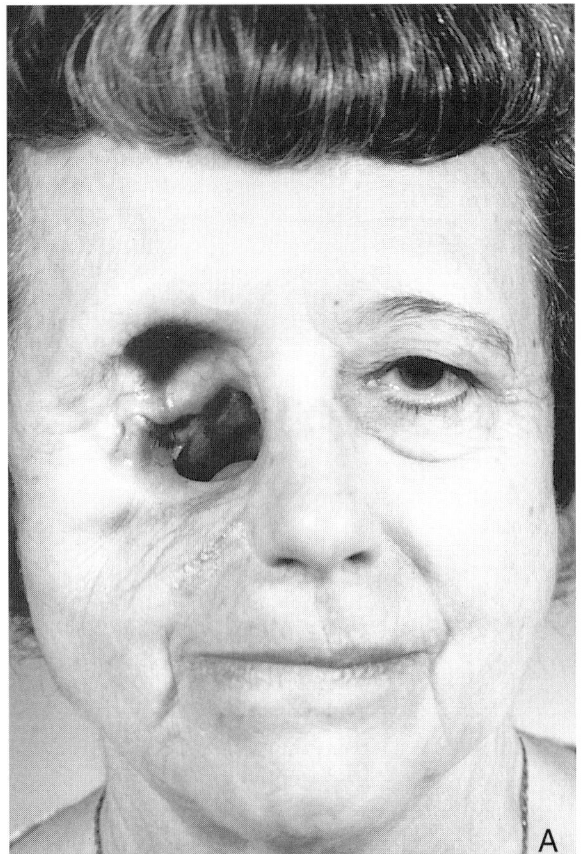

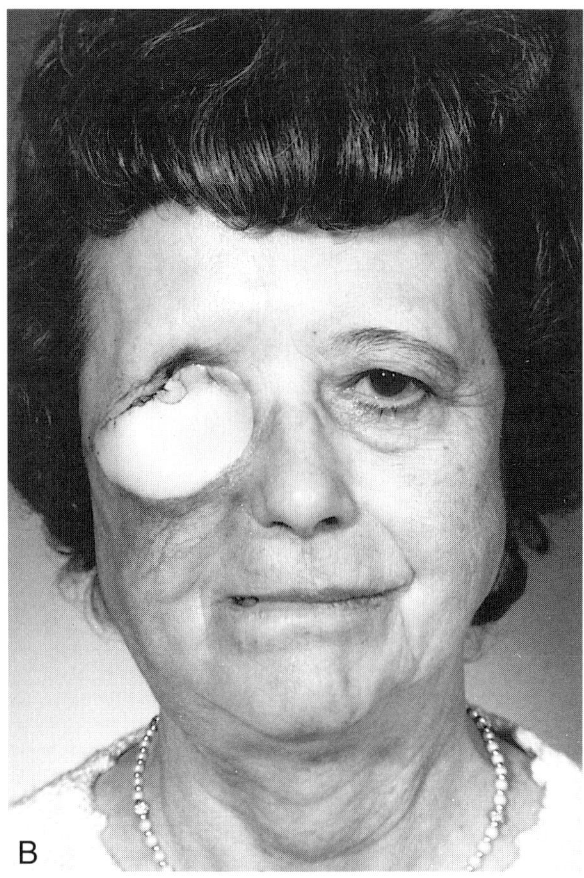

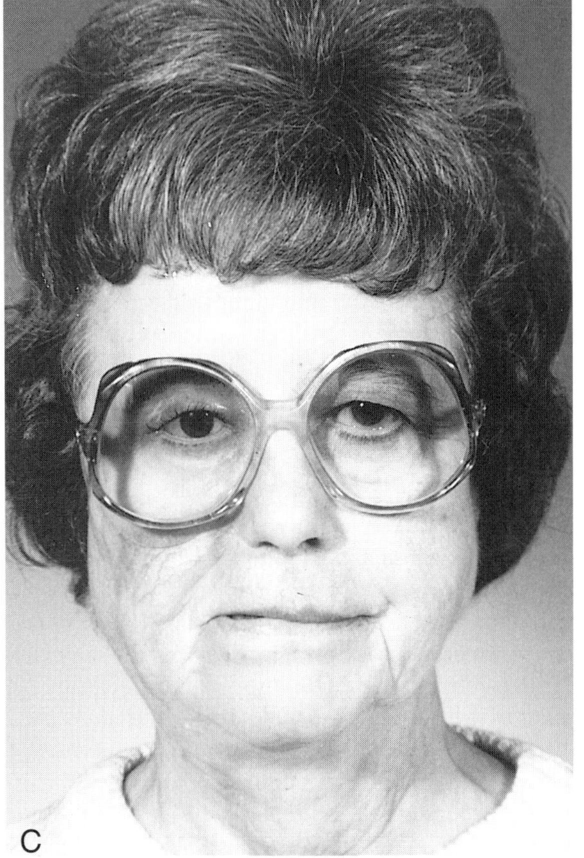

Fig. 20.3 **A.** Five years following surgical resection of squamous-cell carcinoma of the maxilla and orbit. The patient was left with a large orbital–maxillary defect. **B.** The patient was reconstructed with a revascularized latissimus dorsi musculocutaneous flap. The bulky muscle was used to fill the deficient soft tissue of the orbit and cheek. **C.** A concavity created in the vicinity of the orbit provides an excellent fit of an ocular prosthesis. (A and B from Head and Neck Surgery 6: 194 (1984) with permission of the publisher, John Wiley. C from Otolaryngology Head and Neck Surgery, 1989, p 194, with permission of the publisher, C V Mosby.)

The major advantages of microvascular flaps are the ability to transfer far greater quantities of skin, muscle and bone to the face compared to regional flaps, thus providing the surgeon better capabilities of restoring form and function to the patient. Donor site morbidity of most revascularized flaps is acceptable, and most are readily covered by clothing. In addition, reconstruction is generally accomplished in a single-stage procedure.

General disadvantages of revascularized flaps include the need for specialized surgical techniques, and the lengthy surgical procedure. These flaps have the same disadvantages as regional flaps from the standpoint of poor colour and texture match with the skin of the face.

Reconstruction of the nose

Options for reconstructing the nose following surgical

Table 20.3 Reconstruction of nasal defects of tip, columella and ala

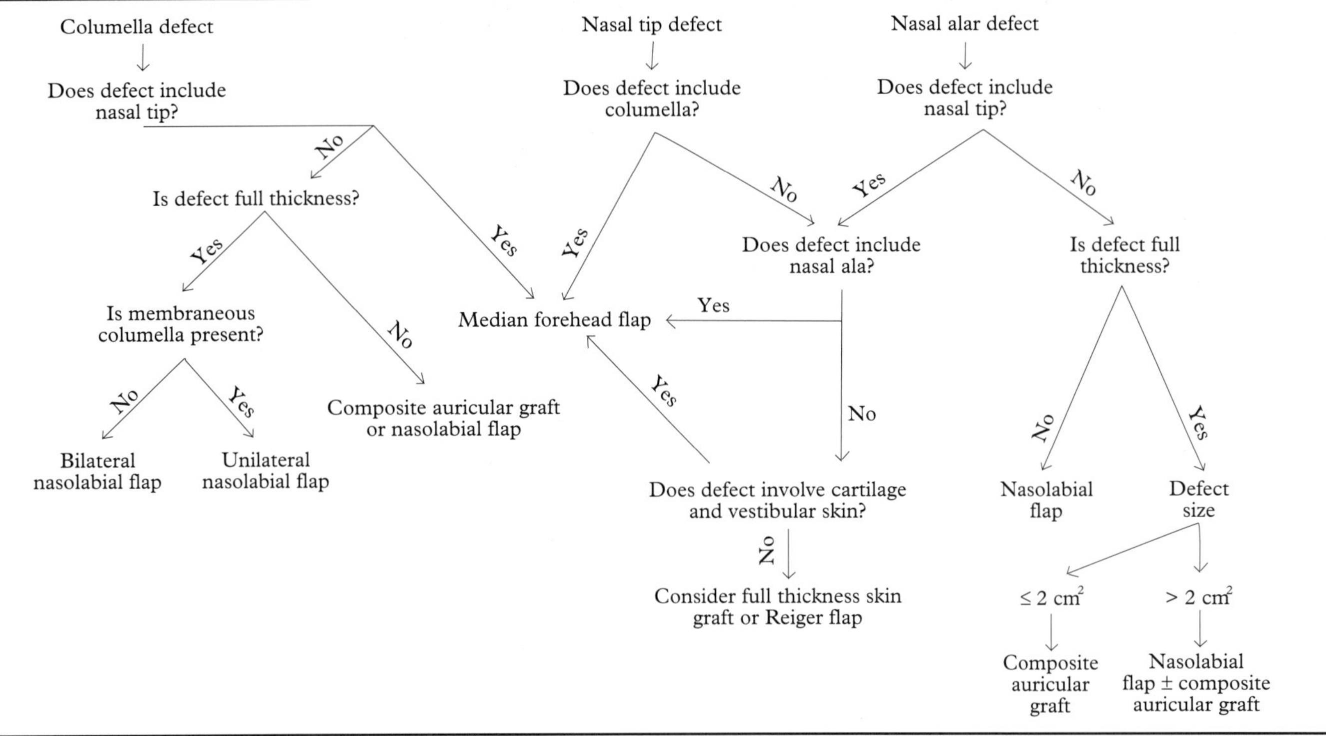

Table 20.4 Reconstruction of nasal defects of dorsum

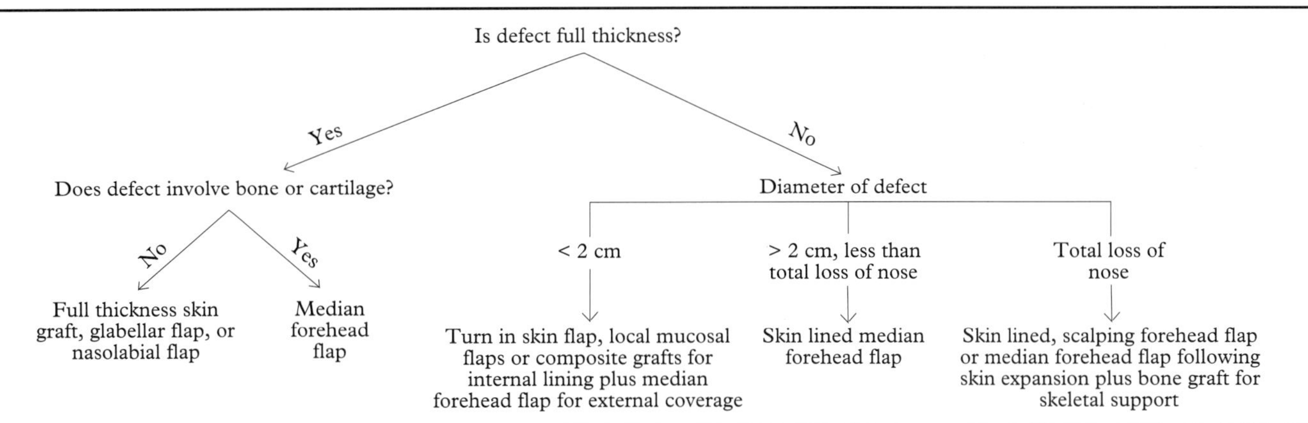

excision of carcinoma have been dealt with previously (see Ch. 18). The author's approach to reconstruction of these important cosmetic and functional units of the nose are outlined in the algorithm listed in Tables 20.3 and 20.4 (Baker 1989).

One area that is particularly difficult in mid-face reconstruction is the columella, and this is worthy of further consideration.

Reconstruction of the columella

Tissue from the nasolabial regions is the most useful source for reconstruction when restoration of full-thickness columella defects is necessary. Nasolabial flaps should be based superiorly and may be tubed or backed with a split-thickness skin graft to avoid tubulation. Such flaps may be tunnelled through the cheek or the nasal base (Heanley 1955) or may be delivered to the columellar region between the superior edge of the upper lateral nasal cartilage and the bony pyriform aperture (DaSilva 1964). These manoeuvres provide a greater useful length to the flap. The pedicle of the flap is then incised transversely 3 weeks later, and the nasocutaneous fistula is closed. Other clinicians lift the ala off its base to accommodate passage to the columella of a superiorly based nasolabial flap (DaSilva 1964). This method is particularly good for concurrent restoration of the columella

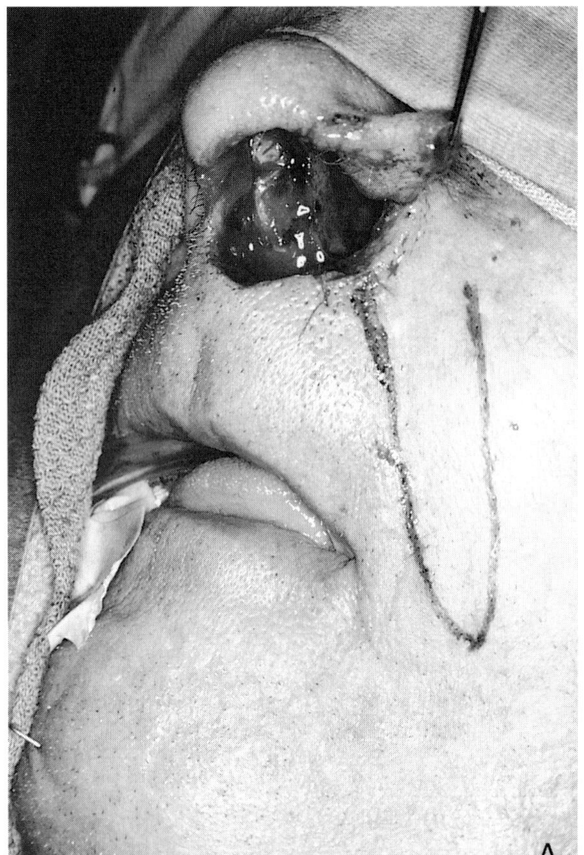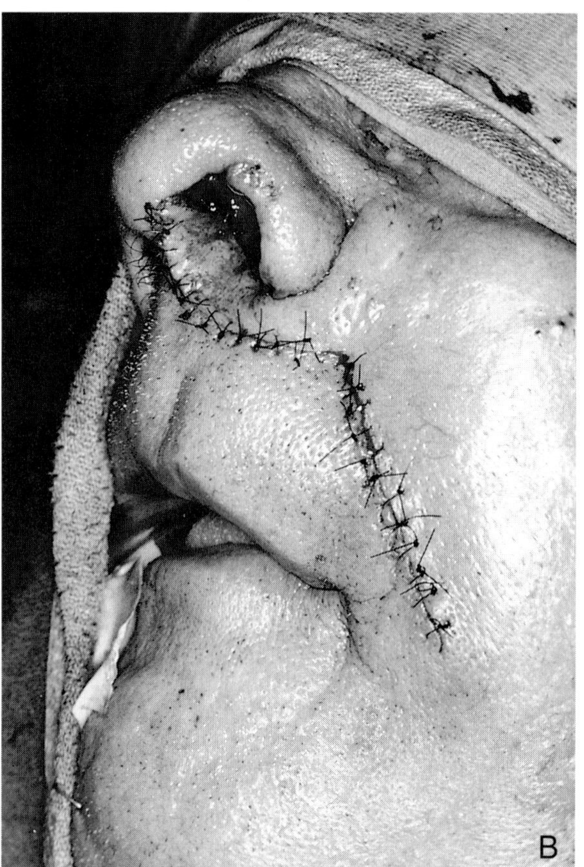

Fig. 20.4 **A.** Loss of nasal columella and portions of sill following resection of malignancy. Superiorly based nasolabial flap outlined for reconstruction. The ala is detached from its base to accommodate passage of the flap to the columella. **B.** Flap transposed. (From Facial Plastic Surgery 2: 412, 413 (1984) with permission of the publisher, Thieme Medical Publishers.)

and nasal sill (Baker & Swanson 1984b) (Fig.20.4). Initially, the wide attachment of the flap must be maintained proximally; however, this causes some residual fullness laterally which necessitates debulking and recontouring of the nasal flap as a second procedure. Re-attachment of the ala to restore a normal anatomical relationship should be accomplished at the time of flap transfer by attaching it to a de-epithelialized region located near the base of the flap.

A single nasolabial flap usually does not provide sufficient tissue for restoration when the entire columella, as well as membranous nasal septum, is absent (Table 20.3) (Baker 1989). In such instances, bilateral nasolabial flaps are useful (Fig. 20.5) (Baker et al 1987). In other instances, the distal portion of a nasolabial flap may be turned on itself to provide an inner lining to the upper portion of the nasal vestibule. In men, it may be necessary to use a higher nasolabial flap than usual to avoid including hair from the beard. A cartilage graft should be inserted in the reconstructed columella to provide nasal tip support.

When defects of the columella extend significantly onto the nasal tip, nasolabial flaps rarely provide sufficient tissue for reconstruction. In these instances, a forehead flap is preferred and usually requires modification to enable the flap to reach the upper lip (Table 20.3) (Baker 1989).

Various modifications of the median forehead flap employed in the original Indian rhinoplasty have been promoted. The medial or mid-line flap remains the most useful of the forehead flaps because the donor site can be closed primarily, leaving a thin mid-line scar on the forehead that is camouflaged relatively easily. This is in contrast to other types of forehead flaps, such as the up-and-down, horizontal supra-orbital, sickle, and scalping flap that may result in the need for split-thickness skin grafts to cover portions of the forehead. The exception to this is the oblique forehead flap (Baker & Swanson 1985) which extends obliquely along the hair-line of the forehead providing additional length for reaching the upper lip in instances where the nasal columella is in need of reconstruction. In many instances, the flap provides sufficient tissue for total reconstruction of the nasal tip and columellar complex (Fig. 20.6) (Baker & Swanson 1984b).

In the majority of cases, the secondary defect resulting

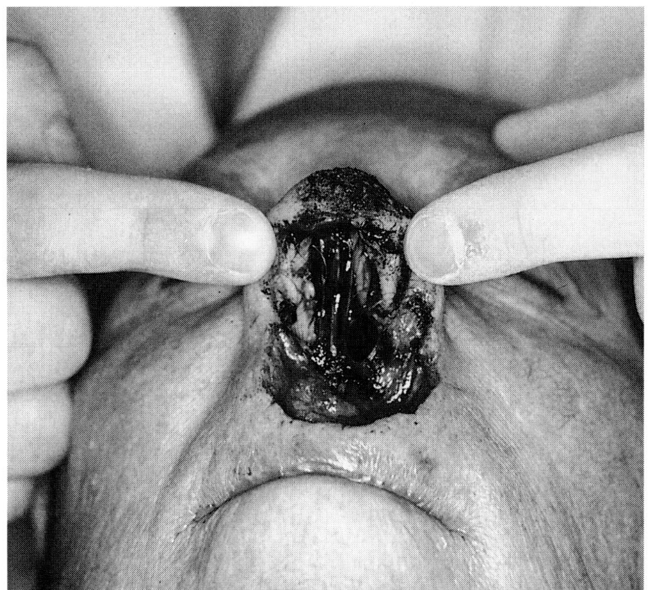
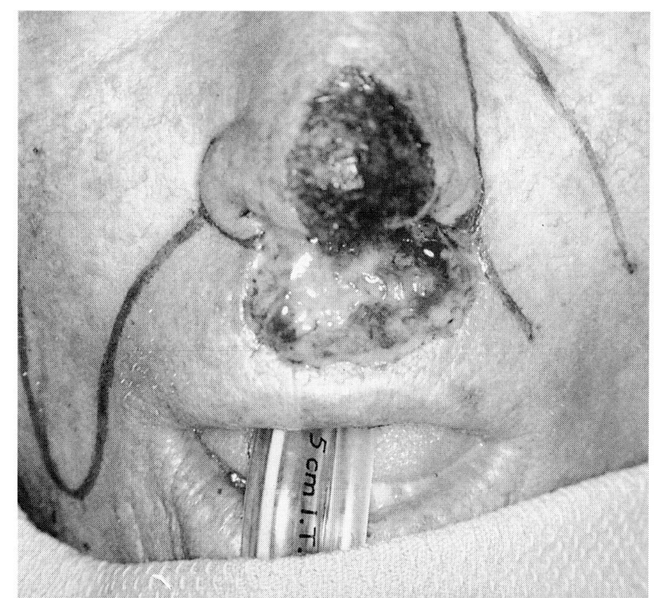
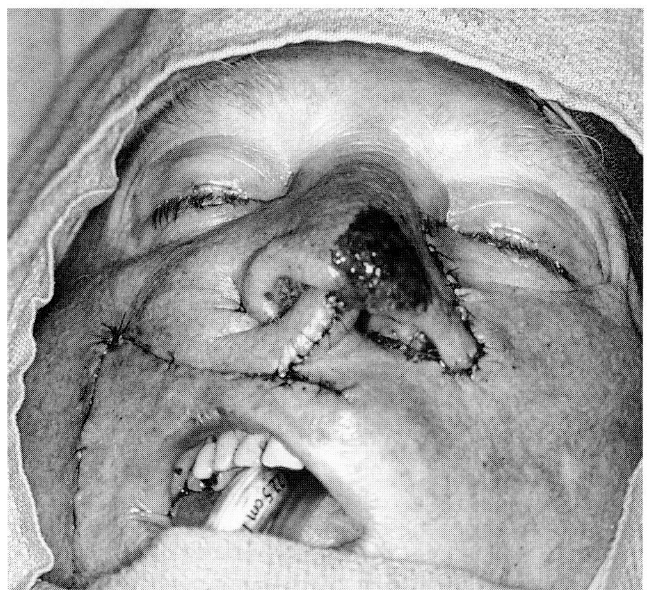
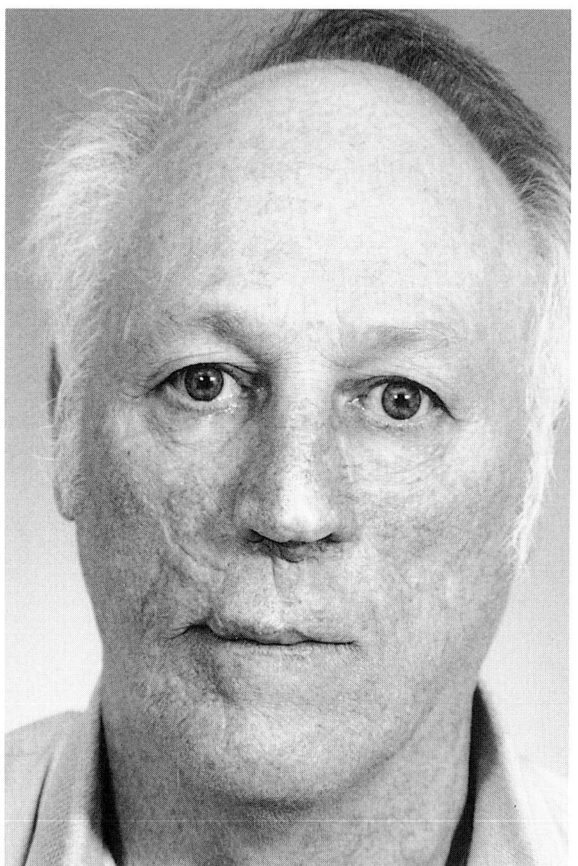
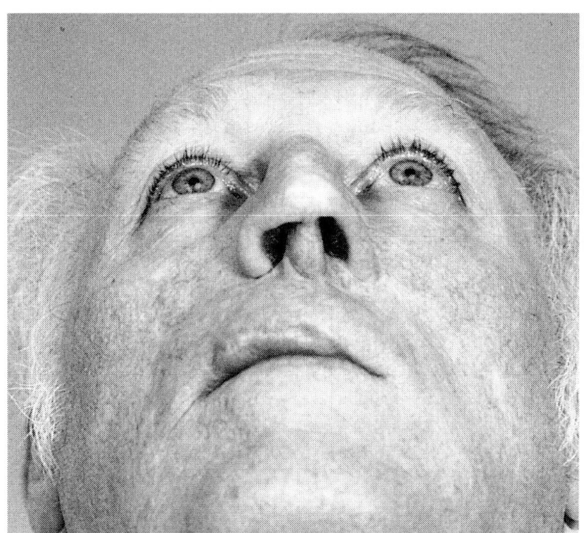

Fig. 20.5 A. Loss of entire membranous septum and columella as well as central portion of upper lip following tumour resection. **B.** Superiorly and inferiorly based nasolabial flaps were used to reconstruct a portion of the upper lip as well as the columella. **C.** Flaps transposed. **D, E.** Nine months postoperative. An Abbe flap from the lower lip was used to further augment the upper lip reconstruction. (From Facial Plastic Surgery 5: 834 (1987) with permission of the publisher, Thieme Medical Publishers.)

from harvest of an oblique forehead flap can be closed primarily. Thus, the flap obviates the need for a scalping flap, which is a surgical procedure of greater magnitude and results in more significant deformity of the skin of the forehead. The major disadvantage of the oblique forehead flap is that it results in an oblique scar on the forehead; however, if designed so that the oblique portion of the flap follows the border of the hairline, the oblique scar is cosmetically as acceptable as the mid-line scar resulting from an extended median forehead flap.

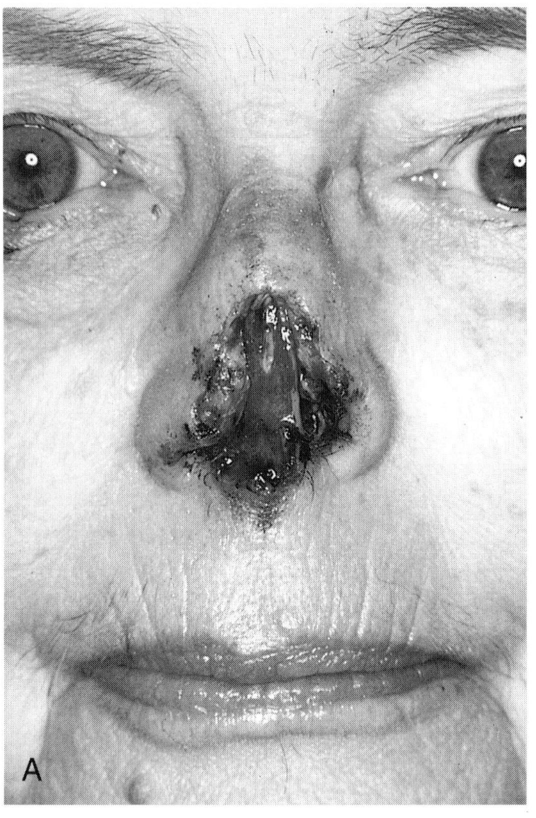

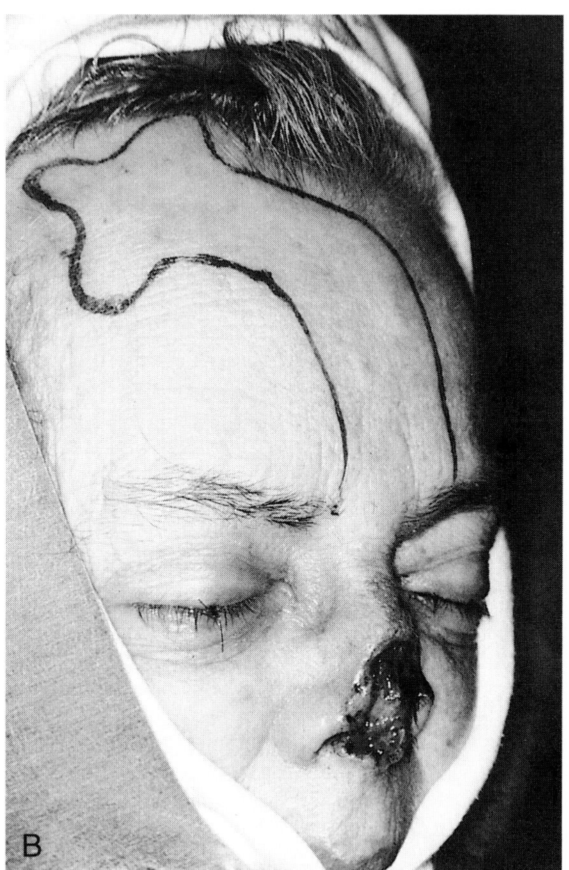

Fig. 20.6

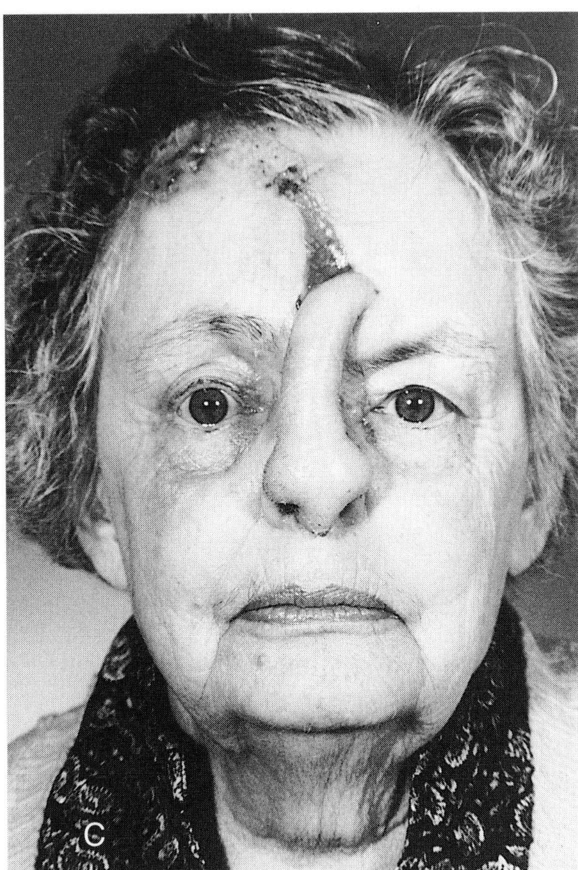
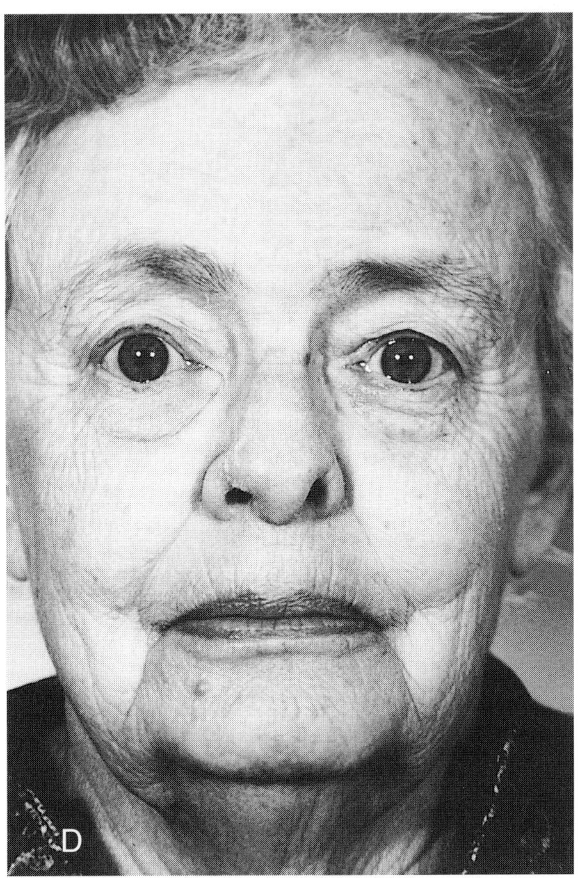

Fig. 20.6 A. Resection of neoplasm resulted in complete loss of the nasal tip and columella. **B.** Oblique forehead flap outlined. **C.** Flap is of sufficient length to reach upper lip and provide for reconstruction of the entire columella. **D.** Twelve months postoperative. (From Facial Plastic Surgery 2: (1984) with permission of the publisher, Thieme Medical Publishers.)

Reconstruction of the orbit

Skin grafts and local flaps

Repair of defects following subtotal exenteration are usually best treated by placing a split-thickness skin graft on the exposed soft tissue of the orbit. Orbital defects following simple orbital exenteration without resection of bone and without bony orbital defects exposing the adjacent sinus may be left to granulate. Conversely, temporalis muscle may be used to fill the orbit in cases of primary tumour of the orbit in which no bone resection is necessary but orbital exenteration is needed. Transposition of the temporalis muscle helps to obliterate the socket, yet allows a shallow depression for the fitting of an ocular prosthesis if desired. The main disadvantage of using a temporalis muscle flap is the possibility of masking a recurrent tumour. There may also be some depression over the temporal fossa. Following exenteration, the temporalis muscle is exposed by extending a 3 cm incision laterally from the lateral canthus. An incision is made to the deep fascia of the temporalis muscle along the lateral border of the orbit, and the muscle, with its fascia, is then freed from the temporal fossa and from under the

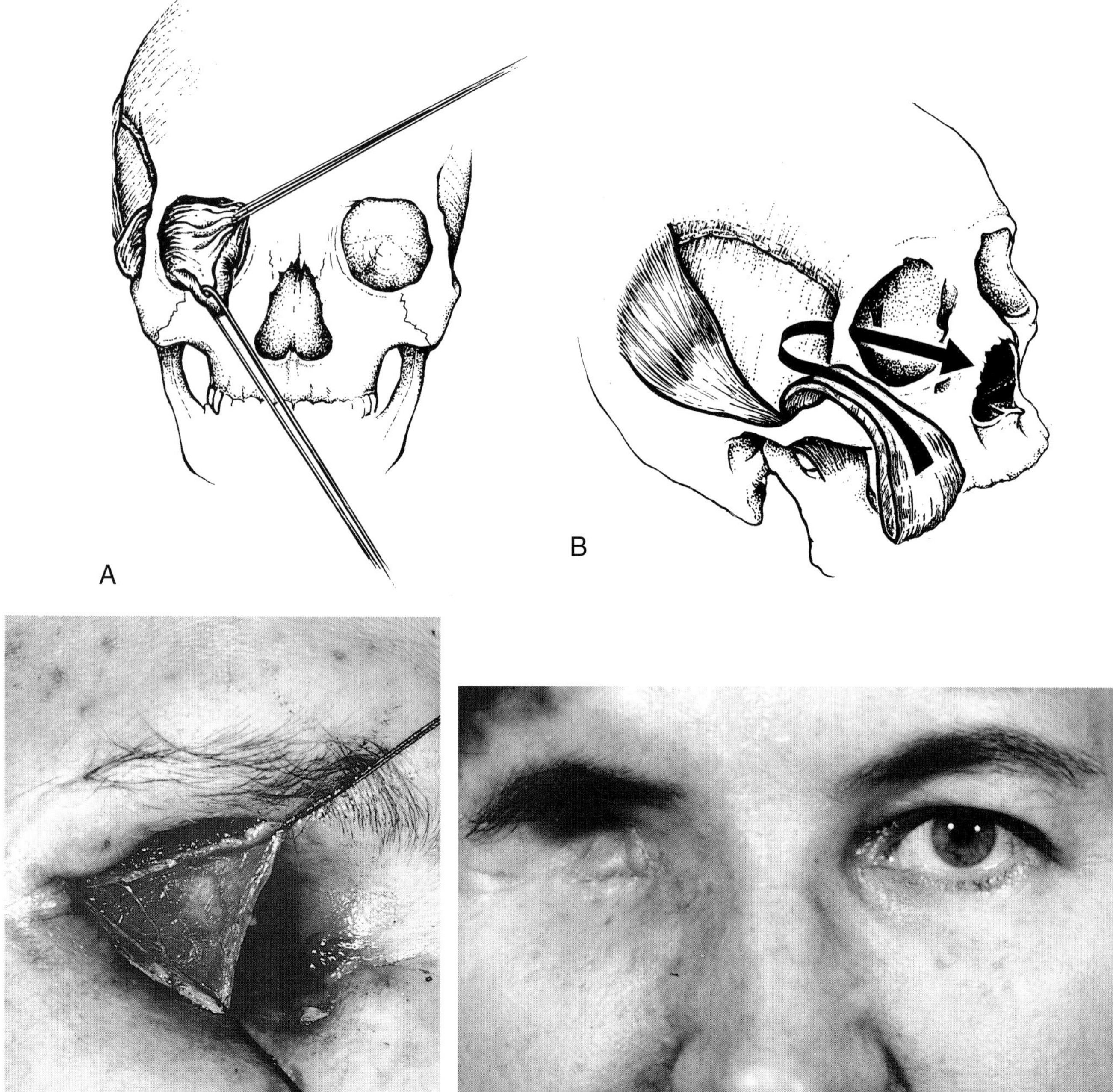

Fig. 20.7 A, B. Portions or all of temporalis muscle may be transposed into the orbit through a surgically created opening in the bony lateral orbit. **C.** Surgical case in which temporalis muscle is transposed to assist in filling the orbital cavity. **D.** Same patient 1 year postoperative. Mild concavity allows fitting with an orbital prosthesis.

zygomatic process all the way to the insertion of the muscle into the coronoid process of the mandible. The muscle must be mobilized sufficiently to allow it to reach the lateral wall of the orbit. A Stryker saw and Rongeur is used to remove the lateral wall of the orbit while maintaining the orbital rim. The temporalis muscle and fascia are passed through the opening into the orbit and sutured to the periosteum remaining along the medial orbital rim (Fig. 20.7). The muscle is fanned out to fill the cavity uniformly. A plastic sphere may be placed in the apex of the orbit and covered by the muscle to help assist in obliteration. When the lids have been preserved they are sutured together. If the lids have been resected with the exenteration, the temporalis muscle may be covered with a skin graft.

In performing a maxillectomy in combination with orbital exenteration the eyelids, conjunctiva and obicularis oculi muscle should be preserved whenever possible. The socket is then reconstructed by directly suturing together the margins of the preserved conjunctiva of the inner aspect of the eyelids to create a new socket. A temporary silastic spacer is placed within the new socket to maintain its shape, and a skin graft is placed on the inner surface of the obicularis oculi muscle and sinus cavity. The medial canthus is secured by a transnasal wire placed through the contralateral lamina papyracea at the appropriate level for the canthus. A maxillary prosthesis augments the cheek, encloses the maxillectomy defect, and helps to support the reconstructed socket.

In instances where the eyelids and conjunctiva must be resected, the orbit is left open, covering the interior of the orbit with a skin graft. The author believes that in such cases the orbit is best rehabilitated by a prosthesis rather than attempting secondary reconstruction which is protracted, multi-staged, and often is not as cosmetically acceptable as a prosthesis.

Although the facial skin and musculature are usually preserved when radical maxillectomy and orbital exenteration are performed, the resulting lack of skeletal support may on occasion lead to breakdown of the skin about the orbit. Skin breakdown in the region of the orbit may lead to progressive enlargement of the opening into the orbital–maxillary defect. If the opening of the orbit enlarges excessively, the patient is troubled with an unsightly appearance. In addition, the defect causes an ill-fitting maxillary prosthesis resulting in difficulties with proper speech and deglutition. Such defects are best reconstructed by a regional or microsurgical flap; however, a local forehead flap may, on occasion, be used for repair. The laterally based forehead flap can be turned upon itself to provide adequate inner and outer cheek coverage in reconstructing large orbital–maxillary defects, or the inner aspect of the flap may be covered by a skin graft. In either situation, the forehead flap usually does not provide sufficient bulk to fill in the orbital defect, and the skin of such flaps tends to be less pliable than adjacent facial skin (Fig. 20.8). For this reason, in addition

to the donor site deformity, the use of a regional flap is preferred.

Regional flaps

Traditional methods of reconstructing large defects of the orbit and maxillary region include the use of the forehead flap, nape of neck flap (shoulder flap), and medially based deltopectoral flap. More contemporary methods of reconstruction include the use of the trapezius or the pectoralis major musculocutaneous flap pedicled on their dominant blood supply. Unsightly donor-site defects are readily visible when the forehead, nape of neck, or superiorly based trapezius musculocutaneous flaps are used. The author's preferred regional flap for reconstruction of orbital–maxillary defects is the pectoralis major or trapezius musculocutaneous flap. Often these flaps can be made sufficiently large to allow the flap to be folded on itself, providing for both external and internal reconstruction of orbital–maxillary defects. The distal portion of the flap is turned inward for intra-oral resurfacing, and the proximal portion of the flap is used for external coverage. The segment of the flap covered by the tissues of the cheek margin is de-epithelialized to prevent burying epidermis and to allow a two-layered internal and external closure.

The luxury of the trapezius, pectoralis, and even the latissimus dorsi musculocutaneous flaps for reconstruction of orbital–maxillary defects is that they usually provide a one-stage reconstruction. These flaps have an added advantage of providing well-vascularized, non-irradiated tissue to repair defects that may have been heavily irradiated. The latissimus dorsi as an island flap offers tremendous size potential, and if designed sufficiently long, can be made to reach the orbital area. The pectoralis major musculocutaneous flap can be used with the patient in a supine position throughout the operative procedure, whereas the use of the latissimus dorsi or trapezius flaps may necessitate repositioning the patient intra-operatively.

The pectoralis major musculocutaneous flap may be expanded to reach the orbital area; however, necrosis of the distal portion of the flap may occur when the cutaneous territory is extended below the sixth rib. This extension is often necessary to gain sufficient length to reach the level of the eyebrow superiorly. Likewise, the trapezius musculocutaneous flap based on the transverse cervical artery and vein or the latissimus dorsi musculocutaneous island flap may be difficult to mobilize sufficiently to reach the forehead, resulting in separation of the suture line at the eyebrow and persistence of the orbital defect (Schuller 1982). The same may be said for the deltopectoral flap. Thus, the most distal portion of these flaps should be delayed prior to their use in reconstructing the orbital area to ensure adequate length and reduce the risks of partial necrosis of the flap.

In instances where a full-thickness defect of the cheek and

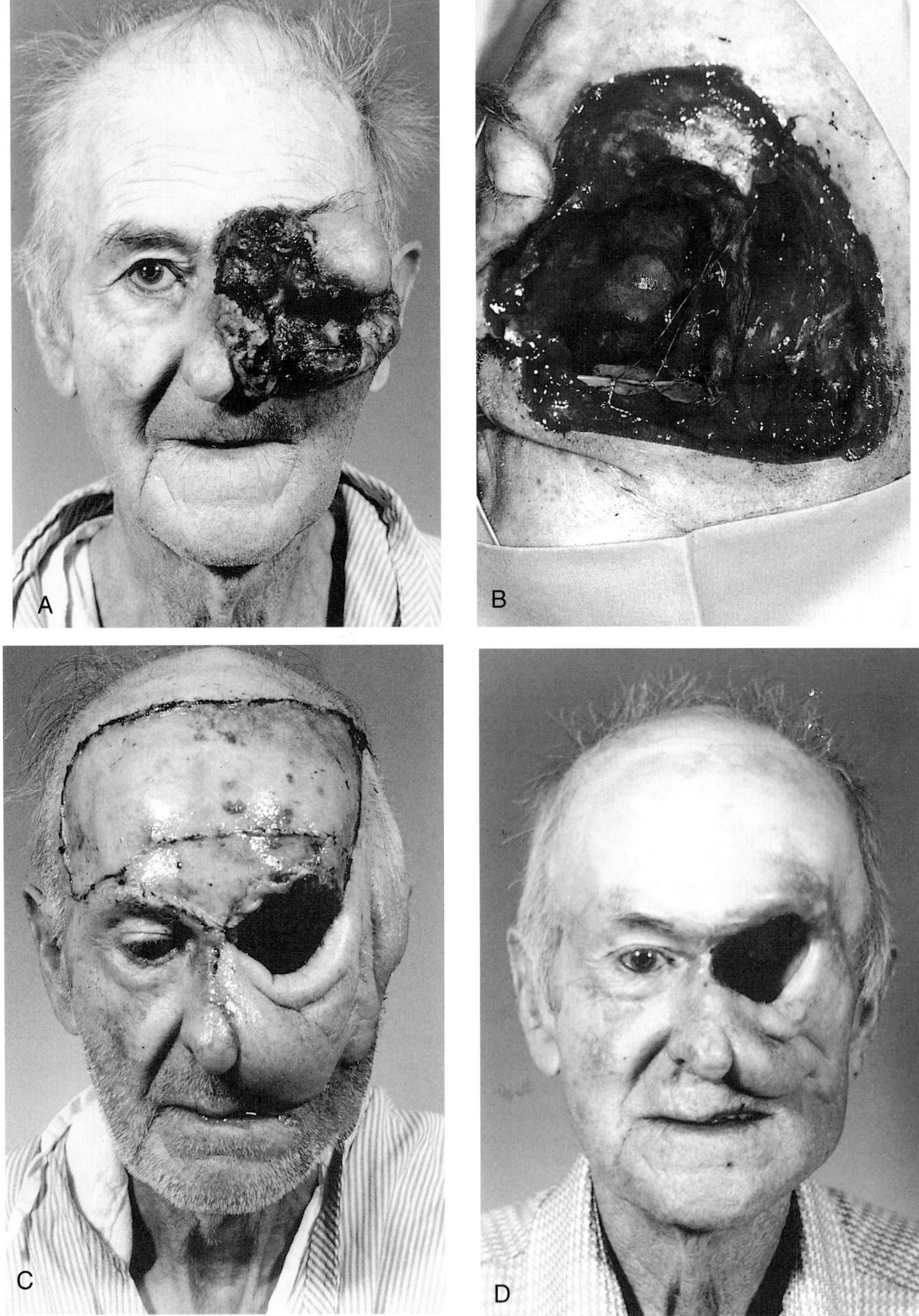

Fig. 20.8 **A.** Large neglected basal-cell carcinoma of mid-face and orbit. **B.** Defect following tumour excision. **C.** Total forehead flap lined with a split-thickness skin graft was used to reconstruct cheek and upper lip. **D.** Four months postoperative.

orbit is of such magnitude that closure with a single regional flap is difficult, a combination of two regional flaps may facilitate closure. Simultaneous temporal and deltopectoral flaps may be utilized to reconstruct full-thickness defects of the orbital–maxillary region. Likewise, the combination of a sternocleidomastoid musculocutaneous flap for intra-oral lining and a pectoralis major musculocutaneous flap for external coverage is possible. A third combination would be to utilize a pectoralis major and trapezius musculocutaneous flap for reconstruction. In most cases where multiple regional flaps are required, the author prefers employing a deltopectoral flap and pectoralis major musculocutaneous flap. The latter flap is transposed over the clavicle and tunnelled subcutaneously to the margin of the defect where it provides an internal lining for the reconstructed defect. The deltopectoral flap is transposed over the top of the intervening cervical skin to provide external coverage. In 3 weeks the pedicle of the deltopectoral flap is divided and the proximal portion of the flap is returned to the donor site.

In some instances, there may be sufficient adjacent tissue to design a local flap that can be used concomitantly with a larger regional flap to reconstruct sizeable orbital–maxillary defects. The local flap may be turned inward in a trapdoor fashion for intra-oral resurfacing, or may simply accompany the regional flap in assisting in the external coverage while a skin graft provides the epithelial covering to the intra-oral aspect of the defect (Fig. 20.9).

Revascularized flaps

In instances where regional flaps are not sufficient or their use significantly impairs form and function, revascularized flaps may be used to repair orbital–maxillary defects. These flaps circumvent many of the disadvantages seen with the pedicle regional flaps discussed. Such flaps can be placed in any location about the head, provided a recipient artery and vein are available in the vicinity. Groin flaps, tensor fascia lata musculocutaneous flaps, gastro-omental flaps, and deltopectoral flaps have all been transferred as microsurgical flaps for the purpose of reconstructing cheek and orbital defects. The latissimus dorsi flap is one of the most useful of the various microsurgical musculocutaneous flaps that can be utilized for orbital reconstruction. The skin of the latissimus dorsi musculocutaneous flap is pliable and its texture is similar to that of the face. The muscle bulk is sufficient to obliterate extensive soft-tissue and bone defects of the orbit and maxilla.

A disadvantage of the latissimus dorsi musculocutaneous flap is that the excessive bulkiness of the flap frequently requires secondary defatting procedures for optimal cosmesis.

Similar to all regional and distant flaps, the colour of the skin of the flap and the skin of the face are often not closely matched. Despite these disadvantages, the latissimus dorsi musculocutaneous flap is particularly suited for reconstruction of large facial soft-tissue defects about the orbit where obliteration of the orbital cavity and restoration of deficient facial skin is desirable (Baker 1984). The skin island flap can be designed anywhere within the musculocutaneous territory. The dominance of the thoracodorsal system allows the entire latissimus dorsi muscle and its overlying skin to be transferred on the thoracodorsal vascular pedicle in a single-stage procedure. To extend the cutaneous portion of the flap beyond the iliac crest, or to harvest a wide segment of distal skin, a preliminary ligation of the intercostal perforators in conjunction with a distal cutaneous delay is helpful. The latissimus dorsi muscle is initially mobilized anteriorly, dissecting in the fascial plane between the latissimus dorsi and serratus anterior muscles. The skin paddle is then fashioned and cut down to the fascia of the underlying muscle. During mobilization, the skin island is secured to the underlying muscle by sutures placed at its periphery. The distal portion of the latissimus dorsi muscle is cut through to allow elevation of the flap superiorly.

Care must be taken to incorporate into the flap the proximal portion of the muscle containing the nutrient vascular pedicle. This is accomplished by making an incision of skin only from the anterior border of the latissimus dorsi muscle to the skin paddle and reflecting the skin and subcutaneous tissue to expose the proximal portion of the muscle. All of the proximal portion of the muscle is incorporated into the vascular pedicle by detaching the muscle from its humeral insertion.

The latissimus dorsi musculocutaneous flap is left attached by its vascular pedicle until the recipient vessels have been prepared. The facial artery and vein are particularly good recipient vessels because their size closely matches that of the thoracodorsal artery and vein. At the time of transfer, the thoracodorsal nerve is severed along with the artery and vein.

The revascularized latissimus dorsi musculocutaneous flap is an effective method of reconstructing large orbital–maxillary defects. The bulk of the flap provides ample tissue to fill the orbital cavity and augment the deficient subcutaneous tissues and bone deficiencies of the maxilla (Fig. 20.10) (Baker 1984).

The donor defect that results from harvesting a latissimus dorsi musculocutaneous flap can be closed primarily in many cases, leaving a secondary deformity that is acceptable and well hidden beneath the arm.

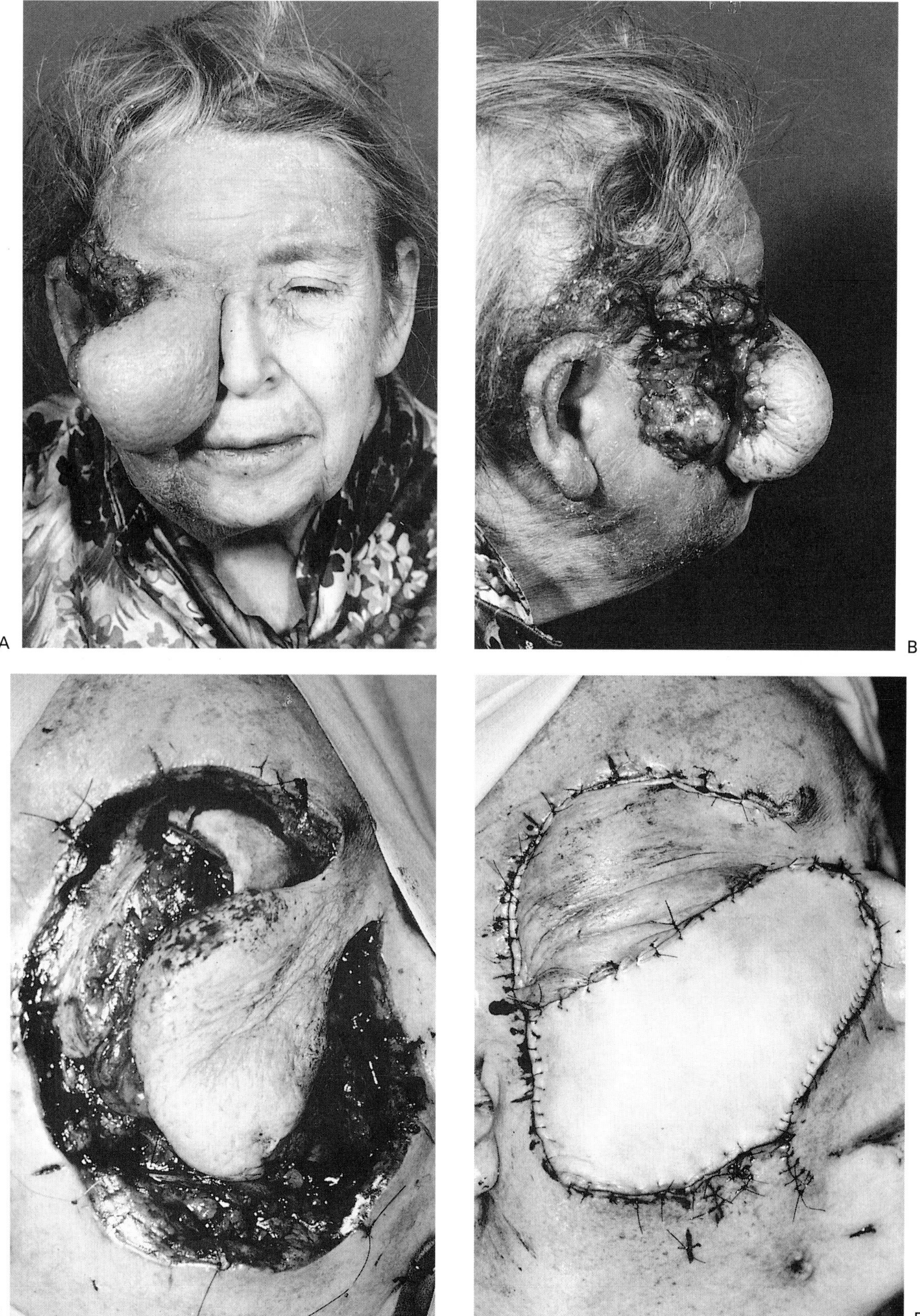

Fig. 20.9 **A, B.** Large neglected basal-cell carcinoma of mid-face and orbit. Chronic lymphoedema has stretched upper eyelid skin. **C.** Surgical defect following orbital exenteration and maxillectomy. Stretched upper eyelid skin was free of tumour and was preserved to assist in reconstruction. **D.** Defect was repaired with remaining upper eyelid skin combined with a pectoralis major musculocutaneous flap.

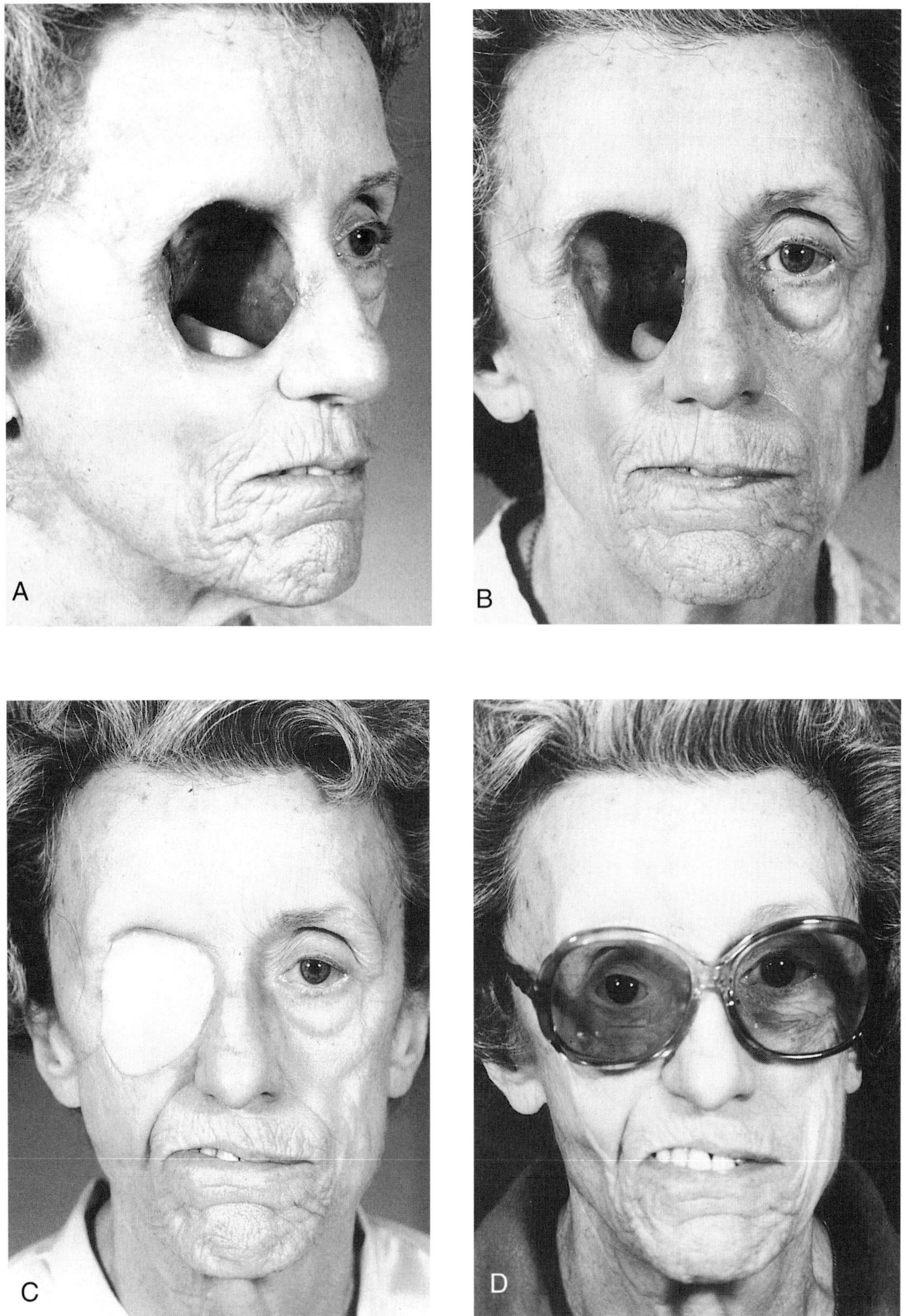

Fig. 20.10 **A, B.** Large orbital–maxillary defect 5 years following maxillectomy and orbital exenteration. Maxillary prosthesis is visible through orbital defect. **C, D.** One year postoperative following reconstruction with a revascularized latissimus dorsi musculocutaneous flap. The flap has provided sufficient tissue for a secure fit of the maxillary prosthesis and a surface area to anchor the ocular prosthesis. (From Head and Neck Surgery 6: (1984) with permission of the publisher, John Wiley.)

PROBLEMS AND COMPLICATIONS

Every surgical procedure has inherent possibilities for complications. Complications may result in immediate or delayed sequelae which may be overwhelming to the patient, resulting in death or severe functional and cosmetic disability. Other complications may be of minor consequence, being only a nuisance to the patient. Some complications are not preventable and may be unpredictable; however, many complications are preventable by careful pre-operative planning, as well as attention to surgical technique.

Paramount to the prophylaxis of complications is the knowledge of factors which influence the success of excision and reconstruction of the orbit and mid-face. These factors include patient selection, selection of appropriate flaps and grafts for the purpose of reconstruction, and surgical technical factors.

Patient selection

Surgery of the mid-face and orbit has been successful in patients ranging in age as young as a few weeks to the eighth and ninth decades of life. Advanced age, however, is often associated with arteriosclerosis and diabetes mellitus which may result in thickening of the walls of small arteries and overall increased fragility and friability of small vessels. This could lead to heightened difficulties with intra-operative bleeding and postoperative healing.

Although age is usually not a major deterrent, there are a number of systemic illnesses that more strongly influence the results of surgery. Patients with blood coagulopathies, collagen vascular disorders and polycythaemia in general are at a greater risk for intra-operative and postoperative complications of all types, including wound infection, haematoma formation, and wound dehiscence.

Obesity may also be a factor influencing successful surgery, particularly when it relates to the transfer of regional flaps for the purpose of reconstruction. The excessive subcutaneous fat makes dissection somewhat difficult and may interfere with proper placement and tailoring of the flap following transfer to the face. This is particularly true when the orbit or a maxillary cavity is the recipient site for the flap. An excessively fatty flap may be defatted at the time of transfer; however, extensive defatting procedures increases the risk of injury to the flap vasculature. Obese patients also have a higher incidence of postoperative wound infection than patients with normal weight.

Previous irradiation to the mid-face or orbit could be influential in the success of surgery performed in this region. Capillaries and arterioles are particularly sensitive to irradiation (Rubin & Cassarett 1968). Late effects of radiation injury to blood vessels include fibrosis and an increase in interstitial connective tissue in the tunica media, along with endothelial proliferation and progressive fibrosis, which further thickens the vessel wall and narrows the lumen to the point of eventual occlusion. Even in cases of slowly progressive vessel fibrosis, the obstructive nature of these changes may severely compromise the vascular supply to an area. These areas may then succumb to necrosis when challenged by an additional injury or increased functional demand. An example of this would be surgical resection of recurrent tumour of the mid-face following a full course of radiotherapy. In such instances, wound dehiscence may occur secondary to necrosis of tissue and result in oral–facial or nasal–facial fistulae.

Flap selection

There are a number of flaps and grafts that the surgeon can select for the purpose of reconstructing the mid-face and orbit. In the case of local and regional flaps, each donor site has advantages and disadvantages from the standpoint of complexity of dissection, colour and texture match with the skin of the face, length and size of the pedicle, and donor site cosmetic and functional disability. Most of these advantages and disadvantages have been discussed in the preceding portions of this chapter. In addition, each donor site has the potential for complications that are specific to the individual donor site.

Surgical technique

Surgical technique and clinical judgement are perhaps the most important factors influencing the success or failure of excision and reconstruction of the mid-face and orbit. The surgeon should exercise prudence in resecting tumours in these regions, taking care to avoid unnecessary trauma to surrounding uninvolved tissues which may result in excessive bleeding, tissue necrosis, or injury to adjacent nerves, vessels or muscles. In the case of surgery in or about the orbit, where exenteration is not planned, protection of the ophthalmic globe and extra-ocular muscles should be of paramount importance. Complications resulting from surgical excision of tumours of the mid-face and orbit are related to the specific site of injury. Excisions of tumours of the skin of the mid-face may result in wound infection and excessive scarring, which in turn may result in impairment of form and function of surrounding structures such as the eyelids, nose or lips. Similarly, surgery of the orbit may result in enophthalmos, diplopia, ectropion, epiphora or blindness, depending on the extent and location of the surgical excision.

The author's approach to reconstruction of the mid-face and orbit has been discussed in earlier portions of this chapter. In instances where a flap is required for reconstruction, the preferred flap is the one that offers the most superior restoration of form and function and at the same time is reliable and results in the least donor site morbidity. Even with careful pre-operative planning and meticulous surgical technique, however, flap necrosis can occur. Partial flap necrosis occurs more frequently than total loss. Partial necrosis is most often due to inadequate cutaneous circulation at the periphery of the flap as a result of excessive surgical trauma or extending the flap beyond the vascular territory of the pedicle vessels. Partial flap necrosis often results in loss of a portion of the skin of the flap while the underlying subcutaneous tissue remains viable. In such instances, healing may occur through secondary intention (Baker 1986).

FUTURE DEVELOPMENTS

Perhaps the most exciting recent development in surgical excision and reconstruction of the mid-face and orbit has been the use of tissue expansion.

Tissue expansion is indicated in the reconstruction of various defects of the mid-face and orbit in instances where there is inadequate adjacent tissue to allow either primary closure of the defect or repair with a local flap (Baker & Swanson 1990a,b). Its use may also be indicated for reconstruction of a defect that can be repaired by local, regional or distant flaps, but at the cost of significant donor or recipient site deformity (Fig. 20.11).

Tissue expansion offers the advantage of increasing locally available tissue with preservation of sensation and adnexal structures. Thus, the missing skin of the defect can be replaced with skin of identical colour, thickness, and appendages (hair growth). This is unlike any other form of reconstruction because there is no need for a secondary defect unless creation of the flap is necessary. Expanded skin can simply be advanced into the defect for primary closure. In instances requiring the use of a flap, the secondary defect can be easily closed because of the additional skin created by the expansion process, thus expansion obviates sacrificing cosmesis of one area to improve that of another.

The use of skin expansion to close large defects of the mid-face and orbit usually eliminates the need for multiple flaps or grafting procedures, thus reducing the overall cost of reconstruction. Tissue expansion is tolerated well by most patients, can be performed in an outpatient setting, and can be accomplished prior to the ablative or reconstructive procedure so that additional tissue will be available at the time of excision and reconstruction. Tissue expanders can also be placed in almost any area of the body.

Flaps harvested from expanded skin have increased vascularity; thus, flaps that would fail as simple primary procedures can be harvested from expanded skin with relative impunity, significantly improving the surgeon's flexibility during reconstructive procedures. This flexibility is enhanced by the fact that expansion can be repeated. That is, the tissue can be re-expanded a second or third time if necessary to achieve the final goals in reconstruction.

The major disadvantage of tissue expansion in reconstruction of the mid-face and orbit is that it involves two surgical procedures: one to implant the expander and the other to remove the expander and perform the reconstruction.

Tissue expansion is labour-intensive in that frequent visits to the office are necessary for the inflation of the implant. This is obviated in some circumstances by training paramedical personnel in the patient's community or a patient's family member to carry out the actual inflation process.

Another major disadvantage of tissue expansion in the head and neck region is the temporary visible deformity that results from expansion, particularly toward the end of the expansion process. This may preclude its use in certain situations where the patient must continue to work in a position that requires interacting with the public. Scalp expansion can be camouflaged by wearing a large hat, and neck expansion can be concealed in part by a turtleneck sweater; however, expansion of the forehead and cheek areas cannot be easily hidden. It is important to ensure that the patient is properly informed concerning the significant but temporary deformity that occurs in the area of expansion.

Tissue expanders are silastic balloons with self-sealing valves or reservoirs that are completely implanted beneath the skin. They are available in many different sizes and shapes such as round, rectangular, and elliptical. Expanders are also available in various volumes ranging from a few cubic centimetres to several thousand cubic centimetres.

Tissue expansion is an extraordinarily simple technique. It allows the surgeon to undertake reconstructive procedures

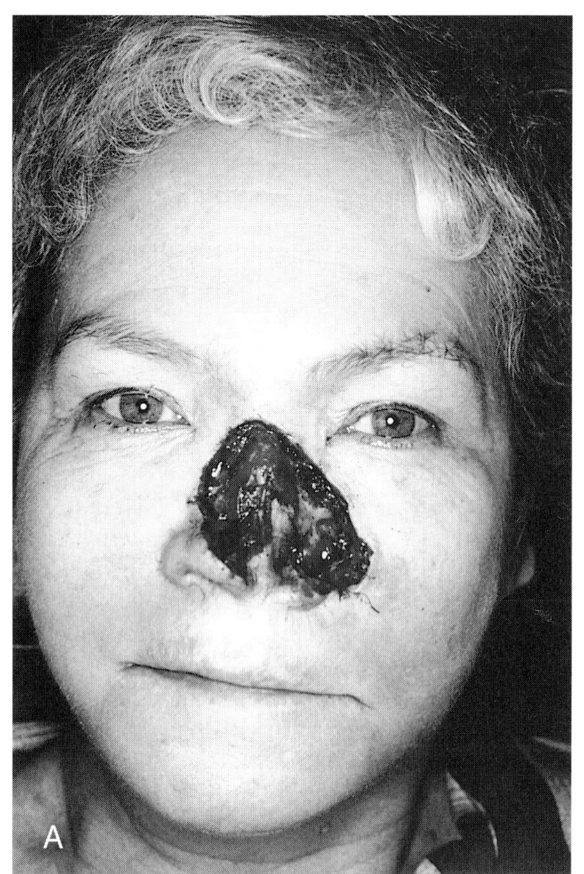

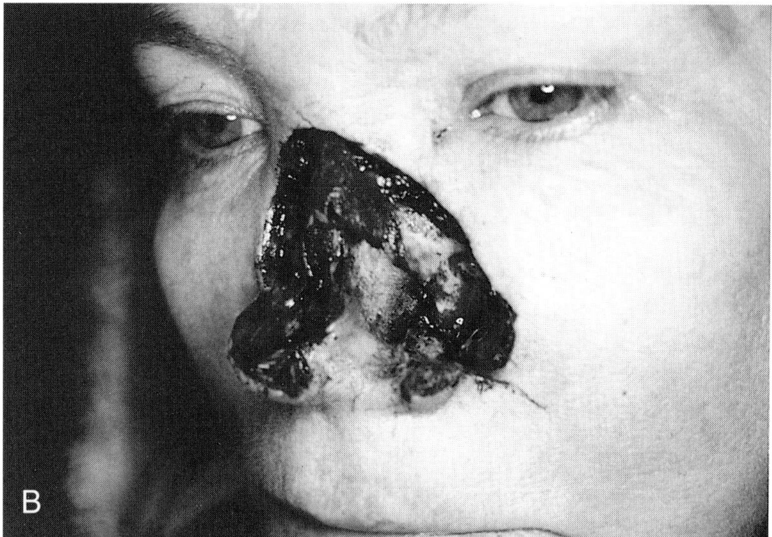

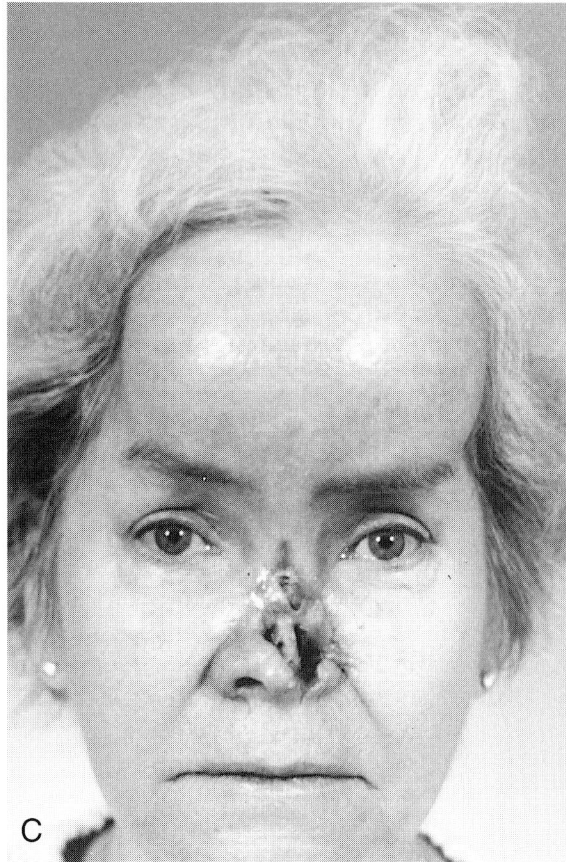

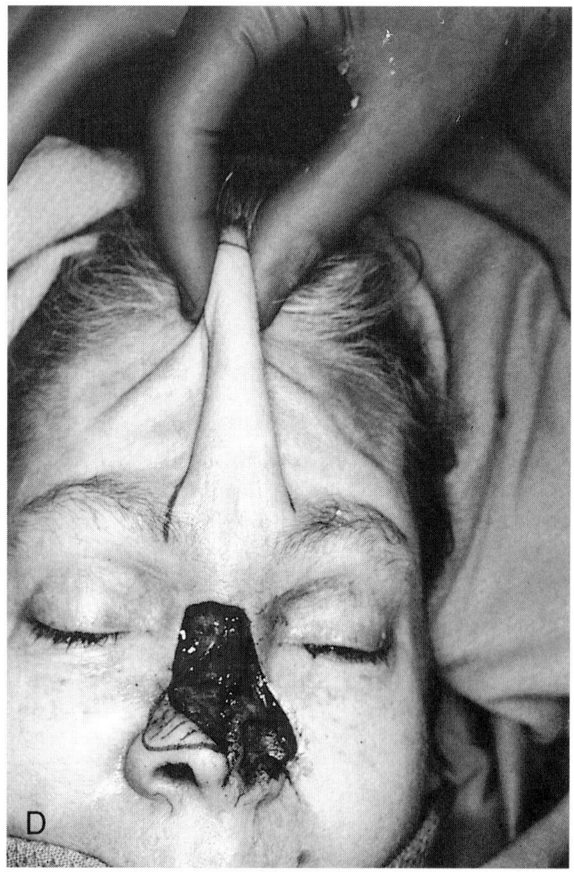

Fig. 20.11

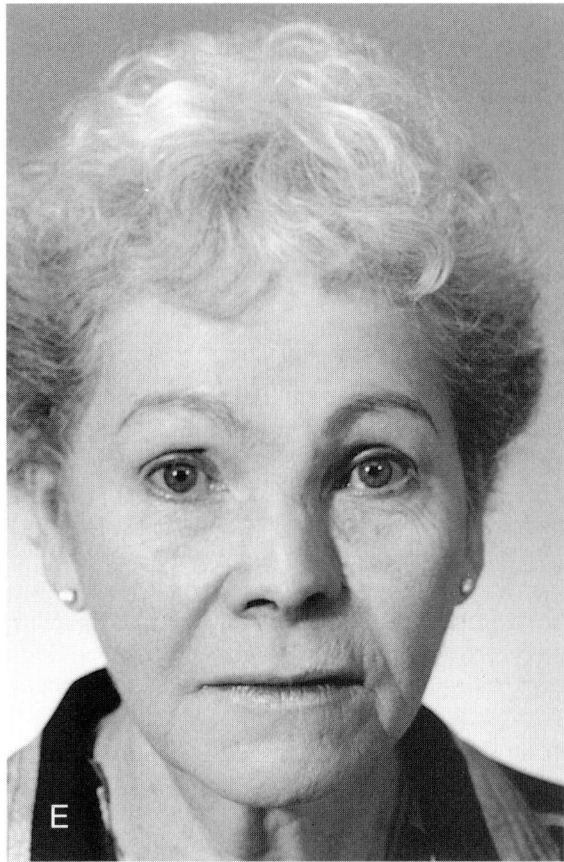

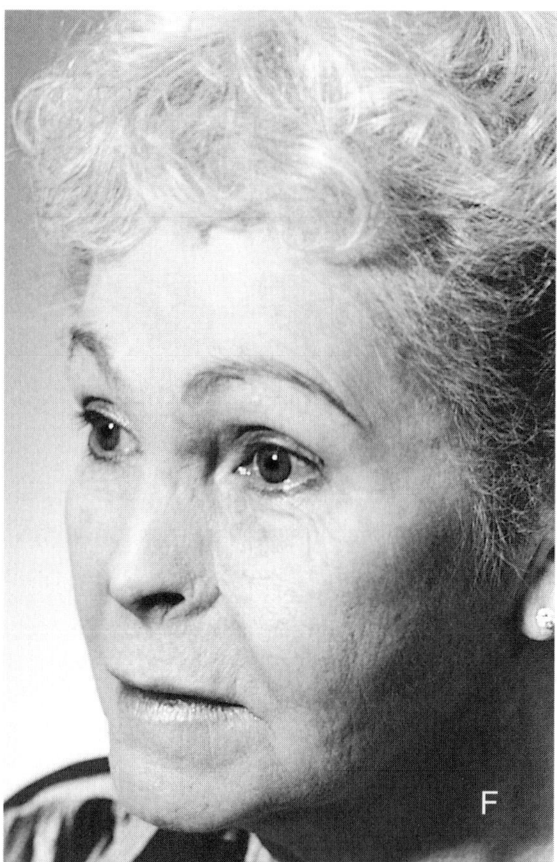

Fig. 20.11 A, B. Large mid-facial defect following removal of an extensive skin cancer. Defect was temporarily repaired with a skin graft. **C.** Tissue expansion of the forehead was performed in anticipation of reconstructing the facial defect with a large mid-line forehead flap. **D.** Tissue expansion provided sufficient tissue for reconstruction of the nose and cheek and allowed primary closure of the donor site. **E, F.** Nine months postoperative following detachment of mid-line forehead flap.

that would have been impossible to accomplish in the past. The applicability of expansion is only beginning to be appreciated and is limited only by the imagination of the surgeon.

Although tissue expansion is simplistic in concept, it does require judgement and in-depth pre-operative planning by the surgeon to ensure optimal results. An accurate analysis of the reconstructive requirements is necessary with respect to expected size of defect and the method of reconstruction. The surgeon must determine pre-operatively whether reconstruction can be achieved by simple advancement of expanded skin or whether some type of pivotal flap will be necessary. This decision will then dictate the location of incisions for implanting the expander. In general, expanders should be located in positions that take advantage of simple advancement or transposition flaps; however, areas of scarring, atrophy, or previously irradiated skin should be avoided.

Incisions for placement of the expander are usually made at the junction of normal tissue and tissue to be replaced. An exception to this rule is at junctions of normal skin and skin grafts. Incisions should be avoided in such junctional zones because of the high risk of dehiscence of the incision during expansion. In such situations, incisions for implantation should be located in skin of normal thickness far removed from the skin graft. Distant incisions allow for more rapid skin expansion without the expander placing excessive forces on the incision. Detailed planning of proposed incisions is important so that the possibility of future flaps or other surgical procedures are not compromised or reconstructive alternatives limited. Consideration should be given to the use of multiple expanders around the defect because it provides for more rapid development of sufficient tissue for reconstruction and at the same time minimizes the visible deformity created during expansion (Argenta & Vanderkolk 1987). Before implanting the expander, prophylactic antibiotics are administered, and the operative site is meticulously scrubbed with a bacteriostatic soap.

In the case of the scalp or forehead, a recipient pocket is created between the periosteum and the galea or deep fascia of the frontalis muscle, respectively. In the neck, a pocket is developed beneath the platysmal muscle. The pocket should be of sufficient size to allow the base of the expander to lie flat without folding or distortion. The injection port should be placed through the same incision as that of the expander, but situated in a separate pocket approximately 6 cm away from the expander. Anchoring sutures to prevent migration of the expander are not necessary if the expander is placed beneath the scalp or forehead skin. Anchoring sutures are recommended to prevent migration of expanders placed beneath the skin of the cheek or neck due to gravitational forces. Meticulous haemostasis must be achieved since drains are not used. The expander is partially expanded (approximately 50 ml for a 250 ml expander) with saline before wound closure to concomitantly obliterate dead space and assist with haemostasis. The incision is closed by layers using permanent suture for approximation of both the subcutaneous and cutaneous tissues.

Inflation begins 2 weeks after implantation of the expander. Saline is infused by percutaneous puncture of the injection port with a 23-gauge scalp needle attached to a 50-ml volume syringe after preparing the injection site with an alcohol swab. The volume of injection depends on the tensile strength and tension of the skin overlying the expander and the amount of patient discomfort. If not precluded by discomfort, the tissue should be expanded until slight blanching is observed in the skin overlying the expander. Saline should then be withdrawn until the blanching disappears. Usually 25 to 50 ml of saline can be injected in to a 250 ml volume expander at a weekly interval. Tightness or pain usually is the limiting factor in preventing further expansion. This discomfort resolves within 24 to 48 hours, and the patient remains comfortable until the next inflation. Inflation is usually conducted as frequently as once or twice a week. More rapid expansion may be possible, but it is associated with a greater risk of expander extrusion (Argenta & Vanderkolk 1987).

The volume of injected saline is recorded. Measurement of the expanded skin is also noted. If weekly visits to the office for inflation are not possible, the patient or a family member of the patient can be taught the inflation technique. In-home expansion is facilitated by a written list of instructions and by marking the injection site with indelible ink or a suture. A small amount of methylene blue dye may be initially injected into the expander. The person performing the inflation may subsequently aspirate a small quantity of saline from the port, prior to injection. If a blue solution is returned, then proper placement of the needle has been achieved.

As expansion proceeds, the dermis becomes thinner and a capsule forms around the expander. This often results in a reversible blue or red discoloration of the expanded skin. Dilated subcutaneous veins are frequently observed, but this is not an indication of cyanosis or infection. Expansion continues until the circumference of the dome of the expanded skin measures two or three times the width of the proposed defect. This usually takes 6 to 8 weeks for the skin of the forehead and neck and up to 12 weeks for the scalp.

The second surgical stage involves removal of the expander and proceeding with reconstruction. We perform acute inflation (booster inflation) of the expander immediately before removal. This may achieve additional tissue expansion. The expander is deflated and removed whether through the original incision used for implanting the device or through one of the incisions used to create a flap. Usually a broad-base pivotal or advancement flap is designed and incised, depending on the size and shape of the defect to be reconstructed. The capsule surrounding the expander provides an excellent blood supply to the flap, and therefore is usually not disturbed unless thinning of the flap is necessary to achieve optimal cosmetic results. A suction drain tube is employed at the donor site. Wound closure and postoperative care are similar to that used for standard flap surgery.

The author believes that the future will see even greater use of tissue expansion as a method of ensuring the surgeon an ample amount of tissue for reconstruction following tumour ablation in the mid-face.

REFERENCES

Argenta L C, Vanderkolk C A 1987 Tissue expansion in craniofacial surgery. Clinics in Plastic Surgery 14: 143–153

Ariyan S, Krizek T J 1977 Reconstruction after resection of head and neck cancer. Cine Clinics Clinical Congress of the American College of Surgeons, Dallas, Texas

Bakamjian V Y 1965 Two-staged method for pharyngo-esophageal reconstruction with a primary pectoral skin flap. Plastic and Reconstructive Surgery 36: 173–184

Baker S R 1981 Free lateral thoracic flaps in head and neck reconstruction. Archives of Otolaryngology 107: 409–413

Baker S R 1984 Closure of large orbital-maxillary defects with free latissimus dorsi myocutaneous flaps. Head and Neck Surgery 6: 828–835

Baker S R 1986 Microvascular surgery. In: Johns M E (ed) Complications on otolaryngology—head and neck surgery. B C Decker, Toronto, vol 2

Baker S R 1989 Options for reconstruction in head and neck surgery. In: Cummings C W, Fredrickson J M, Harker L A, Krause C J, Schuller D E (eds) Otolaryngology head and neck surgery update I. CV Mosby, St Louis, pp 192–248

Baker S R 1991 Malignancy of the lip. In: Gluckman J (ed) Otolaryngology, 3rd edn. W B Saunders, Philadelphia

Baker S R, Swanson N A 1983 Management of nasal cutaneous malignant neoplasms: an interdisciplinary approach. Archives of Otolaryngology 109: 473–479

Baker S R, Swanson N A 1984a Regional and distant skin flaps in nasal reconstruction. Facial Plastic Surgery 2: 33–44

Baker S R, Swanson N A 1984b Complete microscopic controlled surgery for head and neck cancer. Head Neck Surgery 6: 914–920

Baker S R, Swanson N A 1985 Oblique forehead flap for total reconstruction of the nasal tip and columella. Archives of Otolaryngology 111: 425–429

Baker S R, Swanson N A 1990a Tissue expansion of the head and neck—indications, techniques and complications. Archives of Otolaryngology 116: 1143–1153

Baker S R, Swanson N A 1990b Clinical applications of tissue expansion in head and neck surgery. Laryngoscope 100: 313–319

Baker S R, Swanson N A, Grekin R 1987 Mohs surgical treatment and reconstruction of cutaneous malignancies of the nose. Facial Plastic Surgery 5: 29–47

DaSilva G 1964 A new method of reconstructing the columella with a nasolabial flap. Plastic and Reconstructive Surgery 34: 63–65

Heanley C 1955 The subcutaneous tissue pedicle in columella and other nasal reconstruction, British Journal of Plastic Surgery 8: 60–63

Moore C 1980 Changing concepts in head and neck surgical oncology. American Journal of Surgery 140: 480–486

Panje W R, Bardach J, Krause C J, Baker S R 1977 Reconstruction of intraoral defects with the free groin flap. Archives of Otolaryngology 103: 78–83

Rubin P, Cassarett G W 1968 Clinical radiation pathology, vol I. W B Saunders, Philadelphia

Schuller D E 1982 Latissimus dorsi myocutaneous flaps for massive facial defects. Archives of Otolaryngology 108: 414–417

21. The skull base

Ian T. Jackson

INTRODUCTION

Over the past 20 years, skull-base surgery has been evolving into a sub-specialty with more formalization of approaches, methods of excision, prevention of complications and techniques of reconstruction (Jackson & Hide 1981, Shah et al 1987, Janecka & Sekhar 1989). In conjunction with these advances, the results of our surgical endeavours have improved in all ways, both therapeutically, aesthetically and functionally.

Initially surgery of the skull base was hazardous because of prolonged anaesthesia, blood loss, and, especially in the anterior skull-base area, significant life-threatening infections (Ketcham et al 1963). One of the main messages of this chapter will be how to make this surgery efficient and safe.

TYPES OF TUMOUR

It is important that tumours involving the maxilla and all structures cranial to this be considered as potential skull-base problems. In this area, the histology is extremely variable; thus, there is an extensive number of possible tumours, both malignant and non-malignant. Tables 21.1 and 21.2 show the variety of tumours which have been excised over the past 21 years.

INVESTIGATIONS

When the patient presents in the office there may be something to see, such as a mass somewhere in the craniofacial area, displacement of an eye or some other deformity. Apart from the general examination that one would carry out in the head and neck patient, nasendoscopy can be most useful, carefully examining the nasal passage, the nasopharynx, the oropharynx, the larynx and the cords. Evidence suggestive of any neural involvement is significant and may greatly influence the approach to any particular patient. The most common additional investigation is CT scanning with and without contrast. This will help to identify almost all tumours in this area, and for the surgeon is very easy to read and interpret. In selected cases we have been carrying out three-dimensional imaging in an attempt to use this to give us an idea of tumour volume and shape in addition to position and also to do mock surgery on the 3-D images in an interactive fashion on the work station (Fukuta et al 1990). The MRI scan can be useful in some tumours, with or without gadolinium, and in many cases carotid angiography will be carried out in order to see the relationship of the carotid to the tumour—and in some cases, such as neurofibromas and vascular tumours, to assess the vascularity of the tumour. In some, presurgical embolization will be considered. Routine chest X-rays—and any other X-rays which are indicated to look for metastasis—are also carried out.

SURGICAL APPROACH

In the past it was not possible effectively to expose the anatomical regions where these tumours originate; thus, complete resection was impossible and/or hazardous. With experience gained in the surgery for congenital craniofacial anomalies, a more systematic approach to exposure and resection has been developed. There are various combinations of soft tissue and bony exposures (Ketcham et al 1963, Lauritzen et al 1986, Nuss et al 1991). The central concept of these approaches has been to achieve 'extensibility'; this is based on the idea introduced by Henry (1966) in his *Extensile Exposure of the Upper Limb*; in this, he described exposure techniques which could be extended as necessary

Table 21.1 Skull-base tumours (non-malignant)

Fibrous dysplasia
Neurofibroma
Osteoma
Chondroma
Vascular malformations
Non-malignant embryonic tumours
Inverting papilloma
Intradiploic dermoid

Table 21.2 Skull-base tumours (malignant)

Squamous-cell carcinoma	Meningioma
Basal-cell carcinoma	Osteogenic sarcoma
Malignant melanoma	Chondrosarcoma
Dysplastic melanoma	Liposarcoma
Haemangiopericytoma	Fibrosarcoma
Adenocarcinoma	Neurofibrosarcoma
Adenoid cystic carcinoma	Angiosarcoma
Muco-epidermoid carcinoma	Rhabdomyosarcoma
Anaplastic carcinomas	Aesthesioneuroblastoma
Merkel-cell carcinoma	Malignant embryonic tumours
Recurrent retinoblastoma	

to reach every anatomical region in the arm. This concept can be adapted to the head and neck and skull-base area.

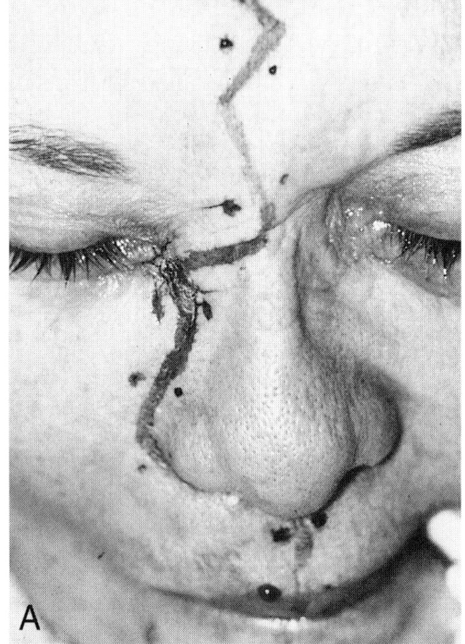

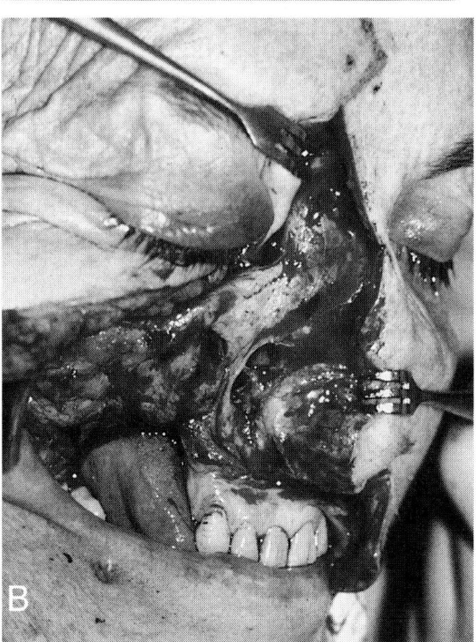

SOFT-TISSUE APPROACHES

These can be classified into limited and extended.

The *limited* approach is best exemplified by the lateral rhinotomy incision to expose the ethmoid sinuses. This is adequate when the tumour is confined to the sinus and does not involve the anterior cranial base or the maxilla. Thus, it is of limited value in this particular group of tumours.

The *Weber–Fergusson* incision is excellent for exposure of the maxilla, nasal cavity and orbit. By itself, however, it does not afford a satisfactory approach to the anterior skull base.

The *facial split* is an extension of the Weber–Fergusson approach using a mid-line forehead incision, which may be a straight line or a W-plasty (Fig. 21.1). This allows effective exposure of the ethmoid sinuses and the anterior portion of the anterior skull base.

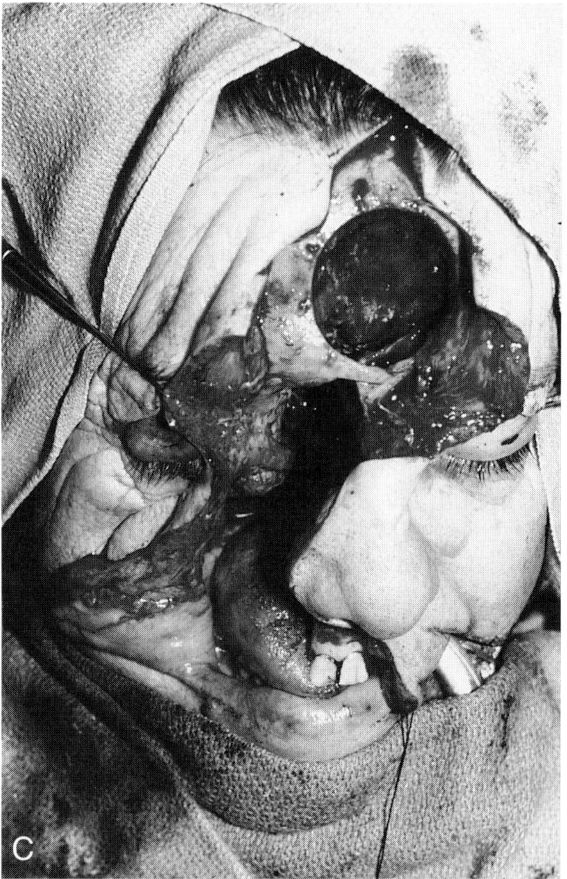

Fig. 21.1 Extended Weber–Fergusson approach—facial split. **A.** The standard Weber–Fergusson incision has been drawn out with a W-plasty extension up onto the forehead in this case of recurrent ameloblastoma. **B.** Maxilla exposed showing previous partial maxillectomy. **C.** The W-plasty extension has been used to perform trephination and allow resection of the anterior skull base, ethmoids and maxilla as a block resection of this recurrent lesion.

CORONAL FLAP

The coronal flap has become the basic soft-tissue approach to the anterior cranial fossa (Fig. 21.2). An incision is made from ear to ear. It should not be brought anteriorly as was favoured by neurosurgeons in the past since this does not increase exposure and frequently results in an unacceptable scar which is difficult to improve. When the cut is made, it should take the line of the hair follicles in order to avoid alopecia along the scar line.

The main portion of the flap is elevated at the subgaleal level. At 1–1.5 cm above the supra-orbital rim an incision is made through the periosteum and further dissection is subperiosteal. The nasal area and the orbits are exposed by elevating the periosteum as required.

There should be no hesitation in using this incision in the bald patient. The scars are usually very good—better than in the patient with hair. If there is only posterior hair, the incision may be placed posteriorly without diminution in exposure.

To gain more exposure in the nasoglabellar area, a vertical incision is made through the turned down periosteum on the under surface of the flap. The edges are spread apart with scissors. The dissection is continued down to the distal edge of the nasal bones. At this point, the periosteum is disconnected from the bone and dissection proceeds under the nasal bones to separate the nasal mucosa from the bone as extensively as possible.

Laterally, the periosteum of the lateral orbital rim is elevated and the dissection over the temporalis muscle is

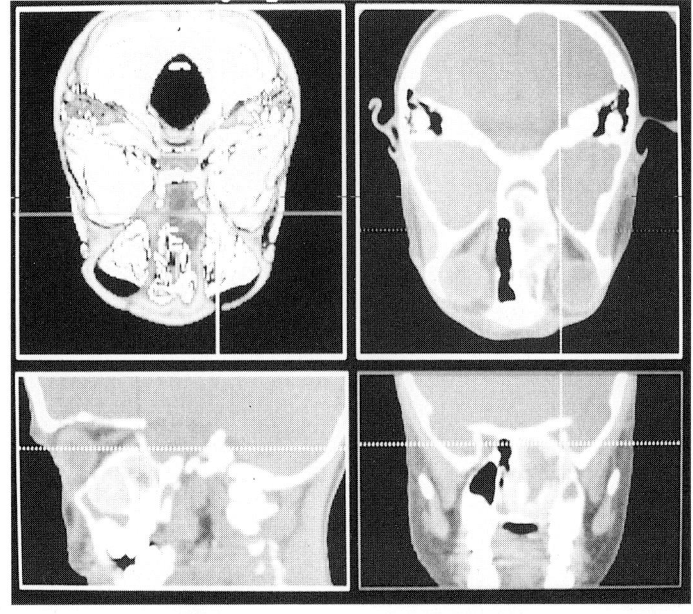

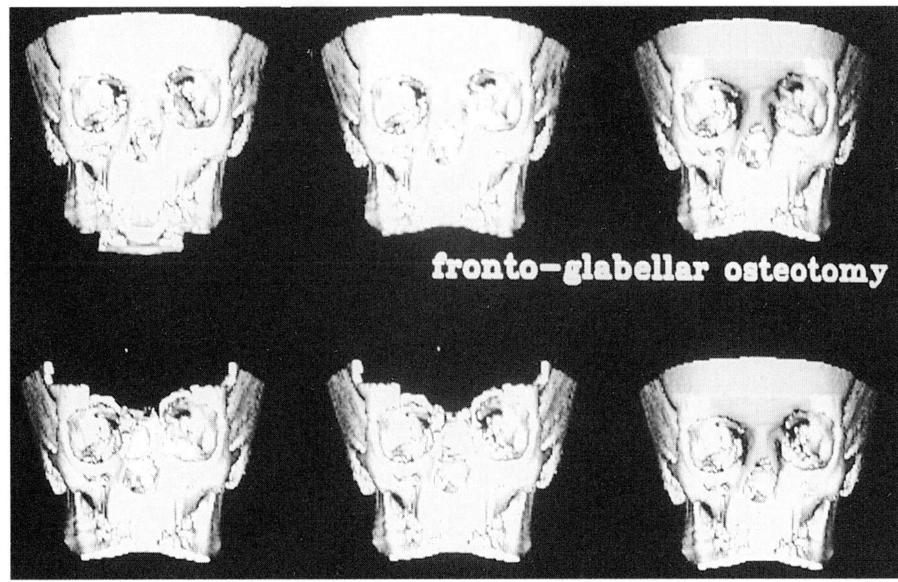

Fig. 21.2

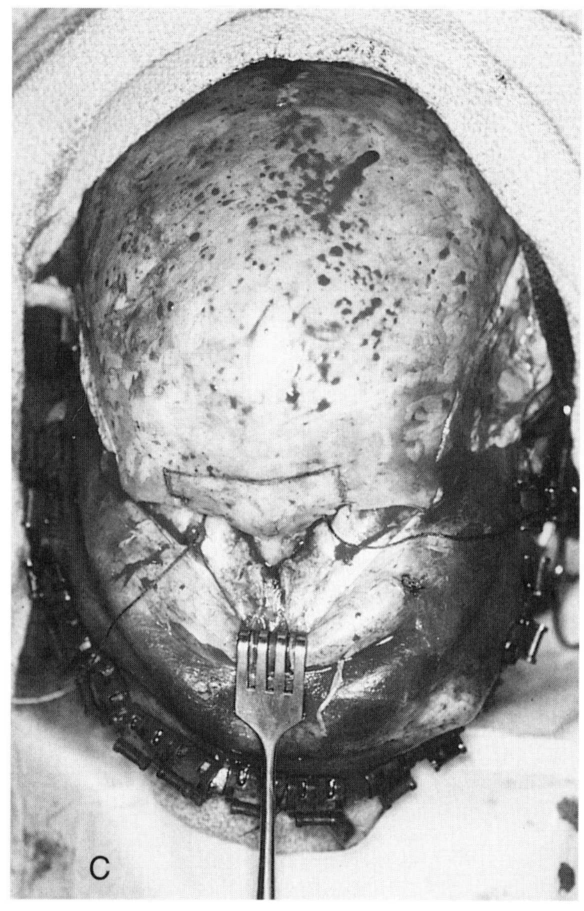

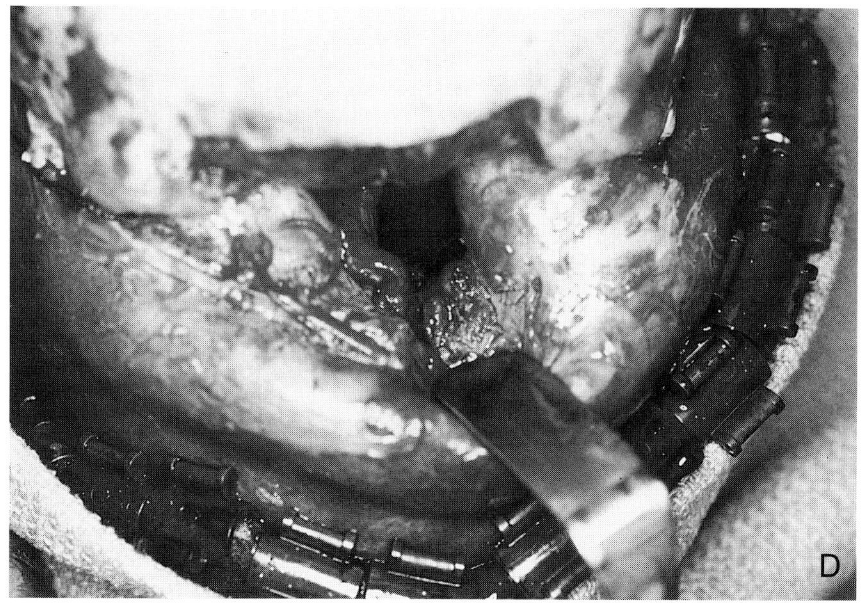

Fig. 21.2

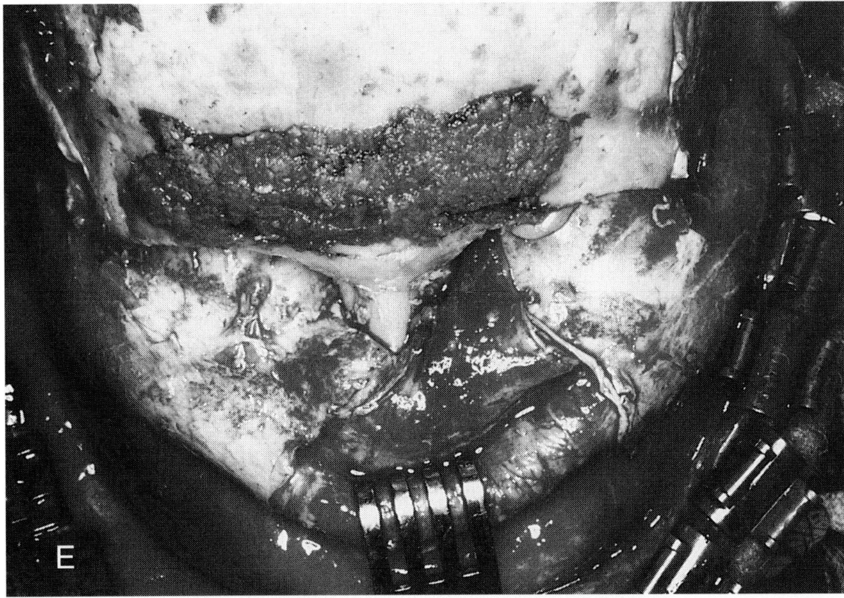
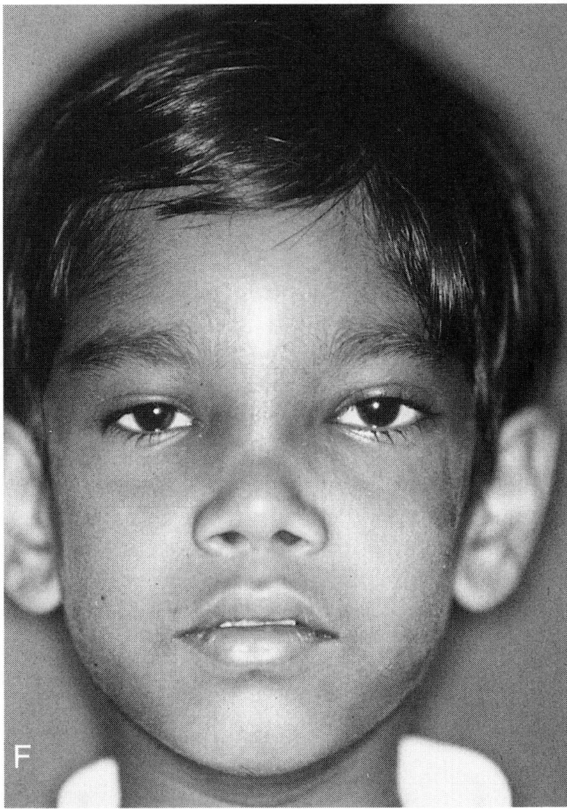

Fig. 21.2   Coronal flap **A.** Three-dimensional CT scan showing fibrous dysplasia involving the nasal cavity and the anterior skull base. **B.** The surgical planning has been formulated on the work station and is displayed in colour. **C.** A coronal flap used to display the fronto-orbitoglabellar area. A glabellar nasal osteotomy will be used to gain access to the lesion. **D.** The lesion has been resected and the defect down into the nasopharynx can be seen. **E.** Osteotomies have been placed back into position. A galeal frontalis myofascial flap has been used to separate the naso-pharynx from the extradural space. Bone dust has been placed over the osteotomy sites. **F.** Patient 1 year after surgery.

performed on the deep temporal fascia; the Faraboeuf periosteal elevator makes this a rapid and safe dissection. During this procedure, it is possible to be too superficial and damage the frontal branches of the facial nerve. From this lateral approach, the lateral peri-orbitum is elevated with division of the orbito-zygomatic vessels; the peri-orbitum of the orbital floor is elevated.

The periosteum of the upper rim of the zygomatic arch is incised and levated from the arch along its entire length. Anteriorly, this leads to the anterior aspect of the maxilla, the inferior orbital rim and the floor of the orbit. A total subperiosteal exposure of the anterior maxilla and orbit is completed by a more extensive medial dissection from the mid-line area. During the course of these manoeuvres, the medial and lateral canthal ligaments are detached. When doing the intra-orbital subperiosteal dissection, it should be remembered that the orbital rim-to-apex distance is at least 4.5 cm.

If the temporal fossa is to be explored or if the temporoparietal area is to be used for access, then the temporalis muscle must be elevated; it is, however, important that this is performed in the correct manner or else

one may be left with a stump of temporalis muscle which is difficult to re-attach at the end of the procedure. When this is the situation, it will result in temporal hollowing.

A sagittal incision is made in the periosteum in the mid-line. This extends to the edge of the intact posterior scalp. It then continues down the edge in a coronal direction bilaterally. Using a Faraboeuf periosteal elevator and copious irrigation, the pericranium can be dissected from the cranium efficiently and effectively. At the level of the temporal crest, the temporalis muscle is elevated from the temporal fossa. Anteromedially, it is stripped from the lateral wall of the orbit. This dissection can be continued down behind the zygomatic arch.

If there is a question of a temporal galeal flap being needed for middle or anterior cranial fossa resurfacing, the superficial temporal vessels should be preserved intact and the dissection over the area of galea required should be at the supragaleal level. It is important to understand that the blood supply of the galea is different from that of the scalp, being axial to the mid-line and random beyond this area.

When a more extensive exposure is required, the coronal flap can be combined with a mid-line forehead split, or a

Weber–Fergusson approach or, if necessary, with a combination of these two approaches.

LATERAL TEMPORAL APPROACH

When the middle cranial fossa, infratemporal fossa and petrous region are to be explored, the lateral temporal approach is used (Fig. 21.3). In this, a hemicoronal or temporal scalp flap is designed; this continues down in the pre-auricular area, as for a face-lift, to the base of the earlobe; it then sweeps anteriorly into the neck under the mandible and then down the neck in a lazy 'S'. The cheek and neck skin can be elevated in the face-lift plane to give extensive exposure. The temporalis muscle is elevated as described previously. If necessary, the parotid gland can be removed completely for exposure with facial nerve preservation, and the masseter can be elevated from the mandible. Frequently, a modified upper neck dissection is used to expose the great vessels for anatomical orientation as the skull base is approached. In some cases, a more extensive dissection is performed to remove cervical lymph nodes for oncological reasons.

BONY APPROACHES

It is also possible to sub-divide the bony approaches into limited and extended. Within the latter is included facial disassembly or exposure osteotomies.

Limited approach

In the exposure of the anterior cranial fossa, once the frontal area is displayed most mid-line lesions can be resected using a limited approach (Fig. 21.4). A central trephine or limited craniotomy is performed. This can be somewhat difficult if there is a large frontal sinus, since both anterior and posterior walls must be cut through. Once this has been achieved, the dura is dissected from the inner aspect of the skull and the floor of the anterior cranial fossa. This now allows an osteotomy to be performed which consists of the medial thirds of the supra-orbital rims and orbital roof, the nasal bones and part of the medial walls of the orbits. These cuts are made with the oscillating saw. Intracranially, the base is cut anterior to the cribriform plate and proceeds laterally into the orbital roofs. This cut is made with a side-cutting

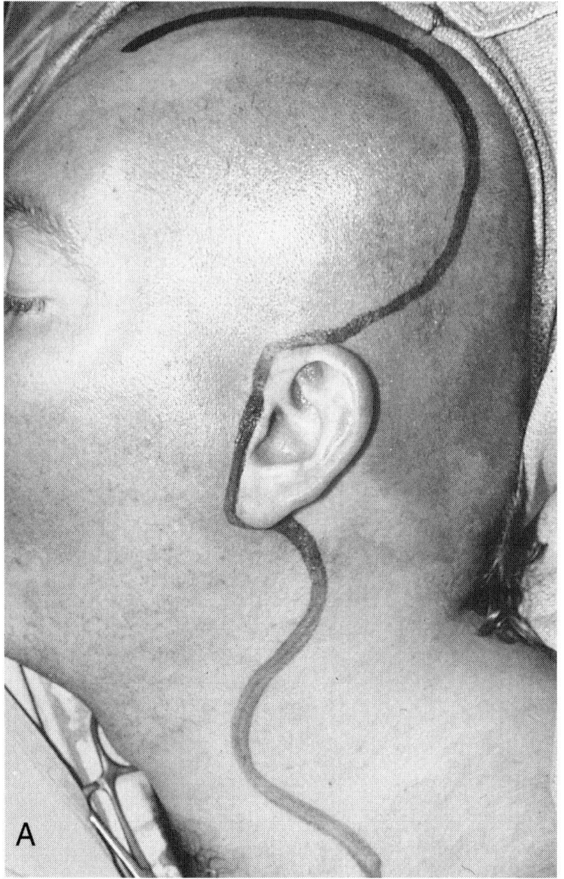
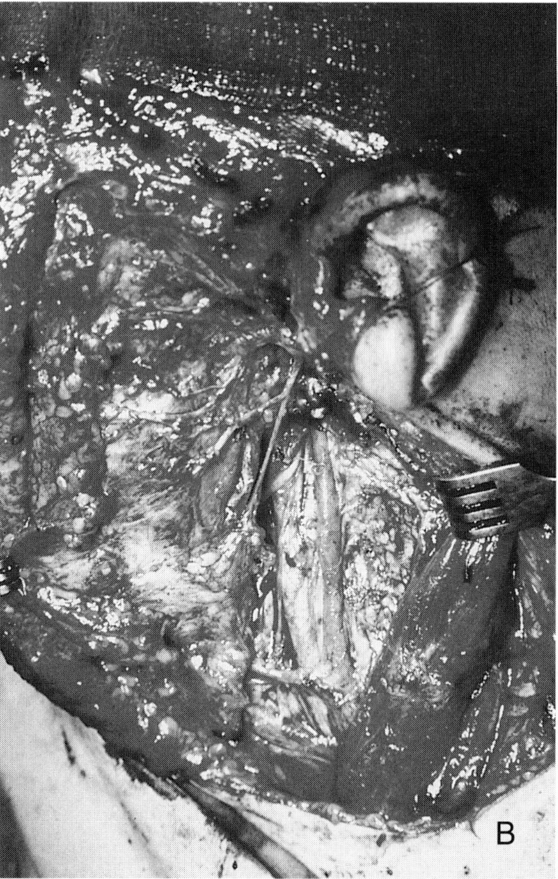

Fig. 21.3 Lateral temporal approach. **A.** The extensive incision for exposure of the temporal area, face and neck has been drawn out. **B.** Superficial parotidectomy has been performed with preservation of all branches of the facial nerve. A neck dissection displays the great vessels passing up to the base of the skull.

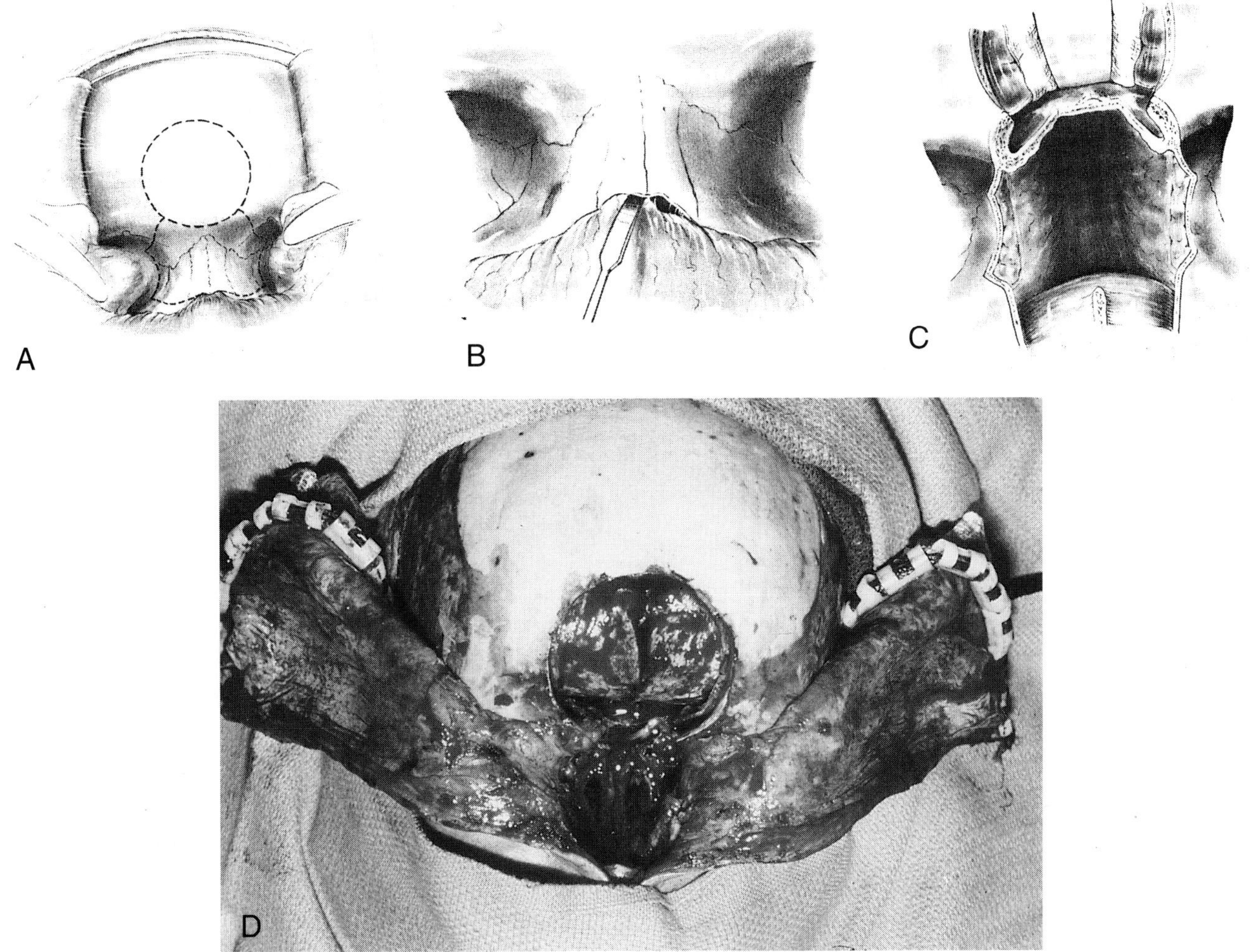

Fig. 21.4 Limited bony approach to anterior cranial fossa. **A.** The trephine together with the glabellar nasal osteotomy is shown **B.** Dissection of the nasal mucoperiosteum from the under surface of the nasal bones. **C.** Resection of the mid-line anterior skull base, nasal septum and medial orbital walls completed. **D.** Exposure and resection displayed in combination with coronal flap and mid-face split.

drill; a small curved osteotome is placed in the mid-line of the intracranial cut and a few taps of the mallet will separate the bony fragment. The nasal mucosa is separated from its under surface and it is removed. From this approach, a resection back to the clivus and down the posterior pharyngeal wall can be achieved; the ethmoid and sphenoid sinuses can be totally resected, as can the medial orbital walls and nasal septum.

The advantage of this limited bony approach is that, should a significant infection occur, only a relatively small amount of bone would be lost, and, consequently, the later reconstruction would be much easier.

Extensive

When the tumour is large or located lateral to the mid-line or in the middle cranial fossa, the approach is consequently more difficult. With the approaches used in the past, the tumour lay at the bottom of a cavity, in effect, in the depths of a cone. The concept now is that, by removing bone, the tumour comes to lie in the surgical field with plenty of room to manipulate instruments and to use the microscope, should this be necessary.

Craniotomy

The frontal or frontotemporal craniotomy allows exposure to lesions which lie in or lateral to the mid-line in the anterior cranial fossa (Fig. 21.5). As necessary, segments of the supra-orbital rim and orbital roof can be removed as described in the previous section. Once again, the concept should be to remove only that amount of bone which is necessary to gain good exposure.

Facial disassembly (exposure osteotomies)

Experience in maxillofacial and craniofacial reconstructive surgery for facial deformity has led to the concept of removal of complex areas of the facial skeleton to provide access to anatomical areas with later replacement of the

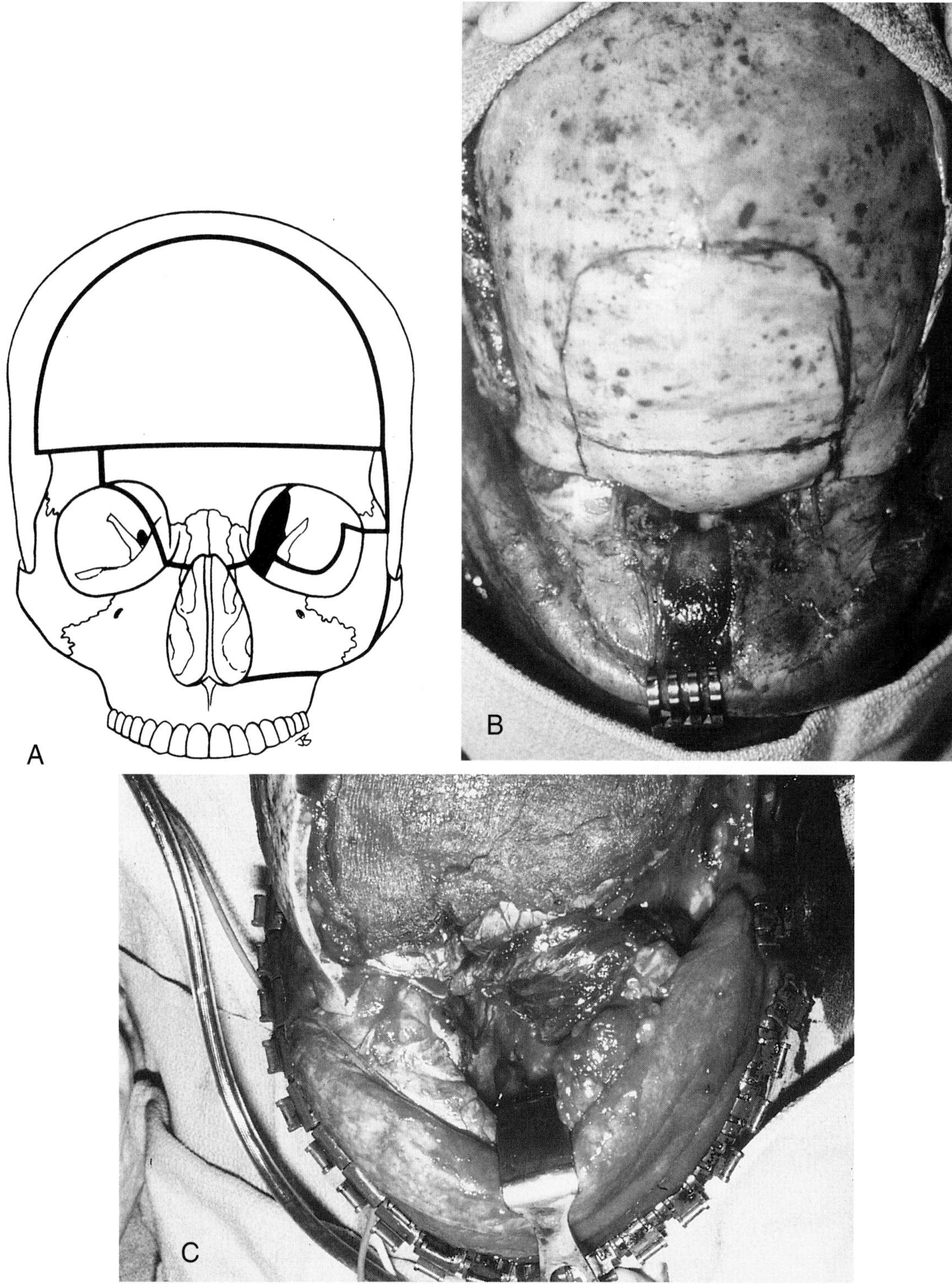

Fig. 21.5 Frontal craniotomy. **A.** Diagram of the frontal craniotomy, together with the glabellar supra-orbital osteotomy is shown. **B.** Frontal craniotomy and glabellar nasal craniotomy being performed on patient. **C.** Resection of recurrent squamous carcinoma of ethmoid sinuses; temporal muscle flap to provide cover for the skull base.

removed bony segments (Jackson 1985, Jackson et al 1986b, Lauritzen et al 1986, Janeka et al 1990, Nuss et al 1991, Jackson 1992).

Le Fort osteotomy

This procedure was initially designed to expose the posterior nasopharynx for tumour resection. It is now used frequently for exposure of clivus lesions. An incision is made bilaterally in the upper buccal sulcus and the periosteum is elevated over the maxilla. The periosteum of the nasal floor and pyriform aperture is elevated as completely and extensively as possible. An osteotomy is made on the front of the maxilla as high as possible from the lateral wall of the pyriform aperture to the pterygoid groove. It continues down the lateral wall of the pyriform aperture. A notched chisel is used to cut the nasal septal area and vomer. If necessary, a submucous resection of septum is performed. Posteriorly, the maxillary tuberosity is disconnected from the pterygoid plate bilaterally with a curved osteotome. The whole lower maxilla can now be dislocated caudally with finger pressure and good exposure gained to the clival area.

At the end of the tumour resection, the maxilla is replaced and stabilized with miniplates placed on the lateral edge of the pyriform aperture and the zygomaticomaxillary buttress.

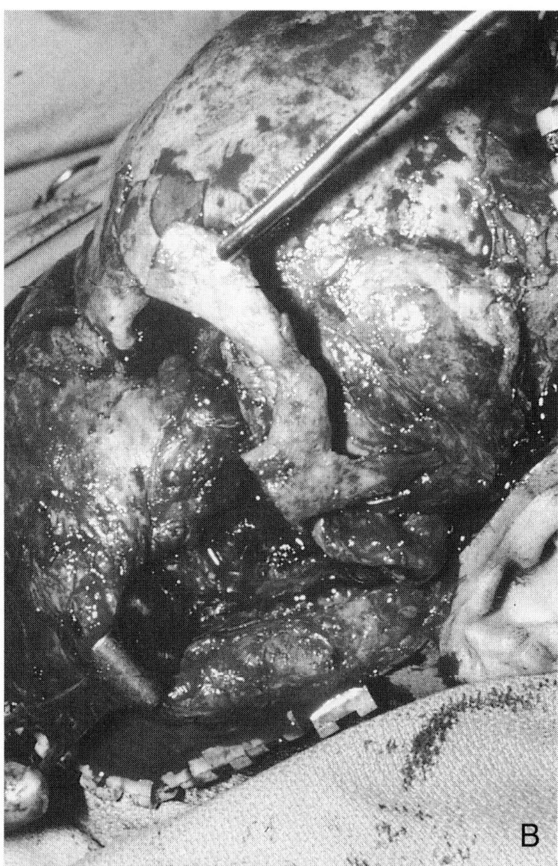

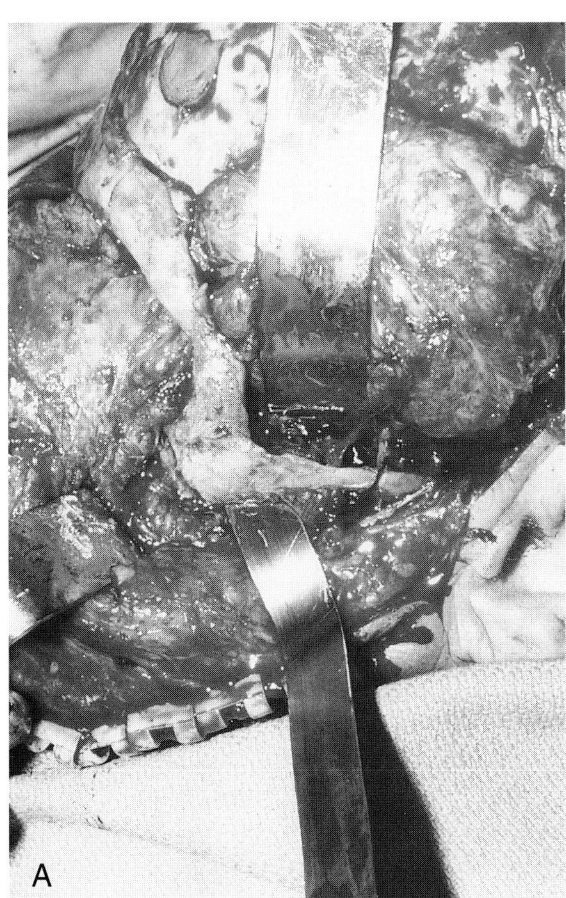

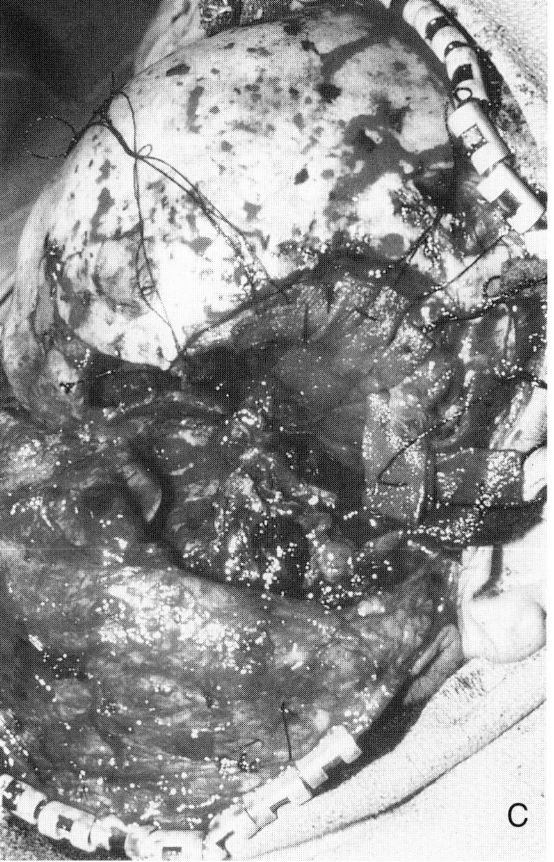

Fig. 21.6 Orbitotemporal exposure. **A.** The osteotomy to remove the zygomatic arch, lateral wall of orbit, orbital roof and supra-orbital rim is shown. The temporal cranium will also be removed. **B.** Removal of osteotomized segment. **C.** Excellent orbitotemporal exposure has been achieved and the meningioma has been successfully resected.

Mandibular swing

This procedure is well described elsewhere in this book (see Ch. 3 and 9). In skull-base surgery, it is used for resection of tumours of the posterior maxilla which penetrate the posterior wall and lie in the pterygoid fossa and may extend into the upper part of the nasopharynx and invade the skull base. In conjunction with a radical maxillectomy with or without an intracranial exploration, the mandibular swing with a mucosal incision which joins the upper buccal sulcus incision posteriorly, provides good exposure in the pterygoid/skull bone area. It is very convenient to add a neck dissection to the maxillectomy skull base pterygoid fossa resection to provide an en bloc clearance.

Orbitotemporal exposure

The first exposure osteotomies were relatively simple in concept. These were for lesions occurring principally in the sphenoid wing and involving the orbit, usually meningiomas or fibrous dysplasia.

The temporal orbital area is exposed using a coronal flap and a lateral frontal and temporal craniotomy performed (Fig. 21.6). Bone in this area is frequently involved by the tumour and is resected. The supra-orbital rim, orbital roof, lateral orbital rim and wall are removed as a block. This gives excellent exposure to the orbital contents, sphenoid wing, anterior and middle cranial fossae, allowing effective tumour resection. The bony segments are replaced and

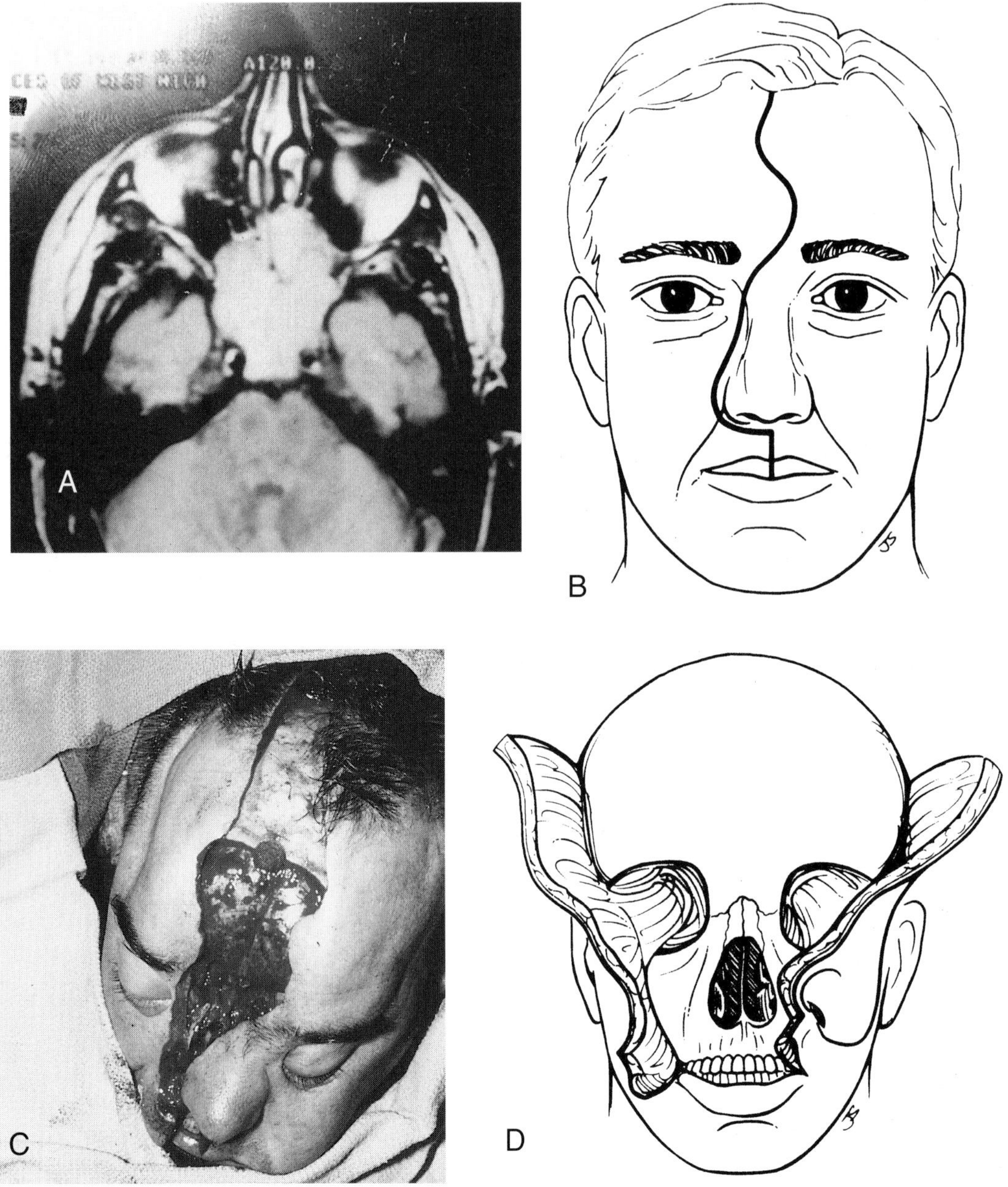

Fig. 21.7

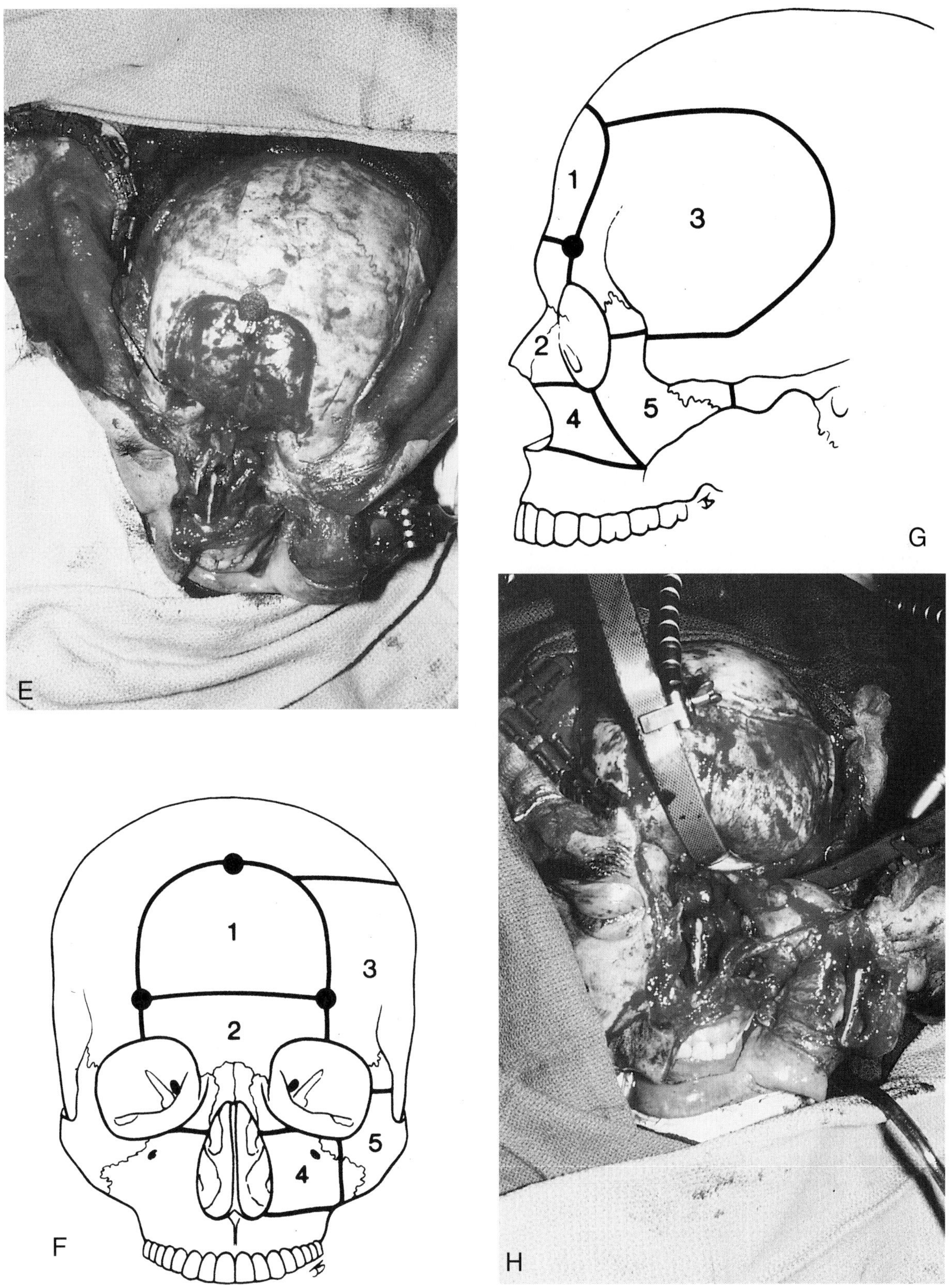

Fig. 21.7

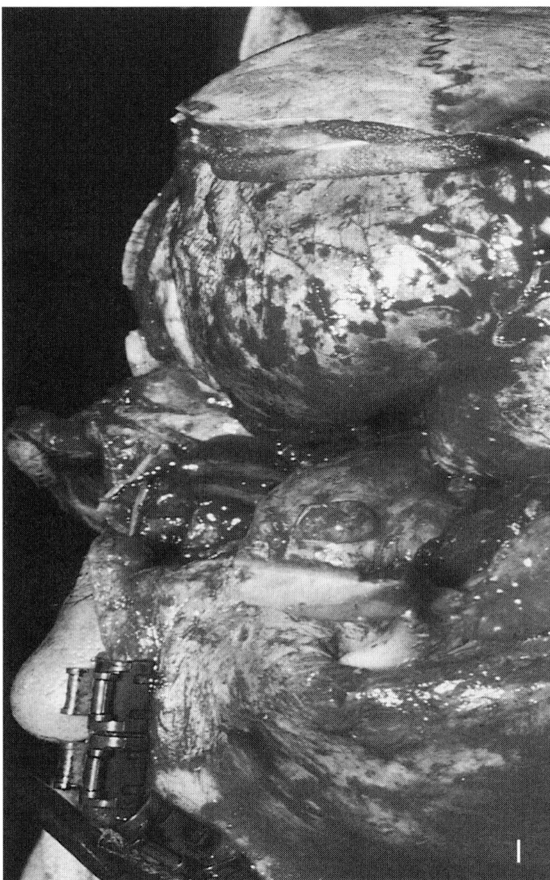

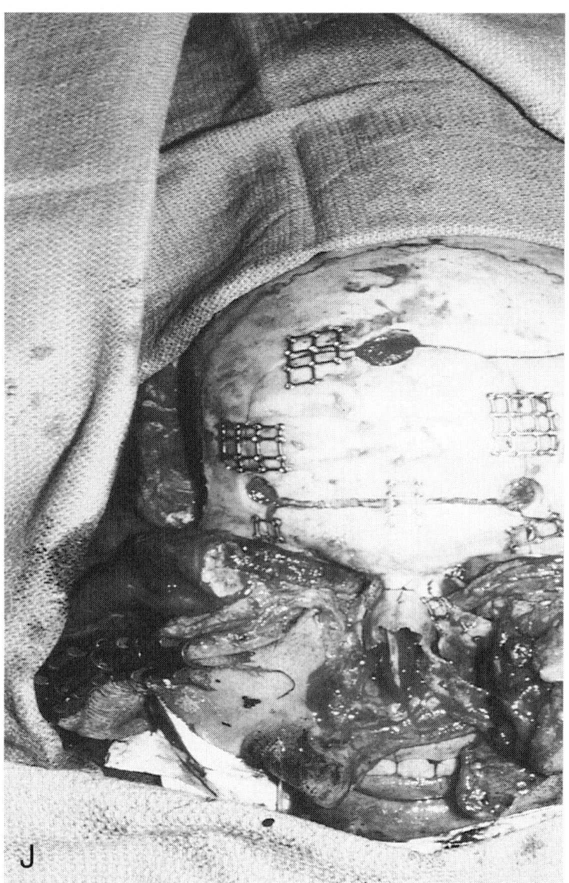

Fig. 21.7   Fronto-orbitonasal approach. **A.** MRI scan showing adenoid cystic carcinoma deep in the anterior cranial fossa invading the middle cranial fossa. **B.** Approach by facial split and coronal flap. **C.** This approach has been used and, together with an osteotomy of the nose, a frontal bone flap will be raised. **D.** Diagram of soft-tissue elevation together with the nose in order to gain good exposure to the mid-face and orbital regions. **E.** This exposure is demonstrated in the patient. **F, G.** The portions of bone have been numbered to give an idea of what was removed for exposure. **H, I.** These give an indication of the excellent exposure that can be achieved, both to the middle cranial fossa and the posterior and central part of the anterior cranial fossa. This allowed the adenoid cystic carcinoma to be removed. **J.** The skeleton has been reconstructed and is shown prior to soft-tissue suturing.

fixed with wires or plates; any bone defects are grafted with cranial bone.

Fronto-orbitonasal approach

With experience in exposure osteotomies, tumours located deeper in the skull base can be exposed in such a manner as to facilitate resection (Fig. 21.7).

The soft-tissue approach is frequently the coronal flap and the facial split. If indicated, the Weber–Fergusson is taken down the side of the nose opposite to the tumour. This allows a coronal osteotomy to be done through the nasal bones and the whole nose can be lifted on the cheek flap as the latter is dissected laterally. If the orbit is to be exenterated, the conjunctiva is cut through at the fornices, which allows a very extensive lateral exposure. Even when the eye is to be preserved, the exposure can be significant by this approach.

The frontal bone flap is removed, as is the upper half of the orbit—medial, supra-orbital roof, lateral rim and wall. It may be necessary, at this point, to remove the temporal bone down to the base of the middle cranial fossa. In some cases, the lower half of the orbit, together with the maxilla down to the tooth roots, is removed as a block. This will usually give excellent exposure to the medial area of the middle cranial fossa, to the apex of the orbit and, of course, to any mid-line structures. In some cases, the oncological treatment may dictate that a maxillectomy be performed.

Side-table assembly

In an effort to reduce time in these lengthy procedures, this technique has been introduced (Jackson et al 1991). While the main procedure is being performed, the bone segments are accurately plated together on a side table (Fig. 21.8). Plates are left protruding from the edges of the re-assembled complex. When this is placed in position, fixation is rapidly achieved placing screws into the protruding plates; frequently, microplates are used in this reconstruction, especially in children.

Lateral temporal approach

When the lateral approach is used, as mentioned earlier, the soft tissue is displaced or resected, as in the case of the parotid gland, to expose the underlying bone. It is routinely planned to expose the temporoparietal area of the skull, the ascending ramus of the mandible and zygomatic arch and lateral orbital wall and lateral orbital rim (Figs 21.3, 21.9).

For the intracranial exposure, the temporoparietal craniotomy is usually taken down to the floor of the middle cranial fossa as a single block. This gives excellent exposure to a large area of the middle cranial fossa base.

To approach the infratemporal fossa, it is often necessary to remove the zygomatic arch and the ascending ramus; these may be pedicled on soft tissue. With the intracranial, neck and subcranial exposure, the tumour can be removed safely. Should the posterior maxilla be involved, or should the tumour be extending more medially, it may be necessary to add an anterior approach to the procedure. In this, a Weber–Fergusson incision is used and, if necessary, a maxillectomy, the extent of which is governed by the tumour, is performed. Often the en bloc specimen is delivered from the temporal area. This combined approach allows resection of very extensive tumours to be accomplished safely and effectively. As experience is gained with fronto-temporo-orbito-maxillary facial disassembly, the combined approach is used less frequently; in fact, the latter is simply an extension of the former.

Petrosectomy

This is purely an operative procedure but none the less can be included in this section because the approach is quite distinct (Fig. 21.10).

Soft tissue

This is very similar to the lateral temporal approach. Depending on the position of the tumour, in relation to the external auditory canal, the ear may or may not be sacrificed. For an external ear tumour growing into the petrous area, the ear is sacrificed totally. Where only the canal is involved, it may be cored out, leaving the greater part of the external ear untouched. In middle ear carcinoma with the lesion confined to that area, the external ear may be raised together with the scalp flap. Thus, the design of the incision varies with the decision as to what must be done with the ear. If it is to be resected, the incision is as for a temporal craniotomy. It then continues downwards, going in front and behind the ear, leaving the latter as an island and

continues downwards into the neck as previously described for the lateral approach. When the ear is to be preserved partially or totally, the incision is taken behind the ear and the latter is raised on the anterior flap; it is cut flush with the external canal if possible, if not, whatever must be taken is left behind on the specimen to be resected. The neck incision is as described above.

Bony approach

A temporal craniotomy is performed to assess operability; if this is feasible, the petrosectomy begins.

A modified neck dissection is useful in that it may be necessary therapeutically but, if not, it allows location of the great vessels up to the styloid process. The ascending ramus of the mandible and the zygomatic arch may have to be osteotomized in some more extensive tumours and the dissection continued up to the skull base. Prior to this, a total parotidectomy with facial nerve-sparing will have been performed. A dissection is made on the base of the skull towards the petrous apex and carotid canal. Posteriorly, the mastoid is dissected and exposure proceeds medially towards the jugular foramen. Intracranially, the temporal lobe is elevated from the skull base to get to the petrous apex. The sigmoid sinus is located and disconnected from the jugular vein. When the latter has been done, the jugular vein can be ligated in the neck. Earlier ligation can lead to dilatation of the sigmoid sinus and the possibility of increased blood loss if this structure is traumatized.

As the dissection continues, it may be necessary to transect the glossopharyngeal, vagus, accessory and hypoglossal nerves. In the total petrosectomy, the facial nerve is also divided since it passes through the specimen.

An osteotomy can now be performed anterior and posterior to the petrous bone; the resection is taken medially to the carotid and jugular foramina. The problem arises in that the carotid canal does not traverse the petrous bone directly and injury to the internal carotid artery is possible. The technique is to gently rock the petrous bone to free it, and, as this is being done, the artery can be protected and dissected out. If tumour is involving the canal, the petrous bone usually fractures in this area, which makes resection much easier but does require a further excision medial to the artery for completeness of resection.

In tumours which are non-malignant and in those in which the facial nerve is not involved, the skin approach is more limited and the bone is removed by the Fisch approach. In this, using the low-speed drill and magnification, the facial nerve is exposed and preserved as is the internal carotid; the tumour is then resected. In this way, vital structures are saved, as is some of the bone of the petrous and mastoid areas; there is less cranial nerve destruction.

Depending on the extent of soft-tissue resection, there may be direct closure of the defect. Local flap or free flap closure, or, in some cases, a split skin graft will be applied

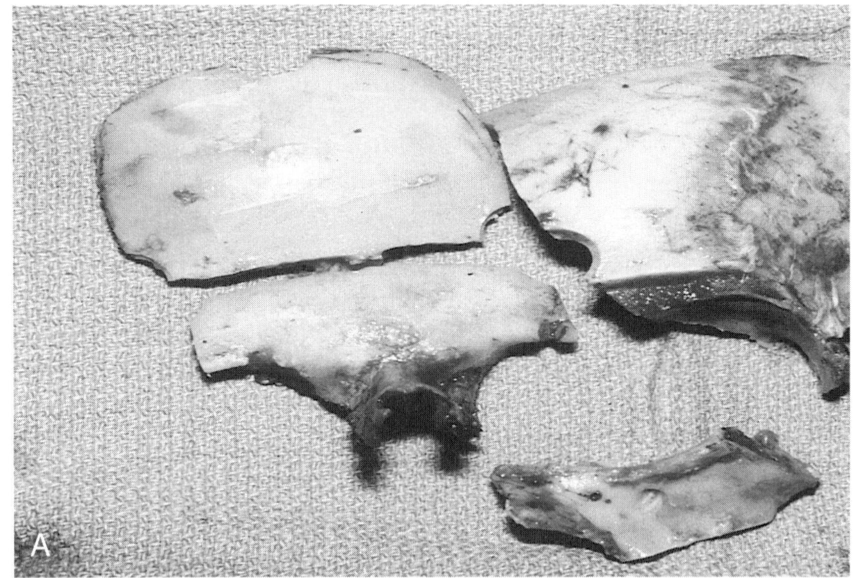

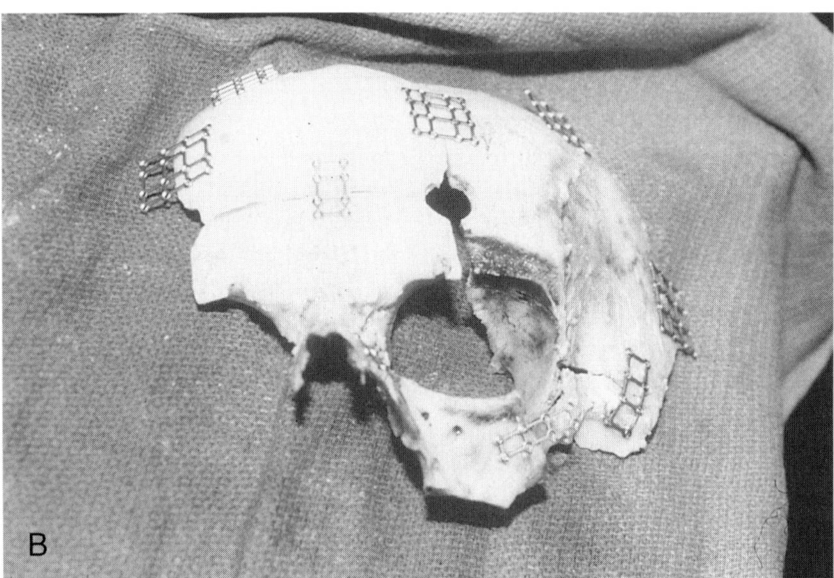

Fig. 21.8 Side-table assembly. **A.** These are the portions of bone removed in the case demonstrated in Fig. 21.7. **B.** Side-table assembly has been completed. There is still one portion of bone to be applied. It is through here that the orbital contents will be introduced into the reconstructed orbit. Note plates overlapping the edge of the specimen for ease of application when returned to the skull and face.

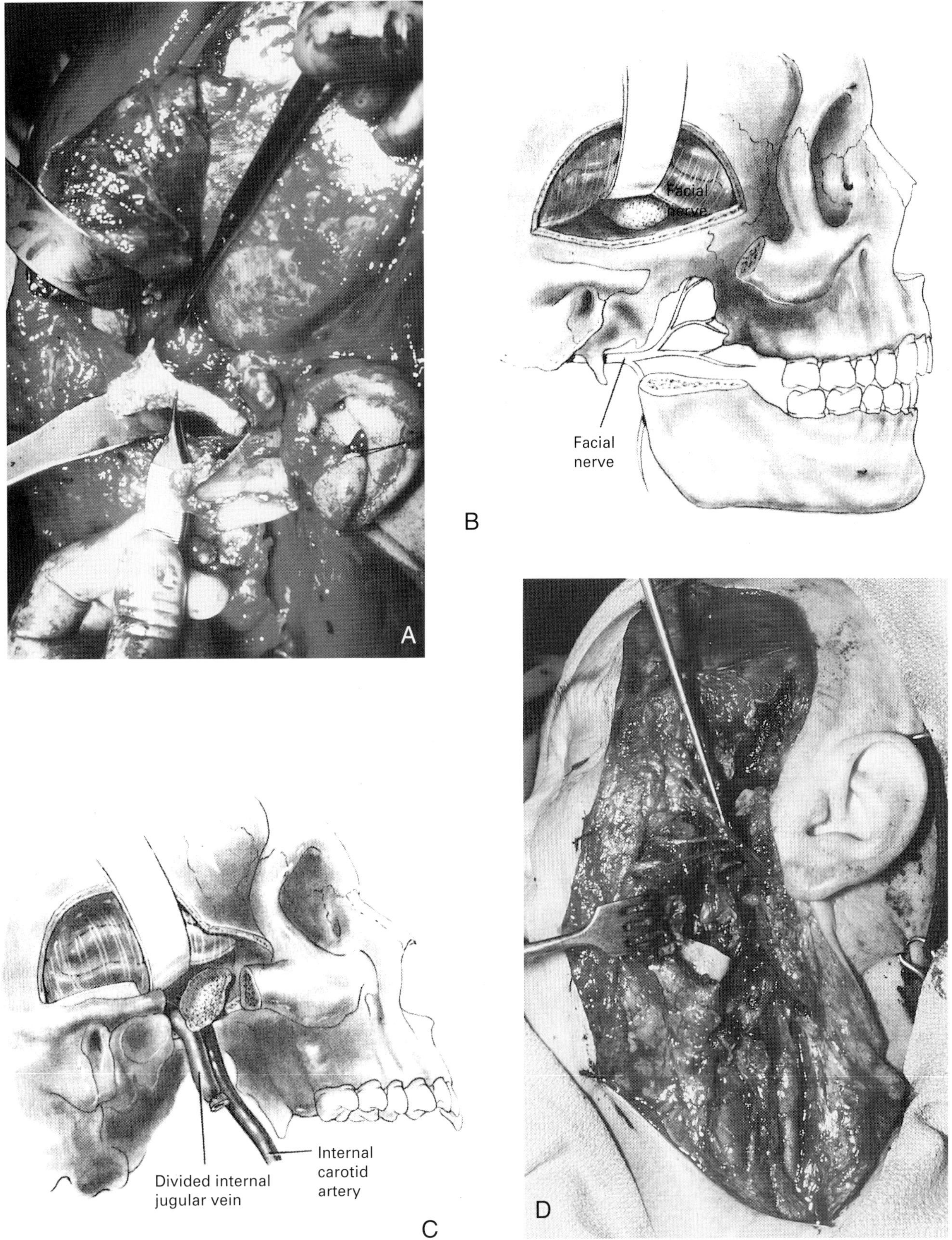

Fig. 21.9 Lateral temporal bony approach. **A.** Removal of zygomatic arch to gain access to infratemporal fossa. **B.** The ascending ramus of the mandible has also been removed. The facial nerve is preserved. The temporal craniotomy has been carried out to display the tumour. **C.** Floor of the middle cranial fossa has been removed in order to resect totally the lesion. **D.** Completion of resection in patient.

Internal carotid
artery
Petrous portion
of temporal bone
Internal auditory
canal
Bone cuts
B

Zygomatic
arch (cut)
Osteotomies
Internal
carotid
artery
Internal
jugular
vein
C

Internal
auditory
canal
D

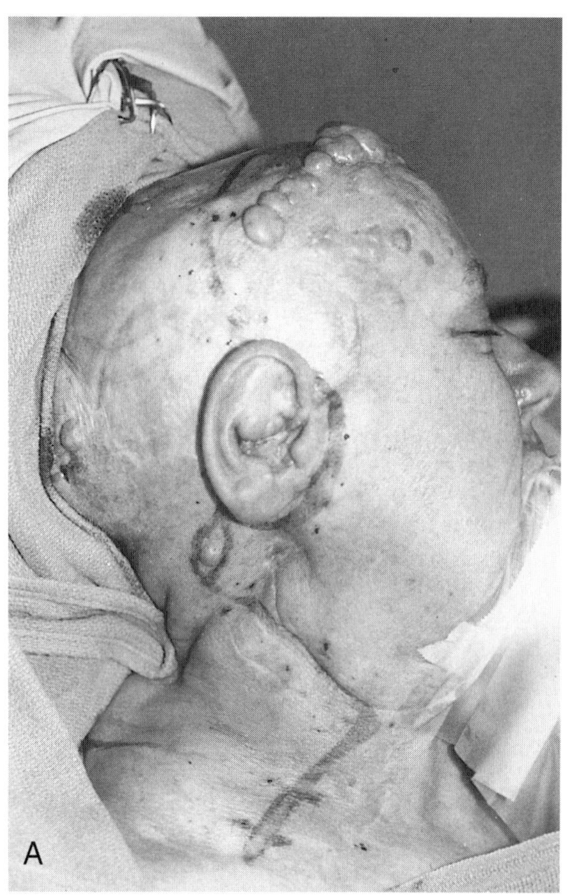

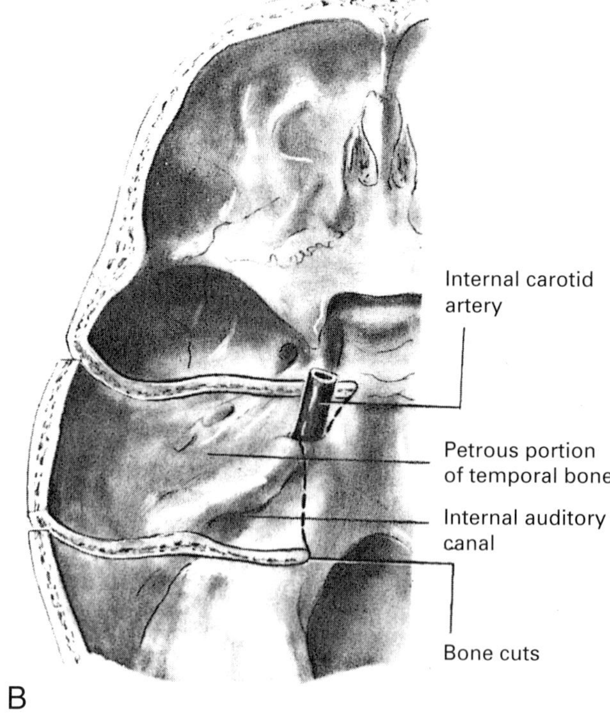

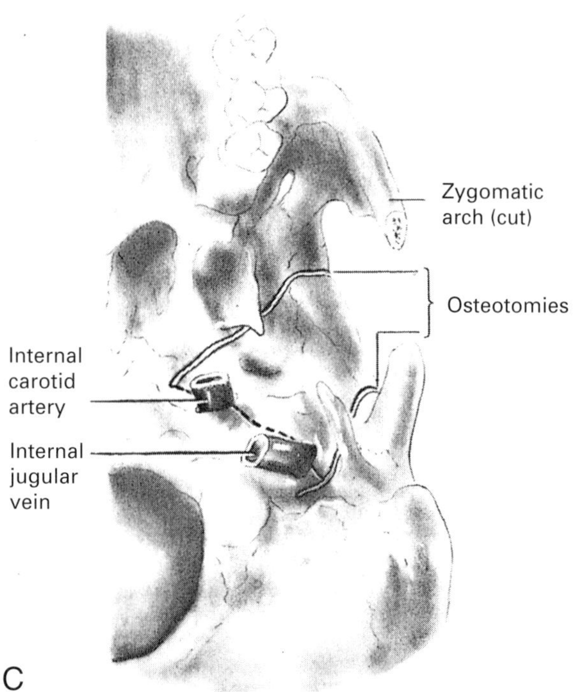

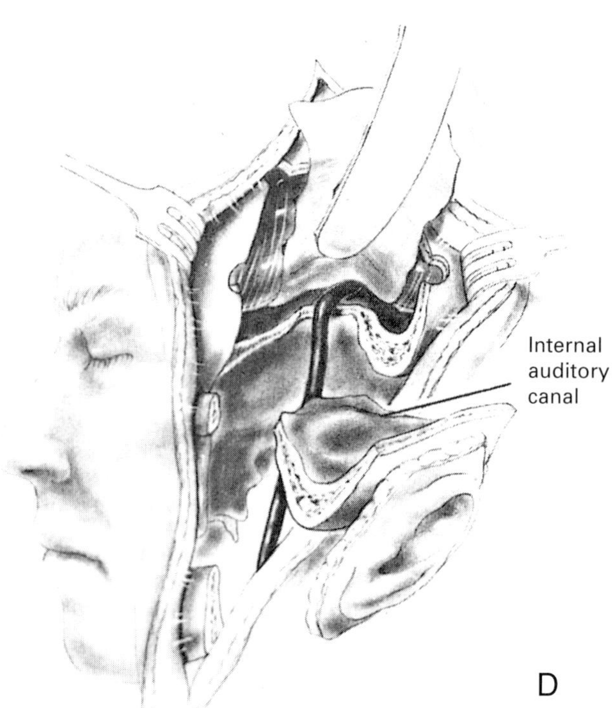

Fig. 21.10

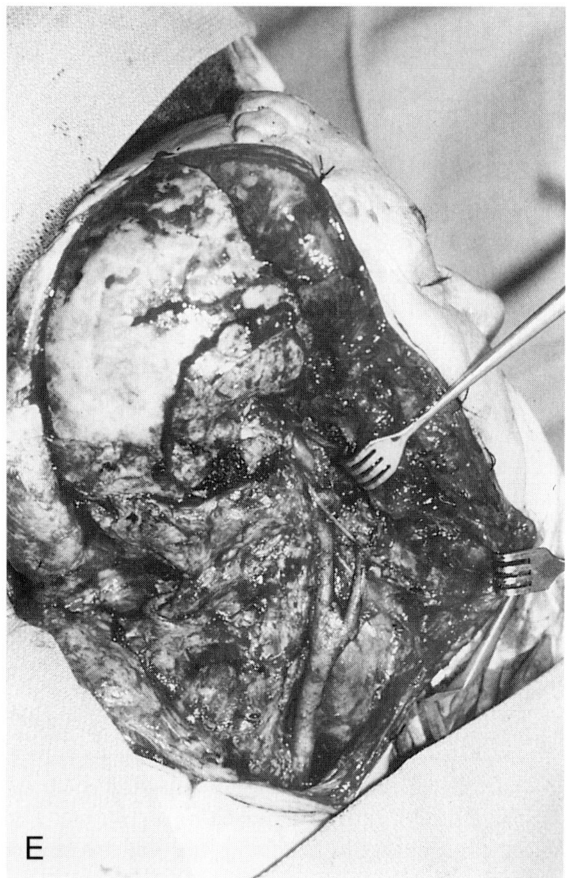

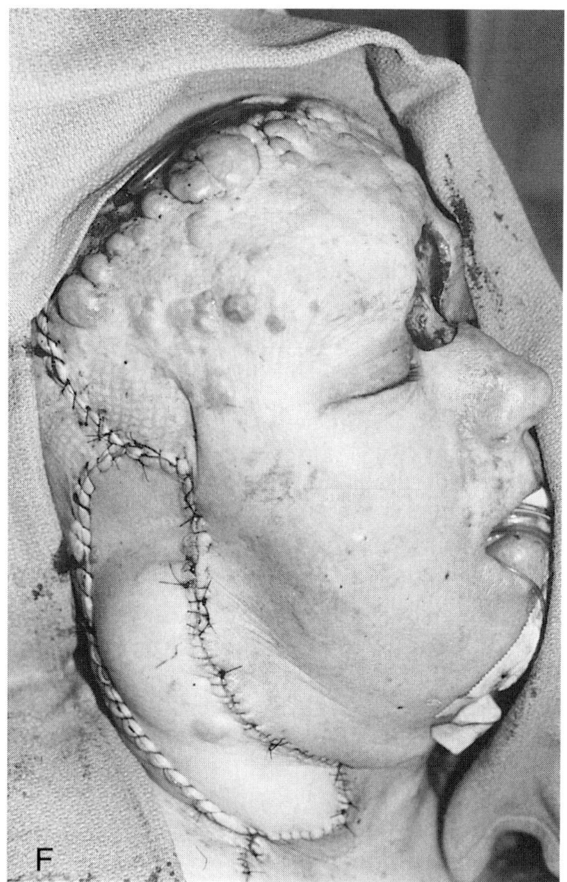

Fig. 21.10 Total petrosectomy. **A.** The skin approach is shown being pre-auricular and coming down into the neck, the latter to display the main vessels as they proceed to the skull base area. **B, C.** These diagrams show the middle cranial fossa base osteotomies from above and from below. **D.** Removal of the total petrous specimen with preservation of the internal carotid artery. **E.** The total petrosectomy has been performed and the bony defect is easily seen. **F.** Reconstruction of soft tissue with pectoralis major myocutaneous island flap.

directly to the temporal bone. As with the orbit, the temporal bone can successfully sustain a free skin graft.

Skull base reconstruction

General principles

In the upper face, there is less necessity for reconstruction than in the lower face. The latter is mobile, and highly involved in function, whereas the former is immobile and less involved functionally. In both, the aesthetic consequences of major resection are very significant.

Undoubtedly, the surgeon's attitude to reconstruction is strongly influenced by the types of cases which are referred to him, and how, in his experience, they have progressed following surgery.

Total reconstruction should be reserved for non-malignant tumours, those malignant tumours with a good prognosis and for which complete excision is not in doubt, and, finally, patients with extremely poor prognosis and a limited life expectancy—they should be given as good a quality of remaining life as possible.

Limited reconstruction should be undertaken in tumours with a good prognosis but where the biological behaviour has been changed by therapy, e.g. surgery and/or radiation therapy. This approach should also be used for aggressive tumours, where completeness of resection is in doubt but where further excisional surgery would be possible, and, rarely, in patients in whom prolongation of surgery is inadvisable.

These are difficult options to consider and difficult decisions to take. Unfortunately, one cannot rely too much on the pathologist because of the anatomical difficulty in interpreting the specimens. Much of the decision making has to be clinical. I have rarely, if ever, regretted the decision to delay reconstruction but I have been very disturbed to have cases of recurrent tumour referred where the best reconstructions have already been utilized.

As will be discussed later, the most disastrous complication, apart from death, blindness and severe haemorrhage in these cases is overwhelming infection which may lead to death. This will be discussed in greater detail later. However, it is an event which can be prevented. The causation of the infection is an intra- and extracranial communication down into the nasopharyngeal area with or without an intracranial dead space.

Techniques have been devised to minimize or, preferably, prevent this disastrous complication and have involved the use of local vascularized flaps or free tissue transfer. It should be noted that reconstruction of the bony skull base is rarely necessary.

SURGICAL TECHNIQUES

Galeal frontalis myofascial flap

This flap, which is a combination of the frontal galea and the frontalis muscle, is the 'workhorse' of anterior skull-base reconstruction (Jackson et al 1986a) (Fig. 21.11). The blood supply is from the supra-orbital and supratrochlear vessels. The flap may contain one or both vessels, and it may be bilateral when required, narrow or broad. The length of the flap is, as yet, undetermined. The flap is raised at the level of the base of the hair follicles in the hair-bearing area of the scalp and is taken down to the supra-orbital or glabellar area where it is based.

This flap can be used to close off securely the intracranial area from the nasopharynx. Drill holes are made at intervals around the bone defect and the flap is sutured using non-absorbable material. The same flap or a second one can be taken down into the nasopharynx to cover a bone graft of the medial orbital wall when this is necessary.

This is an extremely reliable flap and has been used in over 200 skull-base tumours. Apart from one patient with meningitis, who recovered spontaneously, there have been no other significant infections.

There are few complications associated with this flap; occasionally there will be irregularity of the forehead due to loss of bulk in the area of the flap. Sometimes there is a supra-orbital bulge due to the flap base being folded over to place it in the skull-base defect. Lack of forehead movement is much less than one would imagine, and rarely has a patient complained of this. There is a greater intensity of forehead anaesthesia but, again, patients seem to accept this in an uncomplaining fashion.

Temporal galea flap

The temporal galea is a continuation of the superficial temporal fascia; it is supplied by the superficial temporal vessels and can be reliably harvested to the mid-line (Har-Shai et al 1992). The temporal galea flap is used in cases where the galeal frontalis flap is not available. It can be brought through into the frontal area to just beyond the mid-line and is, thus, a reliable cover for this area (Fig. 21.12).

The complications of this technique are few. Alopecia is rare and has occurred, but only partially, in one case, in spite of these flaps being used very frequently, usually for reasons other than skull-base closure.

If the flap is taken anterior to the hair-line, there is a considerable danger to the frontal branch of the facial nerve. Thus, this area should be avoided.

Temporalis muscle

This muscle, which is large and fan-shaped, having its insertion into the coronoid process and ascending ramus of the mandible, is supplied by the superficial temporal vessels posteriorly and deep temporal vessels posteriorly and anteriorly. It can be elevated from the temporal fossa down to its origin with preservation of its blood supply and, depending on how much orbit has been resected, it can be taken into the orbit or across to the mid-line in the subcranial area—the latter can be accomplished only if the muscle is extensively mobilized. This is usually a reliable muscle flap. The complications, apart from muscle necrosis if the mobilization is over-enthusiastic, are few. The hollow in the temporal area is always present and, if the patient wishes, it can be filled with alloplastic material, e.g. methyl-methacrylate, at a later date.

Letter-box technique

In order to use these flaps and reconstruct the bony defects, it is frequently necessary to use this technique (Fig. 21.13). When the galeal frontalis flap is used in the mid-line or the

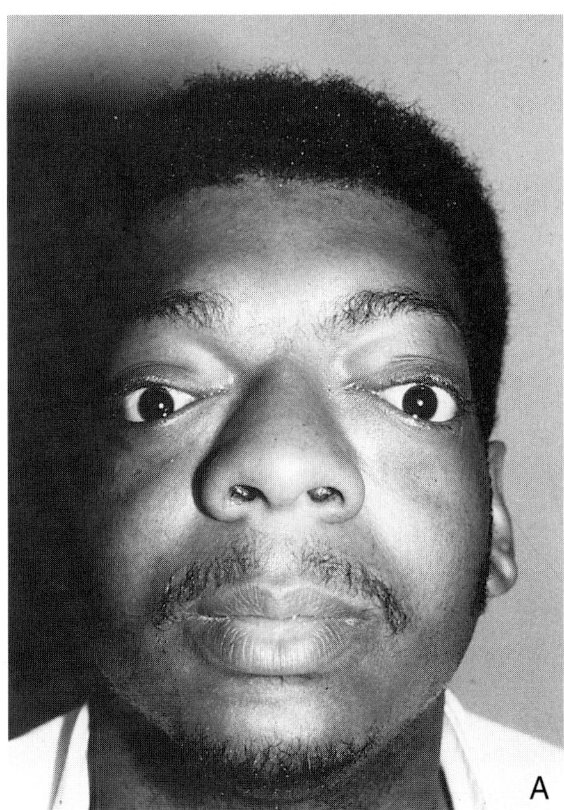

Fig. 21.11

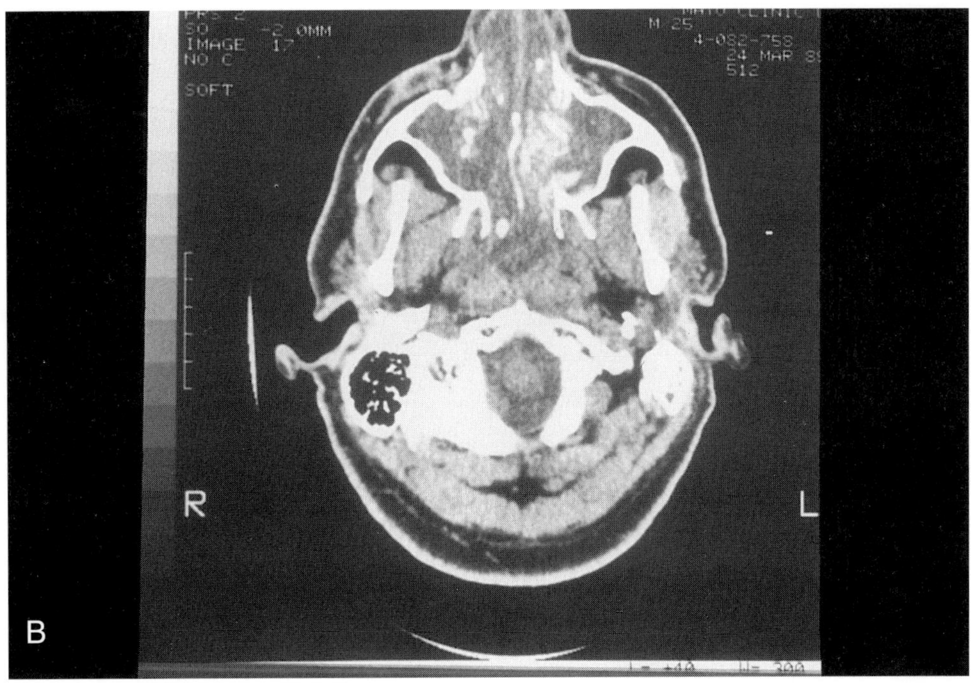

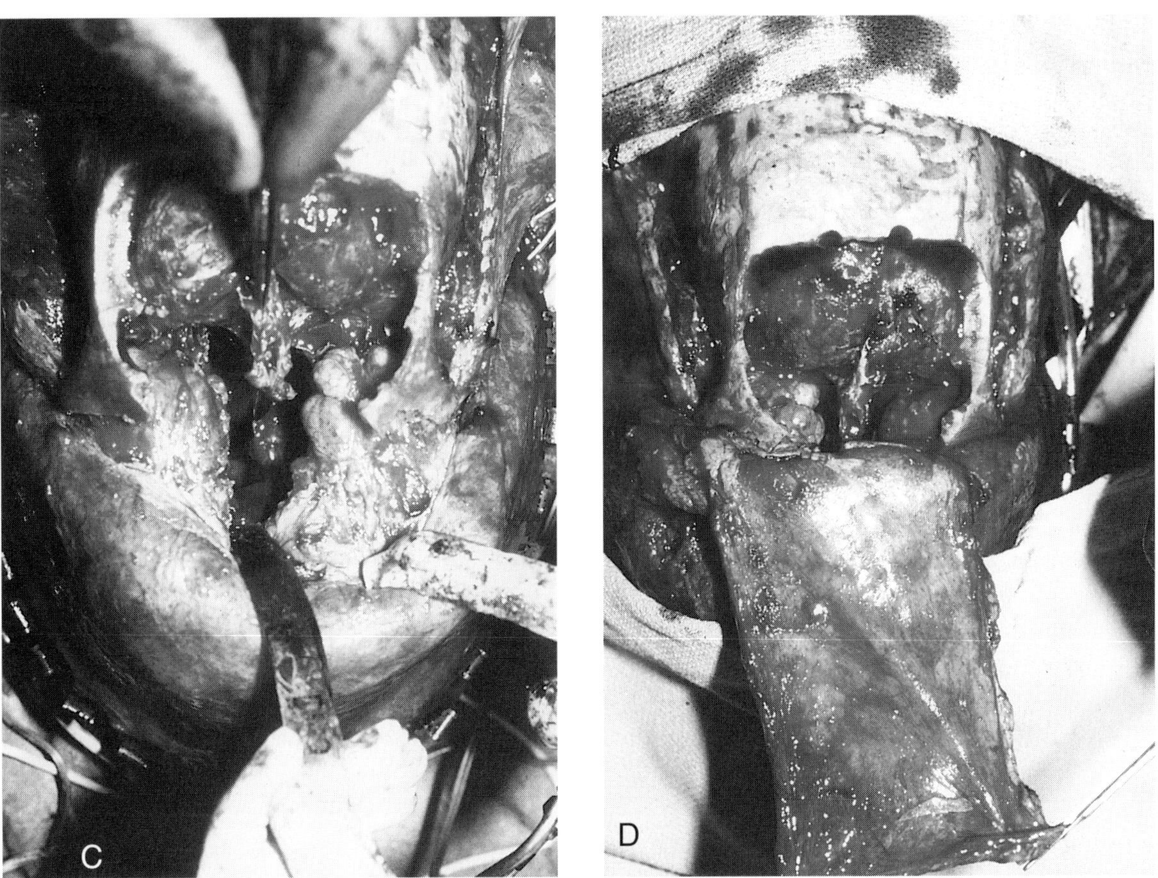

Fig. 21.11

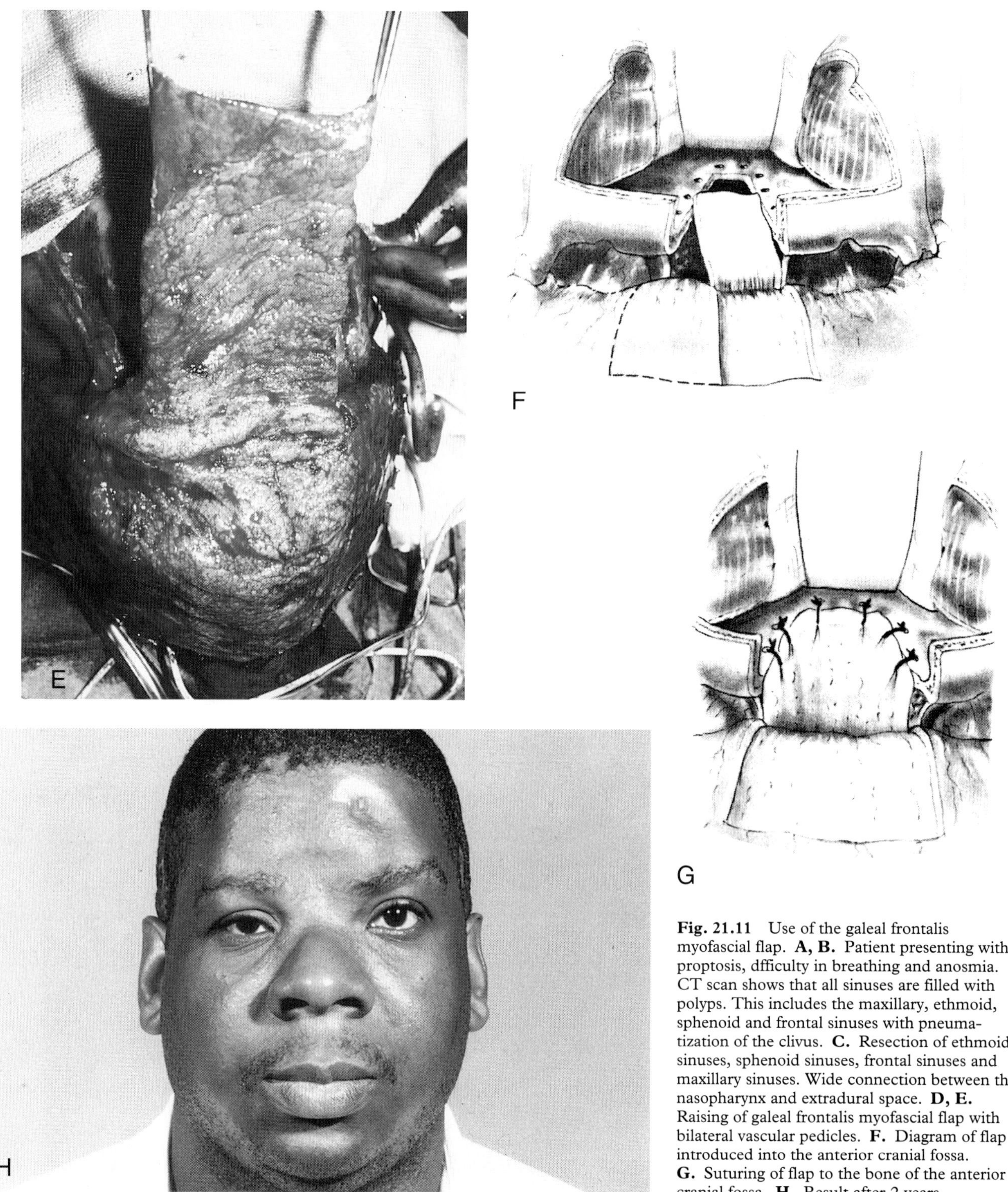

Fig. 21.11 Use of the galeal frontalis myofascial flap. **A, B.** Patient presenting with proptosis, dfficulty in breathing and anosmia. CT scan shows that all sinuses are filled with polyps. This includes the maxillary, ethmoid, sphenoid and frontal sinuses with pneumatization of the clivus. **C.** Resection of ethmoid sinuses, sphenoid sinuses, frontal sinuses and maxillary sinuses. Wide connection between the nasopharynx and extradural space. **D, E.** Raising of galeal frontalis myofascial flap with bilateral vascular pedicles. **F.** Diagram of flap introduced into the anterior cranial fossa. **G.** Suturing of flap to the bone of the anterior cranial fossa. **H.** Result after 2 years.

temporalis laterally, a slot is created by removing bone at the edge of the osteotomies. This should be of sufficient size to allow the flap to be 'mailed' through without constriction of the pedicle.

Similarly, when using the temporalis muscle flap, it is necessary to remove a large part of the lateral orbital wall vertically to allow the bulky muscle passage into or across the orbit.

Free tissue transfer

When there is a chance of an intracranial dead space in addition to a nasopharyngeal connection, the dead space should be obliterated. This is best done using vascularized free tissue transfer (Fisher & Jackson 1989, Jones et al 1986, Jones et al 1987, Guignard et al 1988) (Fig. 21.14). The choice is free muscle, e.g. latissimus dorsi, or omentum. Both have long vascular pedicles, particularly the omentum; this latter is probably the structure of choice. It can be anastomosed to neck vessels; it can be spread around the anterior cranial fossa and the microsurgery is not difficult. The only disadvantage is the need for an intra-abdominal procedure to harvest the flap.

Bone reconstruction

Skeletal reconstruction, when indicated, is usually performed with split skull grafts. These are easily harvested because the skull is in the area of surgery. The usual areas requiring reconstruction are skull, orbit and occasionally the nose. Whenever possible, the grafts are stabilized with plates and screws or, less frequently, wires. If the grafts are exposed into the nasopharynx, they are covered with a galeal frontalis myofascial flap. In the orbit, grafts are frequently covered with temporalis muscle.

Soft-tissue reconstruction

In simple reconstruction, skin cover is frequently obtained using split skin grafts. In the orbit and temporal bones, they can be applied directly to the bone. In other areas, there must be the soft tissue of the area resected or imported galea or muscle as a bed for the graft.

Regional skin or skin muscle flaps can be used. These are best for vertical defects, e.g. the side of the head. The flaps may be rotational from the neck, deltopectoral, pectoralis or latissimus dorsi myocutaneous. These are usually reliable and can be performed rapidly. However, they require two

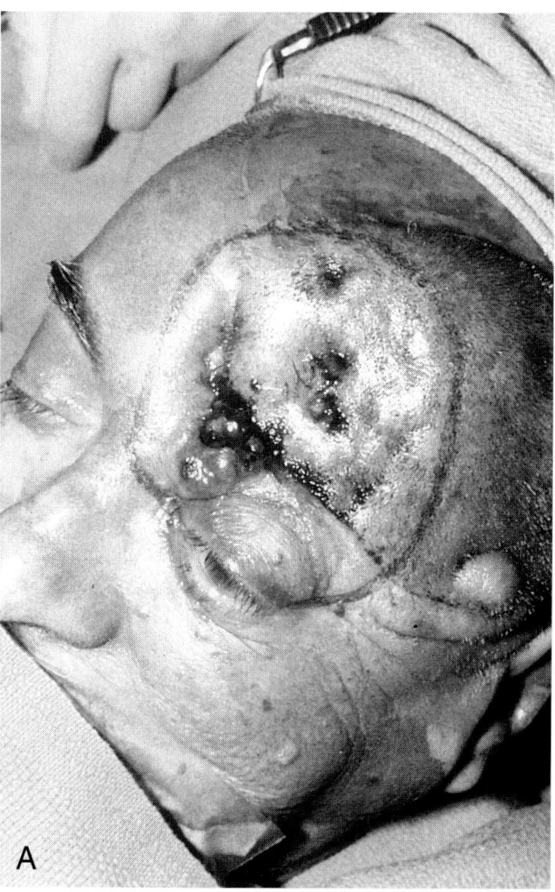

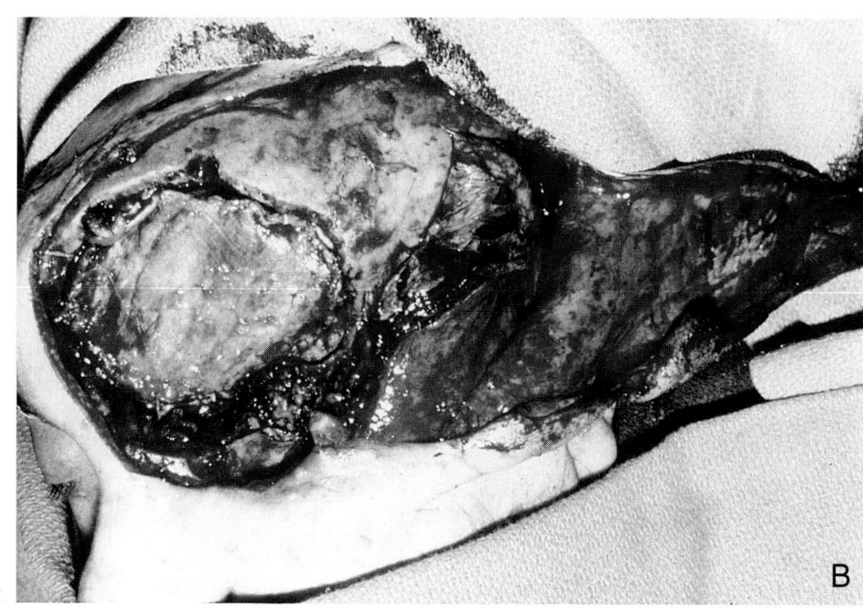

Fig. 21.12

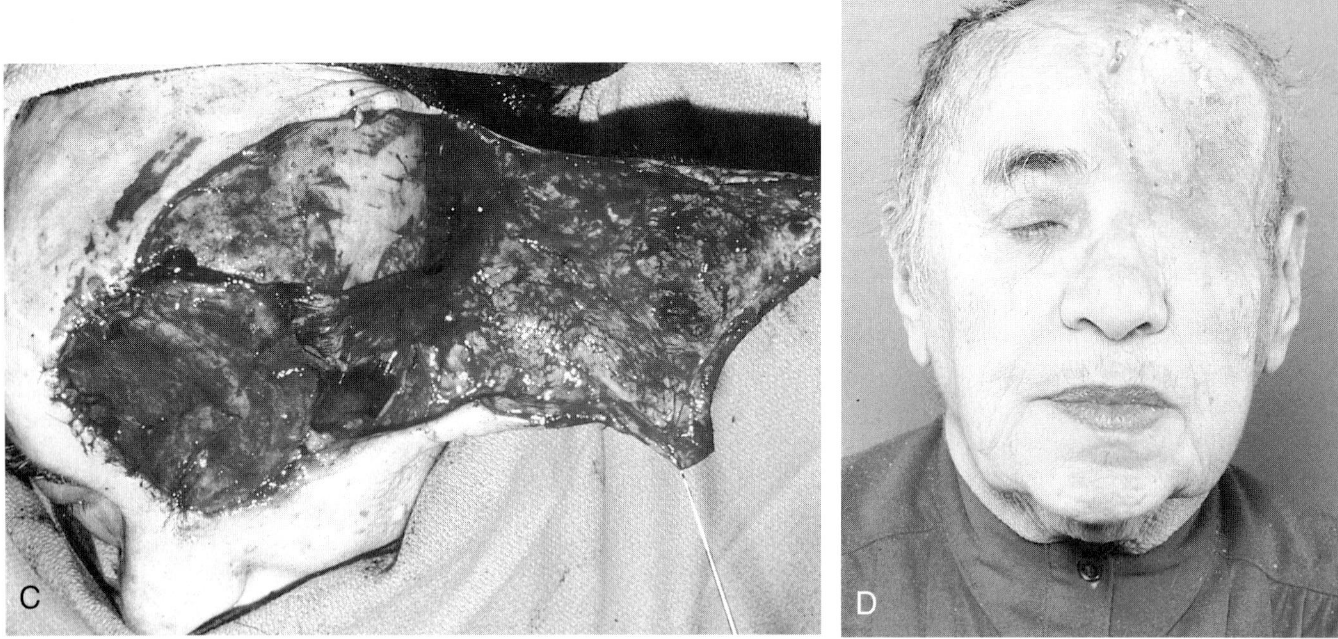

Fig. 21.12 Temporal galeal flap. **A.** Patient with recurrent squamous carcinoma involving left frontal area and orbit. **B.** Resection of lesion with sacrifice of left orbital contents and part of frontal sinus. Defect covered with pedicled temporal galeal flap. **C.** Flap was covered with split skin graft. **D.** Patient 4 years following surgery.

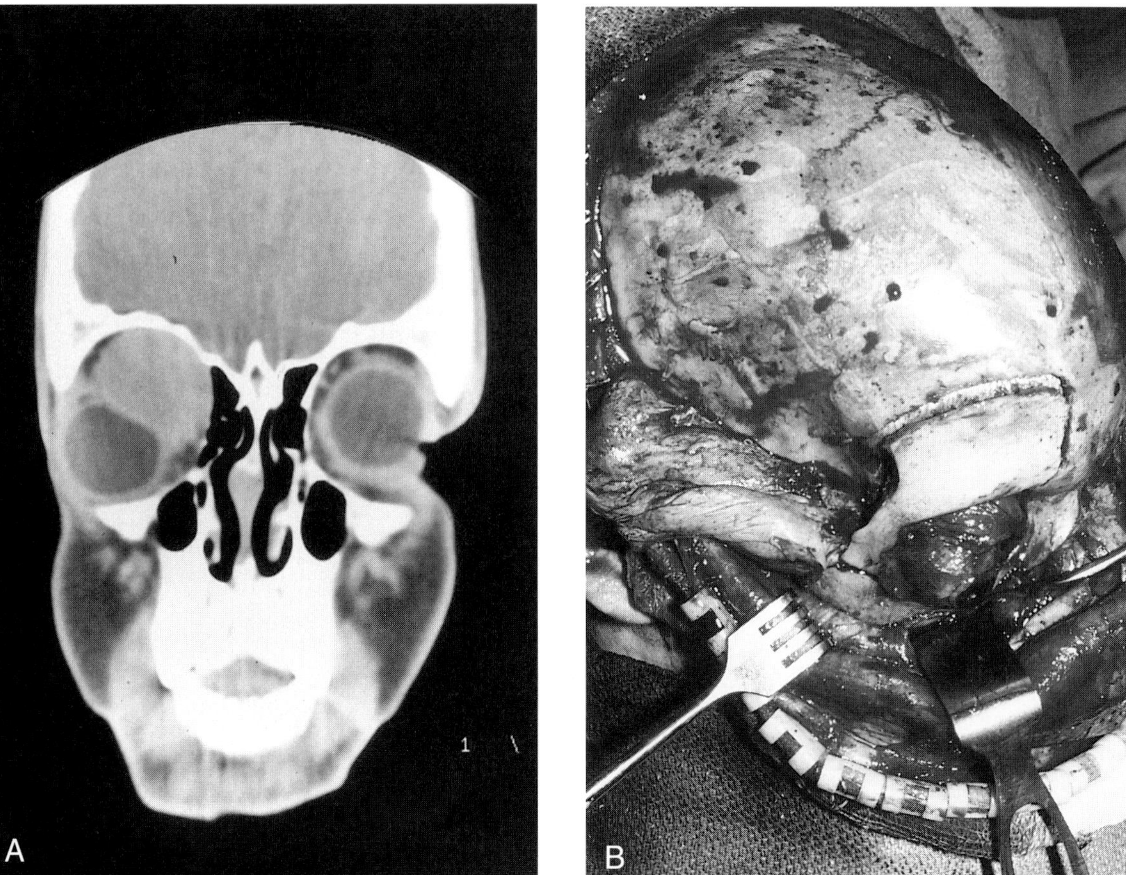

Fig. 21.13

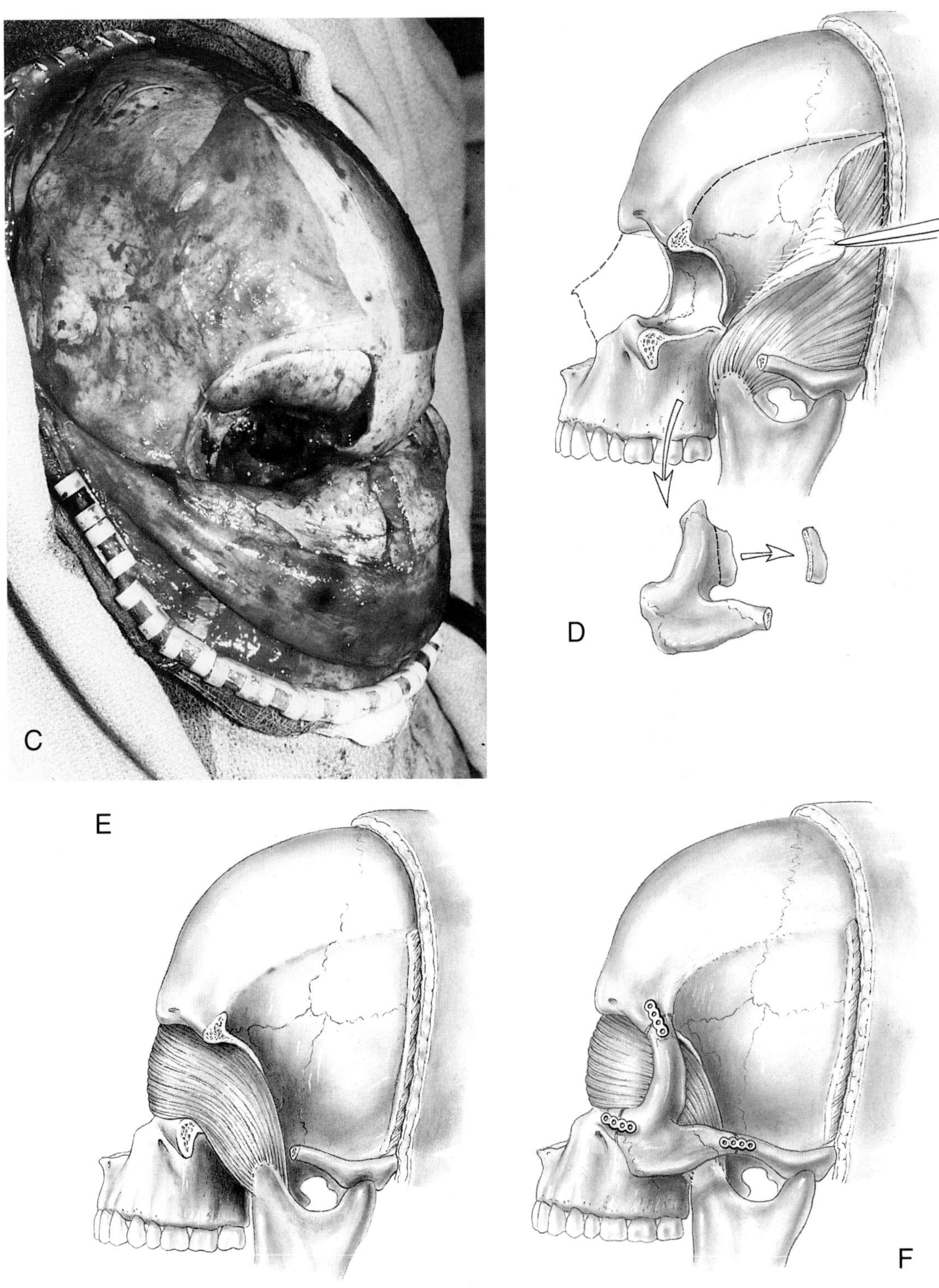

Fig. 21.13

stages, can rarely go above the temporal crest of the skull, and do not always conform as is required.

Free tissue transfer, although involving more time, has the great advantage of being able to be placed anywhere on the head and neck region. It confirms well to all areas and can be used in horizontal defects, e.g. base of skull defects, without problems. It also introduces an excellent blood supply into areas which often have been exposed to radiation therapy. It is possible to transfer composite tissue blocks as required.

These latter two types of reconstruction can also be used when the delayed method is chosen.

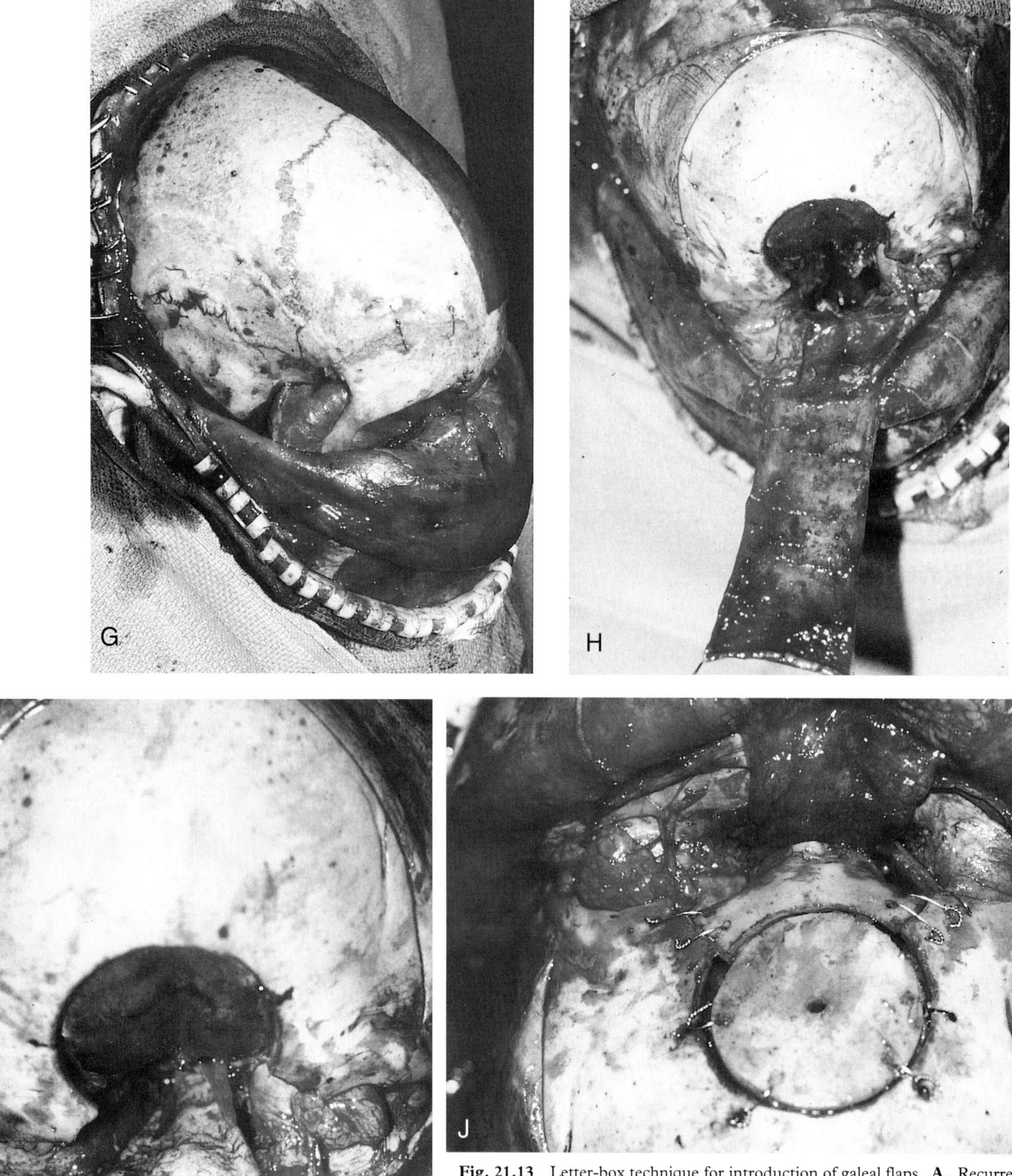

Fig. 21.13   Letter-box technique for introduction of galeal flaps. **A.** Recurrent rhabdomyosarcoma, right orbit. **B.** Osteotomies to remove upper portion of orbit. **C.** Resection of orbital roof, together with orbital contents in order to have complete removal of tumour. **D.** Diagram to show a case where the lateral orbital wall is removed. **E.** Temporalis muscle flap is introduced into the orbit through a defect in the lateral orbital wall. **F.** Modified lateral orbital wall and zygoma, placed in position and stabilized with plates. **G.** Temporalis muscle has been mailed through the letter-box into the orbit. **H.** Galeal frontalis myofascial flap raised. **I.** Galeal frontalis myofascial flap in floor of anterior cranial fossa. **J.** Return of osteotomies with wire stabilization. Note flap being mailed through a slot in the inferior portion of the glabellar osteotomy.

Prosthetics

When there is a defect which has been left for examination, or defies acceptable reconstruction, a prosthesis is used. Now that excellent fixation using the external Branemark system is possible, the results are much more satisfactory, particularly when extra- and intra-oral prostheses which abut on one another are required (French et al 1988). In addition to this, the use of silicone—as opposed to acrylic—has improved the quality of the prosthesis.

COMPLICATIONS

As mentioned previously, the most significant complication

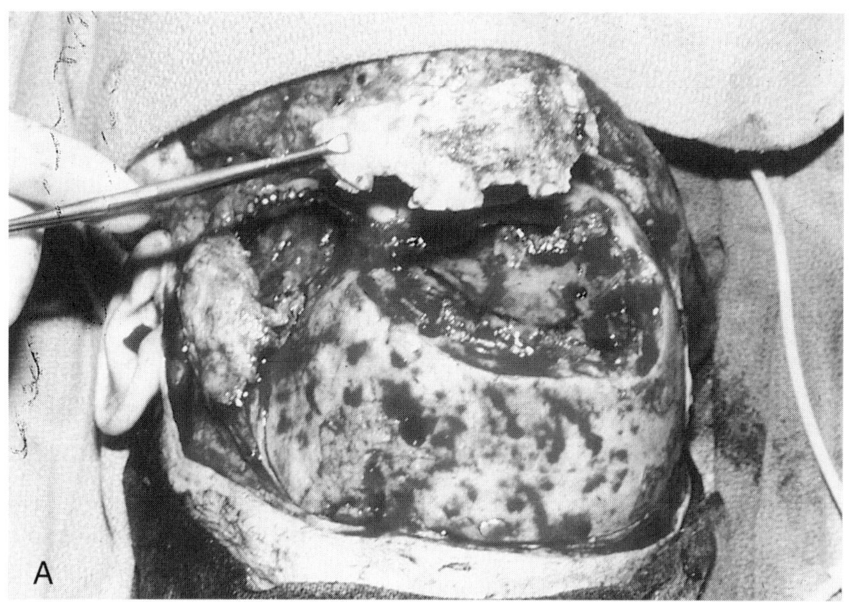

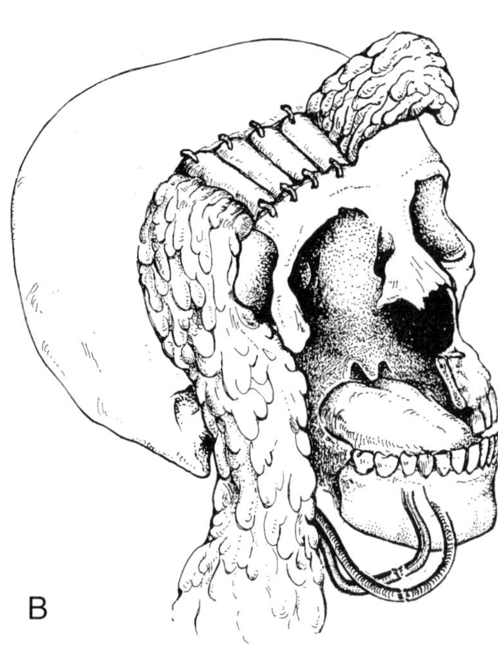

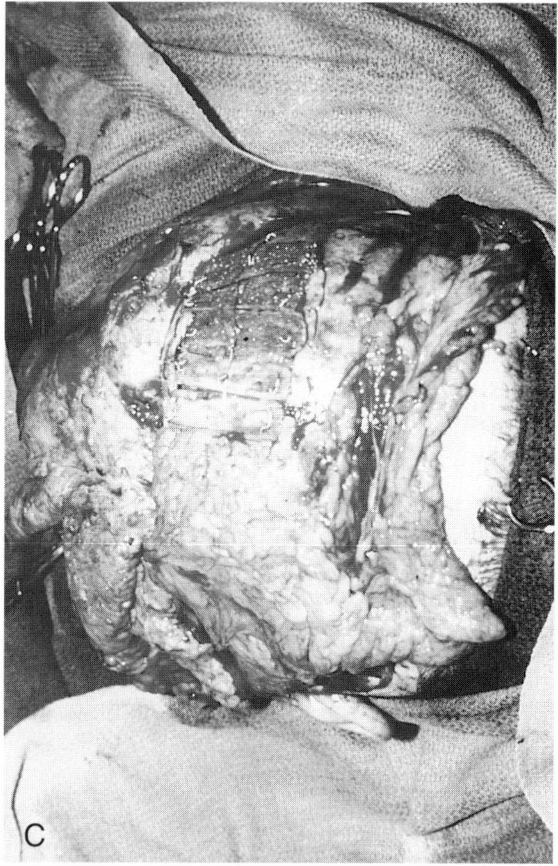

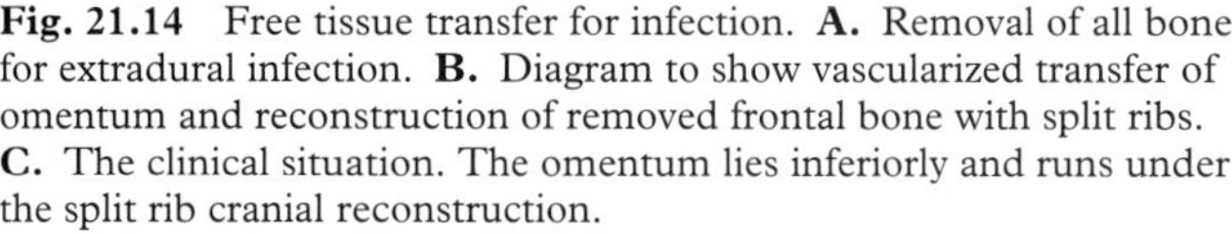

Fig. 21.14 Free tissue transfer for infection. **A.** Removal of all bone for extradural infection. **B.** Diagram to show vascularized transfer of omentum and reconstruction of removed frontal bone with split ribs. **C.** The clinical situation. The omentum lies inferiorly and runs under the split rib cranial reconstruction.

is death. In our series, there has been one early postoperative death at 48 hours. This was due to an intradural venous haemorrhage in an elderly man.

Significant bleeding during surgery is unusual; however, if the tumour is very vascular, a large neurofibroma, fibrous dysplasia or meningioma, highly selective embolization is performed 24 to 48 hours prior to surgery. This has been helpful in reducing blood loss to an acceptable level.

Blindness is a constant worry in many of these cases, whether the surgery is within the orbit or in the posterior central cranial base region. This complication has again been uncommon in our series. In one case of an adenoid cystic carcinoma of the sphenoid sinus with extension beyond the sinus, it was decided, perhaps unwisely, to preserve the orbital contents. There was so much traction on the eye in order to resect this extensive tumour that, in spite of the patient having good vision at the end of the procedure, it deteriorated dramatically over a few hours.

If there is any cause for concern during surgery, e.g. hard globe, proptosis, dilated pupil, the reason for this is determined and dealt with. Should there be no obvious cause, then the steroid/diuretic regime shown in Table 21.3 is instituted. This is not very often necessary and when used has always reversed the problem. It is not possible to state that this is cause and effect, it could simply be a spontaneous resolution.

Other eye complications are those of diplopia and enophthalmus. Diplopia is due either to a change in eye position, extra-ocular muscle change or nerve damage. If the problem is caused by change of eye position, a secondary correction can be performed. This usually involves bone grafting of orbital defects. If muscle and nerve damage is the cause, then muscle surgery may be able to correct the problem. Final correction in some cases will be achieved with prisms inserted into spectacle lenses.

INFECTION

Minor infections are treated in the standard fashion. It is the overwhelming infections that must be recognized early and treated aggressively. As has been stated earlier in this chapter, the causation of this type of infection is a connection between the nasopharynx and the extradural space. This becomes especially significant when there is an extradural dead space with or without a dural repair. The possible results of this type of infection are loss of any osteotomized bone, extradural abscess, subdural or brain abscess and meningitis. Death can result from any of these manifestations of infection.

It is important to recognize early that this situation is developing in order to institute treatment as rapidly as possible. There is the typical abscess temperature chart associated with eyelid oedema which shows no evidence of resolution. Frequently, there is a boggy swelling in the temporal area and the patient is ill. A CT scan showing an anterior dead space with a fluid level confirms the diagnosis.

When this diagnosis has been made, the treatment must be undertaken without delay. It is sometimes possible to explore the area and irrigate and drain the dead space; this may result in a successful outcome. Frequently, all osteotomized bone and bone grafts have to be removed and the overlying scalp falls into and obliterates the dead space.

The most satisfactory solution to the problem is to fill the dead space with material which brings in a fresh blood supply (Fig. 21.14). The most useful filling material is that of free tissue transfer; omentum and latissimus dorsi muscle have been effectively used (Fisher & Jackson 1989). This free tissue transfer is combined with the appropriate intravenous antibiotics.

It is undoubtedly much more satisfactory to prevent infection from occurring at the time of resection as described earlier. This has been our practice and there have been no cases of significant infection apart from a meningitis which responded rapidly to intravenous antibiotic therapy.

RESULTS

The assessment of results in these tumours is difficult. This is because there are few large series of uniform pathology and it is only relatively recently that radical resections have been performed consistently and safely.

Table 21.3 Protocol for suspected raised intra-ocular pressure

1. Immediate ophthalmology consultation for fundoscoy and tonometry

   Steps 2 to 4, inclusive, should be instituted without waiting for the ophthalmology consultation

2. Diamox (500 mg i.v. stat; 250 mg i.v. every 6 hours for 24 hours)
3. Solu-Medrol (1 gm i.v. stat)
4. Mannitol, 20% solution
   2 gm/kg of body weight
   24 hour i.v
   No more than 12.5 gm in 3 to 4 minutes

   If there is no improvement, proceed to step 5

5. Lateral canthotomy
6. Situation desperate—anterior chamber decompression

   Make sure that the medications are present in the operating room at all times

Table 21.4 Analysis of malignant skull-base tumours

	Total	Primary	Recurrent
Anterior cranial fossa	95	20	75
Middle cranial fossa	49	11	38
Petrous area	44	18	26
Posterior cranial fossa	2	2	
Total	190	51	139
		27%	73%

Table 21.5   Malignant skull-base tumours: survival statistics*

	Total	Alive (%)	Alive with disease (%)	Dead (%)
Anterior cranial	95	56 (59)	13 (14)	26 (27)
Middle cranial	49	20 (41)	14 (28)	15 (31)
Petrous area	44	20 (45)	4 (10)	20 (45)
Posterior cranial fossa	2	1	1	
Total	190	97 (57)	32 (17)	61 (32)

* Average follow up: 6.5 years.

In any large referral centre, the pathology of these lesions is very variable. Many are recurrent after surgery and radiation therapy. It is not unusual for them to have been considered to be inoperable by the referring institution. It must be realized, however, that resection cannot always be equated with cure.

In large tumours which may be radiosensitive, it is reasonable to resect as effectively as possible and then present the radiation therapist with a smaller tumour volume to treat. When the tumour recurs and invades bone, it is undoubtedly best to resect surgically and then follow with radiation therapy rather than the other way around. In some cases, interstitial radiation has been employed. Squamous- and basal-cell carcinomas, especially when they invade bone, seem to become more aggressive when given radiation therapy.

In spite of what appears to be a dismal prognosis in malignant skull tumours as they present to a specialist centre, this is not borne out on long-term follow-up, even when the majority of cases are recurrent (Tables 21.4, 21.5). Similar series of assorted cases have suggested hopeful results.

It may be that, with new modalities of treatment, e.g. interstitial radiation, and newer regimes of chemotherapy, these results will be improved. What is very significant is that primary cases referred to a specialized centre have much higher survival rates. It is hoped that this message will encourage earlier referral of primary cases to centres where the appropriate teams are available and where these difficult cases can be assessed in depth, and treated radically and safely.

REFERENCES

Fisher J, Jackson I T 1989 Microvascular surgery as an adjuvant to craniomaxillofacial surgery, British Journal of Plastic Surgery 42: 146–154

French D J, Jackson I T, Toleman D E 1988 A system of osseointegrated implants and its application to dental and facial rehabilitation. European Journal of Plastic Surgery 11: 14–21

Fukuta K, Jackson I T, McEwan C et al 1990 Three dimensional imaging in craniofacial surgery: a review of the role of mirror image production. European Journal of Plastic Surgery 13: 209

Guignard R M, Krupp S, Sauary M et al 1988 Team approach of sinuso-orbital tumours invading the skull base. European Journal of Plastic Surgery 11: 169–174

Har-Shai Y, Fukuta K, Collares M et al 1992 The vascular anatomy of the galeal flap in the interparietal and midline regions. Plastic Reconstructive Surgery 89: 64–69

Henry A K 1966 Extensile exposure, 2nd edn. E & S Livingstone, Edinburgh

Jackson I T 1985 Craniofacial surgery for congenital deformities: its contribution to surgery of the skull. In: Chretien P et al (eds) Head and neck cancer. Decker, Philadelphia, vol 1, pp 263–272

Jackson I T 1992 Tumours involving the anterior and middle cranial fossa. In: McGregor I A, Howard D J (eds) Rob and Smith's operative surgery. Butterworth-Heinemann, Oxford, part 2, pp 593–623

Jackson I T, Hide T A H 1981 Further extensions of craniofacial surgery. In: I T Jackson (ed) Recent advances in plastic surgery. Churchill Livingstone, Edinburgh, ch 16, pp 241–289

Jackson I T, Adham M N, Marsh W R 1986a Use of galeofrontalis myofascial flap in craniofacial surgery. Plastic Reconstructive Surgery 77: 905–910

Jackson I T, March W R, Bite U et al 1986b. Craniofacial osteotomies to facilitate skull base tumour resection. British Journal of Plastic Surgery 39: 153–160

Jackson I T, Fukuta K, Audet B et al 1991 Side table assembly: an adjuvant to craniofacial reconstruction. British Journal of Plastic Surgery 44: 348–350

Janecka A P, Sekhar L N 1989 Surgical management of cranial bone tumors. A report on 9 patients. Oncology 3: 69–74

Janecka A P, Sen C N, Sekhar L N et al 1990 Facial translocation: new approach to the cranial base. Otolaryngology—Head and Neck Surgery 103: 413–419

Jones N F, Sekhar L N, Schramm V L 1986 Free rectus abdominis flap reconstruction of the middle and posterior cranial base. Plastic and Reconstructive Surgery 78: 471–477

Jones N F, Schramm V L, Sekhar L N 1987 Reconstruction of the cranial base following tumour resection. British Journal of Plastic Surgery 40: 155–162

Ketcham A S, Wilkins R, Van Buren J M et al 1963 A combined intracranial facial approach to the paranasal sinuses. American Journal of Surgery 106: 698–703

Lauritzen C, Vallfors B, Lilja J 1986 Facial disassembly for tumor resection. Scandinavian Journal of Plastic and Reconstructive Surgery 20: 201–206

Nuss D W, Janecka I P, Sekhar L N et al 1991 Craniofacial disassembly in the management of skull base tumours. Otolaryngology. Clinics of North America: management of head and neck neoplasms. Otolaryngologic Clinics of North America 24: 1465–1497

Shah J P, Sundaresan N, Attyar R A, Sisson G A 1987 Craniofacial resections for tumours involving the base of the skull. American Journal of Surgery 154: 352

22. Recent trends in maxillofacial prosthetics

Dieter Riediger

INTRODUCTION

Defects in the continuity of the jaws mostly result from surgical tumour resection or less commonly as a result of infection or traumatic bone loss. Such defects can lead to a severe functional deficit in mastication, swallowing, breathing and speaking. Therefore, an osteoplastic bone replacement with the ultimate goal of functional rehabilitation is required as soon as possible. Free autologous bone grafts from the iliac crest have been used in such cases to replace missing jaw bone since their description by Lindemann (1916) and Klapp (1916).

These so-called free, non-vascularized autologous grafts are solely dependent for their vitality on the surrounding soft and hard tissues (Axhausen 1951). Poor recipient sites can, on the one hand, promote infection, and on the other, prolong the process of revitalization of the primarily avital osseous material. This consequently leads to a loss of volume and quantity to a variable degree (Lentrodt et al 1987). This applies to all forms of free bone grafts whether they are of cortico-cancellous or purely cancellous composition. On the contrary, the technique of revascularizing a bone graft via its own vessels, using microsurgical anastomoses, makes it independent in its nutrition and vitality from the surrounding recipient tissues. The nutrition is provided either by the periosteum and attached musculature (vascularized iliac crest) or by vessels entering the medulla directly (vascularized fibula). Due to the persisting vitality of the osseous tissues, such bone transfers should remain structurally unaltered. Complicated resorptive and remodelling processes which have to take place in free bone grafts (Barth 1894, Axhausen 1951, 1952) are not witnessed so that a constant volume of these vascularized grafts may be expected. This is an important prerequisite for the later masticatory load on the jaw-bone.

The frequent contamination with oral bacteria of free grafts used in jaw reconstruction increases the risk of infection. Postoperative antibiotic treatment cannot be expected to reach the free graft in the early phase following transplantation. This may explain why a relatively large percentage of free grafts are lost as a result of infection in the early phase (Holtje & Lentrodt 1972). A constant vascularization, however, allows a continued antibiotic protection of the revascularized bone graft, and the infection rate can be reduced substantially.

The restoration of bone continuity is essential for a functional rehabilitation. Only in a few cases, however, does restoration of bone itself prove sufficient to allow prosthetic dental treatment. Even classical preprosthetic surgical procedures, such as lowering the floor of the mouth, or vestibuloplasty in an attempt to improve the fit of a denture, do not guarantee a successful prosthetic rehabilitation. For these reasons we have developed a new concept in integrating endosseous implants into vascularized cancellous bone reconstructions which seem especially suitable to receive these implants successfully (Riediger et al 1986). Initially, the author chose to implant the Tübingen type aluminium oxide ceramic implants (Frialit®) originally described by Schulte & Heimke (1976).

NEW CONCEPTS IN BONE GRAFTING AND MASTICATORY REHABILITATION

Extended surgical resection in the maxillofacial region leads to considerable functional disturbances, especially when the jaw bones are concerned. Even though an osteoplastic restoration of bone continuity can be achieved and an increased mobility of the tongue might improve speech and swallowing, as well as securing the airway, it remains an exception to restore the masticatory function completely and permit the integration of a functional dental prosthesis. This therefore has become the reconstructive surgeon's ultimate goal.

Definitive improvements have been made using microsurgically revascularized bone graft in combination with endosseous dental implants. This reconstructive regime can set the basis for true restoration of masticatory function. This regime uses special techniques for osteoplastic replacement which first requires a stable bone continuity and the persistence of bone volume even in adverse conditions such as when the local tissues are unfavourable. Secondly, the cancellous bone framework, with its favourably high vascularization, allows the second step towards masticatory restoration using endosseous dental implants. Among the modern scientifically proven dental implants, aluminium oxide ceramic and titanium implants deserve special consideration due to their favourable osseo-integration.

The combined use of free bone transplants and endosseous implants was described by Branemark et al in 1975 and Lindstrom et al in 1981. It is clear, however, that a free bone graft is subjected to bone resorption to an unmeasurable degree. This author employed titanium implants in free non-vascularized bone grafts and had to accept a relatively high degree of bone loss and subsequent rate of complications.

Our own research in Merino sheep demonstrated that endosseous implants in free iliac crest grafts suffered peri-implantal bone atrophy after 4 weeks as well as pronounced resorption after 8 weeks resulting in exposure of implant surfaces and consequent loosening of the implant. On the contrary, revascularized iliac crest grafts demonstrated, over the entire period of up to 12 weeks postoperatively, no signs of either peri-implantal or graft resorption. All these implants remained totally osseo-integrated. The macroscopic results were radiologically verified. In free grafts, incomplete osseous attachment to the implants resulted in a complete peri-implantal radiolucency. The free iliac crest segments showed signs of progressive atrophy demonstrated by increased radiolucency representing a decrease in mineralization compared to their original appearance. Histological examination showed peri-implantal zones of necrotic bone and, using a polarization technique, abundant collagen fibre formation in the experimental implantation into free iliac crest grafts. Osseo-integration did not take place in these implants within 12 weeks because the recipient bone had to be revitalized first. Implants in revascularized grafts from the iliac crest showed giant cells on the implant surface after 2–4 weeks with an osseous attachment and osseo-integration definitely visible after 8–12 weeks. With the periotest technique (Schulte et al 1983) the breaking power of the peri-implantal tissue could be measured using a defined impulse inserted on the implant. The measured value is the breaking time of an impulse exerted on the implant by an electromagnetically accelerated piston. Free bone graft implants showed considerably higher periotest values after 8–12 weeks, expressing their lack of osseo-integration and increased mobility as a sign of graft atrophy. Also, as to be expected, implants and free bone grafts had a lower resistance to exerting forces than did those in a revascularized graft, except for the first week following implantation. Even though single implants in free grafts were able to withstand exerting forces after 8–12 weeks they never matched the values of implants in revascularized bone. This again is an indication of either the lack of or a slow and insecure degree of osseo-integration in free bone grafts. Interestingly, a further improvement of resistance of exerting forces of the implants in revascularized bone was not observed after the eighth week. This perhaps assumes that the osseo-integration is completed at this time.

Furthermore, scintigraphic measurements using bone affinity marking techniques and the uptake of antibiotic agents postoperatively have clearly proven the persistent vitality and biological quality of revascularized bone grafts. These experimental findings stress the fact that revascularized bone grafts have a special place in reconstructive maxillofacial surgery, especially regarding the role of osseo-integration of dental implants in bone grafts and masticatory restoration as well as grafting in difficult local situations.

The results of these investigations persuaded the authors to employ revascularized bone grafts with their superior quality, independent of the recipient site, and osseo-integrated implants initially of the aluminium oxide ceramic type and later titanium implants.

In six of our own patients, bone biopsies were taken from the revascularized iliac crest bone grafts for histological examination either at the time of metal plate removal or at the time of insertion of the implants (Professor Dr C. M. Busing, Pathological Institute, Ingolstadt Hospital). Biopsies varied from 6 months to 17 months following bone transfer. All of the grafts had taken well and were clinically and radiologically stable. At the suture site between mandibular stump and revascularized graft a bony consolidation without callous formation was observed. The biopsies were decalcified and examined by light microscopy. The typical architecture of cancellous iliac crest bone was preserved, and vital osteocytes and spaces filled with adipose tissue and bloodcell generating cells were evident.

PRINCIPLES OF TREATMENT

Excision

The majority of cases requiring reconstruction of the jaw follow resection of a malignant tumour. Squamous-cell carcinoma is the most common malignancy in this area and may require an extensive resection of jaw bone and adjacent oral soft tissues of the cheek, floor of mouth, tongue and palatal regions. A radical tumour resection must adhere to an exactly defined resection margin and, wherever possible, the en bloc resection principle with simultaneous elective or therapeutic lymph node dissection of the neck should be performed. Second to malignant tumours as a cause of major jaw defects requiring reconstruction are benign tumours localized within the jaw bone. Ameloblastomas, for example, often require extended resections because of their locally aggressive behaviour. Rarer conditions, such as traumatic bone loss or chronic infections or osteoradionecrosis, may also require bone and soft-tissue reconstruction simultaneously.

Reconstruction

For soft-tissue reconstruction in the floor of mouth or cheek region the author favours pedicled myocutaneous flaps such as the pectoralis major or latissimus dorsi flap. The latter can also be used as a free flap. For reconstruction of the lateral oral wall, the velar region and the pharyngeal region, the author favours free jejunal transplants. Myocutaneous flaps are used for reconstruction of the tongue, and in cases of total glossectomy a free latissimus dorsi with anastomosis of the thoracodorsal nerve to the hypoglossal nerve is the first choice in an attempt to gain functional rehabilitation.

However, if the plan is subsequently to insert prosthetic devices with the aim of tolerating a masticatory load, the author prefers myocutaneous or osteomyocutaneous or fasciocutaneous flaps which are more robust than the jejunal transplant. If simultaneous reconstruction of soft tissue and bone is required, the composite osteomyocutaneous groin flap is the method of choice when later masticatory rehabilitation is planned. The myocutaneous flap portion is secondarily thinned out and shaped according to classic vestibuloplasty techniques, wherever possible using oral mucosa replacing the skin.

INDICATIONS FOR VASCULARIZED BONE RECONSTRUCTION

As mentioned previously, there are special indications for a revascularized bone graft in the adverse recipient site—such as following radiation therapy, large-scale surgery, chronic infection or trauma, or in extensive scar formation. The common sequelae in these cases is badly vascularized malnourished and biologically inadequate quality tissue in the recipient site. A further indication for using vascularized bone is in cases where there is a need to replace larger quantities of bone and where reconstruction demands the replacement of both soft and hard tissues. In tumour surgery, revascularized bone transfer can be used in primary reconstruction or, more often, in secondary reconstruction following radiation. Other indications for using vascularized bone include failure of conventional free bone grafting osteoplasty techniques or in preprosthetic surgery in extreme cases of alveolar atrophy.

DONOR SITES FOR VASCULARIZED BONE GRAFTS

Basically there are a number of bone grafts that can be used as revascularized bone transfers depending on the specific requirements. These include:

rib graft
fibular graft
iliac crest graft
radial bone graft
ulnar bone graft
scapular bone graft

Among these donor sites, the author favours the revascularized iliac crest graft. It is extremely well suited for mandibular and maxillary reconstruction, and the shape of the pelvis enables voluminous cancellous transplants to be raised and shaped according to the anatomical requirements of the defect.

Iliac crest

Osteomuscular iliac crest grafts consist of the iliac crest bone with its attaching musculature, whereas osteomyocutaneous flaps additionally include a skin portion. Both types of flap may be raised on either the superficial or the deep circumflex iliac artery and vein. The deep circumflex iliac artery (DCIA) is the more reliable vessel concerning bone vascularization (Taylor et al 1979, Taylor 1982). The skin portion in the osteomyocutaneous flap is less reliable, and in approximately 20% of cases the deep circumflex iliac system (DCIA) does not sufficiently vascularize the skin. A safer pedicle for the osteomyocutaneous flap can be raised by including both superficial and deep vessels and anastomosing both systems at the recipient site.

Anatomy

Anatomy of the deep circumflex iliac artery osteomyocutanous groin flap has been described in numerous publications (Taylor & Watson 1978, Taylor et al 1979). The deep circumflex iliac artery (DCIA) originates from the lateral wall of the external iliac artery superior to the inguinal ligament. The artery is usually accompanied by two veins draining into a common trunk and into the external iliac vein. The vessels run superolaterally in connective tissue behind the inguinal ligament. At the level of the anterior superior iliac spine the vascular pedicle crosses the lateral femoral cutaneous nerve, and, in this area, branches are found to the superficial circumflex iliac artery (SCIA) and also to the lateral circumflex femoral artery. Approximately 1 cm medial to the anterior superior iliac spine the DCIA gives a branch to the abdominal wall musculature and skin. This branch is variable and may originate either more proximally or sometimes directly from the external iliac artery. Lateral to the anterior superior spine the DCIA runs along the medial surface of the iliac bone approximately 1–2 cm below the crest and on the fascia of the iliacus muscle. It lies beneath the external oblique, internal oblique and transverse abdominal muscles until approximately half-way along the length of the iliac crest. Here, the DCIA passes superficially to enter the abdominal wall and provides perforators to the overlying skin. During its course, several small perforating branches pass through the abdominal wall and into the subcutaneous tissue approximately 1 cm superior to the iliac crest.

Elevation of the DCIA flap

The course of the femoral vessels and the position of the inguinal ligament, the anterior superior iliac spine and the iliac crest are drawn out. A vertical skin excision starting 4 cm above and extending to 4 cm below the inguinal ligament overlies the course of the femoral vessels. The femoral artery is dissected in a cranial direction and the inguinal ligament divided to expose the external iliac artery. The origin of the DCIA is slightly lateral and cranial to the inguinal ligament and is situated at approximately the same level as the inferior epigastric artery which arises from the medial wall of the external iliac artery. The deep circumflex iliac artery and vein are dissected from the iliac and transverse fascia towards the anterior superior iliac spine. The lateral femoral cutaneous nerve is dissected and protected, and the ascending branch of the DCIA is included in an osteomyocutaneous flap with a large skin portion as planned.

When transferring an osteomuscular flap the skin is incised approximately 1–2 cm from the iliac crest down to the external oblique muscle. The abdominal wall musculature is divided at a distance of 1 cm from the iliac crest. The iliac fascia is often incised at a slightly greater distance from the iliac crest, approximately 2 cm, because closer to the bone lies the epifascial course of the DCIA. Following division of the fascia and the iliacus muscle, dissection is continued down to the iliac bone in an oblique caudal direction. The medial surface of the bone is dissected free. Laterally, the sartorius muscle is separated from the anterior superior iliac spine, and on the outer aspect of the iliac crest the tensor fascia lata, gluteus medius and gluteus minimus muscles are separated from the bone.

The desired shape of the bone graft is created using an oscillating saw directed from the outer to the inner surface. The tip has to be carefully controlled to ensure that the saw perforates the bone inferior to the detached iliac muscle so that damage to the muscle and vascular pedicles is avoided. When the bone cuts are complete, the vascularized bone graft remains attached only by its vascular pedicle.

When raising an osteomyocutaneous flap the vascular pedicle is dissected up to the lateral femoral cutaneous nerve. The skin island is outlined and in such situations the abdominal wall musculature has to be divided at a greater distance from the iliac crest (2–4cm) so as to avoid damage to the cutaneous perforators from the DCIA. Even though these muscular perforators extend into the skin superior to the iliac crest, the skin paddle may extend on both sides of the iliac crest, both superiorly and inferiorly. Inferiorly, the subcutaneous tissues are divided and lifted off the tensor fascia lata fascia up to the iliac crest. After isolating the skin paddle and dividing the abdominal wall musculature slightly more laterally, the flap is raised as described above. Again,

it should be pointed out that a sufficient vascularization of the skin is not completely safe on the DCIA perforators alone.

A further variation arises from the possibility of including a large portion of musculature. Internal oblique musculature can be raised with the ascending branch of the DCIA offering an alternative in reconstructing combined soft-and hard-tissue defects. This has proved useful in obese patients with thick abdominal skin and subcutaneous fat where the bulk of an osteomyocutaneous flap is excessive for the recipient area. This is most often seen in intra-oral reconstruction which can be particularly challenging in obese individuals. In such cases the muscular portion can be used instead of a skin paddle for soft-tissue reconstruction and the muscle subsequently covered with a split-thickness skin graft.

Care should be taken to note any abdominal scars following previous surgery in this area since this might further compromise the perfusion of the skin. Following elevation of the bone there is often strong bleeding from the cancellous bone that is exposed and this can be sealed by using bone wax.

Meticulous wound closure is essential if herniation is to be prevented. The abdominal wall has to be reconstructed in layers. It is important to unite the iliac fascia delicately with the transversus fascia to avoid herniation of abdominal contents. The three flat muscles of the abdominal wall are sutured to the tensor fascia lata and gluteus medius muscles.

In the author's practice, revascularized iliac crest grafts and osteoplastic jaw-bone reconstruction now provide the basis for subsequent endosseous implants.

MANDIBLE RECONSTRUCTION

Mental arch

The bony mental arch of the mandible is of vital importance to maintain a stable base for the floor of the mouth. It is here that the musculature of the floor of the mouth and tongue insert. The curve of the mental arch demands that the bone graft be shaped, contoured and modelled, and this is always necessary. Even though the iliac crest has a natural curvature, this must be increased by fracturing the outer cortex into the inner cortical layer. This fracturing must be performed with the utmost care to prevent damage to the vascularization of the bone. Gaps following these osteotomies can be filled by cancellous bone chips. In composite tissue reconstruction where the soft-tissue defect involves the anterior floor of mouth and tongue region, it is necessary to transplant enough skin to gain a functional vestibulum oris. The vascular pedicle in this type of transfer is normally anastomosed to the upper thyroid or facial vessels (Fig. 22.1).

Mandibular angle and ascending ramus

Reconstruction of the mandibular angle is important for both aesthetics and function (Fig. 22.2). Involvement of the angle region usually denotes an extensive resection where large quantities of bone are required for reconstruction. To maintain function, it is important to gain a broad attachment of the bone to the condylar process and so prevent later pseudoarthrosis. Fixation to the condylar region is usually done by mini-plates or, where this is not possible, by wire osteosynthesis. In such cases a sturdy intermaxillary fixation with wires is mandatory. The shaping of an angled bone graft is eased by the natural curve of the pelvis offering its anterior edge as an ascending ramus and the iliac crest itself

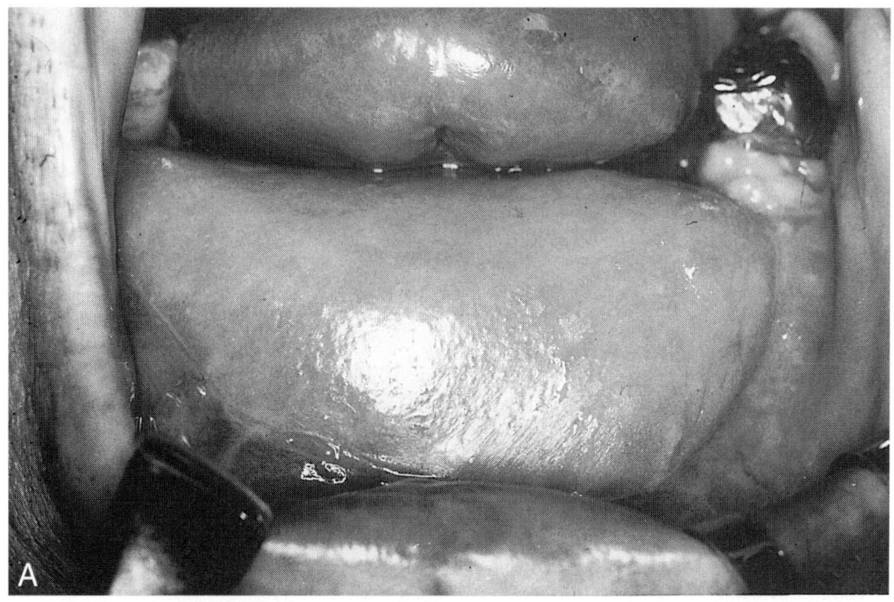

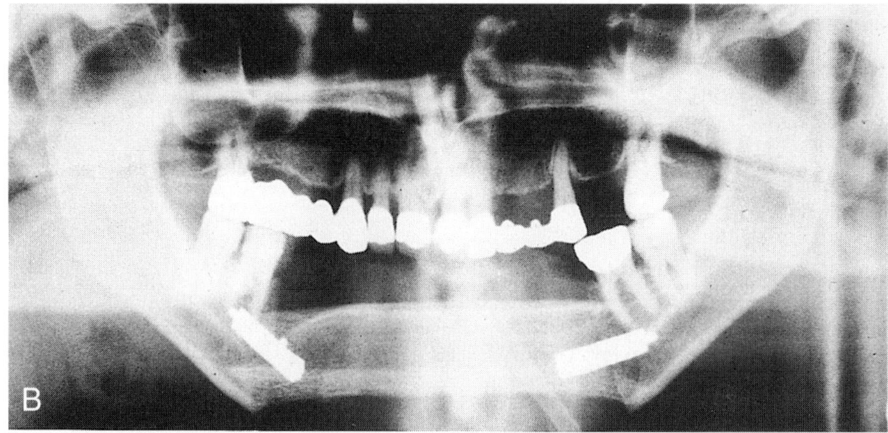

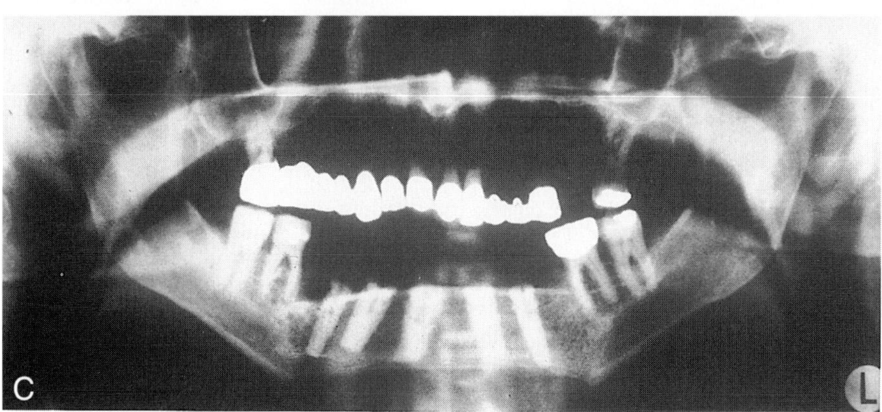

Fig. 22.1

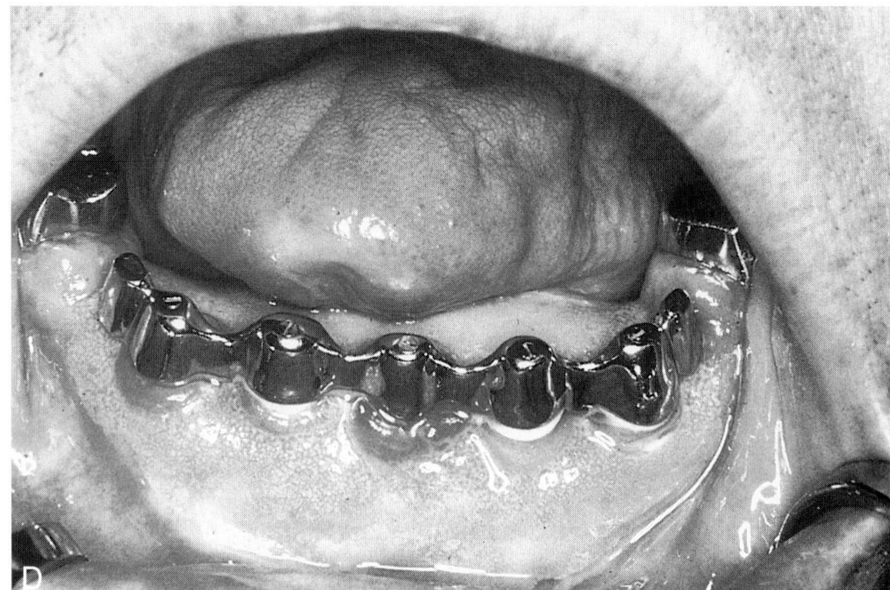

Fig. 22.1 **A.** A 56-year-old patient who underwent excision of a squamous carcinoma of the anterior floor of mouth and symphysis of mandible. The mental arch was reconstructed with an osteomyocutaneous iliac crest flap. The myocutaneous portion replaced the anterior floor of mouth and alveolar mucosa. **B.** The orthopantograph shows the position of the revascularized iliac crest fixed to the mandibular stumps by two miniaturized A0 metal plates. **C.** The grafts survived completely and the plates were removed at 6 months. At this time a vestibuloplasty was performed and 5 Tübingen-type aluminium ceramic implants were inserted. **D.** A prosthetic suprastructure attached to the dental implants allows a removable bridge prosthesis. Restoration and complete masticatory rehabilitation was achieved 15 months following surgery.

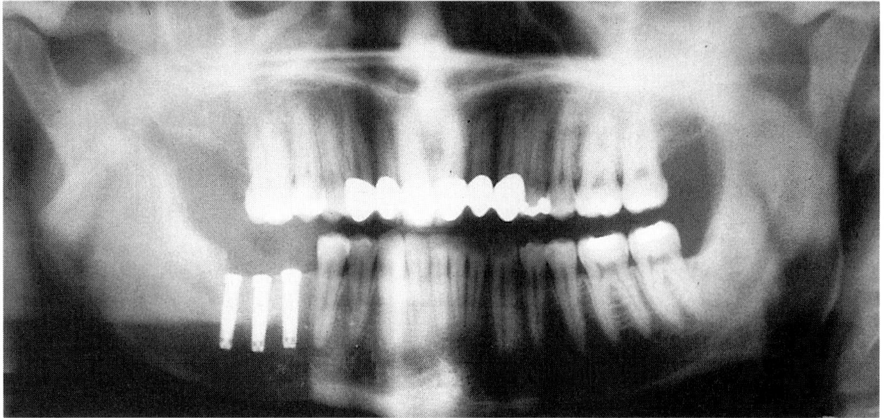

Fig. 22.2 Orthopantogram showing primary reconstruction of the right mandible from the condylar process to the premolar following excision of an ameloblastoma.

as a mandibular body replacement. The vascular pedicle at this site is normally anastomosed to the superior thyroid vessels (Fig. 22.3).

The majority of mandible reconstructions using vascularized bone grafts have used miniaturized plates for bone fixation. All of the prominent brands have been used (A0, LUHR - System, Wurzburg - System). Monocortical plates are preferred in dentulous jaws. Most of the patients were edentulous, or had very few teeth, and no intermaxillary fixation was required. Large-volume reconstruction plates (A0) were used only in subtotal mandible reconstruction with removal of the plates after 6 months.

Maxillary reconstruction

We have performed reconstruction of the maxilla using revascularized bone grafts in six patients. Five cases followed resection of a malignant tumour and the remaining case followed resection of an extensive ameloblastoma. In three of the cases, the vascularized bone graft was used as a secondary reconstruction following previous soft-tissue reconstruction using a latissimus dorsi free flap.

The bone reconstruction was always aimed at subsequent insertion of endosseous implants to facilitate masticatorial rehabilitation (Fig. 22.4).

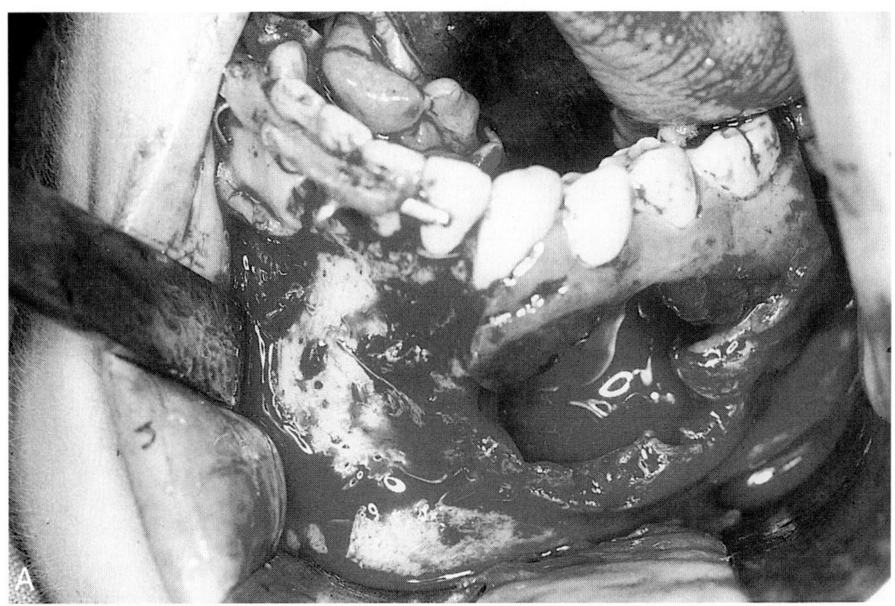

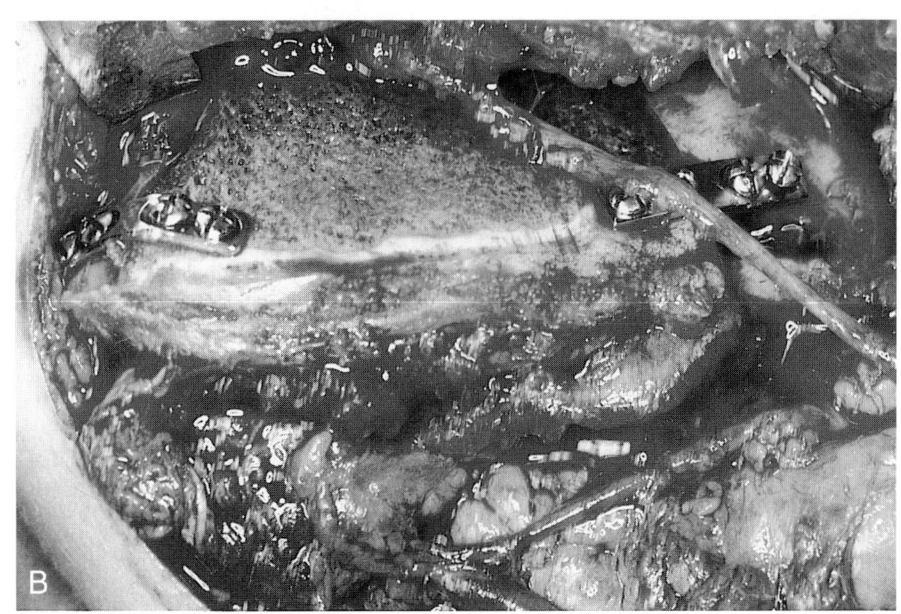

Fig. 22.3

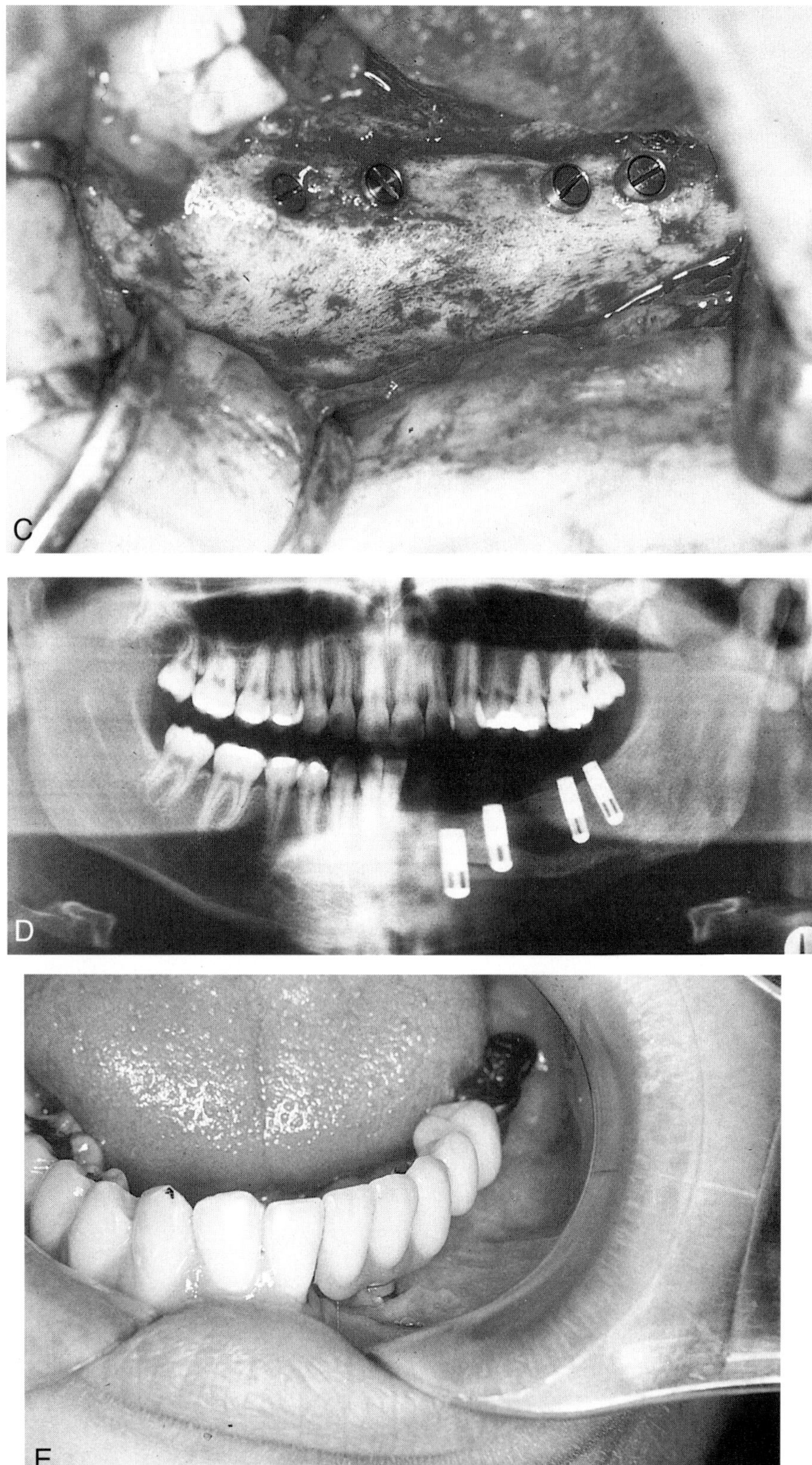

Fig. 22.3 **A.** An ameloblastoma showing destruction of the left horizontal ramus of the mandible in an 18-year-old male. **B.** A DCIA iliac crest vascularized bone graft as used for primary reconstruction with a sural nerve graft to restore the inferior alveolar nerve. Bone fixation utilized A0 mini-plates with the vascular anastomosis performed in the submandibular area. **C.** The metal plates were removed at 6 months, and at 1 year postoperatively four IMZ titanium implants were inserted. **D.** Orthopantogram showing position of the implants and the shape of the reconstructed mandible. **E.** Eighteen months following his primary surgery, the patient was restored to normal masticatory function using a partially removable bridge on the four IMZ titanium implants. Lower lip sensitivity had been regained.

OTHER SITES

The principle of osseo-integrated implants and consecutive loading by a prosthetic suprastructure is not limited to oral rehabilitation but can be used in other craniomaxillofacial areas.

EAR RECONSTRUCTION

In total reconstruction of the external ear autologous grafting does not often give optimal aesthetic results and often an external prosthesis is better. The modern resins allow sufficient shaping and colouring of the prosthesis and an excellent match with the opposite side. The main disadvantage used to be fixation of the prosthesis, but now, using miniaturized titanium screw implants (Branemark) inserted into the mastoid process, fixation can be assured. The method is identical to that used in intra-oral endosseous implants but the ones used for external facial prostheses tend to be smaller.

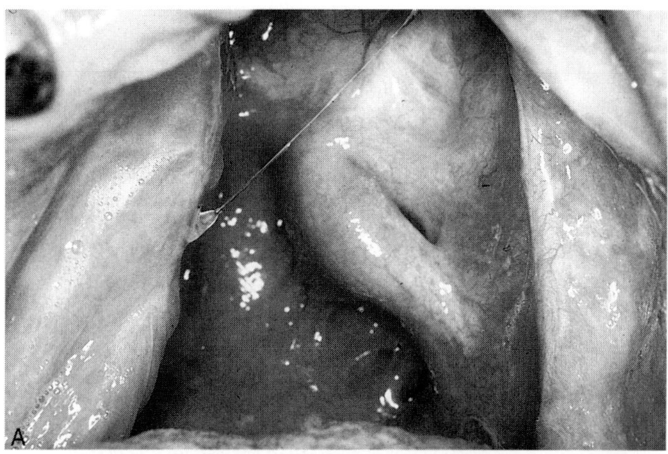

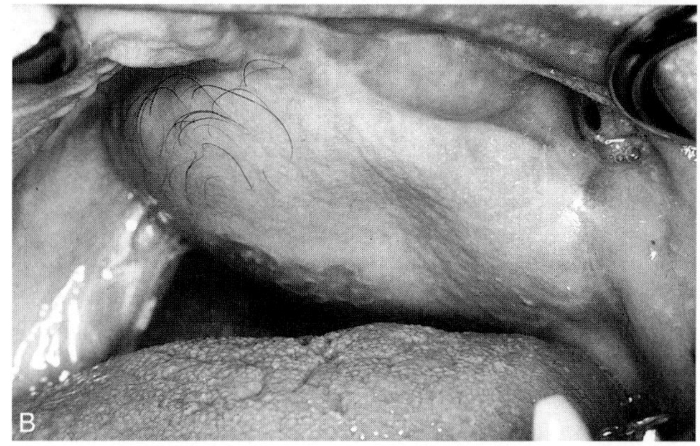

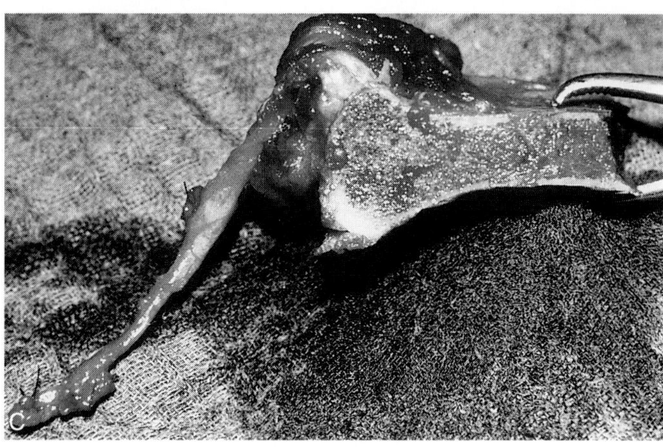

Fig. 22.4

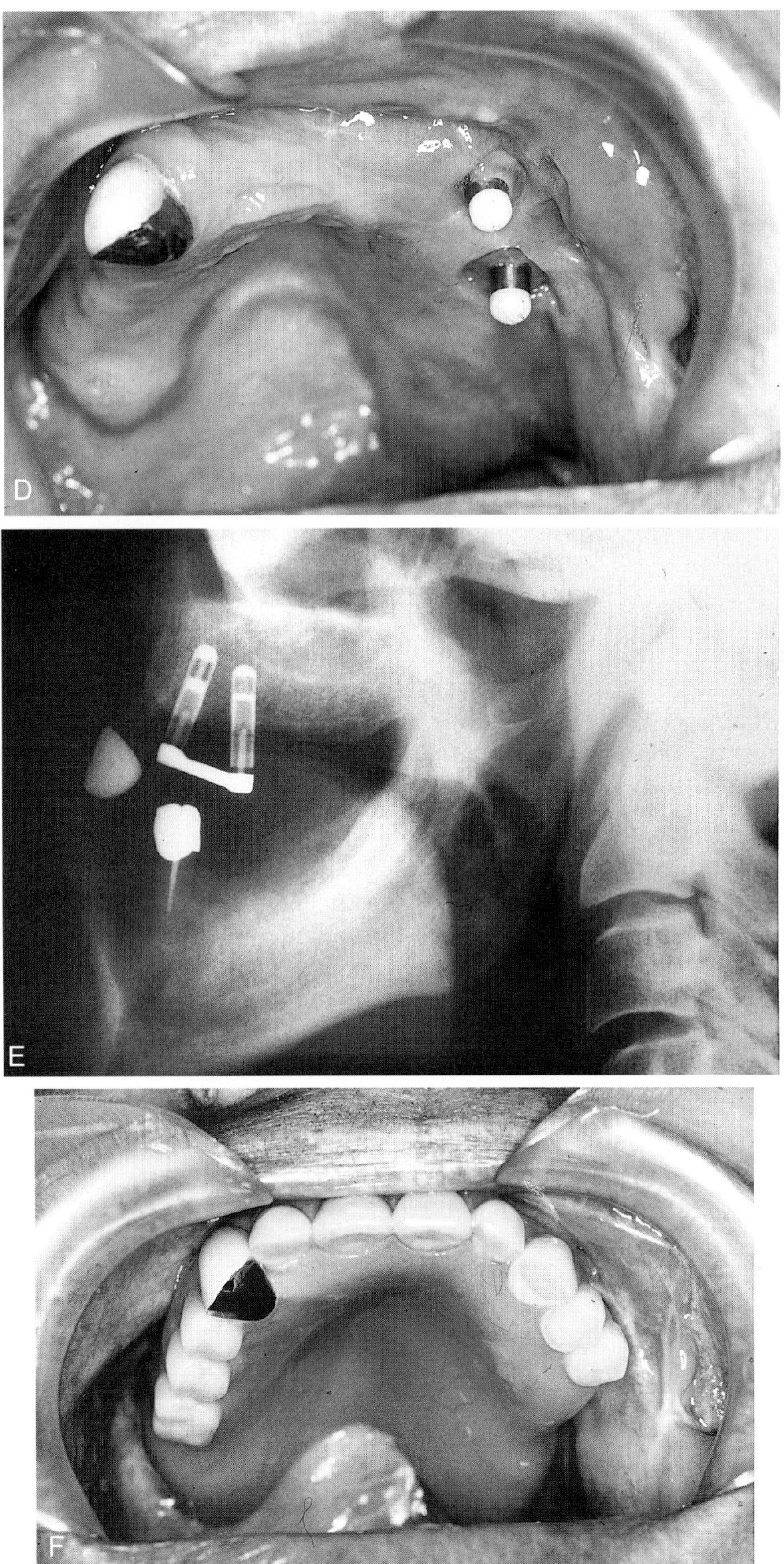

Fig. 22.4

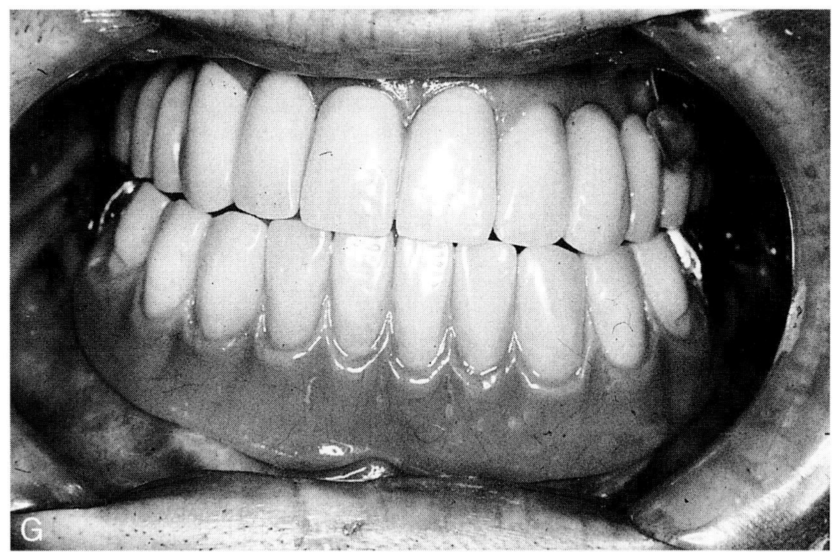

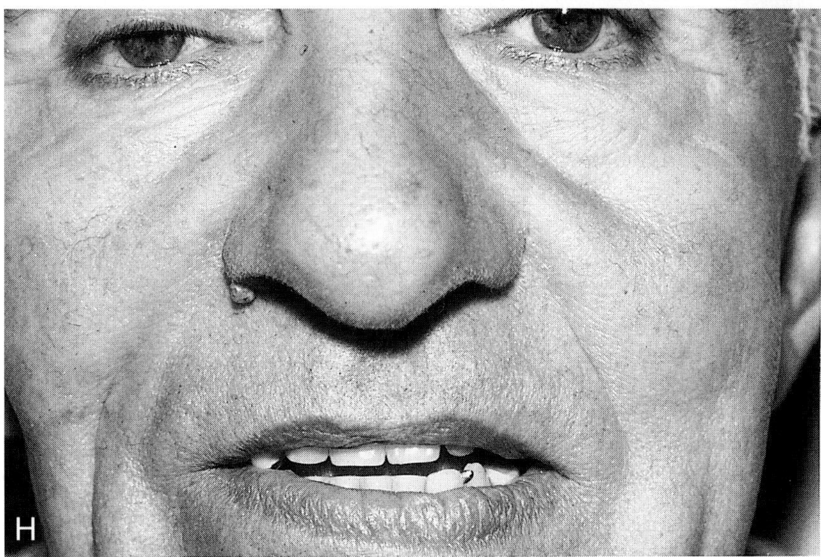

Fig. 22.4 A. A maxillary defect, after resection of an ameloblastoma in a 68-year-old male. **B.** A free latissimus dorsi flap was used to close the soft-tissue defect. **C.** A deep circumflex iliac artery iliac crest bone graft was inserted into the soft-tissue envelope of the latissimus dorsi. Vascular anastomosis was performed to the temporal vessels. **D.** Intra-oral appearance following vestibuloplasty using oral mucosa and the implantation of two IMZ titanium implants. **E.** The lateral radiogram demonstrates the position of the endosseous implants and the extent of the bone graft replacing the left maxilla. A bar suprastructure for subsequent prosthetic dental rehabilitation is in place. **F.** The denture is in place attached to the implant via a bar suprastructure. **G.** A satisfactory occlusion has been achieved. **H.** The extra-oral appearance following prosthetic dental rehabilitation.

Orbital reconstruction

The principle of anchoring an implant and using a supra-structure to fix a prosthesis is also useful in the orbital and nasal areas. For nasal prostheses a triangular position of implants is required bilaterally at the nasal aperture and glabella. For orbital reconstruction there is thick bone available at the frontozygomatic buttress and zygomatic body.

ENDOSSEOUS IMPLANTS

Aluminium oxide ceramic implant—Tübingen type (Frialit®)

This endosseous implant differs significantly in its design from other types. It was designed as a one-stage implant and constructed with a neck-type zone allowing a close attach-ment of the marginal gingiva to protect against risks from a constant break in the ectodermal integrity of the oral mucosa. These risks are mostly of an infectious nature caused by intra-oral debris in the peri-implantal space. The surface size and implant structure were designed as stepped cylinders to achieve a favourable transduction of force into the bone. All edges and bases were rounded to prevent excess force on the bone.

The stepped cylinder brought forward a gradual transmission of force into all different levels of the artificial alveolus as well as the vertical plane. These special advantages were demonstrated by tensionoptic tests. Electromicroscopic examination showed that the cancellous bone adaption to implant surfaces was especially dense in areas of pure pressure. An immediate adaptation of bone to the implant was observed with osteocytes directly on the ceramic surface. To enable an undisturbed integration, a healing phase of 3 months covered by mucosa without any load on the implant is necessary (Schulte & Heimke 1976).

Titanium implants (IMZ®, Branemark®)

The Branemark implant is a screw-shaped pure titanium implant of 3.7 mm with a length of 7–18 mm. Implant and prosthetic supraconstruction are connected by screws that allow later adjustment. The healing period is 3–6 months.

The titanium oxide layer on the implant surface provides one of the most corrosive-resistant metallic surfaces, and this is especially important in the oral cavity. To gain the intended osseo-integration, any premature load must be avoided as this would lead to pseudo-integration with connective tissue interposition and ultimate failure of the implant.

Osseo-integration requires a direct functional and structural connection between living bone tissue and the surface of a loaded implant. It is important to minimize trauma to the tissues, remove minimum bone and preserve the jaw-bone typography. The mechanism of force transmission is also of vital importance. The transmission is possible only because direct contact is established down to the molecular level preventing any relative movement between implant and load-bearing bone.

The screw allows an intimate contact with the bone and a safe direction of force in all directions. A strong prosthetic supraconstruction divides the forces equally onto all implants, and selection of a resin with damping qualities in the supraconstructions crown work reduces the ultimate load on the implants. The Branemark system features a remarkable set of instruments stressing accurate bone preparation in an atraumatic manner.

IMZ implants are also made of titanium and have a plasma flame coating and a cylindrical shape.

Prosthetic supraconstructions

The suprastructure connected to the endosseous implants finalizes the reconstruction. In dental prostheses, occlusion is restored to enable the patient to chew, articulate, regain his defined intra-alveolar distance and facial height and stabilize the stomatognathic system. There are numerous differences between prosthetic dental work on natural teeth and those formed partly or totally on osseo-integrated implants. Peri-implantal tissue conditions, oral hygiene requirements, distribution of load on the implants during occlusion and articulation are decisive factors contributing to their success. Basically, the suprastructure will be a conventional denture secured by implants or, more favourably, a fixed non-removable construction that is carried solely by the osseo-integrated implants. Experienced dental prosthetists must be part of the planning and treating of patients with implants to enable a functional dental restoration that respects the special mechanical and physiological conditions of endosseous implants.

COMPLICATIONS

Restoring masticatory function in a patient who has undergone resection of his jaw with a defect in bone continuity is a complicated and multi-faced process. There are, of course, numerous general and specific risks involved for the patient. It is particularly important, as in all microvascular free tissue transfers, to safeguard the anastomosis as the only supply of blood to the bone graft. It is important to realize that there is a danger of brisk haemorrhage from the cancellous bone graft and the attached musculature and that this might lead to haematoma formation and compression of venous drainage. Close clinical monitoring of the patient is mandatory for the first week since compromise of the vascular anastomosis will result in a conventional free graft which will subsequently demonstrate typical atrophy.

An airway controlled by endotracheal intubation or tracheostomy is important postoperatively. The DCIA osteomyocutaneous flap may suffer partial skin loss but this often concerns only the superficial layers. It is extremely important to avoid any pressure on the mucosa overlying the bone graft and this can be readily achieved by using splints. If an intra-oral dehiscence occurs, the revascularized bone graft is usually well protected against infection, and granulation occurs rapidly with secondary wound healing.

The donor site has a potential for herniation of abdominal contents. Meticulous wound closure is essential together with postoperative bed rest and a compression belt for a few weeks.

Endosseous implantation does not in itself pose any

grave risk to the patient. Inaccurate positioning, however, especially without prosthetic planning, will render the implant useless. Even within the oral cavity the success rate of these implants is well over 90%.

REFERENCES

Axhausen W 1951 Die Quellen der Knochenneubildung nach freier Trasplantation. Langenbecks Archiv Klinische Chirurgie 270: 439

Axhausen W 1952 Die Knochenregeneration—ein zweiphasiges Geschehen. Zentralblatt Chirurgie 77: 435–442

Barth A 1984 Uber Osteoplatik in histologischer Beziehung. Langenbecks Archiv Klinische Chirurgie 48: 466–477

Branemark P I 1975 Reconstruction of the defective mandible. Scandinavian Journal of Plastic and Reconstructive Surgery 9: 116–128

Holtje W J, Lentrodt J 1972 Experimentelle Grundlagen zur Verhutung von postoperativen Infektionen nach autologen Knochentransplantationen in der Kieferchirurgie. In: Kirsch T (ed) Chemotherapie in der Zahn-Mund und Kieferheilkunde. 2 Norddeutsche Therapiegesprache. Bad Pyrmont, Thieme, Stuttgart

Klapp R 1916 Uber die chirurgische Behandlung der Kieferschussbruche. Zeitschrift Arztliche Fortbildung 13: 225–232

Lentrodt T J, Fritzemeier C U, Bethmann J 1987 Erfahrungen bei der osteoplastischen Unter Kieferrekonstruktion mit autologen freien Knochentransplantaten. In: Kasterbauer E, Wilmes K, Mees K (eds) Das Transplantat in der plastischen Chirurgie. Sasse, Rottenburg, pp 59–61

Lindemann A 1916 Uber die Beseitigung der traumatischen Defekte der Gesichtsknochen. In: Bruhn C Die gegenwartigen Behandlungswege der Kieferschussverletzungen. HIV–VI Wiesbaden, pp 243–328

Lindstrom I, Branemark P I, Albrektsson T 1981 Mandibular Reconstruction using the preformed autologous bone graft. Scandinavian Journal of Plastic and Reconstructive Surgery 15: 29–38

Riediger D, d'Hoedt B, Pielsticker W 1986 Implantation nach mikrochirurgischer Beckenkammtransplantation. Deutsche Zeitschrift Zahnarztliche Implantologie 2: 9–10

Schulte W, Heimke G 1976 Das Tubinger Sofortimplantat. Quintessenz Zahnarztlicher Literatur 27: 5456

Schulte W, d'Hoedt B, Lukas D, Muhlbradt L, Scholz F, Brettschi I, Frey D et al 1983 Periotest—ein neues Messverfahren der Funktion des Parodontiums. Zahnarztliche Mitteilungen 73: 1229

Taylor G I 1982 Reconstruction of the mandible with free composite iliac bone grafts. Annals of Plastic Surgery 9: 361

Taylor G I, Watson N 1978 One stage repair of compound leg defects with free vascularised flaps of groin skin and iliac bone. Plastic and Reconstructive Surgery 61: 494

Taylor G I, Townsend P, Corlett R 1979 Superiority of the deep circumflex iliac vessels as the supply for free groin flaps. Plastic and Reconstructive Surgery 64: 595

23. Management of parotid malignancy

Paul. J. Donald

INTRODUCTION

Malignancies of the parotid salivary gland are challenging lesions. The gland is separated into a superficial and deep lobe by the facial nerve and abuts a host of vital anatomical structures. To spare this important nerve, the gland must be removed piecemeal: a violation of the standard oncological philosophy of en bloc resection. A variety of tumours arise in the gland, usually from the ductal epithelium, but occasionally from the glandular parenchyma and even, rarely, from the glandular stroma. Their protean behaviour will invoke a variety of surgical solutions covering a spectrum of aggressiveness. Adapting a radical posture towards the more malignant varieties will ensure the greatest chance of success.

SURGICAL ANATOMY

The first anlage of the salivary glands appear as epithelial invaginations growing into the mesoderm of the peristomadeal tissues at 6.5 weeks of gestation. These buds intrude themselves into the loose undifferentiated mesodermal tissue and then branch. These arborizations are destined to be the ductal system of the fully developed embryo. Mesodermal elements coalesce around the primitive ductal system to form the acini.

The parotid gland is a J-shaped organ with a tail that extends over the mastoid tip of the temporal bone and a superior extension that arises over the zygomatic processes of the temporal bone. The main body of the gland overlies the masseter muscle and extends inferiorly to the angle of the mandible. Its anterior limit is variable, but usually covers about 75% of the masseter muscle. Stensen's duct exits the hilum of the parotid at this extremity of the gland and runs a course roughly on a line joining the auricular tragus and the mid-point between the ala of the nose and the angle of the mouth. The duct sweeps around the anterior border of the masseter, pierces the buccopharyngeal fascia and the buccinator muscle, then enters the oral cavity through the buccal mucosa at the level of the second maxillary molar tooth.

The so-called deep lobe of the parotid gland hooks around the posterior border of the mandible to lie deep to the mandibular ramus and, in part, up against the medial surface of the medial pterygoid muscle. This lobe lies up against the stylohoid membrane and styloid musculature in the parapharyngeal space and is thus closely related to the contents of the carotid sheath. It lies directly behind the faucial tonsil.

The facial nerve exits the stylomastoid foramen to enter the deep surface of the superficial lobe of the parotid gland. It loops forward posterolaterally to the styloid process. In the parotidectomy operation, the dissection of the facial nerve is the key manoeuvre. Its position relative to the skull base and course through the gland merits close study because, even in many malignant parotid tumours, the nerve trunk and most or all of its branches can be spared. The nerve ascends from the skull base into the gland. Within millimetres, it splits into usually an upper and lower main division. There may be three branches. After the initial bifurcation, the nerve splits into its peripheral branches supplying the muscles of facial expression. This branching pattern is highly variable. The branches of VII are related to key surface anatomical landmarks. The frontal branch traverses the upper one-third of the face to supply the frontalis portion of the occipital frontalis muscle. This branch begins approximately 1.5 cm anterior to the auricular tragus and ascends in a curvilinear fashion to a point 2 cm superior and parallel to the lateral one-third of the eyebrow. This finding, originally described by Pitanguy & Ramos (1966) was further elaborated by Bernstein & Nelson (1984) in their dissections where they discovered a highly variable branching pattern of this nerve. In some instances, the nerve was looped around the superficial temporal artery.

The zygomatic branch is by far the most vital branch of the facial nerve. It supplies the orbicularis oculi and, as such, is responsible for lid closure and corneal protection. Loss of zygomatic branch function is a severe functional as well as cosmetic defect. The nerve leaves the upper main division, crosses the anterior one-third of the zygoma and enters the orbicularis oculi. It may begin as a single branch and ramify to two, or emerge from the upper main division as two separate branches.

The buccal branch has a variable origin either from the upper or lower main divisions, or both. The buccal branch travels along an imaginary line that roughly connects the tragus of the ear to a point midway between the ala of the nose and the lateral angle of the mouth. It runs a course that is within 1 cm of Stensen's duct and parallel to it. The elevators of the angle of the mouth and orbicularis oris are innervated by the buccal branch.

The ramus mandibularis is the most commonly injured branch of the facial nerve. It exits the lower main division and descends in an anteroinferior direction over the lateral surface of the inferior one-fifth of the masseter muscle. It crosses superficially to the posterior facial vein, and can run into the upper neck below the inferior border of the posterior aspect of the mandibular ramus as far as 2 cm. Dingman & Grabb (1962) found that the course of the nerve is highly variable and can remain exclusively in the face or dip down into the neck. When the latter situation exists, this branch crosses the ramus to re-enter the face at a point where the facial artery crosses the anterior border of the masseter muscle. They concluded from their dissections that the ramus could not be damaged by a high cervical incision made anterior to the facial artery. This branch supplies the depressors of the mouth.

PATHOLOGY

Most of the tumours arising from the parotid gland (Table 23.1) take origin in cells of the ductal system, especially cells of the intercalated ducts. Tumours also arise from the acinar cells. The connective tissue, neural, vascular and lymphoid elements produce tumours, as do inclusions. There are lymph nodes with the gland that serve as metastatic sites in cases of malignancy of the upper facial skin and ear canal.

The commonest tumours are benign, making up approximately 80% of all parotid masses. The commonest among these is the benign mixed tumour or, more accurately, the pleomorphic adenoma. These tumours have a mixed composition of stellate cells, a loose mesenchymal matrix, chondroid sometimes with chondrocytes, mucous glands, epithelioid cells, myoepithelial cells and lymphocytes. The tumours present with variable size, but rarely if ever with a facial palsy. The tumour may comprise a single morphological cell type, which, in this instance, is called a monomorphic adenoma. The biology and pathogenesis of this type of tumour differs little from the pleomorphic variety. These tumours possess numerous bosselations upon their cell surface, a finding made by Eneroth (1965) after doing serial histological sections of a number of these tumours. He dispelled a notion previously held that these tumours possessed satellite lesions which explained their frequent recurrence (often >30%) following 'lumpectomy'.

The next commonest tumour is the papillary cystademoa

Table 23.1 Histological classification of salivary gland tumours

1. Adenomas
   Pleomorphic adenoma
   Myo-epithelioma (myo-epithelial adenoma)
   Basal-cell adenoma
   Warthin tumour (adenolymphoma)
   Oncocytoma (oncocytic adenoma)
   Canalicular adenoma
   Sebaceous adenoma
   Ductal papilloma
   Inverted ductal papilloma
   Intraductal papilloma
   Sialadenoma papilliferum
   Cystadenoma
   Papillary cystadenoma
   Mucinous cystadenoma

2. Carcinomas
   Acinic-cell carcinoma
   Muco-epidermoid carcinoma
   Adenoid cystic carcinoma
   Polymorphous low-grade adenocarcinoma (terminal duct adeno-carcinoma)
   Epithelial–myo-epithelial carcinoma
   Basal-cell adenocarcinoma
   Sebaceous carcinoma
   Papillary cystadenocarcinoma
   Mucinous adenocarcinoma
   Onocyctic carcinoma
   Salivary-duct carcinoma
   Adenocarcinoma
   Malignant myo-epithelioma (myo-epithelial carcinoma)
   Carcinoma in pleomorphic adenoma (malignant mixed tumour)
   Squamous-cell carcinoma
   Small-cell carcinoma
   Undifferentiated carcinoma
   Other carcinomas

3. Non-epithelial tumours

4. Malignant lymphomas

5. Secondary tumours

6. Unclassified tumours

7. Tumour-like lesions
   Sialadenosis
   Oncocytosis
   Necrotizing sialometaplasia (salivary gland infarction)
   Benign lympho-epithelial lesion
   salivary gland cysts
   Chronic sclerosing sialadenitis of submandibular gland (Küttner tumour)
   Cystic lymphoid hyperplasia in AIDS

lymphomatosum: so-called Warthin's tumour or adenolymphoma. It is generally found in the tail of the parotid gland in elderly males. It is distinctly rare in females and is almost never seen in young patients. The origin of this tumour is thought to be the oncocyte, a cell of the intercalated interlobular ducts first described by Schaffer & Beitragelzur in 1897. This cell is a sign of ageing and is rarely seen in the ducal system in patients under the age of 50 years. Histologically, it has a pathognomonic appearance. It comprises cysts of varying sizes filled with an eosinophilic amorphous material. The lining epithelium comprises mainly two layers: the outer, a cubiodal cell, and the inner, a columnar cell that is commonly ciliated. Between each cyst are lymphocytic aggregates. There is a definite capsule around the tumour, making it one of the few tumours that can be actually shelled out of the gland. There is about a 5–10% incidence of bilaterally occurring tumours and a significant incidence of concomitant or eventual lymphoma.

Oncocytomas are uncommon and are solid tumours composed of a monotonous array of oncocytes that possess that same coarse granularity seen in the basal layer of the Warthin's tumour. These granules correspond to mitochondria, indicating a high degree of metabolic activity of these cells.

Adenomas of both serous and mucous glands are extremely rare. The so-called clear tumour is also rare; it is made up of solid aggregates of an inner layer of intensely eosinophilic cells of intercalated duct derivation surrounded by glycogen-rich clear cells of myo-epithelial origin. There have been some reports of malignant behaviour, so they are sometimes classified as clear-cell tumour rather than adenoma (Thackray & Lucas 1974). Sebaceous adenomas are unusual, benign, well encapsulated tumours that arise from the sebaceous cell proliferations often seen at the end of intralobular ducts. They comprise cysts of squamous epithelium and sebaceous cells, some of which may secrete keratin into the cysts' lumen. Often aggregates of lymphocytes are present—thus the common appellation 'sebaceous lymphadenoma' (Peel & Gnepp 1985).

Most malignant parotid tumours arise in the body of the gland. They are only occasionally seen in the tail and rarely in the deep lobe. The commonest malignant tumour is muco-epidermoid carcinoma, constituting 30% of the malignancies of the parotid. The tumour has a variable histology that closely matches the clinical behaviour. The most benign form of the disease is characterized by nests of benign-appearing squamous cells that are well differentiated, showing little or no mitotic activity, and a regular and relatively uniform morphology. Cysts of mucoid-containing material are surrounded by cells containing pale reticulated cytoplasm interspersed with squamous cells. There are no intermediary cells. These tumours have limited local invasiveness and rarely, if ever, metastasize. Some individuals even consider them benign, but most consider all muco-epidermoid tumours to be malignant. The more intermediate grade of muco-epidermoid tumour has squamous cells showing pleomorphism and mitotic figures with nuclei that tend to be hyperchromatic. There are irregular mucus-containing cells and fewer cysts. There are some aggregates of intermediary cells. These cells are smaller than the mucous or squamous cells with intensely staining nuclei and very scant cytoplasm. They closely resemble a large lymphocyte, and there appears to be a relationship between malignant activity and their numbers.

The behaviour of this tumour resembles that of a well-differentiated squamous-cell carcinoma. The most malignant variety has poorly differentiated squamous cells with numerous mitotic figures and considerable pleomorphism.

There is a dense infiltration of intermediary cells and scant mucous elements. The clinical behaviour of this tumour is that of a high-grade malignancy, and invasion of local tissues may be extensive. Regional metastasis is common.

Adenoid cystic carcinoma is next commonest, comprising up to 20% of the malignancies of the parotid. It is a tumour with an unpredictable behaviour and protean manifestations. There are basically three histological types: cribrose, tubular and solid. Perzin et al in 1978 did a study attempting to correlate histological appearance and biological behaviour. They found that the cribrose pattern had the most benign behaviour and the best prognosis, and the solid pattern the worst. The tubular had an intermediate activity. The cribrose is characterized by small epithelial-like cells arranged in cysts. The histology looks something like Swiss cheese. The tubular has cords and strands of cells that, in cross-section, have a tubular configuration. The solid pattern, although possessing microscopic spaces, has solid sheets and nests of cells. Lymphocytic infiltration is common to all forms. Often the forms are mixed, with biological behaviour corresponding to the predominant pattern. Any significant amount of a solid pattern usually denotes a poor prognosis.

Adenoid cystic carcinoma has a highly invasive quality although, conversely, it may remain quiescent for a long period of time. Such tumours may be present for 10 to 15 years and demonstrate little evidence of growth, then suddenly and extensively infiltrate adjacent tissues. An affinity for travel along perineural planes, although not unique to this tumour, is characteristic of it. An unusual feature of this property is the finding of skip areas: regions along an affected nerve that appear tumour-free, but which, many millimetres—and even a centimetre—further, show evidence of tumour. The wide skip areas seem to disappear once the neural invasion becomes intracranial. The reason for this finding is unclear.

Tumour metastasis to regional lymphatics is uncommon, but late blood-borne metastases to various organs outside the head and neck is agonizingly common. The lung is particularly vulnerable to this process. Patients often do not develop distant metastases until diagnosis.

Only about 20% of squamous-cell cancers of the parotid metastasize to the neck. However, facial skin secondaries to the gland should have a radical neck dissection because the lesion is the first nodal station of a possible cascade of cervical lymphatic metastasis. Some of these cutaneous metastatic lesions are tumours with neurotropic potential. Coman (1990) from Brisbane, Australia, has noted this, and it is not an uncommon finding in my experience.

Adenocarcinoma arises primarily from the secretory element of the parotid gland. It is an aggressive lesion with both lymphatic and blood-borne metastatic potential. The histological appearance resembles a bowel carcinoma with glandular structures possessing much pleomorphism, frequent mitoses and lymphocytic infiltration.

Acinic cell carcinoma is an intermediate-grade malignancy with infrequent lymphatic metastasis, but occasional late distant metastasis. This tumour, like adenoid cystic carcinoma, is unpredictable but not with the same frequency or virulence. They are usually solid and rarely cystic. Histologically, the cells are the malignant counterpart of the glandular acinar cell. They rarely metastasize, but may have perineural spread.

Sebaceous carcinoma is a rare tumour that takes origin from the intralobular duct epithelium. It presents as a painful mass and commonly invades the skin.

Lymphoma of the parotid is not uncommon in elderly males. It is seen in 5–10% of patients with Warthin's tumour.

Malignant mixed tumours may arise de novo or as a focus of carcinomatous degeneration within a pre-existing benign pleomorphic adenoma. The metastatic lesions resemble the malignant counterpart and none of the benign component. Eneroth & Zetterberg (1968) resolved the dilemma concerning the nature of the origin of malignancy within a pleomorphic adenoma. Their studies with cellular DNA showed that these malignancies began within benign pleomorphic adenoma and did not exist without the initial emergence of this benign lesion. They also demonstrated that the longer a pleomorphic adenoma is present, the greater the chance of malignant degeneration.

True malignant mixed tumours can be detected by virtue of the malignant appearance of their epithelial or stromal elements, or finding of normal pleomorphic adenoma cells in metastatic sites such as bone or lung. This latter presentation is exceedingly rare.

DIAGNOSIS (TABLE 23.2)

The usual presentation of a patient with a parotid neoplasm is a lump in the neck or a mass in the posterior cheek. Most often the mass is painless, even in malignancies. Pain in the gland is a warning sign of possible malignancy. The duration of the mass and rapidity of growth is important. Slow-growing masses of long standing tend to be benign. The history of excision of cutaneous malignancy such as squamous carcinoma, malignant fibrous histiocytoma, or melanoma, coupled with the finding of a parotid mass, suggests the possibility of intraglandular metastasis. The history of prior excision of a parotid tumour is important—often the patient will know the diagnosis of the prior lesion. This should obviously be confirmed by microscopic examination of the previous specimen when obtainable. Too often in these cases an inadequate resection has been done, leaving behind microscopic and even gross tumour, often in the name of facial nerve presentation. The concept of risking tumour recurrence and possible death for the sake of the reasonably satisfactory reconstructible and rehabilitable problems left as the residual of facial nerve sacrifice defies logic.

Facial nerve paralysis is an ominous sign, not only just

Table 23.2   Investigation and diagnosis of parotid tumours

Clinical	History
	Examination
Radiological	Sialography
	Contrast sialography + CAT scan
	CT scan
	gadolinium contrast
	MRI scan
Pathological	FNA
	Frozen section
	Fixed section

denoting probably malignancy but also portending a grave prognosis. Facial nerve paralysis is almost never seen in benign disease processes of the parotid. In Conley's (1975) series of 35 patients presenting with VII nerve paresis and salivary gland cancer, 67% were dead of tumour at 5 years.

Skin involvement and fixation is a sign of malignancy. Certainly, any lesion breaking the skin surface is cancerous. Deep fixation is common because the gland is tethered to the underlying structures by its fascial envelope. Benign tumours are generally firm, but not rock hard. Cystic degeneration is not helpful because it may be the result of necrosis of the avascular centre of a malignant lesion. Pus or blood from Stensen's duct is a sign of malignancy, but is an extremely uncommon finding.

The presence of an adjacent rock hard, painless lymph node makes one highly suspicious of malignancy. Nodal metastasis is uncommon in parotid cancer, but does occur.

Advanced malignancies may present with invasion of the temporomandibular joint, a mass in the external auditory canal, or involvement of the mandibular branch of the trigeminal nerve. The latter is especially true in cancers of the deep lobe of the gland. Trismus is a sign of advanced disease into the masticatory muscles.

Deep lobe tumours may present with dysphagia or the sensation of a foreign body in the oropharynx. Examination may reveal bulging of the lateral pharyngeal wall or the soft palate. The commonest tumours are pleomorphic adenomas. Dumb-bell tumours originating in either lobe with extension into its fellow must be borne in mind. Palpation with one finger against the lateral pharynx and the other in the deep neck often confirms the tumour origin and its extent.

Traditionally, the definitive diagnosis of parotid salivary gland tumours has been made by superficial parotidectomy. Incisional biopsy is to be decried for two reasons. Spillage of carcinoma or pleomorphic adenoma into the tissues sets the stage for rapid local recurrence and, secondly, the facial nerve is at risk when not properly identified. Early attempts at diagnosis by sialography helped to differentiate benign from malignant tumours on the basis of the findings of ductal erosion, cavitary sialectasis, or the extravasation characteristic of malignancy. Sialograms were helpful only when these features were demonstrated. Numerous false negatives were unfortunately seen. Tc^{99m} scanning was initially thought to be positive only for Warthin's tumour. Although this finding was characteristic of this lesion, too many false-positives were seen.

With the advent of the CAT scan, the parotid could be displayed using soft-tissue windows. Rice et al (1980) popularized the use of contrast sialography and CAT scanning. This helped to localize lesions and especially to characterize those of the deep lobe in contrast to other parapharyngeal space neoplasms. This technique was helpful due to the poor resolution of the early scanners. With the advent of modern CT and MRI, especially with the enhancement lent by gadolinium contrast, contrast sialography has become, along with plane film sialography, mostly a thing of the past.

Lajicek & Eneroth in 1970 introduced the notion of wide-bore needle biopsy for the diagnosis of salivary gland tumours. Although this was the state of the art in Sweden, this technique was largely decried by American surgeons. They were concerned, not only with the accuracy of diagnosis, but also with the problem of seeding of tumour along the needle track. In the 1950s, fine-needle aspiration cytology (FNA) was being used extensively in Europe, and only lately was accepted as a routine procedure in the USA (Abele & Miller 1985). The technique employs a fine-gauge (usually #22) needle which is passed into the tumour a number of times and then removed, the contents being deposited on a glass slide and then smeared like a haemotology slide when done for morphology. The slide is dried, fixed and stained, and cellular morphology is elucidated. For many head and neck neoplasms, such as those of the thyroid gland, or suspected metastasis to the lymph nodes, this has become standard practice in many parts of the world. However, it presumes an individual who can accurately and adequately sample the lesion and a skilled cytopathologist who can read the slide. A negative biopsy is of little value, but a positive one is of great worth. The use of this modality in salivary gland tumours is still highly controversial among surgeons and only the test of time will establish its definitive use. At UCDMC, this procedure has been extremely valuable and is used in every case. There is an extremely high correlation between FNA and final diagnosis. The utility of having the luxury of being able to define more clearly the therapeutic options to the patient, thereby adequately obtaining informed consent from the patients, is of great value. It is still important to avoid proceeding with a radical cancer operation until a definitive frozen-section diagnosis is made at the time of surgery, but it still helps a great deal in the pre-operative planning.

The frozen-section diagnosis at the time of surgery often presents a dilemma if the pathologist equivocates even slightly; a superficial lobe parotidectomy should be done and a more definitive procedure should be delayed until a final fixed-section diagnosis has been established. If the pathologist is solidly behind his frozen-section diagnosis, then the definitive procedure can be done. The surgeon must combine the information he has accrued from history and physical examination, the radiological and FNA results, and finally the sum of his own acumen and experience in making his decision whether or not to proceed on the basis of the frozen-section diagnosis. The advice of Dr John Conley is, I believe, very sound: look the pathologist in the eye and ask him to imagine that his mother or close relative is on the operating table and that, if the diagnosis is cancer, then the gland, possibly the mandible, the facial nerve and part of the temporal bone will be resected; if the pathologist remains resolute in his diagnosis then the surgeon should proceed with the definitive procedure. If, however, wavering and equivocation by the pathologist follows this admonition, then curtailment of the major procedure and delay until the definitive diagnosis can be established is the wisest course.

EXCISION

Parotidectomy for benign tumours is a well standardized procedure. The author's minor variations on this procedure and high points are presented. The approach to malignant tumours is radical, mainly because of the poor surgical results of more conservative resections. In squamous-cell carcinoma, the more malignant muco-epidermoid tumours, and adenocarcinoma postoperative irradiation with 6500 to 7000 centiGy to the primary and 4000 to 5000 centiGy to the neck is routinely given.

Recurrent pleomorphic adenomas are treated in a special way. Once conservatively resected and recurrent, these lesions appear to take on an aggressive and pernicious quality (Fig. 23.1). The patient in Figure 1A had had 17 prior resections over a 19-year period. I did the 18th and 19th procedures, the last one 3 weeks after the first because of positive margins. She is now 18 years without further recurrence. The patient in Figure 1B had had 15 operations in the preceding 20 years, and had had brain stem invasion at the time of her first visit to our clinic. She had intractable pain and was inoperable. Both patients had histology that was 'benign' recurrent pleomorphic adenoma. There is nothing benign about the course of this disease in the recurrent phase. It must be treated like a low-grade malignancy. There are reports of response of this tumour to radiation therapy. Unfortunately, I have seen too many refractory cases who did not respond to this modality to maintain any enthusiasm for its use in recurrent pleomorphic adenoma.

OPERATIVE TECHNIQUES

Superficial lobe parotidectomy

The standard procedure described by McCabe & Work in 1967 is hard to improve upon. A modified Blair incision is used (Fig. 23.2). It begins at a point at the superior

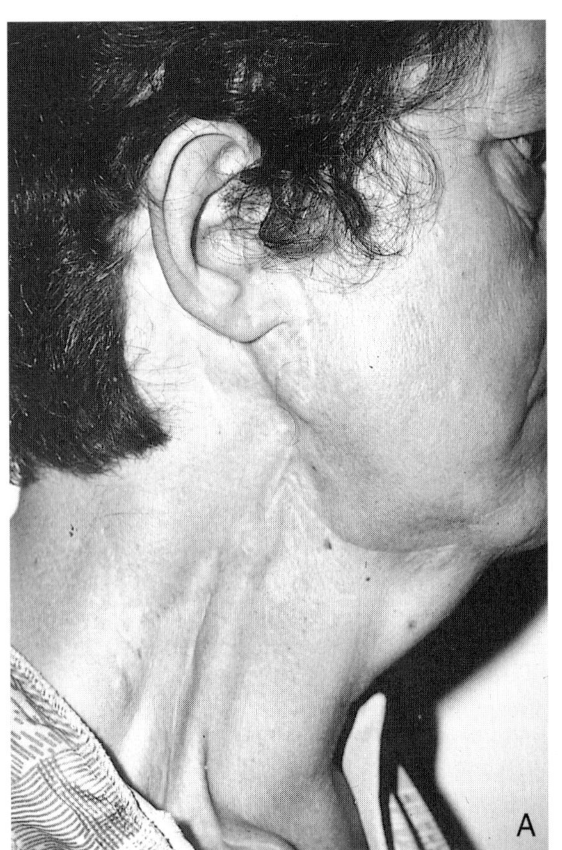
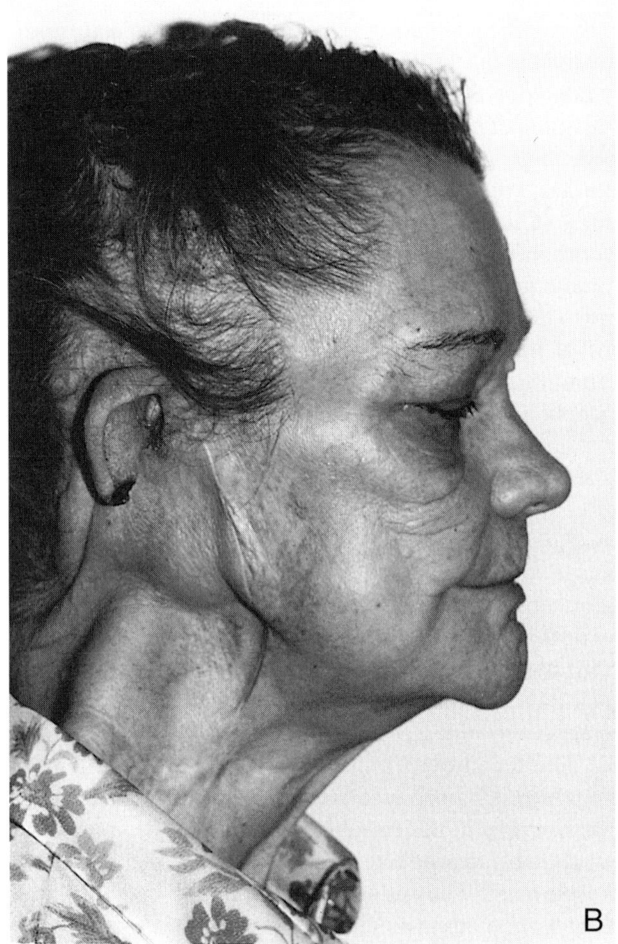

Fig. 23.1 **A.** Woman with 19 resections over a 19-year period for 'benign' pleomorphic adenoma. **B.** Woman who had 15 operations over a 20-year span for pleomorphic adenoma. Visible mass in temporal bone defect was attached to the brain stem. (From Donald P J 1984 Head and neck cancer: management of the difficult case. W B Saunders, Philadelphia, p 263.)

attachment of the auricle and traverses inferiorly in a pre-auricular crease, making a small incursion toward the pinna just above the tragus, then back out into the pre-auricular crease again. The incision loops under the ear lobe, arches over the mastoid tip and dips anteriorly into a cervical crease toward the greater cornua of the hyoid bone. The incision is carried through the subcutaneous fat and the superficial aponeurotic muscular system until the tan colour of the parotid lobules is seen. The skin is elevated anteriorly over the gland almost to the anterior limit of the masseter muscle. The small skin flap over the mastoid tip is elevated over the sternocleidomastoid muscle (SCM) to the level of the mandible. Care is taken to avoid, when possible, cutting the greater auricular nerve as it obliquely crosses the upper one-third of the muscle.

The parotid gland is then separated from the temporal bone. The first step is identification of the posterior limit of the tail of the gland over the mastoid tip and upper aspect of the SCM. The investing facia is incised and the tail elevated to the anterior border of the SCM. Although care is taken to avoid cutting the greater auricular nerve, in many cases the nerve is intimately associated with the gland and cannot be separated from it. It is important not to cut across the posterior facial vein at this stage as it causes the gland to become engorged with venous blood. Haemostasis should be performed with #4-0 catgut or the bipolar cautery. The regular cautery should be avoided. Once the glandular tail is freed, attention is turned to that portion of the gland over the cartilaginous and bony external auditory canal. Blunt dissection with a fine mosquito haemostat is done between the gland and the ear canal. Small perforating vessels are coagulated with the bipolar cautery or fine ligatures. The perichondrium is assiduously maintained intact as accidental incision and cartilaginous exposure predisposes the patient to perichondritis. At this point, a silk retention suture is placed through the cut surface of the ear lobule and anchored to the head drape.

Before the last manoeuvres are done to identify the facial

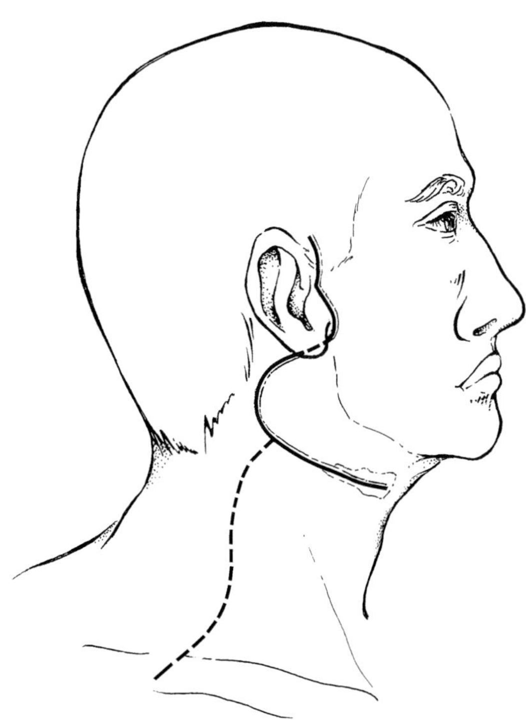

Fig. 23.2 Modified Blair incision for parotidectomy. (From Donald P J (1984) Head and neck cancer: management of the difficult case. W B Saunders, Philadelphia, p 263.)

nerve, the superior-most aspect of the gland is dissected off the zygomatic root. With this portion and the tail of the gland mobilized, the remaining separation of the gland from the bony external auditory canal is facilitated. The next step is to identify the facial nerve. The optimal circumstances for this manoeuvre include the use of a headlight, good haemostasis and suction. The assistant stands across the table from the surgeon and with a curved deep retractor, such as the Sewell, retracts the gland taking care to toe in its tip adequately. The tragal pointer is identified at the deep extent of the cartilaginous canal. The facial nerve is approximately 1 cm deep to this key landmark. Progressively deeper separation of gland from bone is done over as wide a field as possible. The facial nerve is seen as a thick white band coursing around the styloid process posteriorly after exiting the stylomastoid foramen. The nerve runs a short horizontal course and then ascends to enter the gland between the superficial and deep lobes of the gland. Careful dissection with a finely pointed haemostat or the McCabe facial nerve dissector separates the fine fibrous connective tissue that binds the parotid to the bony external auditory canal. The dissection is done in a plane paralleling the course of the nerve. A progressively deeper dissection is carried out over a relatively wide plane in order to avoid working in a deep narrow hole. Thick bands of connective tissue may be misconstrued as the facial nerve trunk. Close

inspection usually provides the differentiation, but further reassurance is provided by the use of the disposable facial nerve stimulator. With counter traction on the gland, the nerve can sometimes be palpated as a tight band. Occasionally either by virtue of tumour size and position, or by the fibrosis secondary to past surgery, the nerve may be difficult to find. One of the simplest methods of identification is by doing a complete mastoidectomy. The Fallopian canal is skeletonized and the facial nerve readily identified at the foramen as the digastric ridge expands in a fluted fashion at its anterior termination. Alternatively, the various branches can be traced from their site of distal identification, then followed proximally in a retrograde fashion. The simplest to identify is the ramus mandibularis that is picked up either as it crosses the posterior facial vein or in its close association with the posterior belly of the digastric muscle.

Once the main trunk of the facial nerve has been identified, it is dissected from the overlying parotid by taking advantage of the perineural space surrounding the nerve. With a gentle dissecting lifting motion, the tines of the forceps engage the perineural space on the lateral surface of the nerve. The tines are separated and the scissors or a #12 scalpel blade inserted along the tine of the forceps away from the tumour. A full-thickness cut of the parotid is done down to the forceps tip as long as the scissors tip remains in view. The sides of the cut are clamped by a haemostat placed parallel to the course of the nerve and rolled outwardly. This provides not only haemostasis, but improved exposure.

From the first branchings of the main trunk of the facial nerve, i.e. the pes anserinis, the main divisions and then the principal branches are dissected to the point of termination of the gland. Care is taken to direct the cuts away from the tumour so that it will not be violated and contaminate the wound with tumour spill.

If a branch is close to a benign tumour it should be dissectable from the tumour. Careful retraction with a nerve hook may be required in order to separate completely the nerve from the lesion. The only exception to this situation in benign tumours is in cases of recurrent pleomorphic adenoma where the nerve is commonly bound down by fibrous tissue and encased in tumour and inseparable from the neoplasm. In these instances, I agree with the advice of Work & Hecht (1980) that the best course is to resect nerve with tumour and then perform a cable graft to bridge the gap. An alternative is to leave tumour behind and irradiate. In my experience the latter approach has resulted in further recurrence and the increased difficulty of repeated resection, usually of a more radical type, with the usual morbidity attendant on radiation failure.

With the facial branches completely dissected to their exit from the gland, the intervening portions of gland and the tumour itself can be easily excised. If the deep lobe is uninvolved, and the tissue diagnosis is benign, only the superficial lobe need be removed. Small parotid remnants do not present a problem and will atrophy with time.

Closure is done with multiple small subcutaneous absorbable sutures with fine #5-0 or #6-0 nylon to the skin. Suction drainage is used and antibiotic ointment applied to the wound. If a significant depression is left, this can be partially effaced with a fat dermis graft. The dermis is tacked to the edges of the wound to stretch it into the defect, thus eliminating much of the depression left by the excision. This also helps to eliminate Frey's syndrome. Frey's syndrome, or gustatory sweating, is occasionally seen following parotidectomy. Unfortunately, few permanent solutions are available. The placement of a dermis fat graft under the skin may ameliorate the condition. Tympanic neurectomy of the tympanic plexus through a transaural approach gives only temporary relief in most instances. Excellent palliation is achieved by applying an antiperspirant over the affected skin and is usually the best solution.

Deep-lobe tumours

Excision of benign and low-grade malignant tumours of the deep lobe begins with a superficial lobe parotidectomy. Most of these tumours are pleomorphic adenomas and

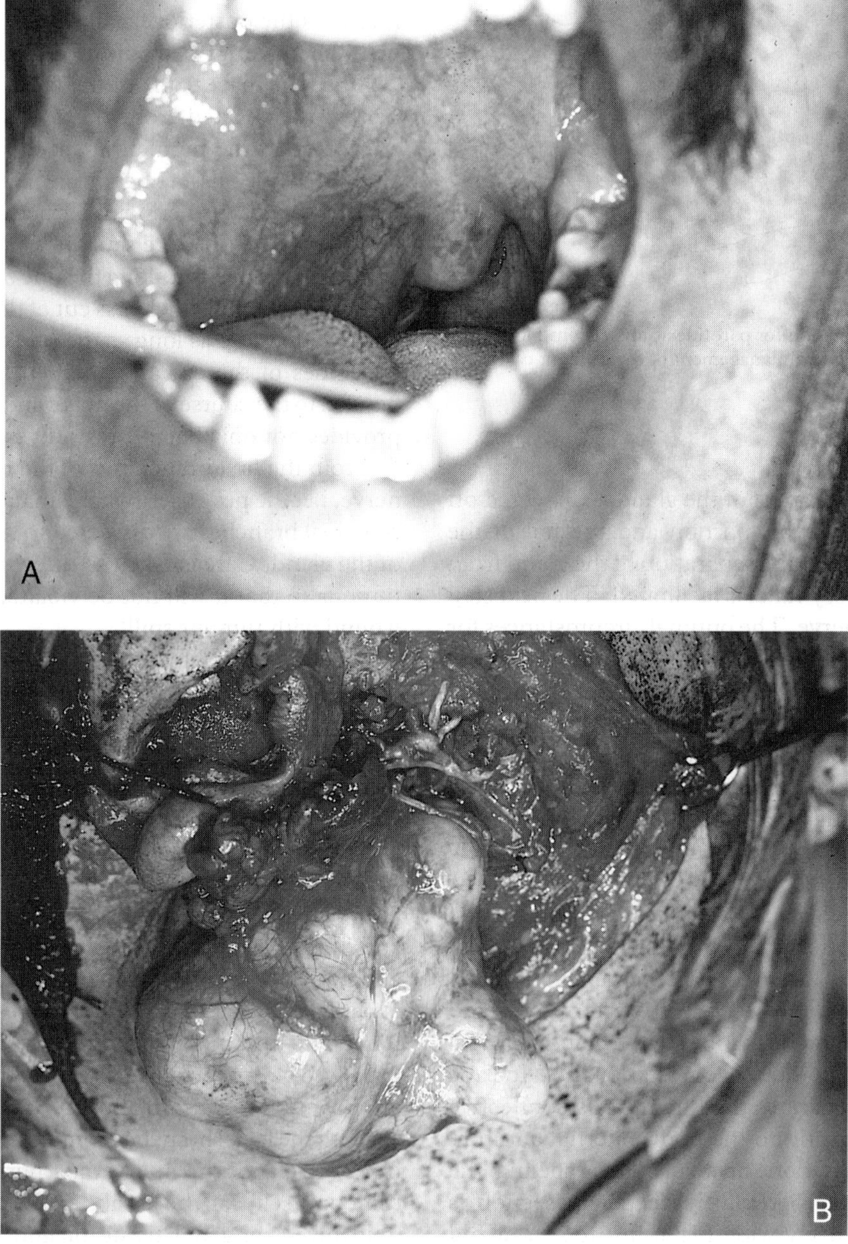

Fig. 23.3 Large pleomorphic adenoma of deep lobe of parotid. **A.** Intra-oral view showing bulging of the tonsillar fossa. **B.** Intra-operative view.

many of them have a component in the superficial lobe in a 'dumb-bell configuration' (Fig. 23.3). Because the lesions often reach considerable size prior to diagnosis, the tumours are jammed between the ramus of the mandible and the cervical spine, making extirpation en bloc a difficult chore. For pleomorphic adenomata, tumour spillage risks local recurrence. Care must be taken to remove the neoplasm in a single piece; transoral, alone or combined with transcervical excision, is to be decried because the exposure is poor, there is no control of the carotid artery, the facial nerve cannot be dissected or seen, and incomplete excision commonly occurs. Proximity of the tumour to the carotid sheath mandates adequate control of these vital structures during resection. In some instances, usually with small tumours, vigorous retraction at the angle of the mandible with a bone hook will provide enough exposure. The facial nerve is retracted gently with a nerve hook and the tumour is shelled out.

For larger lesions, a mandibular osteotomy may be required. A stair-step osteotomy executed from the coronoid notch to the angle behind the entrance of the inferior alveolar nerve will spare the nerve and preserve normal lower lip sensation. The degree of retraction is not as liberal as a transverse osteotomy at the mandibular angle. The latter procedure is quick and easy, but obviously compromises the nerve. The tumour is dissected from the posterior belly of the digastric muscle, the stylohyoid and styloglossus. Care is taken to preserve cranial nerve XII and especially cranial nerve IX. The glossopharyngeal nerve runs just inferior to the stylopharyngeus muscle which it supplies. These structures are near the tonsillar bed at its inferior pole against which the deep surface of the tumour usually rests. In addition, the deep aspect of the tumour is often against the medial pterygoid muscle and the superior constrictor of the pharynx. At the completion of the tumour excision, the jaw is re-approximated by a mandibular plate. A 2–3 week period of intermaxillary fixation is recommended until the jaw begins to stabilize. Suction drainage is applied to the wound, and the closure done in the usual fashion.

Malignant tumours

The degree of radicality of resection of parotid gland neoplasms is dependent on histological type, tumour location relative to adjacent structures, evidence of seventh or fifth nerve involvement, and the presence of metastatic neck disease. Low-grade malignancies, such as low-grade mucoepidermoid carcinoma, are not as aggressively attached as squamous-cell carcinoma or adenocarcinoma. Metastasis to parotid lymph nodes from cutaneous cancers have usually breached the capsule of the node and are treated liked squamous-cell primaries of the gland. En bloc resection is attempted only if all or part of the facial nerve is to be excised. By the nature of facial nerve dissection, some degree of piecemeal resection may be required. Still, a vigorous attempt is made to stay completely clear of the tumour during facial nerve trunk identification and branch dissection.

In most parotid malignancies, a radical approach is taken. The gland is completely excised, and all facial nerve branches invaded by neoplasm or within 2 to 5 mm of the tumour are resected. A lateral temporal bone resection just lateral to the tympanic annulus—and sometimes including the mandibular condyle—is done. Masseter muscle, ramus of mandible, zygomatic arch and temporalis muscle are resected if invaded by tumour. A radical neck dissection is done only if lymph nodes are palpable in the neck or if involved in the juxtaparotid area. The exception to this is in those instances when the tumour is metastatic in the parotid lymph nodes from a cutaneous primary. A radical neck dissection is done rather than a modified one because high nodes near the emergence of the spinal accessory nerve are commonly involved. Invasion of the temporal bone per se requires complete temporal bone resection. Invasion of the foramen ovale is an indication for a combined infratemporal fossa–middle fossa approach

The modified Blair incision is made in a similar fashion to the operation for benign disease. Skin invasion demands a wide margin of excision (Fig. 22.4). A liberal margin of as much as 3–4 cm is taken, especially if there is skin penetration with ulceration, and most especially if there is a surrounding area of erythema. The skin is left attached to the bloc as dissection proceeds.

Proximity of tumour to the cartilaginous and bony external auditory canals (EAC) is very common, and lateral temporal bone resection is the rule rather than the exception because of the possible spread of tumour through the fissures of Santorini in the cartilaginous EAC. The nice avascular plane between the gland and the EAC, usually afforded in benign disease, would carry the dissection directly through tumour in malignant cases. The approach to the facial nerve trunk must be done then from below. The tail of the gland is elevated off the SCM and dissection along the undersurface of the temporal bone proceeds to the styloid process. Nodes are sampled and sent for frozen section diagnosis. If tumour is also in the tail, then one proceeds with a mastoidectomy. When the trunk of the nerve is difficult to identify, separation of the origin of the SCM, and then high transection of the posterior belly of the digastric muscle, will open the region of the stylomastoid foramen. The occipital artery is deep to the digastric groove and usually requires ligation.

Once the trunk of the nerve has been identified, dissection is carried out as far as safe proximity to tumour will allow. This may permit exposure of only a portion of the trunk, the bifurcation into upper and lower main trunks, or even out to individual branches. All involved nerve is sacrificed.

During the dissection of the nerve, the degree of invasion

of the underlying structures such as masseter, temporo-mandibular joint, zygoma, temporalis, or even mandibular ramus, begins to become apparent. The definitive cutting down on these structures is delayed until the mastoidectomy has been done.

A complete mastoidectomy is carried out with careful skeletonization of the digastric ridge, the Fallopian canal, the attic, and the facial recess. In most instances, amputation of the bony EAC can be carried out just lateral to the tympanic annulus and thereby lateral to the Fallopian canal. The tympanic bone is deeply notched with the cutting burr to later facilitate fracture with the osteotome. The mastoid tip is removed to the digastric ridge.

If the tumour is adjacent to, or invading, the temporomandibular joint, a condylectomy is necessary to remove all the soft tissue in the joint's proximity. Mandibular condylectomy is done by first incising the temporal mandibular ligament and underlying joint capsule with the cutting cautery. The superior joint space is the easiest to enter. Periosteum is stripped down the mandibular neck and a subperiosteal dissection carried deep to this structure. This is a key, moreover, to avoid injury to the underlying middle meningeal artery. The periosteal pocket must be

wide enough to permit the insertion of a malleable retractor. The power saw is used to incise the condylar neck and the condyle is removed. Often, at least part of the meniscus is left behind in this manoeuvre. The soft tissue in the region of the joint, often including the insertion of the lateral pterygoid muscle on the anteriomedial surface of the condylar neck and adjacent joint capsule, also becomes part of the bloc. This tissue will be attached to the glenoid fossa and come away with the temporal bone in the final stages of the procedure.

At this point, all deep structural involvement with tumour is incised. If the zygoma is invaded, the arch is cut through anteriorly and the posterior portion will be removed with the temporal bone. Temporalis muscle invasion is managed by incision down to calvarium.

The final stage of temporal bone removal is accomplished by the placement of the osteotome lateral to the tympanic annulus and driving through to the anterior canal wall. The canal wall skin is cut circumferentially just lateral to the annulus. Superiorly, the bone cut joins the atticotomy to the glenoid fossa through the zygomatic root. If zygoma is involved, the osteotomy is driven straight into the infratemporal fossa. Occasionally some middle fossa dura

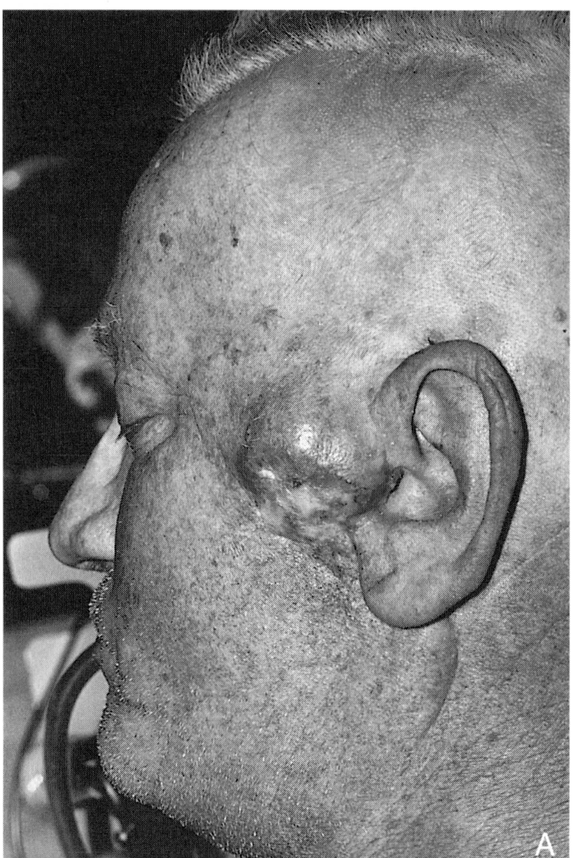

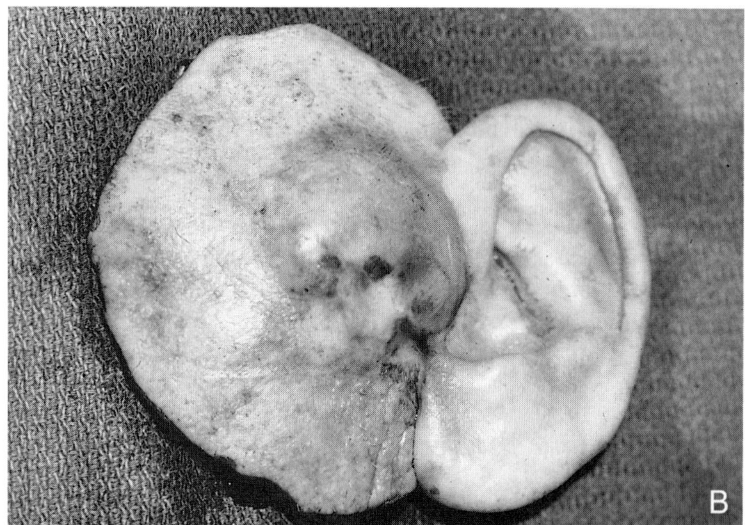

Fig. 23.4 A. Large metastatic malignant fibrous histiocytoma of the parotid gland with extensive skin involvement. **B.** Tumour with margin of adjacent healthy skin. (From Wallis A, Donald P J 1988 Lateral face reconstruction with the medial-based cervicopectoral flap. Archives of Otolaryngology—Head and Neck Surgery 114: 731.)

will be exposed. This is because the vault of the glenoid fossa is one of the thinnest areas of the middle fossa floor. Inferiorly, the osteotome is driven through the tympanic bone lateral to the styloid process (Fig. 23.5). This incision also ends up in the glenoid fossa. The anterior canal wall is cut or is fractured in the process, and the bony attachments become free from the remaining temporal bone but are still connected to the tumour specimen. At this point, some minor final soft-tissue attachments are severed. Not uncommonly the distal portion of the external carotid artery is cut and requires suture ligation.

The resected specimen is checked to ensure that an adequate cuff of normal-appearing soft tissue has been included around the tumour. Areas of questionable involvement are biopsied and sent for frozen section analysis. An area that occasionally escapes attention is the soft tissue of the infratemporal fossa. Tumour proximity to the mandibular branch of the trigeminal nerve requires nerve biopsy and, if positive, the bone around the foramen ovale bone should be removed with a cutting burr. The nerve trunk is severed flush with the dura and submitted for pathological examination. If tumour is still present at this site, a combined infratemporal fossa/middle cranial fossa approach will be needed to effect complete tumour excision.

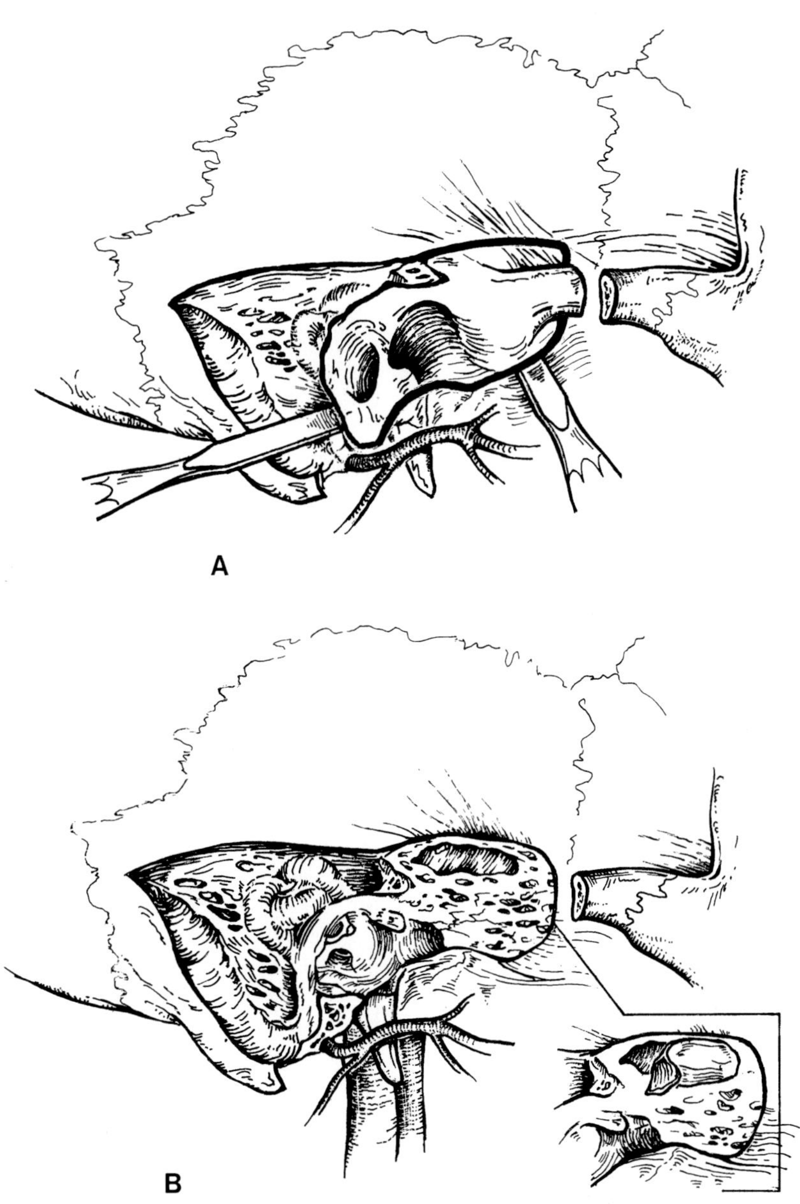

Fig. 23.5 Lateral temporal bone resection. **A.** Single mastoidectomy done, lateral temporal bone excision outlined. **B.** Lateral temporal bone excision completed. Inset: note exposed middle fossa dura. (From Donald P J 1984 Head and neck cancer: management of the difficult case. W B Saunders, Philadelphia, p 238.)

RECONSTRUCTION

The resection of a wide margin of skin is mandatory when parotid tumours break through. One of the most challenging problems in this group of patients is their closure. Because such defects are so obvious, a good cutaneous colour and texture match is essential. This is best provided by a cervicothoracic rotation flap. Since this flap carries adjacent facial and cervical skin into the defect, these two aesthetic requirements are adequately fulfilled. An incision is carried from the edge of the defect around under the ear, along the anterior border of the trapezius muscle, or even as much as 2 cm behind it (Fig. 23.6). The incision is carried down to the base of the neck and then continued in a horizontal fashion just above the clavicle or, if a larger flap is required, it is curved onto the chest at the level of the second or third intercostal space. The modified Blair incision is obviously abandoned at the outset of the case if the flap is contemplated.

The flap is elevated in the 'face lift' plane just under the

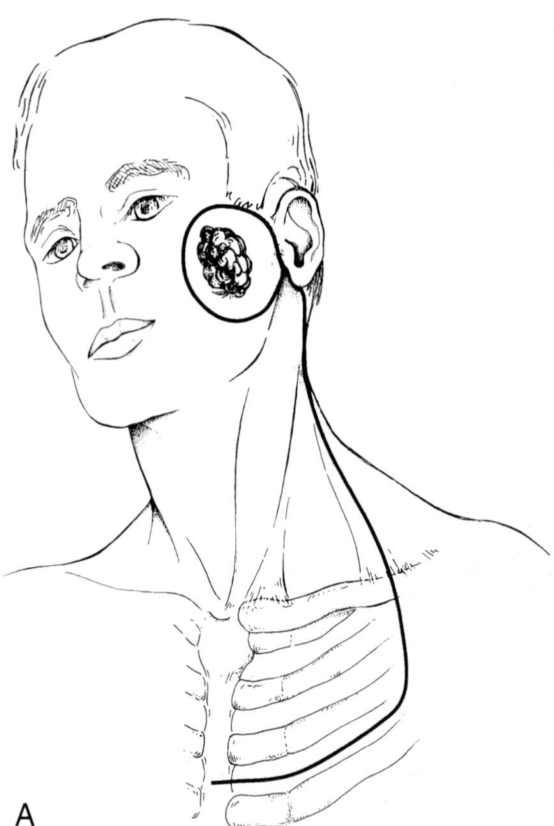

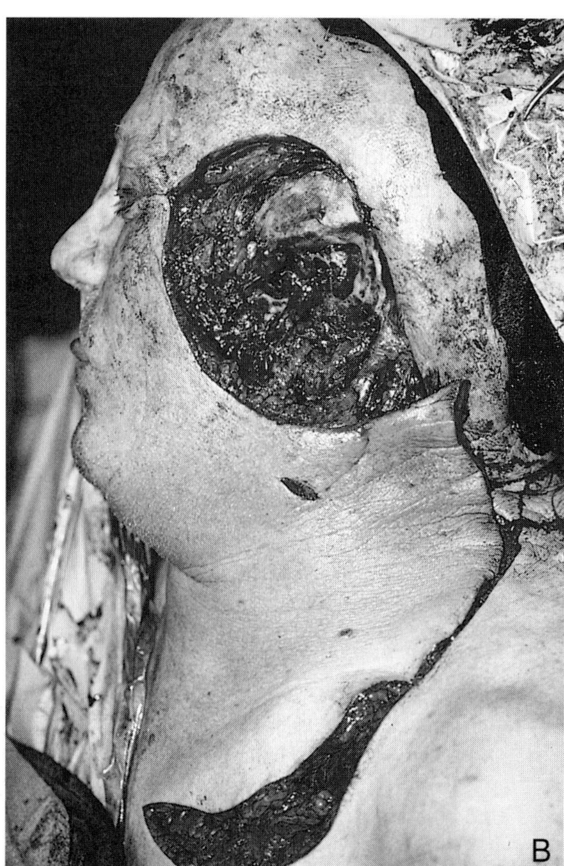

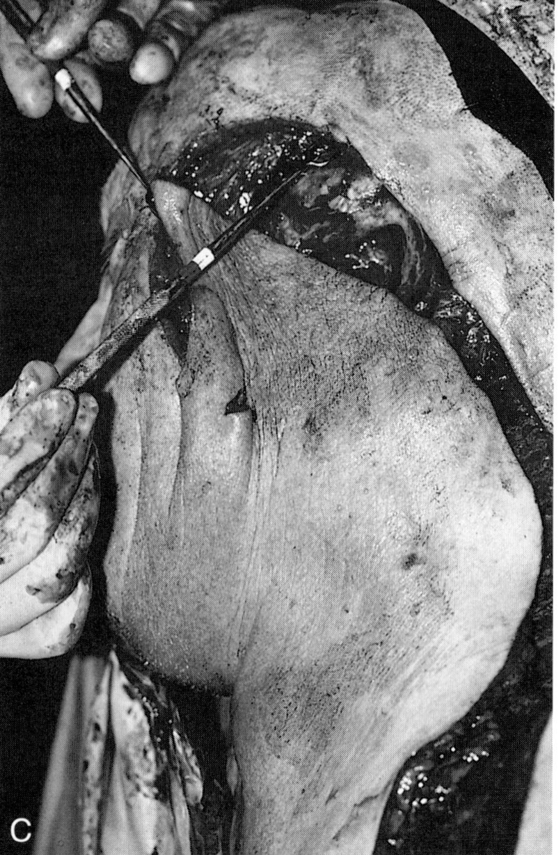

Fig. 23.6 Cervicothoracic rotation flap. **A.** Flap outline. **B.** Defect following skin excision, auriculectomy, parotidectomy, condylectomy, resection of lateral temporal bone, zygoma and masseter and temporalis muscles. **C.** Flap rotated into position. (From Wallis A, Donald P J 1988 Lateral face reconstruction with the medial-based cervicopectoral flap. Archives of Otolaryngology—Head and Neck Surgery 114: 730, 732.)

subcutaneous fat of the face. In the neck, a subplatysmal plane ensures the best blood supply. Care is taken to avoid injury to the ramus mandibularis, if still intact. The flap is rotated into the defect and carefully sutured into position after placing an underlying suction drain. The tension on the flap is evenly distributed along the cervical closure line. In larger defects that necessitate extension of the incision onto the chest, occasionally a donor defect may arise that will need a split-thickness skin graft to close. In these instances, serial excisions at a later date can eliminate the graft site. The cervicopectoral flap is best applied to those defects anterior to the auricle.

Alternatives to closure are the superior-based trapezius flap (Fig. 23.7) and the pectoralis major myocutaneous flap. These flaps are more suitable for those defects left by the lateral temporal bone resection because they are more strategically placed and their bulk helps to efface the volume deficit secondary to the tumour excision. They are especially applicable when the pinna requires resection and the deep cavity of the temporal bone is exposed. The trapezius flap with its superior pedicle as described by McCraw et al (1979) and Donald & Chole (1984) or in its inferior pedicle as described by Netterville & Wood (1991) are good choices.

If these flaps are contemplated, the patient should have the surgery performed using a Mayfield head rest. If the inferior pedicle is used, the extended trapezius flap will be necessary in order to reach the top of the defect. The patient will then need to be rolled onto the lateral position and even a second surgical prep done in order to accomplish this flap. The extended trapezius flap is pedicled on the subscapular artery and if the rhomboids are cut will easily reach the furthest superior extent of the exenteration.

The pectoralis major musculocutaneous flap (Fig. 23.8) is preferred because it is quick and easy. Additional length can be gained by resecting the anterior one-third of the clavicle. This also prevents vascular compression of the pedicle which may ensue in asthenic individuals or those who have had a prior neck dissection, especially if they have had postoperative irradiation. The flap, however, may not be able to gain the most superior extent of the resection site because of the length of the patient's thorax. Adding a random pattern type extension to the end of the flap to bridge this gap seriously jeopardizes the repair and has not been a wise choice in my experience. Careful pre-operative planning will establish the feasibility of this flap.

An alternative method of wound closure is the vascularized

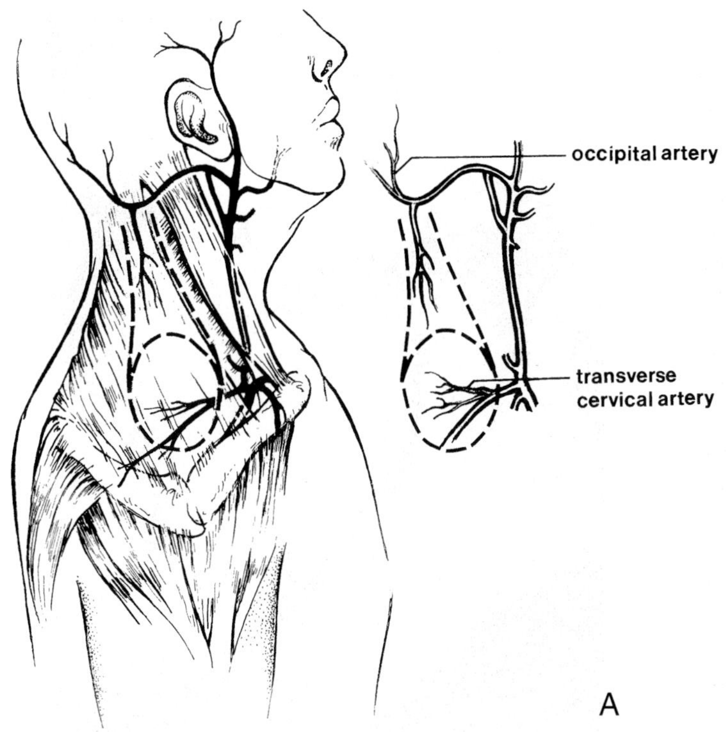

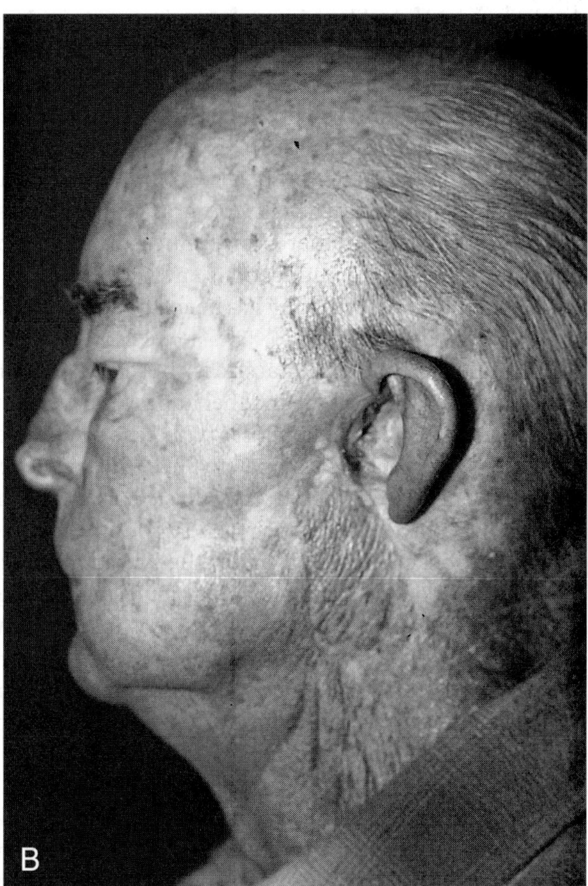

Fig. 23.7 A. Superiorly based trapezius flap. **B.** Parotid and overlying cutaneous defect filled in with superior based trapezius flap. (From Donald P J, Chole R A 1984 Superior based trapezius flap. Laryngoscope 94: 969, 972.)

free flap. The groin or parascapular areas are preferred donor sites. These flaps suffer from the problems of markedly prolonging operative time and the provision of a flap with poor colour and texture match.

In the bulky flaps, especially the pectoralis flap, the force of gravity adds much tension to the superior suture line. This may cause the flap to pull away from its superior attachment. Prevention may be afforded by large support sutures from the scalp to the flap, secured to tie-over bolsters.

The least aesthetic reconstructive alternative for cutaneous loss is the application of a split-thickness skin graft. It is, on the other hand, the method by which the early identification of local recurrence can be most easily detected. These grafts have poor take over bare bone and are not recommended in a patient who has had prior radiotherapy to the area.

Facial nerve deficits are the most troublesome problems for the patient and their solution is one of the most demanding in reconstructive surgery. Facial nerve rehabilitation is both a functional and an aesthetic challenge. The primary consideration is eye closure and corneal protection. Inadequate corneal coverage may lead to keratitis, corneal scarring and blindness. These are completely preventable complications and assiduous attention to eye care is an essential aspect of postoperative management.

If the zygomatic branches are compromised in any way, adequacy of lid closure is assessed on a daily basis. Taping the eye at night, the liberal use of eye ointment, or the use of a moisture chamber, are all good prophylactic measures. The insertion of a gold weight varying between 0.8 and 1.2 grams in the upper lid will produce almost normal closure in almost all patients. This is an excellent procedure for a patient with a permanent VII nerve paralysis or as a temporizing measure until a facial nerve graft re-innervates. The palpebral spring is another choice, but is more technically difficult, has serious complications and the results are more unpredictable. Tarsorrhaphy has been abandoned in favour of the gold weight.

The gold weight of optimal size is chosen pre-operatively by having the patient sit up and then taping the weight to the upper eyelid. When the lid closes with ease and the levator muscle is strong enough to open the eye, the correct choice of weight has been made. An incision is made in the supratarsal crease of the upper eyelid about the width of the cornea. A pocket is created under the pretarsal orbicularis oculi muscle down to the lid margin. A gold weight of previously determined appropriate size is inserted into the pocket. One or two anchoring sutures of #5-0 or #6-0 absorbable suture are placed through the holes in the implant and sutured to the fibrous tissue on the outside of the tarsal plate. The incision is closed with #6.0 nonabsorbable suture.

Restoration of nerve function is optimally undertaken at the time of primary exenterative surgery. If a nerve branch is sacrificed, it is replaced with the cable graft of greater auricular nerve, usually taken from the opposite neck. A skin crease incision is made over the SCM at Erb's point: a point along the muscle one-third away from the mastoid tip to the clavicular head. Careful dissection of the branches of this nerve are done and the trunk is dissected to its point of emergence from the cervical plexus. The cable is sutured in with fine sutures of #10-0 nylon using a 75μ needle under microscopic control (Fig. 23.9). The sutures are placed just through the epineurium, occasionally taking a little perineurium with the needle. A main division or the whole trunk of the nerve may be replaced with a cable graft. If the greater auricular will be too short or unavailable, the sural nerve provides a good alternative.

If the nerve needs to be approximated in the Fallopian canal, one or two sutures are all that are needed for approximation. In the main trunk ten sutures are commonly used and, in a main division, six to eight. Often only four or five can be placed in a branch. When multiple branches need anastomosis, the cervical and often the frontal are omitted. Occasionally tumour will be so extensive that resection out to the facial muscles may be the only way of ensuring a safe

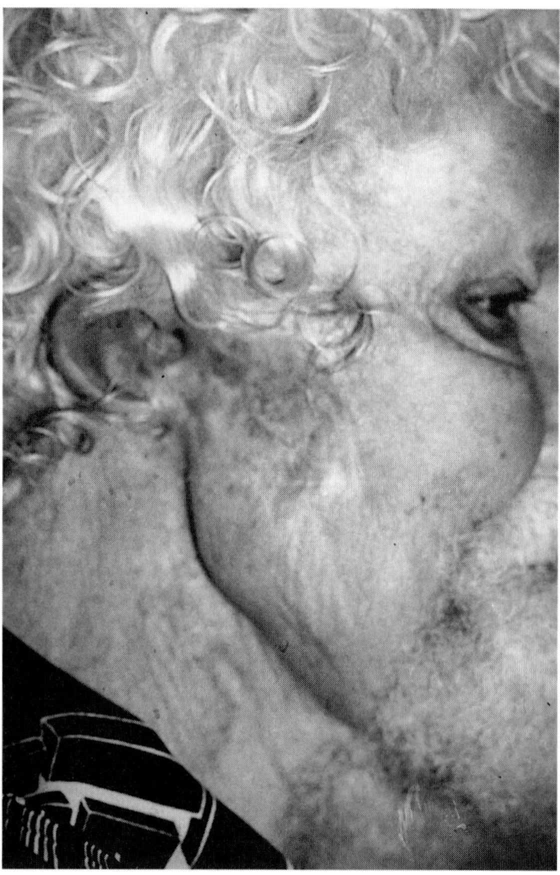

Fig. 23.8 PMC flap in place and healed. Patient is 24 months status post-resection of parotid, masseter muscle, mandibular condyle and lateral temporal bone for adenocarcinoma of the parotid.

margin. In these instances, a facial nerve cable graft can be implanted directly into the muscle. Often this procedure will need to be supplemented by either a static or dynamic sling procedure.

When the entire temporal bone is resected and the facial nerve is sacrificed in the petrosal part, intracranial to extracranial grafting can be done. An alternative to this is a hypoglossal to VII cross-over anastomosis. The latter is much quicker and less technically demanding.

If the facial nerve function does not recover as anticipated, a host of reconstructive techniques are available. None, however, restore the symmetry and function of the normal nerve. For the eye, brow ptosis is a vexing problem, especially in the elderly, often requiring taping of the brow for reading. A carefully executed unilateral brow lift can alleviate this problem. The procedure should be done in the sitting position under local anaesthesia. One must be most careful to avoid over-zealous resection of skin that would subsequently preclude complete lid closure facilitated by the prior placement of the gold weight. A modified tear-drop-shaped excision of skin and orbicularis oculi just above the eyebrow is followed by meticulous closure with interrupted fine suture.

With time, especially in the elderly, the gradual onset of lower-lid ectropion may occur. This eversion of the lid is not only unsightly, but may be uncomfortable because of secondary inflammation of the conjunctiva. In addition, epiphora may result from the lack of approximation of the lacrimal punctum to the laca lacrimalis. A lid-shortening, modified lower blepharoplasty, and lateral canthopexy resolves the problem in most cases (Fig. 23.10). A subcilliary incision is made from the lacrimal punctum and swept up approximately 2 cm lateral and superior to the outer canthus of the eye. A skin muscle flap is developed to a point a few millimetres below the tarsal plate. A pentagonal excision of the lower eyelid in a position just lateral to the corneal limbus is taken through the palpebral conjunctiva and adjacent tarsal plate. A scimitar-shaped portion of the skin muscle flap is excised from its most lateral extremity.

Closure is preceded by first taking one or two bites of suture in the lateral canthal tendon of the eye, then fixing to the orbital periosteum above its usual insertion. Following this lateral canthopexy, the conjunctiva is closed with interrupted #6-0 catgut sutures. This closure is usually best preceded by placing two parallel sutures of #6-0 silk in the lid margin that exactly approximate it. These are left long as traction sutures and enable more accurate placement of those in the conjunctiva. Few, if any, sutures are needed in the tarsal plate. The lower lid skin-muscle flap is advanced laterally. Most of the skin trimming is done from its lateral part. It is closed like a blepharoplasty incision. The long tails of the lid margin sutures are gently taped to the facial skin to avoid corneal irritation. Sutures are removed at the fourth to fifth day.

Dynamic slings of temporalis and masseter muscle or static slings of fascia lata looped around the zygomatic arch

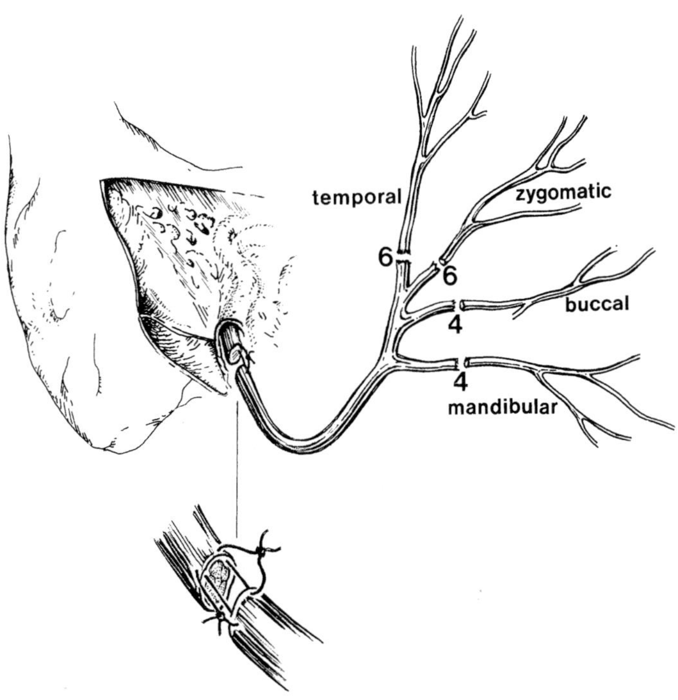

Fig. 23.9 Facial nerve graft is sutured into place.

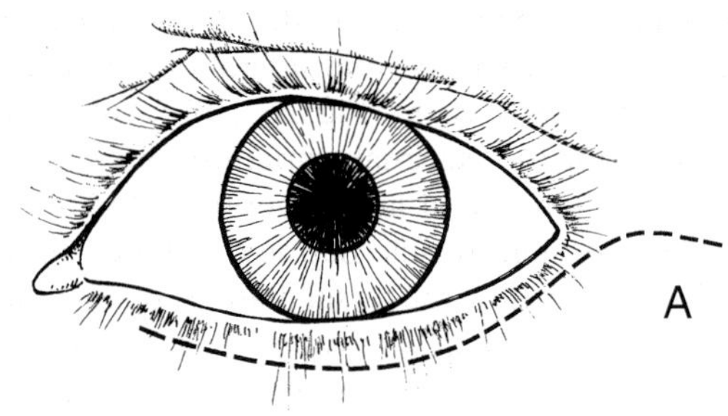
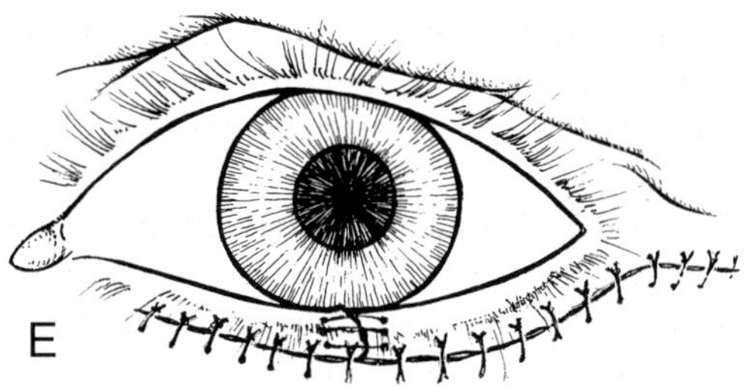
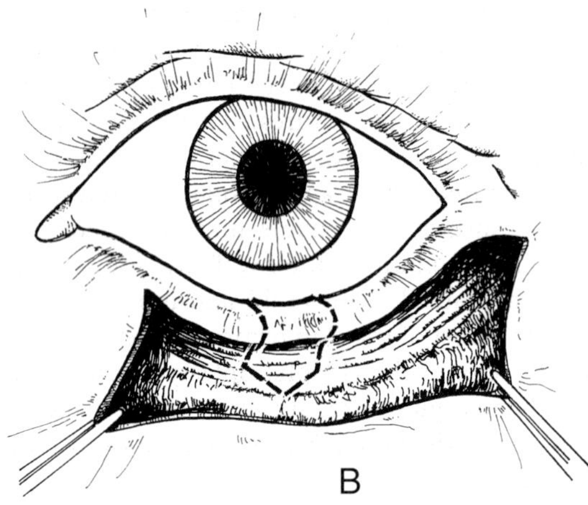
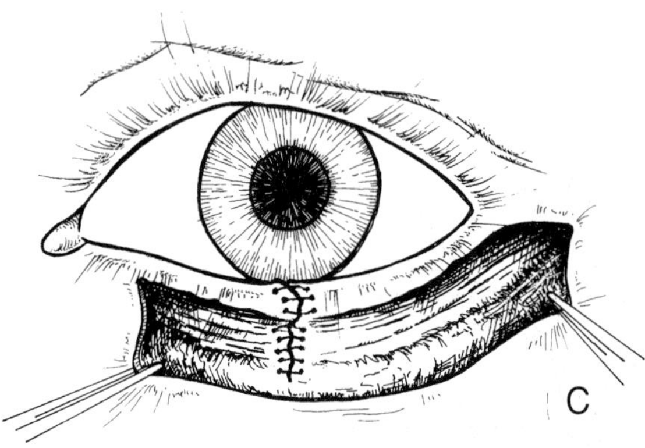
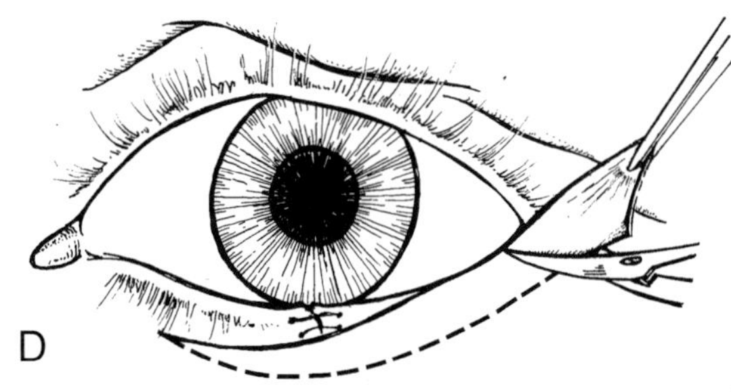

Fig. 23.10 Lid shortening, lower blepharoplasty and canthopexy for lower lid ectropion following facial paralysis. **A.** Skin incision marked out. **B.** Pentagonal excision lower lid. **C.** Lid shortened. **D.** Skin excess trimmed. **E.** Wound closure. (From Smith B C, Nesi F A 1981 Practical techniques in ophthalmic plastic surgery. C V Mosby, St Louis, p 125.)

and knitted into the upper and lower lip as well as oral commissure provide some support for the mouth (Fig. 23.11).

Cross-over facial nerve grafts may be used. Free muscle transplants with baby-sitter hypoglossal to facial grafting can then be re-innervated by cross-nerve grafts at a second

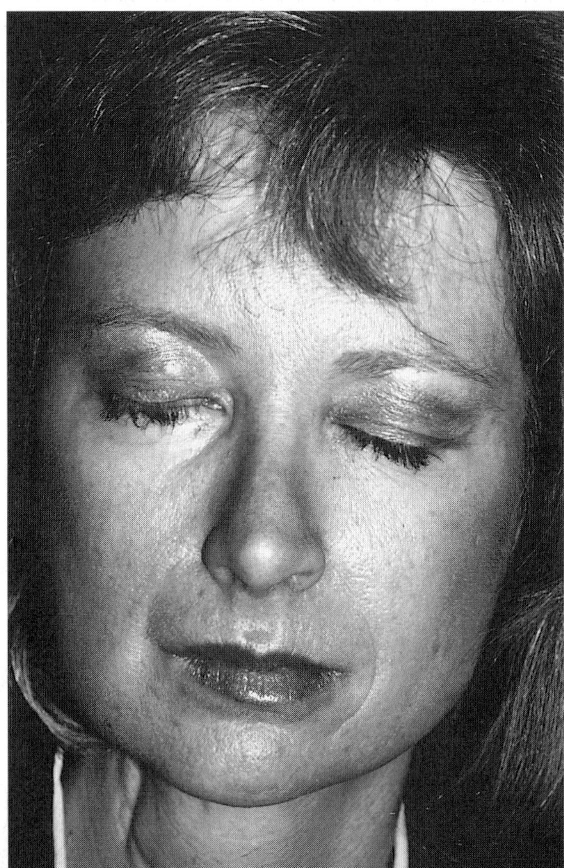

Fig. 23.11 Patient with gold weight in upper lid, static fascial sling and partial return of lower face following XII to VII anastomosis 2 years after skull-base surgery for massive intracranial–extracranial glomus tumour.

stage as described by Ferreira (1987). This is a remarkable procedure, but extremely labour-intensive and often reserved for the most difficult cases.

Filling in of the large defect left by prior radical parotidectomy still defies satisfactory solution. The use of muscle in the form of pedicle or free flaps has the unfortunate sequela of atrophy. Free fat–dermis grafts have an unpredictable absorption rate. Omental free flaps as described by Harii (1978) maintain their original bulk, but because of a dearth of innate stiffness tend to sag with gravity.

CONCLUSIONS

The appropriate management of parotid neoplasms requires a detailed understanding of the pathophysiology of the manifold types of tumour to which the parotid falls ill. Anticipating their behavioural pattern, an appropriate surgical procedure can be designed for their exenteration. Benign tumours demand careful preservation of facial nerve integrity. Malignant tumours should be addressed in a radical fashion, and involved facial nerve branches must be sacrificed. In the author's experience, this approach has resulted in over 90% local control of disease and an approximately 70% 5-year tumour-free survival rate.

Reconstruction employs the judicious use of grafts and flaps to restore function and maintain the best aesthetic result possible. Assiduous attention to eye care is the most important aspect of postoperative management.

REFERENCES

Abele J S, Miller T R 1985 Fine needle aspiration of the thyroid nodule: clinical applications. In: Clark O H (ed) Endocrine surgery of the thyroid and parathyroid glands. C V Mosby, St Louis, ch 10, pp 293–366

Bernstein L, Nelson R H 1984 Surgical anatomy of the extraparotid distribution of the facial nerve. Archives of Otolaryngology 110: 177–183

Coman W B 1990 Perineural infiltration and skull base tumours. Panel presentation made at the Sisson Head and Neck Course, Steamboat Springs, 7 March

Conley J J 1975 Salivary glands and the facial nerve. Grune & Stratton, New York, pp 197–199

Dingman R O, Grabb W C 1962 Surgical anatomy of the mandibular ramus of the facial nerve based on the dissection of 100 facial halves. Plastic and Reconstructive Surgery 29: 266–272

Donald P J, Chole R A 1984 Superior based trapezius flap. Laryngoscope 94: 969–973

Eneroth C M 1965 Mixed tumours of major salivary glands: prognostic role of capsular structure. Annals of Otology, Rhinology and Laryngology 74: 944

Eneroth C M, Zetterberg A 1968 Malignancy in pleomorphic adenoma. A clinical and microspectophotometric study. Acta Otolaryngologica 77: 426–492

Ferreira M C 1987 Cross-facial nerve grafting. In: Terzis J K (ed) Microreconstruction of nerve injuries. W B Saunders, Philadelphia, ch 43, pp 601–605

Harii K 1978 Clinical application of free omental flap transfer. Clinics in Plastic Surgery 5: 273

Lajicek J, Eneroth C M 1970 Cytological diagnosis of salivary gland carcinomata from aspiration biopsy smears. Acta Otolaryngologica 262: 183

McCabe B F, Work P W 1967 Parotidectomy with special reference to the facial nerve. In: English G M (ed) Otolaryngology. Harper & Row, Hagerstown MD, vol 4, p 39

McCraw J B, Magee W D, Kalwaic H 1979 Uses of the trapezius and sternocleidomastoid myocutaneous flaps in head and neck reconstruction. Plastic and Reconstructive Surgery 63: 49–57

Netterville J, Wood D 1991 Lower trapezius flap: vascular anatomy and surgical technique. Archives of Otolaryngology 117: 73–76

Peel R H, Gnepp D R 1985 Diseases of the salivary glands. In: Barnes L (ed) Surgical pathology of the head and neck. Marcel Dekker, New York, vol 1, ch 13, pp 559–562

Perzin K H, Gullane P, Clairmont A C 1978 Adenoid cystic carcinomas arising in salivary glands. Cancer 43: 265

Pitanguy I, Ramos A S 1966 The frontal branch of the facial nerve: the importance of its variations in face lifting. Plastic and Reconstructive Surgery 38: 352–356

Rice D H, Manusco A A, Hanafe W N 1980 Computerised tomography with simultaneous sialography in evaluating parotid tumours. Archives of Otolaryngology 106: 472–473

Schaffer J, Beitragelzur 1897 Histologie menschlicher organe, IV. Zurge V, Mundhohle-Schundkopf, VI, Oesophagus VII, Cardia Sitzungsb. K. Akod. Wissensch. Mathnaturw Cl. Wein PT-3 106: 353–355

Thackray A C, Lucas R B 1974 Atlas of tumour pathology : Fasicle 10. Tumours of the major salivary glands; AFIP, Bethesda MD, p 53

Work W P, Hecht D W 1980 Tumours and cysts of major salivary glands. In: Shumrick D A, Paparella M M (eds) Otolaryngology, 2nd edn. W B Saunders, Philadelphia, vol 3, p 2244

24. The skin

David S. Soutar   Rammohan Tiwari

INTRODUCTION

The surgical treatment of malignant tumours involving the skin of the head and neck poses considerable problems for the head and neck surgeon. On the one hand, the skin can be affected by a wide variety of pathologies which may be primary to the skin or the result of secondary infiltration of the skin from an underlying tumour. The commonest primary cutaneous malignancies include basal-cell carcinoma, squamous-cell carcinoma and malignant melanoma. In addition, there are a wide variety of malignant skin appendage tumours (adnexal tumours) and malignancies affecting specific cells of the skin and subcutaneous tissue, e.g. Merkel-cell tumours, lymphomas and sarcomas.

Secondary infiltration of the skin from underlying tumours is most commonly seen in the neck in advanced cervical metastasis with extranodal spread and in stomal recurrence from laryngeal carcinoma. In the face, local infiltration can occur in advanced parotid malignancy, and advanced carcinomas of the maxillary antrum and oral cavity. Inappropriate biospy of a lump in the head and neck prior to referral to a specialized head and neck service can often result in infiltration and fixation to the overlying skin. This can be complicated by secondary infection which serves only to increase the area affected, thus requiring a larger excision. Less commonly, distant metastasis, e.g. renal-cell carcinoma can present as an infiltrative tumour involving the skin.

These widely differing pathologies can often complicate surgical excision, but equally there are problems in reconstruction. The skin of the head and neck is not a uniform structure. It varies in colour, thickness and texture in differing sites within the same individual and varies between differing individuals with regard to genetic composition, race, age and obesity. The skin of the neck in the mid-line, for example, and the paramedian area is thinner and has fewer sebaceous glands than does the skin over the posterior triangles and the nape of the neck. There are significant differences in colour and texture in various sites within the face, the most obvious being between hair-bearing and non-hair-bearing skin. At certain sites, the skin is very specific—such as in the upper and lower eyelids. It is often very difficult, if not impossible, to replace like tissue with like and so obtain the ideal reconstruction. A good colour and texture match for reconstruction of the skin of the head and neck remains one of the greatest problems.

The head and neck is visible to the public at large and the majority of primary cutaneous malignancies present with a noticeable blemish on the skin surface. A large proportion of these patients do not consult the surgical oncologist or the head and neck surgeon in the first instance but present to a wide variety of medical specialties including beauty specialists, dermatologists, radiotherapists and facial plastic surgeons. Unfortunately it is only when the tumour has recurred and grown that the head and neck surgeon is consulted. In addition, the face and neck is exposed to the damaging effects of exposure to sunlight and there is little doubt that in many areas of the world the incidence of primary carcinoma of the skin is increasing (Silverstone & Searl 1970, Emmett & O'Rourke 1991). It is estimated that nearly 300,000 whites develop skin cancer every year in the United States of America alone, and the incidence is equally high in countries such as Australia and New Zealand. Similarly, in Scotland, there has been an increasing incidence in all forms of cutaneous malignancy, particularly noticeable in malignant melanoma (MacKie et al 1992). A similar increase in incidence of both melanoma and squamous-cell carcinoma has been reported in the United States (Glass & Hoover 1989).

Although ultraviolet radiation is the most common aetiological factor in primary skin cancer, it is important for the head and neck surgeon to consider other significant aetiologies. In particular, Roentgen-radiation-induced carcinoma of the skin should be identified. It is occasionally encountered in individuals around 50 years of age or over who have a history of radiation in the early years of life, e.g. for tuberculous lymph nodes or patients who were unfortunate enough to be treated for ringworm or acne by radiation. Immunosuppression is also an important factor in the development of skin cancer (Hardie et al 1980). With the improved success and survival of transplantation patients this is becoming an increasingly significant aetiological factor as is the emergence af AIDS.

PATHOLOGICAL CONSIDERATIONS

The increasing incidence of primary cutaneous malignancy mainly relates to the three commonest pathologies, namely, basal-cell carcinoma, squamous-cell carcinoma and malignant melanoma. For this reason, it is worth considering these three conditions in more detail.

Basal-cell carcinoma

Basal-cell carcinoma is the commonest skin cancer encountered in clinical practice (Emmett & Broadbent 1981, Goldberg et al 1983, Proper et al 1990). The West of Scotland Regional Plastic Surgery Unit currently deals with over 1000 patients with basal-cell carcinoma each year. A study to monitor the natural history of basal-cell carcinoma has recently been completed (El-Sheemy 1991). This study looked at 357 patients who underwent surgical treatment for basal-cell carcinoma in 1982. At the time of presentation in 1982, 70.3% of the patients had a single lesion, the remainder having two or more lesions. Overall, there was no significant difference in incidence between males and females (Fig. 24.1).

The study has identified a group of patients who have gone on to develop a second basal-cell carcinoma during the follow-up period, (Fig. 24.2). This occurred in 92 patients (25.6%). Furthermore, 3.2% of patients with new primary tumours and 14.3% of patients with recurrent disease developed recurrence during the time of this study. This is in keeping with other published series which report a recurrence rate of 5–10% following primary surgical treatment (Koplin & Zarem 1980, Richmond & Davie 1987) and 15–25% following surgery for recurrent disease (Hayes 1962, Richmond & Davie 1987).

Although the recurrence rate is lower than might be expected following incomplete excision (Taylor & Barisoni 1973) our series showed a recurrence rate of 1.9% for completely excised basal-cell carcinomas compared to a recurrence rate of 24.1% following incomplete excision. It is now our practice to advocate further treatment following a report of incompletely excised basal-cell carcinoma, and this policy is supported by other published data (Gooding et al 1965, Pascal et al 1968, Richmond & Davie 1987).

A wide variety of clinical and histological types of basal-cell carcinoma have been described (Emmett & O'Rourke 1991). Certain types with well defined edges, such as papulonodular basal-cell carcinomas or cystic basal-cell carcinomas, can be removed with a 2–3 mm margin. Larger lesions and those with indistinct margins require a 4–5 mm margin of clearance.

The most difficult types of basal-cell carcinoma are the sclerosing or morpheic, the infiltrating basal-cell carcinoma and the metatypical basal-cell carcinoma which histologically shows squamous differentiation.

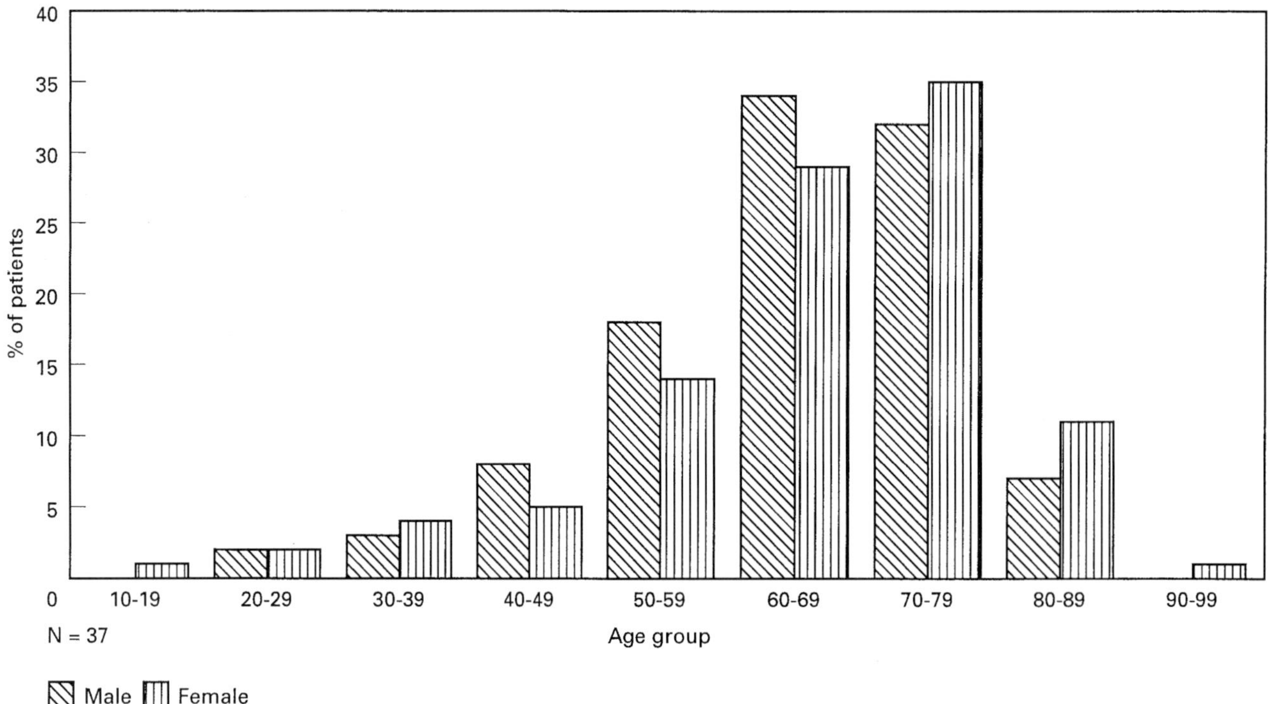

Fig. 24.1 Basal-cell carcinoma—age and sex distribution. (Mean age for males 64.9 yrs; for females 66.2 yrs.)

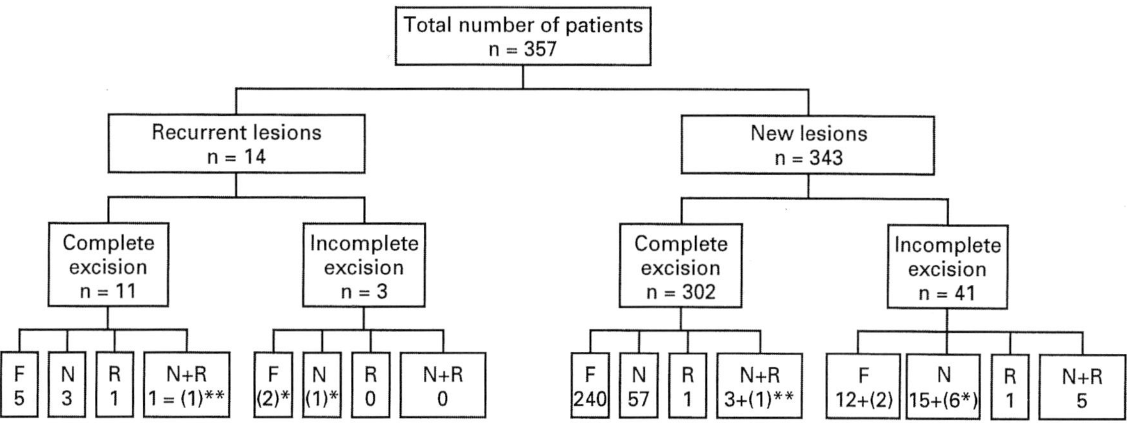

Fig. 24.2 Natural history of basal-cell carcinoma.

In our recent study, the histological type of basal-cell carcinoma was divided into two main groups. The more benign group was characterized by the presence of well-defined large aggregates of cells showing marked peripheral pallisading and a mucoid stromal response. The more aggressive type of basal-cell carcinoma showed small cell aggregates with an infiltrative pattern and a desmoplastic stromal response with little evidence of pallisading. This latter picture was seen in morpheic, sclerosing, infiltrative and metatypical basal-cell carcinomas. In keeping with other published series (Emmett & Broadbent 1981, Hauben et al 1982, Dellon et al 1985), recurrence was more common in basal-cell carcinomas showing a more aggressive histological pattern.

Surgery as a primary treatment for basal-cell carcinoma is associated with cure rates of about 95%, and for recurrent disease gives cure rates of 75–85% (Koplin & Zarem 1980, Richmond & Davie 1987). Identifying patients at risk of developing recurrence is therefore important, and our series supports the view that high-risk patients include those who already present with recurrent basal-cell carcinoma, basal-cell carcinomas showing an aggressive histological pattern, and those lesions presenting in sites where tissue is scarce. Furthermore, additional treatment is required in cases where the pathologist reports incomplete excision.

The major problem with basal-cell carcinoma is local because of its infiltrative and destructive nature. Danger sites include the alar crease of the nose, the external auditory meatus and the inner canthus of the eye. At these sites, infiltration can progress fairly rapidly and destructively into the facial skeleton and eventually erode through the cranial base to the brain. Metastasis from basal-cell carcinoma is exceedingly rare (Weedon & Wall 1975) and mostly affects the regional lymph nodes, but metastasis to lung, liver and bone have been reported (Cranmer et al 1970, Sakula 1977). Basal-cell carcinomas that are reported to have metastasized are usually of the metatypical type showing squamous differentiation and have often been present for many years (Cranmer et al 1970) or have a history of repeated recurrence following previous treatment.

Squamous-cell carcinoma

Squamous-cell carcinoma occurs at any site on the exposed areas of the head and neck but is found relatively infrequently on the scalp (Harris 1976). As with other skin cancers, exposure to sunlight is a major aetiological factor and the incidence of squamous-cell carcinoma is increasing (Glass & Hoover 1989). In addition to exposure to sunlight, the increased survival of patients on immunosuppression therapy, the emergence of AIDS and patients with chronically damaged skin as the result of previous radiotherapy, trauma or burns has further increased the incidence of squamous-cell carcinoma of the skin.

As with basal-cell carcinomas, there is a wide variation in the clinical presentation of squamous-cell carcinoma of the skin. It may appear as a patch of hyperkeratosis in an area of actinically damaged skin. Removal of the crust will show an ulcerated base, and clinical palpation will show a degree of induration and infiltration. Solar radiation can also give rise to an intra-epidermal squamous-cell carcinoma known as Bowen's disease.

Another non-invasive squamous-cell carcinoma is the keratoacanthoma which histologically expands the dermis but does not penetrate deep to the sweat glands. Keratoacanthoma is a clinical rather than a histological diagnosis and classically occurs in adults over the age of 50. It has a rapid growth phase extending for a period of approximately 6 weeks and subsequently undergoes cellular regression or apoptosis and appears to resolve but always leaves a permanent scar on the skin surface (Fig. 24.3). There remains considerable debate surrounding the malignant potential of keratoacanthoma and there is a significant risk of inappropriate treatment being instituted and an aggressive malignant squamous carcinoma being missed.

To avoid the potential dangers of adopting a wait-and-see policy in keratoacanthoma, McGregor (personal communication) has advocated shave excision of these lesions and close monitoring of the wound postoperatively. If the lesion is truly a keratoacanthoma the skin will heal within a matter of weeks, giving a relatively normal appearance. Wounds that fail to heal satisfactorily are indicative of an invasive tumour and should be treated by more radical excision.

Although shave excision provides a specimen for histological diagnosis, it is often impossible for the pathologist to differentiate between keratoacanthoma and an early invasive well-differentiated squamous-cell carcinoma. Multiple keratoacanthomas can also occur, and here the condition has to be differentiated from the multiple primary self-healing squamous epithelioma of Ferguson Smith. However, these cases have a confirmed hereditary basis, with patients confined to the West of Scotland and a few emigrants from this area (McGregor & McGregor 1986).

It appears that squamous-cell carcinomas arising in actinically damaged skin on a basis of actinic keratosis behave in a more benign fashion than those arising de novo with an accelerated growth phase. Furthermore, there appear to be danger sites for the development of rapidly growing squamous-cell carcinomas, and these include the lip, the columella of the nose and the ear. The surgeon should adopt a high index of suspicion in tumours arising at mucocutaneous junctions, in otherwise normal undamaged skin, and in tissues scarred by trauma, chronic sepsis, burns or irradiation (Moller et al 1979).

The extent of excision will vary according to the TNM staging, the anatomical site of the lesion and the histological appearance of the tumour. Some centres use Broder's classic grading from 1 to 4 to help determine prognosis. Tumours that exhibit perineural invasion histologically have been reported as indicating a poorer prognosis (Goepfert et al 1984, Mendenhall et al 1989).

In contrast to basal-cell carcinoma, where metastasis occurs in long-standing tumours, it is often the rapidly growing infiltrative squamous-cell carcinoma with a short

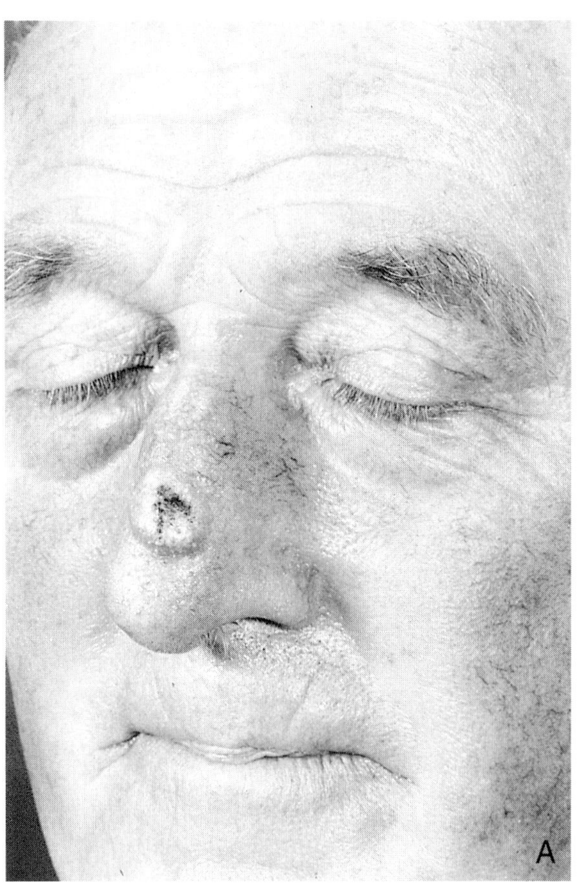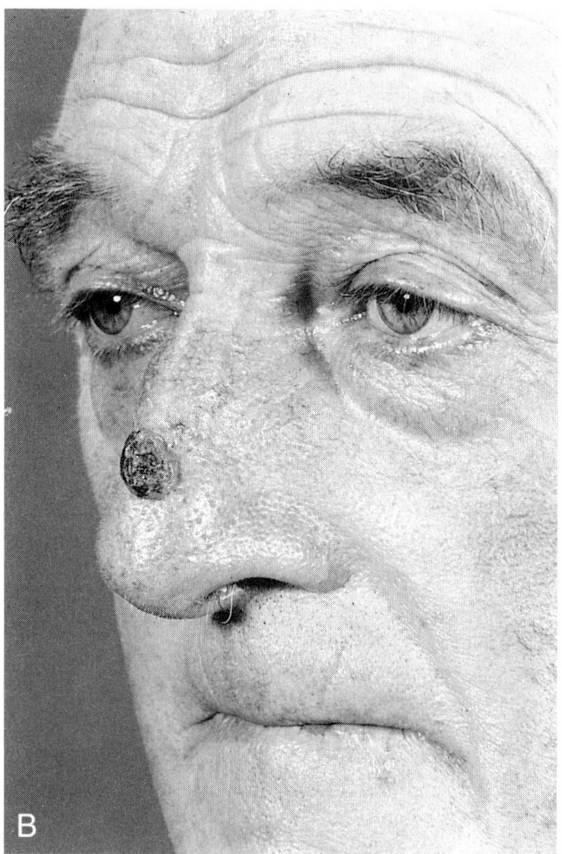

Fig. 24.3

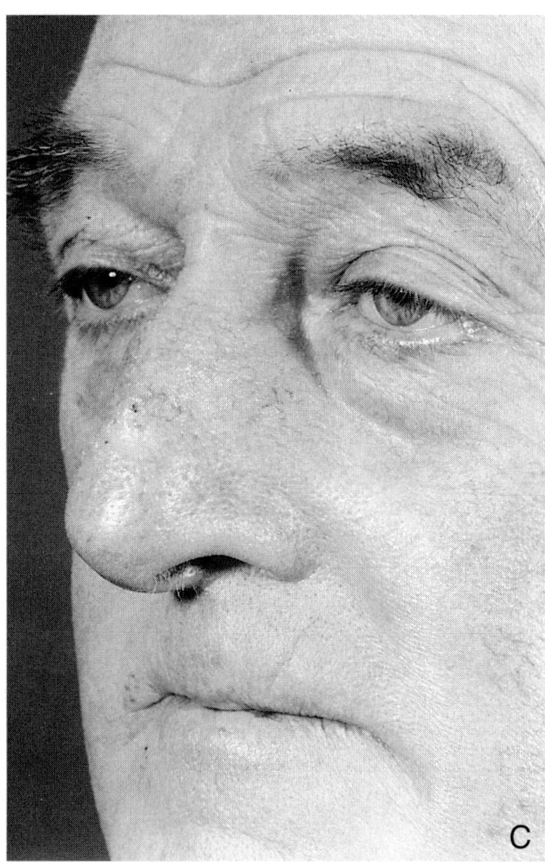

Fig. 24.3 **A.** The appearance of a keratoacanthoma with a 6-week history. **B.** Appearance 3 weeks later showing partial involution. **C.** One month later the lesion has almost totally regressed.

history which metastasizes to the regional lymph nodes. Metastasis from squamous-cell carcinomas arising in solar-damaged skin, on the other hand, is relatively infrequent (Lund 1965, Weedon 1982).

Malignant melanoma

As with basal-cell carcinoma and squamous-cell carcinoma, exposure to sunlight is widely thought to be a major factor in the aetiology of malignant melanoma. However, there is a wide disparity in incidence depending on geographical site, and the incidence is much lower in heavily pigmented races. An autosomal dominant disorder known as the 'dysplastic naevus syndrome' is associated with a high risk of developing malignant melanoma. Patients with first-degree relatives with malignant melanoma are twice as likely to develop the disease when compared with members of the general population (Woods 1989).

Unlike squamous-cell carcinoma and basal-cell carcinoma, malignant melanoma is a disease which can affect young people and can arise in congenital pigmented naevi. This is often associated with a poor prognosis (Reed et al 1965, Trozak et al 1975). Queensland, Australia, was once notorious for its high incidence of malignant melanoma in

the population (Davis et al 1976). Nowadays the incidence of malignant melanoma is found to be increasing in virtually every country where it is under investigation (Osterlind et al 1988, Glass & Hoover 1989, Magnus 1991, MacKie et al 1992).

In Scotland, the trends in malignant melanoma have been studied since 1979 when the Scottish Melanoma Group (SMG) was established. The primary aim was to gather accurate and detailed information about the mortality and incidence of malignant melanoma and relate this to clinical features, pathology and management (MacKie et al 1985). More recently the SMG has reported its findings on patients registered between January 1979 and December 1989 (MacKie et al 1992). A total of 3903 patients resident in Scotland were registered during this time, showing a progressive increase in incidence of 7.4% per year (Fig. 24.4). The 5-year survival data for 1661 patients registered between 1979 and 1984 (Table 24.1) was 71.6% (77.6% for women, 58.7% for men). The survival advantage for women persisted even when appropriate statistical adjustment was

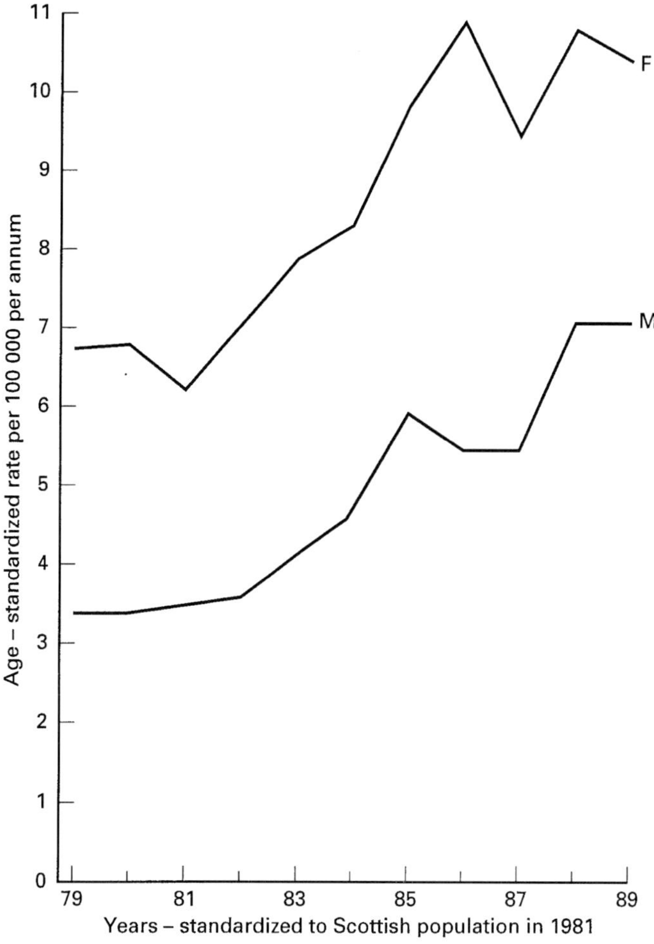

Fig. 24.4 Melanoma incidence in Scotland 1979–1989. (Reprinted from Lancet 339: 971 (1992) with permission from the publisher.)

made for thickness, ulceration and histogenetic type. Melanoma of the head and neck accounted for 25.5% of all melanomas in men and 19.7% in women.

The Scottish Melanoma Group (SMG) has adopted the following classification for malignant melanoma.

Superficial spreading melanoma (SSM)

This is the most common type of melanoma both in Scotland and in other areas of the world. It has a radial growth phase prior to developing a vertical growth phase which is clearly invasive.

Lentigo maligna melanoma (LMM)

This lesion often develops in an area of lentigo maligna (Hutchison's freckle). A true lentigo maligna, however, should not be regarded as a more benign form of melanoma. Its behaviour is identical to that of other classified melanomas when comparing thickness for thickness. The incidence of lentigo maligna melanoma in Scotland is higher than in many other areas in the world and accounts for 50% of all melanomas in the head and neck (Cox et al 1987).

Nodular melanoma (NM)

Nodular melanoma has an immediate vertical growth phase without any accompanying intra-epidermal or radial growth phase. They can therefore be fairly thick at the time of presentation and have a relatively poor prognosis.

Table 24.1   Scottish Melanoma Group survival data (1979–1984)

	Breslow thickness		
	0.1–1.49 mm	1.5–3.49 mm	>3.50 mm
Sex			
Female	95.4 (459)	77.1 (333)	52.9 (36)
Male	84.9 (172)	61.8 (149)	38.1 (199)
All	92.5	72.6	48.0
Histogenic tpye			
SSM	92.8 (448)	74.9 (253)	47.0 (146)
LMM	93.3 (117)	82.5 (53)	67.2 (41)
Nodular	88.9 (20)	68.3 (123)	49.4 (244)
Acral	92.8 (29)	54.2 (31)	34.6 (44)
Other	87.8 (17)	69.5 (22)	27.5 (40)
Site			
Face, head and neck	92.0 (152)	77.0 (89)	60.1 (114)
Trunk	88.5 (131)	65.7 (89)	36.2 (110)
Arm	97.3 (75)	70.1 (52)	58.2 (61)
Leg	94.0 (224)	79.0 (188)	55.9 (123)
Other (mucosal, subungual, palm and sole)	91.1 (46)	57.3 (63)	27.3 (106)

* Figures in parentheses are the numbers of patients in each category.

Reprinted from Lancet 339: 971 (1992) with permission from the publisher.

Acral lentiginous melanoma (ALM)

They occur on the palms of the hand or the soles of the feet and often have an irregular border. Particularly on the feet, they can be aggressive with a tendency to metastasize.

Other melanomas

This group compromises the rarer melanomas including subungual melanoma, desmoid or desmoplastic melanoma, mucosal melanomas and melanomas which are difficult to classify in a particular sub-group.

In malignant melanoma size alone is not indicative of prognosis or of the extent of surgical excision. Lentigo maligna melanoma (LMM), for example, can present as a very extensive lesion in the head and neck but on histological examination can show limited depth of invasion.

It is the thickness of the tumour and the depth of invasion that appears to correlate best with prognosis. The depth of invasion of melanoma into the dermis and subdermal tissue is the basis of the classification developed by Clark et al (1969). A more reproducible measurement of the thickness of melanomas was described by Breslow (1970) where the actual thickness of the melanoma is measured from the top of the granular layer of the epidermis to the deepest level of invasion of melanoma cells. The actual thickness of melanoma appears to correlate well with prognosis and the incidence of lymph node metastasis. The TNM classification adopted by AJCC uses a combination of Clark levels and Breslow thickness (AJCC 1980).

The importance of the thickness of melanoma in prognosis has led to a change in attitude with regard to surgical excision. Wide local excision with a minimum of 5 cm margins, as advocated by Handley (1907), and popularized by Petersen et al (1962) has given way to more tailored excisions depending on the pathological features of the melanoma. Where the tumour has a Breslow thickness of less than 0.7 mm a tumour clearance of 1 cm appears to be adequate (Breslow & Macht 1977). The effectiveness of simple excision in thin melanomas has been confirmed by other authors (Naruns et al 1986, Veronesi et al 1988, Evans & McCann 1990). The debate continues, however, as to adequate margins of excision in slightly thicker melanomas (Goldman & Byrd 1988), and there are a number of prospective randomized trials currently in progress. Balch et al (1985) has demonstrated a fall in survival rate with respect to tumour thickness which ranges from 98% for lesions of less than 0.76 mm thickness to 55% for those greater than 4 mm in thickness. This group has also shown the significance of lymph node metastasis with an overall actuarial survival for stage II disease of 28% at 5 years compared to only 8% at 2 years for stage III melanoma. Many studies have confirmed the poor prognosis in patients with regional lymph node metastasis with 5-year survival rates varying from 13% (Das Gupta 1977) to 38% (Goldsmith et al

1970). Woods (1989) believes that the presence or absence of nodal metastasis is the single most important determinant in outlook for melanoma and states that, when nodal metastases are present, patient survival may be less than half that of patients without nodal involvement. This poor prognosis has led surgeons to consider the role of elective regional node dissection (ERND). Much of the work has been done in melanomas involving the trunk and limbs, and several prospective randomized studies have failed to show any benefit (Veronesi et al 1977, Sim et al 1978). However, there remains debate as to whether ERND may prove useful for intermediate thickness lesions (Milton et al 1982, Reintgen et al 1983, O'Brien et al 1992).

In the West of Scotland it is not our practice to carry out elective regional lymph node dissections for melanoma because of the morbidity involved. Modified neck dissection to minimize morbidity has been advocated in head and neck malignant melanoma (Byers 1986) but this has rarely been justified in our experience. The problem with advocating function-preserving neck dissections for malignant melanomas in the head and neck relates to the site of the lesion and the lymphatic drainage. Lesions in the upper part of the face, particularly the temple, forehead and scalp, may well require clearance of the parotid group of lymph nodes. More posteriorly situated lesions will require clearance of the posterior triangle of the neck, and lesions involving the ear require extensive neck dissection, including excision of the postmastoid skin.

Certainly, where the nodes are clinically involved then a neck dissection is performed with frozen section confirmation of the diagnosis. The neck dissection in such cases has to be tailored to the site of the primary lesion and its lymphatic drainage.

SURGICAL MANAGEMENT

It is clear from the above discussions that there can be no hard and fast rules for excision of malignant lesions involving skin. It is advisable for the head and neck surgeon to adopt a routine when assessing patients with skin tumours to help design appropriate surgical treatment.

Clinical examination

There is no substitute for experience, and many clinicians in differing specialities are highly accurate in the clinical diagnosis of primary cutaneous malignancy. The review of basal-cell carcinoma in the West of Scotland Regional Plastic Surgery Unit (El-Sheemy 1991) showed that the diagnosis of basal-cell carcinoma was made clinically in 90.6% of cases and a biopsy was deemed necessary prior to definitive treatment in only 9.4%. Of those diagnosed purely on clinical grounds, basal-cell carcinoma was confirmed on histology in 98.2% of the cases. Less-experienced practitioners, perhaps with a lower index of suspicion, are much less accurate in their clinical diagnosis—often leading to inadequate surgical excision (Cox et al 1992).

Good lighting is an essential aid to the diagnosis of primary cutaneous lesions, and this is greatly assisted by the use of magnification, either in the form of a magnifying glass, or loupes. Stretching of the skin can sometimes help identify indistinct tumour margins. Gentle palpation is also required to determine the depth of invasion and infiltration, and palpation of the regional lymph nodes is mandatory where malignancy is suspected.

The importance of obtaining an accurate clinical history cannot be over-emphasized. The development of the lesion, time interval, exposure to sunlight and other aetiological agents, the presence of symptoms and associated diseases can all provide valuable information.

PATHOLOGICAL DIAGNOSIS

Although a histological diagnosis prior to surgical intervention may appear ideal this not always necessary or indeed desirable. Where there is a high index of clinical suspicion as to the nature of the lesion, and excision and closure can be performed with minimal disfigurement, excisional surgery is performed at a single stage. When malignant melanoma is suspected, an excisional biopsy is always carried out. Such treatment is often curative, but should the histological report show incomplete excision or pathology that warrants further surgical treatment the initial procedure is regarded as if it were an incisional biopsy.

Incompletely excised basal-cell carcinoma, for example, or evidence of perineural spread from a malignant skin tumour or an unsuspected pathological diagnosis or malignant melanoma where the thickness of the tumour is greater than was expected, all warrant secondary definitive excisional surgery.

Incisional biopsy as a diagnostic aid prior to definitive surgical treatment is reserved for cases where the clinical diagnosis is in doubt or where excision of the tumour may well require major reconstruction. Alternatively, frozen section diagnosis can be obtained at the time of excisional surgery.

SPECIAL INVESTIGATIONS

Extensive skin tumours and cases in which there is skin involvement from underlying neoplasms warrant more detailed investigation of the head and neck, including X-rays, CT scans and MRI scans where appropriate (Fig. 24.5). Lesions with a known propensity to metastasize should also have a routine clinical work-up, including chest X-ray and, where appropriate, abdominal ultrasound or MRI scan. As a general rule, the more major the surgery proposed as a form of treatment the more essential it is to ensure that there is no gross evidence of metastatic disease which would negate the effects of radical surgery. The rare instances of

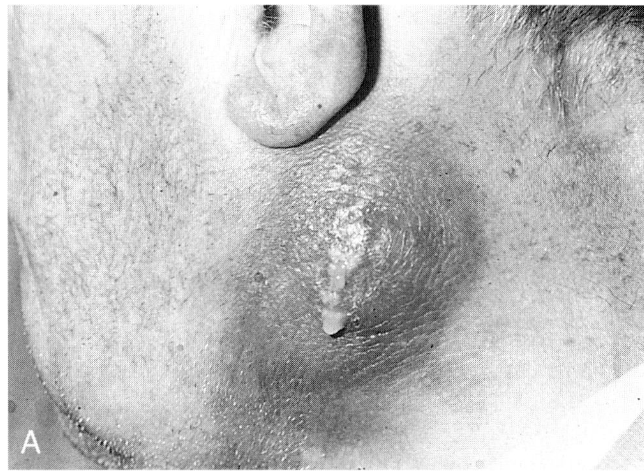

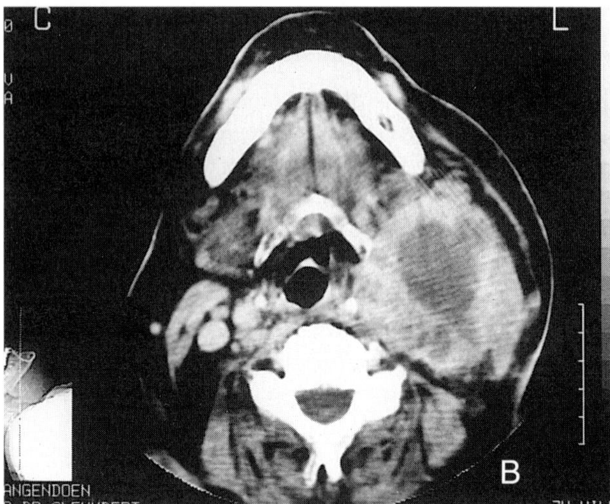

Fig. 24.5   A. Neck node metastasis from a head and neck primary involving the superficial skin (N3). **B.** CT scan showing extent of extracapsular invasion with evidence of central necrosis.

metastatic disease affecting the skin of the head and neck may well require special investigations to hunt for the primary following histological diagnosis of the cutaneous deposit.

EXCISION

As mentioned previously, many superficial skin tumours can be curatively excised and the defect either closed directly or a simple method of reconstruction used without the necessity to embark on any detailed pre-operative investigations. More complicated lesions with indistinct margins or in areas of damaged tissue, or recurrent tumours, or large tumours may well require a different approach. Where the aim is to excise the tumour totally it is mandatory that this be completed prior to reconstruction. On the other hand, there are cases where no attempt is made to excise the

tumour totally, and a major reconstruction is performed. This is usually in patients who present with foul-smelling ulcerated painful lesions and palliative surgery is carried out to improve the quality of life.

In the majority of cases, however, the surgeon is aiming for complete excision of the tumour. In the United States, many surgeons have adopted the policy of obtaining confirmation of tumour clearance in the operating room. The initial stimulus for this arose from the work of Mohs (1941) who originally described a multi-staged technique which proved a very effective method for dealing with difficult tumours (Robins 1981). Mohs' idea of horizontal sections was subsequently used in frozen section diagnosis (Tromovitch & Stegman 1974, Swanson & Taylor 1982) and has proved a major advance. Traditional frozen section analysis of tumour margin clearance has the disadvantage of tumour sampling since only 0.1% of the surgical margins are examined when the tissue is sampled vertically (Davidson et al 1984). The horizontal section allows the whole specimen, particularly the base of excision and its lateral margins, to be examined and, to a certain extent, diminishes the problems associated with sampling error. One major problem of using frozen section diagnosis as an immediate method of estimating tumour clearance is that it is suitable only for soft tissue and that any bone or cartilage excision has to await formal histology on the fixed specimen. McGregor & McGregor (1986) have pointed out the dangers of using frozen section as an excuse for cheese-paring surgery or as a scapegoat when recurrence appears. Perhaps the major disadvantage of frozen section when used to assess tumour clearance, especially when multiple biopsies are taken, is that this can add significantly to the operating time.

In the United Kingdom there has been less use of frozen section and a greater reliance placed on histological examination of the fixed specimen. In difficult cases it is the practice of one of the authors (DSS) to excise the lesion completely according to clinical examination and seal off the wound with a vaseline gauze pack and await the full report from the fixed histological specimen. These reports can usually be obtained within a matter of days and the patient at the second operation undergoes either further excision, if deemed necessary, or reconstruction. Although this may require several operations, the excisional operations are generally short and there is minimal wastage of operating time. This technique also allows full histological examination of both soft and hard tissue and minimizes sampling errors associated with frozen section. The technique, however, is suitable only where vital structures—such as major vessels and nerves—are not exposed as a result of the excision. In these cases, reliance has to be placed on frozen section clearance since immediate reconstruction is mandatory to protect these vital structures.

One further technique that is available to the surgeon is to use a temporary method of wound closure such as a split-thickness skin graft, leaving all available tissues intact for secondary reconstruction. Such reconstruction can be delayed for several months to ensure that there is no recurrence of disease.

The surgical management of tumours involving the skin therefore demands planning of both surgical excision and reconstruction. Ideally, the histopathological diagnosis should be established and the tumour staged on clinical grounds. Clinical staging furnishes the surgeon with information about the size and depth of infiltration as well as the possibility of regional spread and distant metastasis. For the same TNM staging the extent of excision varies with the histopathology of the tumour and the anatomical site of the lesion. It is clear that one can extend to the upper limits of excision, where ample tissue is available, but may need to stay within the lower limits where more radical excision would sacrifice more vital structures and impose serious disability or disfigurement. Wherever doubt exists as to the radicality of excision, frozen section can be employed or reconstruction delayed. It is vital to mark specimens clearly for proper orientation by the histopathologist. The same applies when skin excision is part of a larger specimen as, for example, after neck dissection for N3 neck node metastasis or when skin excision accompanies excision of an organ such as larynx or trachea as in the case of extensive laryngeal cancer or a stomal recurrence.

RECONSTRUCTION

The ideal reconstruction should provide an adequate amount of the correct type of tissue or tissues with a good colour and texture match of the skin and minimum morbidity. Unfortunately, as mentioned previously, the head and neck is made up of a variety of different types of skin and subcutaneous tissue and it is often not possible to reconstruct like with like. However, there are a wide variety of methods that are available for reconstructing soft-tissue defects in the head and neck.

Skin grafts

Split-thickness skin grafts do not provide the necessary thickness, colour or texture match and their use is therefore restricted. They may be used as previously mentioned as a temporary measure or, in elderly patients, as a simple method of reconstruction. Because of the tendency of split-thickness skin grafts to contract they are most useful when applied over fixed surfaces—such as the forehead and scalp where they can give satisfactory results in the elderly patient.

Full-thickness grafts can be used at specific sites in the face to good effect. Skin defects of the lower eyelid, for example, can often be reconstructed using a full-thickness graft obtained from the upper eyelid, and this provides an excellent colour and texture match. The postauricular Wolfe graft can provide a good colour and texture match but is sometimes rather thin for some defects. An alternative is to use a pre-auricular full-thickness skin graft which is somewhat thicker. The supraclavicular skin similarly provides a good colour match where a larger amount of skin is required.

Local skin flaps

There are a wide variety of local skin flaps available, some of which have been mentioned in other chapters (see Chs 2, 9 and 18). Local flaps often provide the best colour and texture match for reconstruction in the face. It is important to remember when designing local flaps that the incisions must be maintained as far as is possible in the lines of election so that scarring is kept to a minimum. It is not within the remit of this chapter to identify all the possibilities in local flap design and usage, as this subject is dealt with in other texts. However, there are two local skin flaps which are used for larger defects and are worth considering. The first is the superiorly based or laterally based cheek flap, sometimes known as the cervico-facial flap (Kaplan & Goldwyn 1978). This flap allows elevation of the whole of the cheek via an incision in the nasolabial crease extending down into the neck. It is supplied by branches arising from the facial artery and is designed as a rotation flap utilizing the laxity of the skin in the neck (Fig. 24.6). This flap is extremely useful in dealing with large defects of the cheek, including exenteration, and the flap will rotate up to the level of the eyebrow. The second flap, the cervico-occipital flap, has recently been described for the specific purpose of resurfacing large areas of cervical skin after surgery for head and neck cancer (Tiwari 1988, 1991). The flap makes use of the skin of the scalp as a paddle based on the nape of the neck (Fig. 24.7). The nape of the neck is supplied by musculocutaneous perforators from the deep cervical artery (Taylor & Palmer 1987). The deep cervical artery is a branch of the costocervical trunk which is a branch of the second part of the subclavian artery. After its origin it runs between the transversus process of the seventh cervical vertebra and the neck of the first rib. From here, the artery runs between the semispinalis capitis and cervicis muscles deep to the scalenes and anastomoses with the descending branch of the occipital artery. Because of its protected course, the deep cervical artery is not encountered in a neck dissection and is safe. The dermal–subdermal plexus of the skin of the nape of the neck and the scalp is in continuity, and skin of the occipital parietal region can survive even when the occipital artery is ligated. This provides the anatomical basis for the cervico-occipital flap.

To raise this flap, an incision is made in the retro-auricular sulcus and extended superiorly over the cranium. The base of the flap is located at the junction of the nape of the neck and the scalp. The required length of the flap is therefore measured cranially from this point and may extend up to the occipital parietal suture depending upon the required length. The breadth of the flap is from the

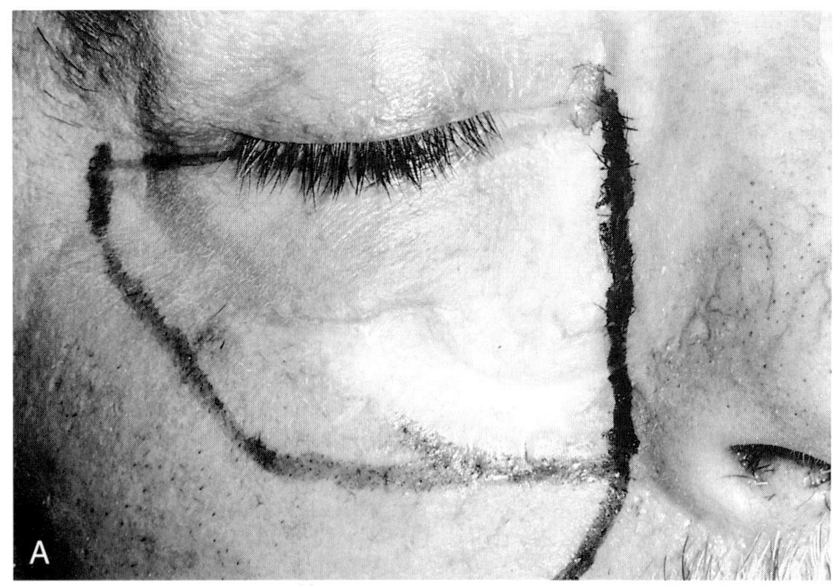

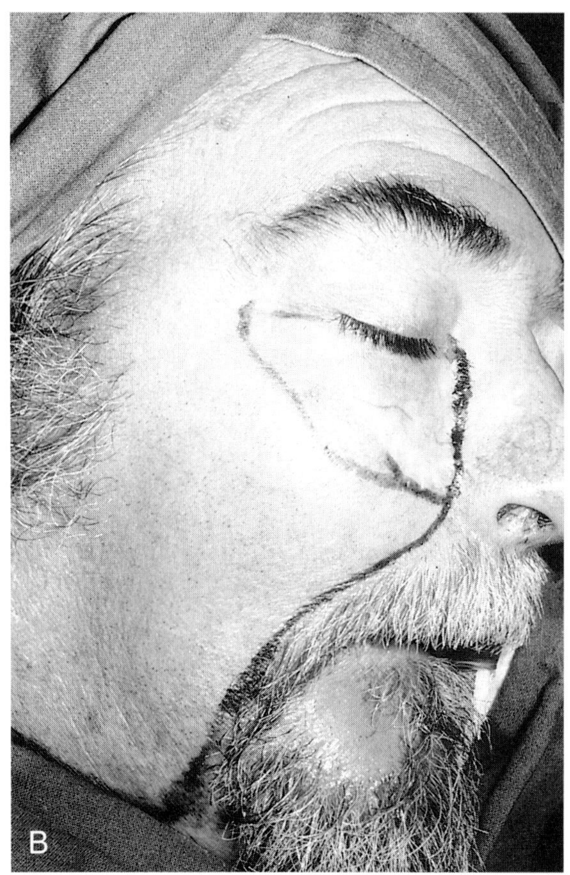

Fig. 24.6

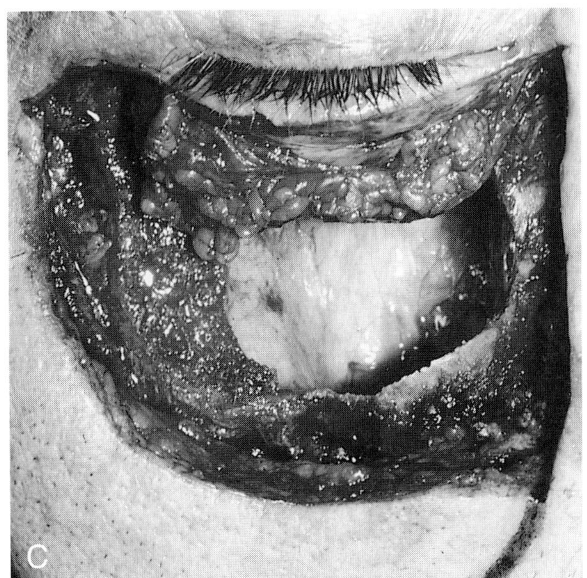
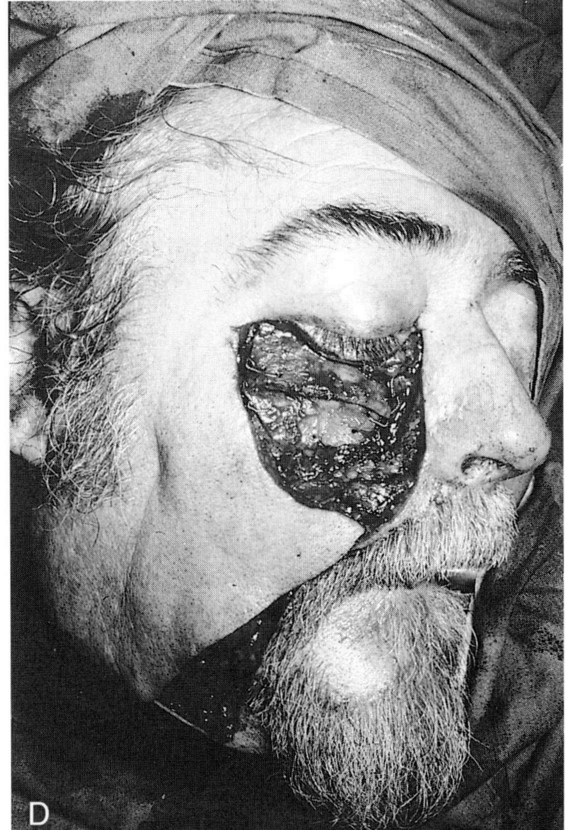
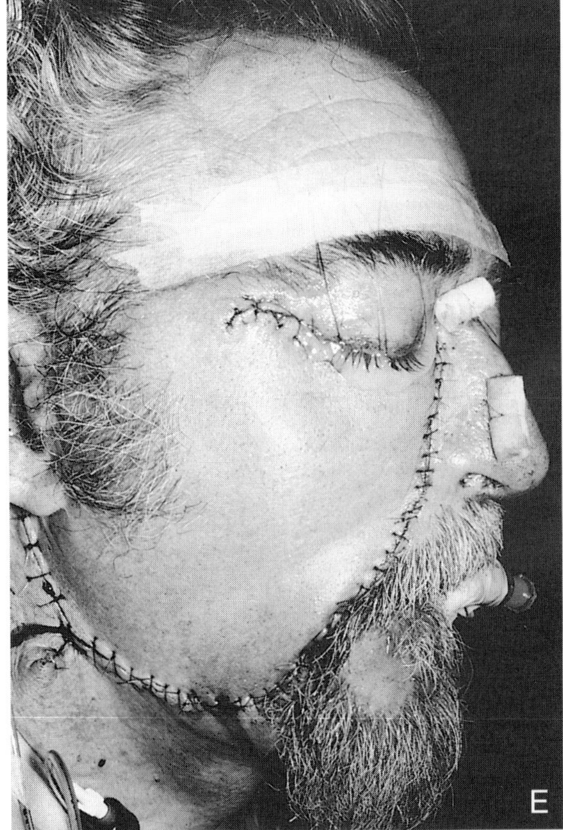
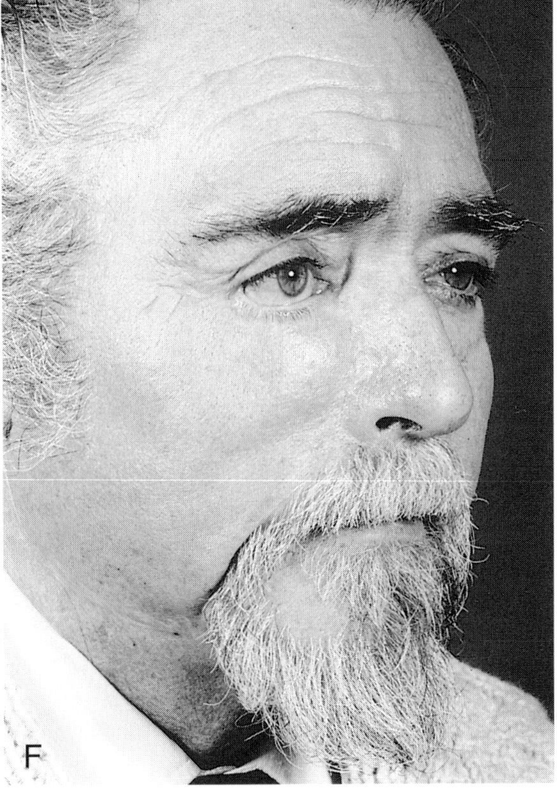

Fig. 24.6 **A.** Recurrent basal-cell carinoma presenting in a skin graft.
B. A wide radical excision is outlined with a cervico-facial flap for
reconstruction. **C.** Excision involved the anterior wall of the maxilla
and floor of orbit. **D.** The maxilla and floor of orbit were reconstructed
with rib grafts. **E.** Cervico-facial flap is transposed and all wounds
closed directly. **F.** The appearance at 5 years postoperatively is shown.
The patient remains disease-free 10 years following surgery.

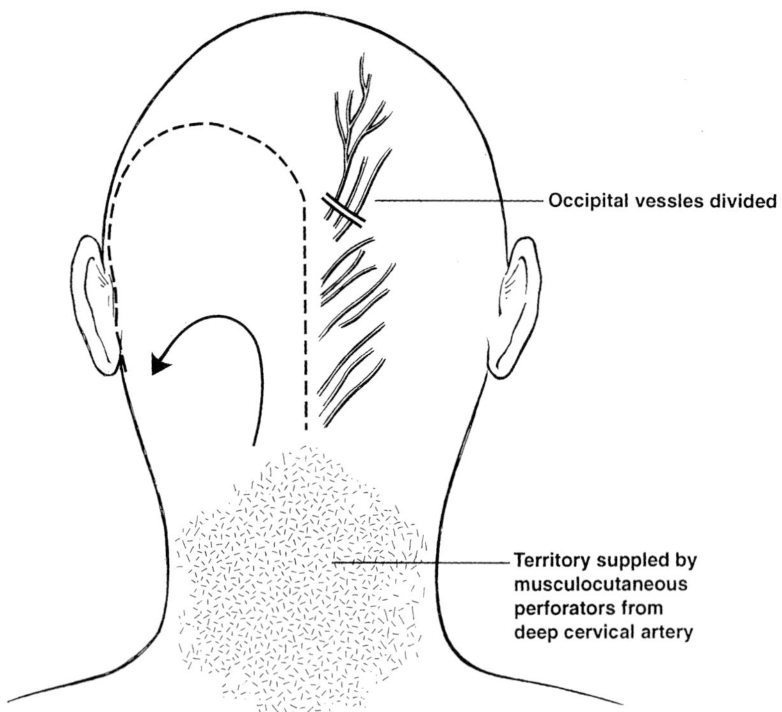

Fig. 24.7   Surgical anatomy of the cervico-occipital flap. (Reproduced with kind permission of B C Decker, Philadelphia, from Plastic and Reconstructive Surgery of the Head and Neck (Proceedings of the Fifth International Symposium)

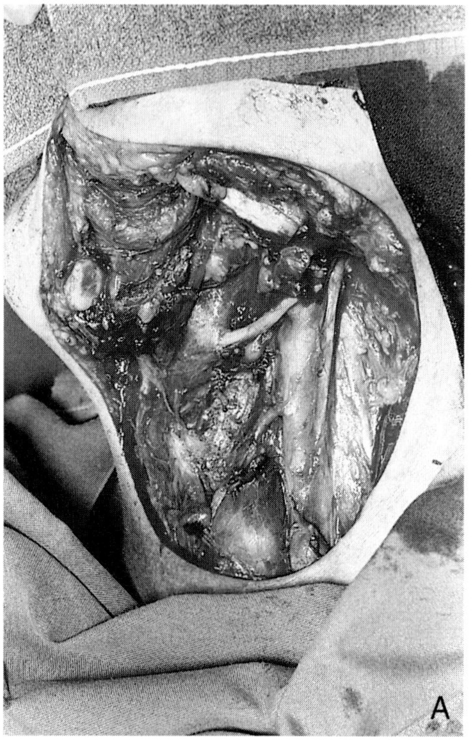
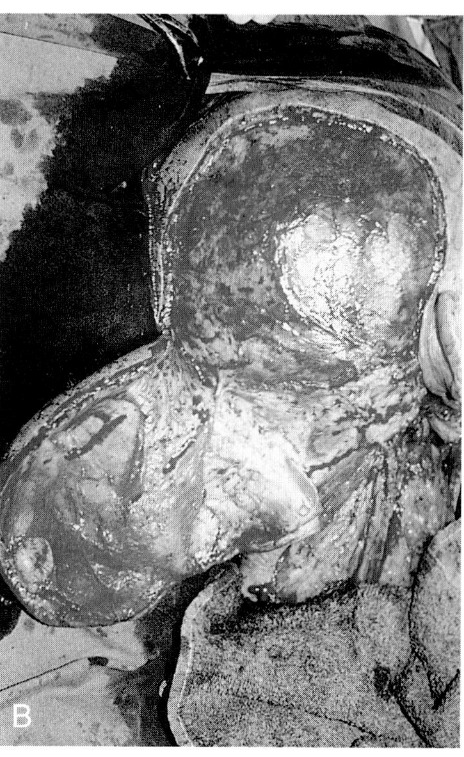

Fig. 24.8

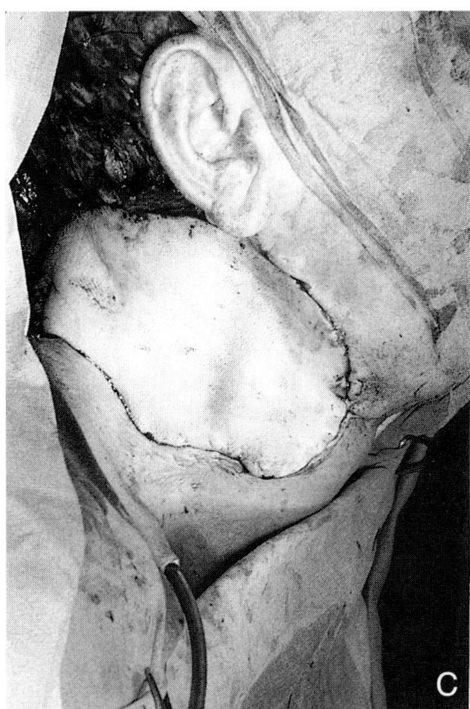

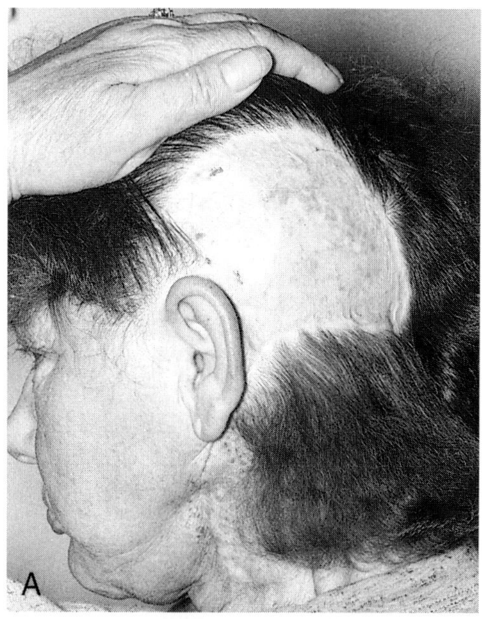

Fig. 24.8 A. Defect following a radical neck dissection with sacrifice of the overlying irradiated skin. **B, C.** A cervico-occipital flap is raised and transposed to cover the defect.

postauricular sulcus to the mid-line and may be extended beyond this point. The flap can be extended superiorly but it is important to leave its attachment to the nape of the neck untouched. The pericranium is preserved and the flap is harvested between the pericranium and the galea. Laterally, it may encroach on the temporal area where it is harvested superficial to the temporal fascia. The occipital artery is ligated and divided allowing the flap the necessary mobility to be rotated laterally into the defect (Fig. 24.8).

The donor area is skin grafted and is concealed by hair growth (Fig. 24.9). The flap provides the correct thickness required for reconstructing defects in the neck. The galea, in addition, provides an excellent thin layer of muscular aponeurosis to protect vessels and nerves. Healing by primary intention is the rule, and this is very helpful since these individuals often require postoperative radiotherapy which must commence within 6 weeks of surgery (Vikram et al 1984). The presence of hair on the flap is at first sight a drawback, but following radiotherapy this does not pose any problem. As a result, the flap can safely be used in women as well as men.

Basic research continues on the viability and design of local skin flaps. In designing skin flaps, attention must be paid to their retraction if tension and subsequent complications are to be avoided. The experiments of Stell, both on animals and humans, showed that flaps perpendicular to tension lines do not retract, whereas flaps parallel to these lines retract as much as 30% (Stell 1980). The increased risk

of flap survival in irradiated tissues has been well documented, and a complication rate up to 43% has been reported (Rudolph 1982). Surgical delay seems to increase the chance of survival of such flaps (Fischer et al 1984). There is also experimental evidence that smoking has a detrimental effect on flap survival (Reus et al 1984, Nolan et al 1985).

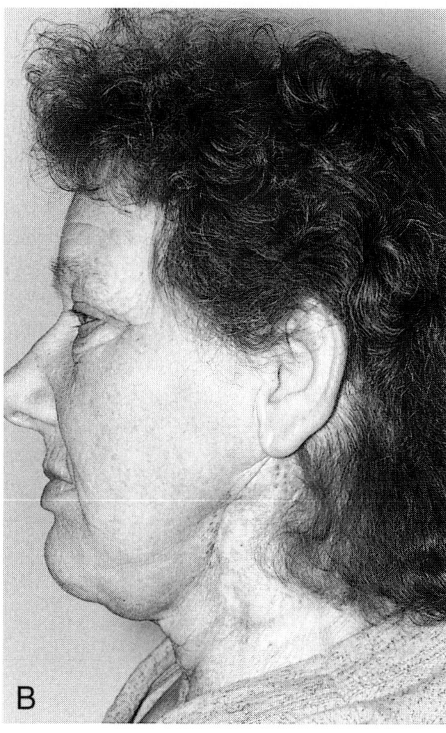

Fig. 24.9 A. A patient 4 years following reconstruction using a cervico-occipital flap showing the defect which has been skin grafted. **B.** The normal growth of hair adequately covers the secondary defect.

The introduction of controlled tissue expansion has been a significant step in reconstructive surgery (Argenta 1984). However, the use of tissue expansion in cancer reconstruction is limited because it is often preferable to carry out an immediate—and preferably one-stage—method of reconstruction. However, tissue expansion can be used to effect in secondary reconstruction to provide a better colour and texture match for facial reconstruction.

Regional flaps

The deltopectoral flap described by Bakamjian (1965) has been used for over two decades. It provides excellent colour, texture and thickness match for defects in the cervical skin. It can also be used in lateral cheek defects overlying the parotid area. In the neck, it can sometimes be used as a single-stage procedure. For defects more cranially a two-stage procedure is required and the donor defect skin grafted. The deltopectoral flap will satisfactorily reach defects only up to the level of the zygomatic arch and there remains a significant complication and failure rate (Krizek & Robson 1972, Mendelson et al 1977, Gilas et al 1986). Friedman applied the concept of a bilobed flap to prevent the sacrifice of vessels to the supraclavicular area (Friedman et al 1987). This provides a good alternative for replacement of cervical skin loss.

The advent of myocutaneous flaps has increased the role of regional flaps in cervical facial reconstruction (Fig. 24.10). The pectoralis major myocutaneous flap (Ariyan 1979) has been extensively used in the last decade. It is a reliable flap with a dependable blood supply and provides a muscle layer as well as skin coverage. However, there are several drawbacks to this flap when applied to resurfacing cervical defects (Schuller 1980). This flap is best used in combination with a neck dissection and is rarely indicated for reconstructing defects where the neck has not been entered. Although the muscle tissue of the flap atrophies, the fatty tissue does not and is often too thick, and under the influence of gravity it can sometimes cause an unsightly deformity. Secondary debulking is therefore often necessary. To overcome this problem a pectoralis major muscle flap with a split skin graft on the outer surface can be used. This can give a very satisfactory appearance in the neck but cannot be used in facial reconstruction because of the poor texture match and the paucity of muscle at this level. The pectoralis major myocutaneous flap will extend to above the zygomatic arch but becomes less reliable for reconstructing more cranial defects. The scar on the chest wall, however concealed, may create physical and psychological problems— especially in women, and the colour match of the skin is not ideal.

The trapezius myocutaneous flap is not usually a first choice for reconstruction of cervical defects since the position of the patient may require to be changed on the operating table. However, it is a versatile flap and can be

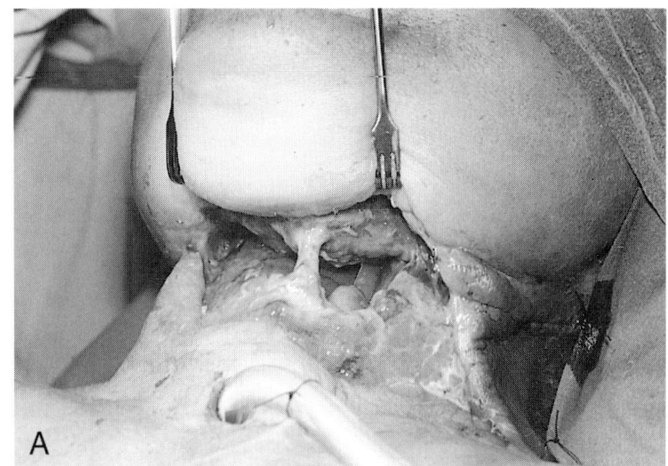

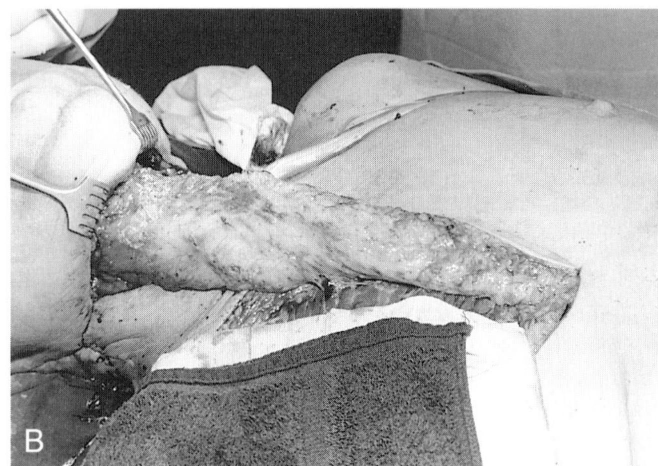

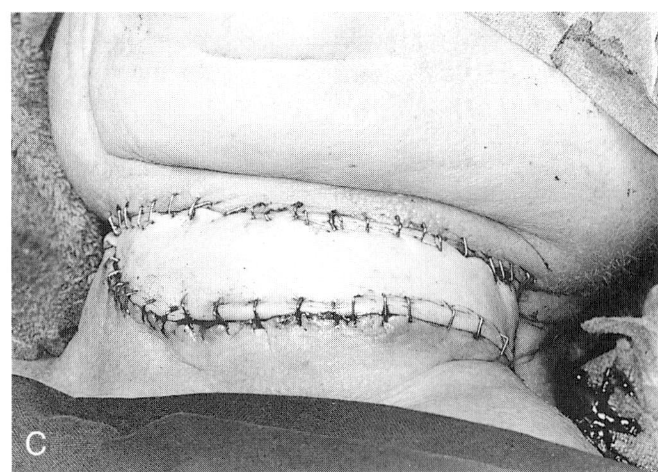

Fig. 24.10 A. A through and through defect of the pharynx following breakdown of a supraglottic laryngectomy. **B.** The inner lining is created with a deltopectoral flap in two stages. **C.** External skin cover is obtained using a pectoralis major myocutaneous flap.

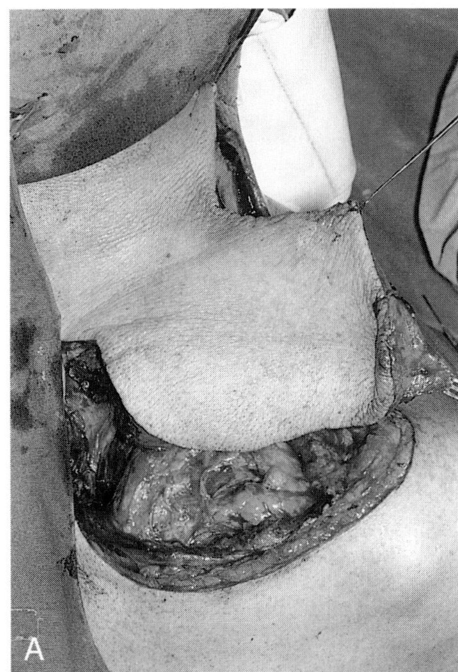

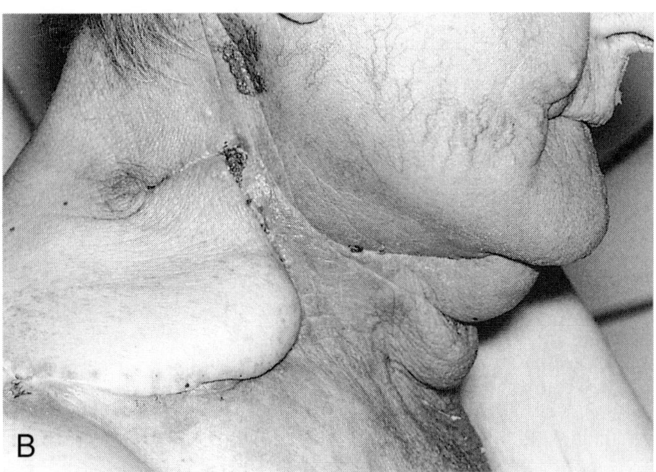

Fig. 24.11 **A.** A lateral trapezius flap from the shoulder is prepared and transposed to cover a defect in the anterior supraclavicular area (**B**).

used in a variety of ways because of its vascular anatomy (Demergasso & Piazza 1979, Guillamondegui & Larson 1981, Netterwille et al 1987). The most useful flap is the lateral trapezius myocutaneous island flap (Fig. 24.11) based on the transverse cervical artery and vein. This has been used effectively for reconstructing defects in the anterior part of the neck almost up to the mid-line (Tiwari & Snow 1983). It has an excellent arc of rotation, but care should be exercised to avoid kinking of the vessels. The vein is the more delicate of the two vessels and there is some variability in the vascular pedicle. In a small percentage of

cases (4%) the vessels run deep to the brachial plexus in which case the flap cannot be used. The donor area is either closed primarily or grafted with split skin. This flap usually does not require a change in the position of the patient on the operating table. The second most useful trapezius flap is the lower myocutaneous island flap which is based on the descending branch of the transverse cervical artery. This flap can turn 180° and is useful particularly for posterior defects of the skull and nape of neck and also for lateral defects of the cheek.

The latissimus dorsi myocutaneous flap is another large musculocutaneous flap which is available for head and neck reconstruction. It is not a technique favoured by the authors, primarily because of the difficulty of bringing this bulky flap into the head and neck region. To avoid stretching the pedicle it is best to bring this flap under the clavicle, but, because of the bulk, this is often extremely difficult. Although the muscle atrophies, the skin and subcutaneous tissue is too thick for cervical or facial reconstruction. It provides a large volume of tissue but is more useful as a free flap rather than a pedicled flap in head and neck reconstruction (Fig. 24.12).

One further myocutaneous flap which does provide a good colour match is the platysma island musculocutaneous flap (Futrell et al 1978). The situation of the donor site in the neck, however, excludes its use in irradiated patients (Coleman et al 1982). Furthermore, it is not oncologically safe to enter the cervical tissues in patients with head and neck cancer, and the platysma island musculocutaneous flap is of only limited use in specially selected cases.

The major problem with pedicled flaps, whether cutaneous or myocutaneous, is that vital tissue is often wasted in the pedicle and not used primarily to reconstruct the defect. The myocutaneous flaps in particular have a problem of gaining access to the defect unless a neck dissection or radical exposure of the neck is performed. A further disadvantage of most pedicled flaps lies in their inability to reach cranially beyond the zygomatic arch with safety and reliability. With the increasing reliability of microvascular surgical techniques there have opened up new possibilities in soft-tissue reconstruction in the head and neck.

Microvascular free flaps

There is now a wide variety of donor sites available for free tissue transfer offering different types of tissue with regard to colour, texture and thickness. This tissue can be used to reconstruct defects in isolation without the necessity of opening up planes of dissection—such as the neck—to allow access for pedicled flaps. They have the great advantage of being able to be placed anywhere in the head and neck, particularly to reconstruct defects above the zygomatic arches beyond the reach of pedicled flaps. One of the most consistently reliable and useful free flaps in reconstruction of the cervical skin has proved to be the radial forearm flap

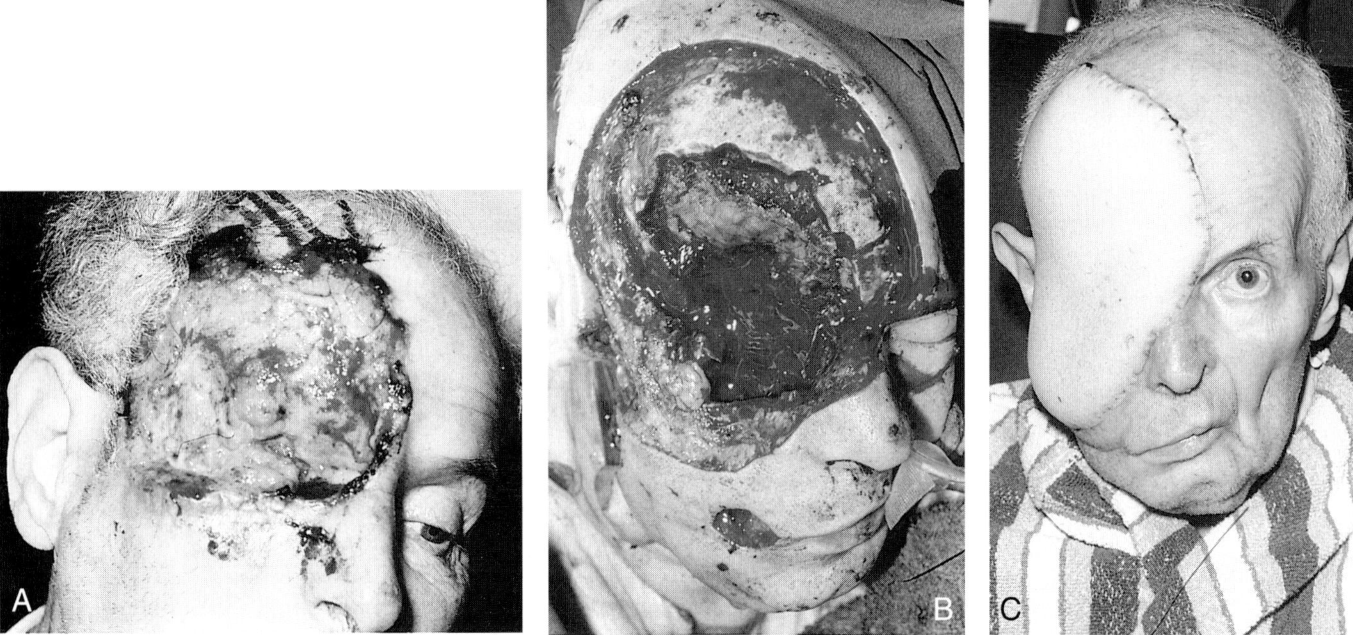

Fig. 24.12 **A.** An extensive basal-cell carcinoma involving the orbital and frontal areas. **B.** Defect following radical excision resulting in exposure of the dura and a direct communication with the oro and nasopharynx. **C.** A latissimus dorsi myocutaneous flap was used to reconstruct the defect to allow skin closure and obliterate the cavity and protect the brain from ascending infection.

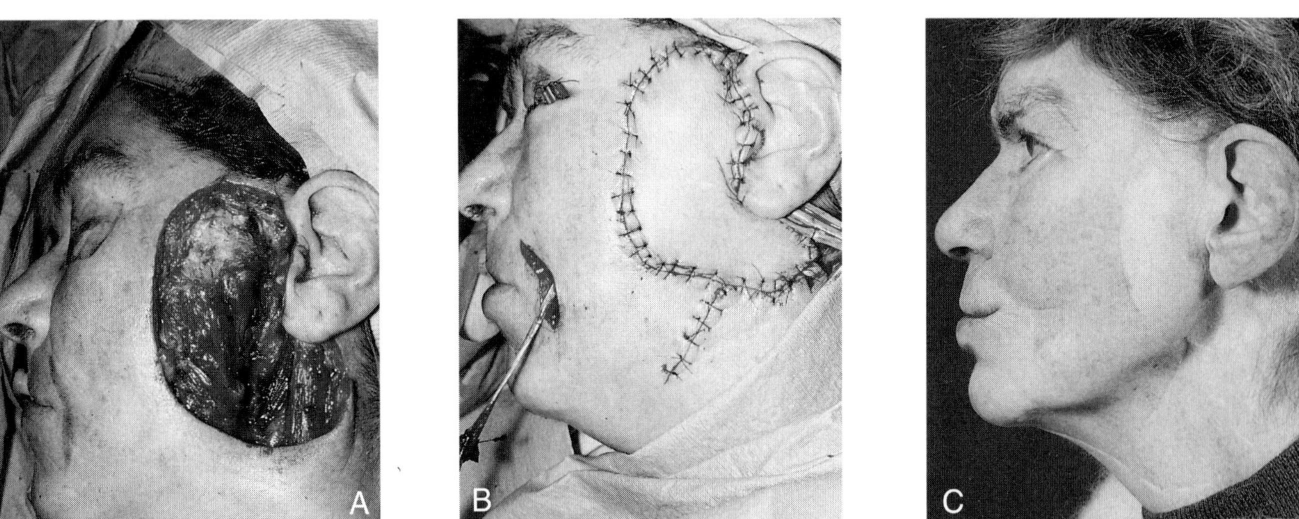

Fig. 24.13 **A.** A radical parotidectomy has been performed including facial musculature and overlying skin. **B.** A free radial forearm flap incorporating a vascularized palmaris longus tendon was used for reconstruction. The tendon provided a reconstructive sling for the oral cavity. A lateral tarsorrhaphy has also been performed. **C.** The patient underwent radical postoperative radiotherapy and the appearance at 5 years postoperatively is shown. The patient remains disease free at 8 years. The angle of the mouth has been retained in a good position, and oral competence is maintained. (See also colour plate section.)

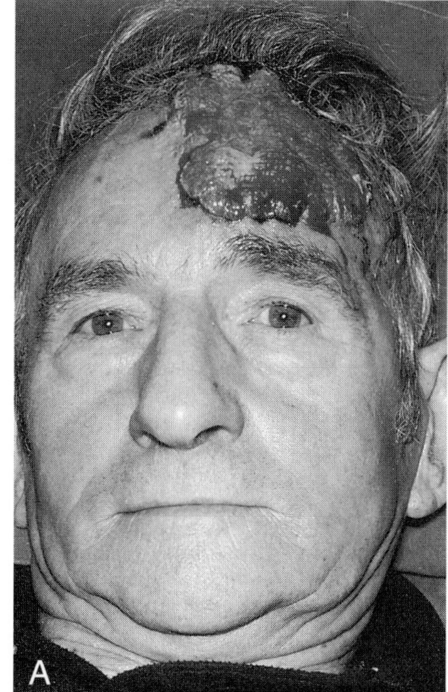

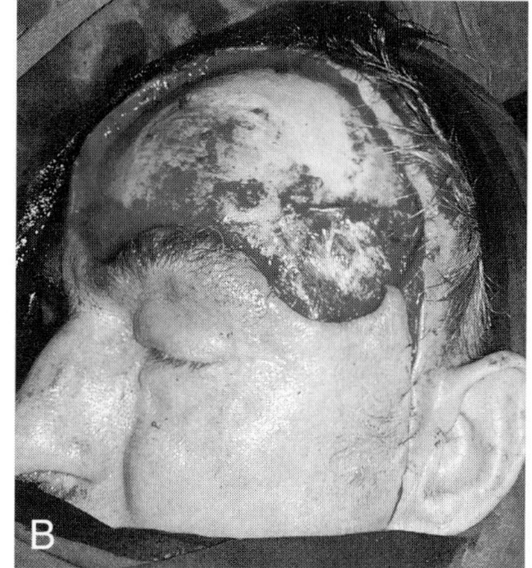

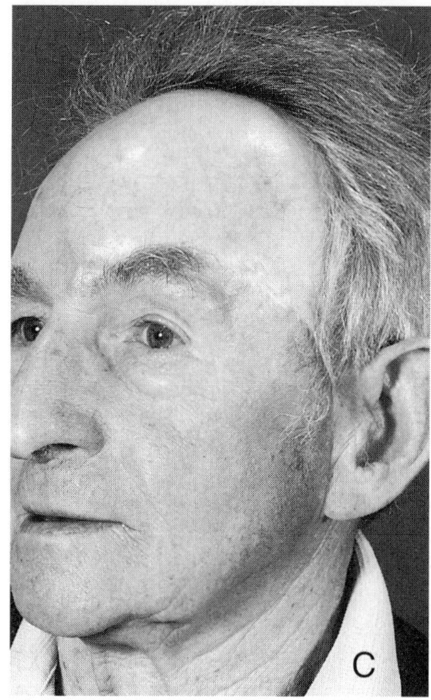

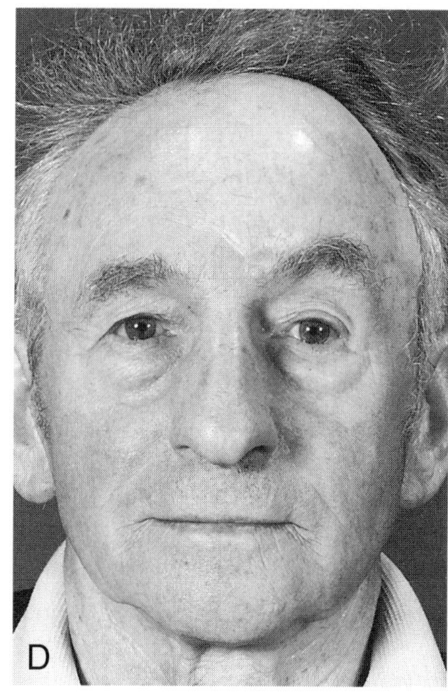

Fig. 24.14 A. A metatypical basal-cell carcinoma of the forehead in a patient aged over 70 years. **B.** Excision involved removal of the periosteum and exposure of bare cranial bone. **C, D.** The appearance following reconstruction with a scapular flap which required one thinning procedure. The patient remains alive and free of disease 8 years following surgery. Contour has been satisfactorily achieved, but the colour and texture of the skin are not ideal. (See also colour plate section.)

(Yang et al 1981, Song et al 1982). The flap provides a good texture and thickness match for both cervical skin and cheek skin (Fig. 24.13).

Free flaps can now be tailored very accurately to suit individual defects, but skin colour and texture match remain the major problem (Fig. 24.14). In experienced centres microvascular free tissue transfer is very competitive with pedicled techniques, reporting equal success rates in excess of 90%.

Free tissue transfer using microvascular techniques, however, becomes the first method of choice in very complex reconstructions. Such free flaps can allow greater freedom with regard to both excision and reconstruction (see Ch. 26).

REFERENCES

American Joint Committee on Cancer 1980 Staging of cancer of head and neck sites and of melanoma. p 51.

Argenta L C 1984 Controlled tissue expansion in reconstructive surgery. British Journal of Plastic Surgery 37: 520

Ariyan S 1979 The pectoralis major myocutaneous flap: a versatile flap for reconstruction in the head and neck. Plastic and Reconstructive Surgery 63: 73

Bakamjian V Y 1965 A two-stage method for pharyngo-oesophageal reconstruction with a primary pectoral skin flap. Plastic and Reconstructive Surgery 36: 173

Balch C M, Urist M M, Maddox W A et al 1985 Melanoma in the southern United States: experience at the University of Alabama in Birmingham. In: Balch C M, Milton G W (eds) Cutaneous melanoma: clinical management and treatment results worldwide. J B Lippincott, Philadelphia, p 397

Breslow A 1970 Thickness, cross-section areas and depth of invasion in the prognosis of cutaneous melanoma. Annals of Surgery 172: 902

Breslow A, Macht S D 1977 Optimal size of resection margin for thin cutaneous melanoma. Surgery, Gynecology and Obstetrics 145: 691

Byers R M 1986 The role of modified neck dissection in the treatment of cutaneous melanoma of the head and neck. Archives of Surgery 121: 1338

Clark W H, From L, Bernardino E A et al 1969 The histogenesis and biologic behaviour of primary human malignant melanoma of the skin. Cancer Research 29: 705

Coleman J J, Nahai F, Mathes S J 1982 Platysma musculocutaneous flap. Clinical and anatomic considerations in head and neck reconstruction. American Journal of Surgery 144: 477

Cox N H, Jones S K, MacKie R M 1987 Malignant melanoma of the head and neck in Scotland: an eight year analysis of trends in prevalance, distribution and prognosis. Quarterly Journal of Medicine, New Series 64 244: 661

Cox N J, Wagstaff R, Popple A W 1992 Using clinical pathological analysis of general practitioner skin surgery to determine educational requirements and guidelines. British Medical Journal 304: 93

Cranmer C, Raingold I M, Wilson J W 1970 Basal cell carcinoma of skin metastatic to bone. Archives of Dermatology 102: 337

Das Gupta T K 1977 Results of treatment of 269 patients with primary cutaneous melanoma. A five year prospective study. Annals of Surgery 186: 201

Davidson T M, Nahum A M, Haghighi P et al 1984 The biopsy of head and neck skin cancer. Archives of Otolaryngology 11: 193

Davis N C, McLeod E R, Beardmore G L et al 1976 Primary cutaneous melanoma. A report from the Queensland melanoma project. Cancer 26: 80

Dellon A L, De Silva S, Connelly M, Ross A 1985 Prediction of recurrence in incompletely excised basal cell carcinoma. Plastic and Reconstructive Surgery 75: 860

Demergasso F, Piazza N 1979 Trapezius myocutaneous flap in reconstructive surgery for head and neck cancer: an original technique. American Journal of Surgery 138: 533

El-Sheemy M A 1991 The surgical management of basal cell carcinoma: an analysis of 563 lesions. MSc thesis, Glasgow University

Emmett A J J, Broadbent G 1981 Basal cell carcinoma in Queensland. Australia and New Zealand Journal of Surgery 51: 576

Emmett A J J, O'Rourke O (eds) 1991 Malignant skin tumours, 2nd edn. Churchill Livingstone, Edinburgh

Evans J, McCann B G 1990 A new protocol for the treatment of stage I cutaneous malignant melanoma: interim results of the first 806 patients treated. British Journal of Plastic Surgery 43: 426

Fischer J C, Hurn I, Rudolph R et al 1984 The effect of delay on flap survival in an irradiated field. Plastic and Reconstructive Surgery 73: 99–102

Friedman M, Toriumi D M, Grybauskas V 1987 The bilobed deltopectoral advancement flap. Archives of Otolaryngology Head and Neck Surgery 113: 612

Futrell J W, Johns M E, Edgerton M T et al 1978 Platysma myocutaneous flap for intraoral reconstruction. American Journal of Surgery 136: 504

Gilas T, Sako K, Razack M et al 1986 Head and neck reconstruction with deltopectoral flaps. American Journal of Surgery 152: 430

Glass A E, Hoover R N 1989 The emerging epidemic of melanoma and squamous cell cancer. Jama 262: 2097

Goepfert H, Dichtel W J, Medina J E et al 1984 Perineural invasion in squamous cell skin carcinoma of the head and neck. American Journal of Surgery 148: 542

Goldberg L, Stall S, Spira M 1983 Recognition and treatment of recurrent basal cell carcinoma. Annals of Plastic Surgery 11: 313

Goldman L I, Byrd R 1988 Narrowing resection margins for patients with low risk melanoma. Surgery 155: 242

Goldsmith H S, Shah J P, Kim D H 1970 Prognostic significance of lymph node dissection in the treatment of malignant melanoma. Cancer 26: 606

Gooding C A, White G, Yatsuhasi M 1965 Significance of marginal extension in excised basal cell carcinoma. New England Journal of Medicine 273: 923

Guillamondegui O M, Larson D L 1981 The lateral trapezius musculocutaneous flap: its use in head and neck reconstruction. Plastic and Reconstructive Surgery 67: 143

Handley W S 1907 The pathology of melanotic growths in relation to their operative treatment. Lancet 1: 927, 996

Hardie I R, Strong R W, Hartley L C J et al 1980 Skin cancer in caucasian renal allograft recipients living in a subtropical climate. Surgery 87: 177

Harris T J 1976 Skin cancer in sunny Queensland. British Journal of Plastic Surgery 29: 61

Hauben D J, Zirkin H, Mahler D et al 1982 Biological behaviour of basal cell carcinoma. Plastic and Reconstructive Surgery 69: 103

Hayes H 1962 Basal cell carcinoma. The East Grinstead experience. Plastic and Reconstructive Surgery 30: 273

Kaplan I, Goldwyn R M 1978 The versatility of the laterally based cervicofacial flap for cheek repairs. Plastic and Reconstructive Surgery 61: 390

Koplin L, Zarem H A 1980 Recurrent basal cell carcinoma. Plastic and Reconstructive Surgery 65: 656

Krizek T J, Robson M C 1972 Potential pitfalls in the use of the deltopectoral flap. Plastic and Reconstructive Surgery 50: 326

Lund H Z 1965 How often does squamous cell carcinoma of the skin metastasise? Archives of Dermatology 92: 635

McGregor I A, McGregor F M 1986 The skin of the face. In: McGregor I A, McGregor F M (eds) Cancer of the face and mouth. Churchill Livingstone, Edinburgh

MacKie R M, Smyth J F, Soutar D S et al 1985 Malignant melanoma in Scotland 1979 to 1983. Lancet ii: 859

MacKie R M, Hunter J A A, Aitchison T C et al 1992 Cutaneous malignant melanoma, Scotland, 1979 to 1989. Lancet 339: 971

Magnus K 1991 The nordic profile of skin cancer incidence. A comparative epidemiological study of the three main types of skin cancer. International Journal of Cancer 47: 12

Mendelson B C, Woods J E, Masson J K 1977 Experiences with the deltopectoral flap. Plastic and Reconstructive Surgery 59: 360

Mendenhall W M, Parsons J T, Mendenhall M P et al 1989 Carcinoma of the skin of the head and neck with perineural invasion. Head and Neck 11: 301

Milton G W, Shaw H M, McCarthy W H et al 1982 Prophylactic lymph node dissection in clinical stage one cutaneous malignant melanoma: results of surgical treatment in 1319 patients. British Journal of Surgery 69: 108

Mohs F E 1941 Chemosurgery: a microscopically controlled method of cancer excision. Archives of Surgery 42: 279

Moller R, Reymann F, Hou-jensen K. 1979 Metastasis in dermatological patients with squamous cell carcinoma. Archives of Dermatology 115: 703

Naruns P L, Nizze J A, Cochran A J et al 1986 Recurrence potential of thin primary melanomas. Cancer 57: 545

Netterville J L, Panje W R, Maves M D 1987 The trapezius myocutaneous flap. Dependability and limitations. Archives of Otolaryngology—Head and Neck Surgery 113: 271

Nolan J, Jenkins R A, Kurihara K, Schultz 1985 The acute effects of cigarette smoke exposure on experimental skin flaps. Plastic and Reconstructive Surgery 75: 544

O'Brien C J, Gianoutsos M P, Morgan M J 1992 Neck dissection for cutaneous malignant melanoma. World Journal of Surgery 16: 222

Osterlind A, Engholm G, Moller Jensen O 1988 Trends in cutaneous melanoma in Denmark 1943 to 1982 by anatomic site. APMIS 96: 953

Pascal R R, Hobbie L W, Lattes R et al 1968 Prognosis of 'incompletely excised' versus 'completely excised' basal cell carcinoma. Plastic and Reconstructive Surgery 41: 328

Petersen N C, Bodenham D C, Lloyd O C 1962 Malignant melanomas of the skin Part 2. British Journal of Plastic Surgery 15: 97

Proper S A, Rose P T, Fenske N A 1990 Non-melanomatous skin cancer in the elderly: diagnosis and management. Geriatrics 45: 57

Reed W B, Becker S W Sr, Becker S W Jr et al 1965 Giant pigmented naevi, melanoma and leptomeningeal melanocytosis: a clinical and histopathological study. Archives of Dermatology 91: 100

Reintgen D S, Cox E D, McCarty K S et al 1983 Efficacy of elective lymph node dissection in patients with intermediate thickness primary melanoma. Annals of Surgery 198: 379

Reus W F, Robson M C, Zachary L, Heggers J P 1984 Acute effect of tobacco smoking on bloodflow in the cutaneous micro circulation. British Journal of Plastic Surgery 37: 213

Richmond J D, Davie R M 1987 The significance of incomplete excision in patients with basal cell carcinoma. British Journal of Plastic Surgery 40: 63

Robins P 1981 Chemosurgery: my 15 years of experience. Journal of Dermatology Surgery and Oncology 7: 779

Rudolph R 1982 Complications of surgery for radiotherapy skin damage. Plastic and Reconstructive Surgery 70: 179

Sakula A 1977 Pulmonary metastases from basal cell carcinoma of skin Thorax 32: 637

Schuller D E 1980 Pectoralis myocutaneous flap in head and neck cancer reconstruction. Archives of Otolaryngology 109: 185

Silverstone H, Searle J H A 1970 The epidemiology of skin cancer in Queensland: the influence of phenotype and environment. British Journal of Cancer 24: 235

Sim F H, Taylor W F, Ivins J C et al 1978 A prospective randomised study of the efficacy of routine elective lymphadenectomy in management of malignant melanoma: preliminary results. Cancer 41: 948

Song R, Gao Y, Song Y et al 1982 The forearm flap. Clinics in Plastic Surgery 9: 21

Stell P M 1980 Retraction of skin flaps. Clinical Otolaryngology 7: 45

Swanson N A, Taylor W B 1982 Commentary: the evolution of Mohs surgery. Journal of Dermatology, Surgery and Oncology 8: 650

Taylor G A, Barisoni D 1973 10 years experience in the surgical treatment of basal cell carcinoma. A study of factors associated with recurrence. British Journal of Surgery 60: 522

Taylor G I, Palmer G B 1987 The vascular territories of the body. Experimental studies and clinical applications. British Journal of Plastic Surgery 40: 113

Tiwari R M 1988 Cervico-occipital flap for replacement of neck skin. Journal of Laryngology and Otology 102: 341

Tiwari R M 1991 Cervico-occipital flap. A new reliable technique for resurfacing of defects of the neck. In: Stucker F J (eds) Plastic and reconstructive surgery of the head and neck. Proceedings of the Fifth International Symposium. B C Decker, Philadelphia, p 515

Tiwari R M, Snow G B 1983 Role of myocutaneous flaps in reconstruction of the head and neck. Journal of Laryngology and Otology 97: 441

Tromovitch T A, Stegman S J 1974 Microscopically controlled excision. Archives of Dermatology 110: 231

Trozak D J, Roland W D, Hu F 1975 Metastatic malignant melanoma in prepubertal children. Paediatrics 55: 191

Veronesi U, Adamus J, Bandiera D C et al 1977 Inefficacy of immediate node dissection in stage one melanoma of the limbs. New England Journal of Medicine 297: 627

Veronesi U, Cascinelli N, Adamus J et al 1988 Thin stage I primary cutaneous malignant melanoma. Comparison of excision with margins of 1 or 3 cms. New England Journal of Medicine 318: 1159

Vikram, B, Strong E W, Shah J P, Spiro R 1984 Failure in the neck following multimodality treatment for advanced head and neck cancer. Head and Neck Surgery 6: 724

Weedon D 1982 Pathology—squamous cell carcinoma. In: Emmett A J J, O'Rourke M G E (eds) Malignant skin tumours. Churchill Livingstone, Edinburgh

Weedon D, Wall D 1975 Metastatic basal cell carcinoma. Medical Journal of Australia 2: 177

Woods J E 1989 Malignant melanoma: an update. Advances in Plastic and Reconstructive Surgery 5: 1

Yang G, Chen B, Gao Y et al 1981 Forearm free skin flap transplantation. National Medical Journal of China 621: 139

25. Management of head and neck tumours in childhood and adolescence

Bryan J. Michelow   Ronald M. Zuker   Jeffrey C. Posnick

INTRODUCTION AND HISTORICAL REVIEW

Tumours of the head and neck in children span a spectrum of conditions ranging from developmental malformations and dysplasias of embryonal remnants to benign and malignant neoplasms. Common adult malignancies such as lung, breast, gastrointestine and skin cancers are rare in children and are replaced by reticulo-endothelial, central nervous and mesenchymal tumours (Altman & Schwartz 1983). According to Altman & Schwartz (1983), less than 1 in 600 children will develop a malignancy before their fifteenth birthday. Leukaemia is the commonest malignant tumour in children, while vascular malformations account for the majority of the benign tumours (Altman & Schwartz 1983). Dermoid and epidermoid cysts are the most frequently seen of the developmental conditions (Rapidis et al 1988); these authors noted that 7.8% of childhood tumours were located in the head and neck region.

Although the Smith Papyrus (2300 BC) describes wounds of the head, and the Ebers Papyrus (1500 BC) mentions an 'eating ulcer' of the gums (Rush 1983), it was Celcus who, according to Martin, first described cancers of the face (Martin 1940). In the treatise *The Surgery of Theodoric*, Campbell & Colton (1955) illustrate the clear understanding of cancer possessed by Theodoric in AD 1267, but could find no mention of treatment of this problem. Galen, according to Rush (1983) popularized the concept that cancer was a systemic disease which therefore required systemic treatment 'to balance the constitution by bleeding and purging'.

Surgery for the management of cancer evolved slowly. The various stages included the ability to differentiate cancer from chronic infection, the understanding of the primary origin and secondary spread of cancer, and the advent of anaesthesia and microscopic pathology in the mid-1800s. During the pre-antibiotic era, the operations for cancer were not only disfiguring, but were fraught with complications. Cellulitis, abscess formation, septicaemia and pneumonia were common sequelae following cancer surgery, and mortality rates exceeded 50% (Rush 1983).

Patients who survived excision of the primary lesion, frequently developed tumour in the regional lymph nodes. Crile, at the turn of the century, being influenced by this observation, popularized radical neck dissection as a means of improving local control of the disease (Rush 1983).

Largely due to the mutilating nature of the surgery and the inability to reconstruct the resulting defect, radiation therapy was introduced as an alternative treatment. Radiation was not without morbidity, but this improved when radium therapy was replaced by external beam radiation and fractionated therapy replaced single-dose treatments. Radiation therapy remained the treatment of choice until the end of the 1930s when metastatic spread was shown to respond better to surgery than to radiation. The combination of surgery with pre-operative radiation therapy, aimed at improving survival, has not proved effective (Luce 1986).

Improved chemotherapy protocols have not only aided control of systemic disease, but also facilitated modification of radical surgical procedures (Luce 1986). When given pre-operatively to selected patients, chemotherapy has also improved resectability of the primary tumour (Posnick et al 1992d).

Presently, pioneering work is influencing the trend in the management of head and neck tumours. Surgical extirpation followed by immediate reconstruction has become possible. Recent advances in craniofacial surgery and free tissue transfer have made this feasible. The coronal scalp incision provides wide exposure of both the mid-face and skull regions. An intracranial, extracranial or combined intra- and extracranial approach to the lesion affords excellent exposure, thus allowing accurate resection of the primary lesion (Posnick 1992). The bony defects are reconstructed with calvarial bone grafts, stably fixed with mini- or microplates and screws. Immediate bony restoration is covered with suitable soft tissue, facilitated by the use of free-tissue transplantation. This option has enhanced successful immediate reconstruction, particularly after extensive surgical resection in irradiated beds (Zuker & Posnick 1992).

PAEDIATRIC CONSIDERATION IN THE MANAGEMENT OF HEAD AND NECK TUMOURS

An understanding of the differences between child and adult physiology is important if morbidity and mortality is to be reduced. The increased metabolic processes in neonates, the greater need for temperature control and the newborn's reduced ability to combat infection must be addressed (Izant 1987). Providing appropriate nutritional support and maintaining precise fluid balance are essential basic skills required in the management of these patients. A knowledge of embryology promotes an understanding of the aetiology of congenital anomalies. Prenatal and perinatal events are important, therefore, when assessing congenital abnormalities.

The child's height, weight and head circumference should be periodically assessed and compared to standardized growth charts with age-adjusted norms (Hamill et al 1979). Any visual field, hearing, speech or dental occlusion abnormality requires pre-operative assessment by the appropriate specialist. Questions about excessive bleeding or bruising should be asked.

The pre-operative laboratory investigations should include: complete blood count, electrolyte analysis, coagulation profile and urine analysis. If a malignancy is suspected or possible, tests to evaluate the existence of metastases should be performed. These include some or all of the following: chest radiograph or tomogram; ultrasound; liver, spleen and bone scan; bone marrow biopsy and cerebrospinal fluid cytology (Posnick et al 1992d). Head and neck tumours that may be malignant should be assessed by a multidisciplinary team of oncologist, radiation therapist and oncological and reconstructive surgeon to provide a treatment plan that takes into consideration the various management alternatives. In this way, control of both local and systemic disease can be maximized (Posnick et al 1992d).

Psychological considerations in the pediatric surgical patient must not be ignored. Campis et al (1990) have deftly defined the developmental influences on adjustment of children to hospitalization. According to these authors, conceptual (cognitive) understanding and the level of psychological (emotional) development of the child will determine how he or she experiences hospitalization:

1. During the first year of life, infants establish a secure and trusting relationship with parents or guardian. Interruption of this developmental milestone may lead to distress. Robertson (1958) described 'protest, despair and detachment' in infants after a few days of hospitalization. Regression to more immature behaviour may occur.

2. Pre-school children, 1–4 years old, begin to develop a sense of independence and self reliance. Illness, therefore, may be perceived as punishment for bad behaviour which results in feelings of defencelessness and of being deserted by parents (Campis et al 1990).

3. School-age children between 5 and 12 years experience

the rewards of self achievement and learn to value personal skills (Erickson 1950). Pain from surgical procedures may be misunderstood, manifesting as one of a variety of behavioural responses such as anxiety, regression, depression or aggression (Melamed & Siegel 1975).

4. Adolescents strive for independence from family as they learn to develop relationships with peers. Defiance of authority makes hospitalization difficult for this group. Surgery, too, generates concerns for their body image (Campis et al 1990).

Tumours of the head and neck in children can be considered according to the following categories:

Congenital
Present at birth or shortly after
Developmental
Benign
Malignant

Acquired
Benign
Malignant

For the purposes of this chapter, the common tumours of childhood will be discussed under 'Benign and Malignant'.

BENIGN TUMOURS

Vascular lesions

Vascular birthmarks should be classified into one of two major categories, namely, haemangiomas or vascular malformations (Mulliken & Glowacki 1982). A haemangioma is a mass or proliferation of endothelial cells with or without lumena, while vascular malformations are abnormal, enlarged vascular channels which may be arterial, venous, capillary or lymphatic in origin.

Haemangiomas

Characteristics. Of the vascular tumours affecting children, haemangiomas are the most common. The haemangioma is present at birth in only 40% of patients. In the remaining 60%, the haemangioma appears within 2 to 4 weeks after birth as a tiny macular telangiectasia or a pale spot (Krafchik 1989). They grow rapidly until the child reaches 6 to 8 months of age (proliferation phase) and then slowly regress by adolescence (involuting phase) (Williams 1980, Krafchik 1989). The head and neck regions are commonly affected, although any area of the body may be involved. By the age of 5 years 50% will have regressed, by the age of 7 years, 75%, and by the age of 9 years 95% will have regressed (Margileth & Museles 1965). Females are three to five times more frequently affected than males (Mulliken 1988, Krafchik 1989).

The majority of haemangiomas (50–60%) are superficial, arise as bright red areas of discoloration in the papillary dermis and were previously termed 'capillary haemangiomas'. In 15% of cases, haemangiomas are deep, developing within the reticular dermis or subcutaneous fat. Being deep, they are less well defined, may give the overlying skin a blue tinge and are compressible. Previously termed 'cavernous haemangiomas', these haemangiomas, apart from being deep, are essentially no different from their superficial counterparts. Because the terms 'capillary' and 'cavernous' haemangioma cause confusion, they should be replaced by the more useful descriptive terms of 'superficial' or 'deep' haemangioma (Mulliken 1988). Both superficial and deep haemangiomas may be present in the same patient in 30% of cases (Krafchik 1989).

Superficial haemangiomas tend to disappear completely over a period of time, while deep haemangiomas may have some residual fatty parenchymal tissue remaining.

Occasionally, a giant haemangioma may trap circulating platelets, sequestrating them from the intravascular system. A systemic coagulopathy follows; this is known as the Kasabach–Merritt syndrome (Warrell & Kempin 1985, Larsen et al 1987, El-Dessouky et al 1988). The presence of proliferating endothelial cells and mast cells seems to be an important factor in this phenomenon which is therefore less frequently seen in vascular malformations.

Congenital subglottic haemangiomas, although rare, may present with life-threatening airway obstruction during the first 6 months of life. Holinger & Brown (1967) reported 13 such patients in a sample of 846 cases of congenital laryngeal anomalies. Deviation of the trachea occurs as the subglottic haemangioma progressively enlarges (Burrows et al 1983).

Haemangiomatous involvement of the soft tissues around the orbit can threaten visual development. Eyelid involvement with lid closure and consequent obstruction to vision may cause sensory deprivation amblyopia (loss of vision) if present for a week or more (Thomson et al 1979, Garcia & Dixon 1984). Intra-orbital haemangiomas may produce pressure on the globe causing refractive errors (anisometra) and astigmatism. With more extensive involvement strabismus and proptosis may occur.

Compression of the optic nerve will lead to optic atrophy and blindness (Pasyk et al 1984).

Diagnosis. It is important to distinguish between haemangiomas and vascular malformations. Unlike vascular malformations, haemangiomas involute spontaneously with time. Accurate historical data, thorough examination and a study of newborn and infant photographs are important aids in making the distinction (Bartlett et al 1988, Garfinkle & Handler 1980).

Like all benign tumours, haemangiomas frequently have distinct margins, feel spongy or firm on palpation, and in children 8 months of age or older, often show signs of involution (small, central areas of grey colour change). Deeper haemangiomas soften and slowly shrink, occasionally leaving a fibro-fatty mass.

Radiology. Plain X-ray often demonstrates a soft-tissue mass. Ultrasonography can determine the vascular nature of the lesion, but cannot differentiate between a haemangioma and a vascular malformation. Endoscopy is indicated if involvement of the air passage is suspected.

Angiography is indicated when the diagnosis cannot be made on the characteristic clinical features or when therapeutic intervention is required. It typically demonstrates a well circumscribed mass with feeding arteries from adjacent vessels, a transient soft-tissue flush in the capillary phase and a longer-lasting venous phase blush. The adjacent vessels are normal and usually discrete (Burrows et al 1983).

Computerized tomography (CT scan) following intravenous administration of contrast medium reveals a uniformly enhanced mass if the haemangioma is in the proliferative phase. Dense enhancement with shadows from fatty locules are seen in the involution phase (Burrows et al 1983). Nuclear magnetic resonance scan (NMR) may show the feeding vessels.

Treatment. In the majority of cases, a conservative approach, with patient and family counselling, is indicated. Since these lesions involute spontaneously before puberty, the patient and family require reassurance and periodic reassessment (Garfinkle & Handler 1980, Krafchik 1989). Serial photographs are helpful in providing objective evidence of involution to support this conservative approach. Haemangiomas which are extensive and limit function or threaten to cause airway or visual obstruction require intervention. When intervention is indicated, successful treatment modalities include one or a combination of the following:

1. Steroid therapy. Systemic administration of steroid has been successful in shrinking haemangiomas (Zak & Morin 1981, Argenta et al 1982). A dose of 2–3 mg/kg/day of prednisone may have to be given for long periods (up to 18 months) for the effective treatment of giant haemangiomas (Zarem & Edgerton 1967, Bartoshesky et al 1978). Steroid therapy is indicated for the treatment of extensive lesions. It is particularly useful when the potential for airway compromise exists, or where eyelid lesions threaten to obstruct vision or produce pressure on the globe. The mechanism of action is not known, but theories include (i) steroid-induced increased sensitivity of the terminal vessels to vasoactive substances (Edgerton 1976) and (ii) a steroid block of the uptake of oestradiol at the increased oestrogen receptor sites in proliferating haemangiomas (Krafchik 1989). Administration of systemic steroids for prolonged periods in children has the disadvantage of growth delay and cushingoid characteristics.

Intralesional injection of long-acting Triamcinolone (40 mg) with short-acting dexamethasone (4 mg), betamethasone or methyl prednisolone (20 mg), directly into and around the haemangioma has also been successful (Kushner 1982). Repeated doses may be required. Intralesional therapy has proved useful for eyelid lesions with obstruction or pressure on the globe. It has numerous advantages over systemic therapy. It is simple and safe with none of the systemic complications, has a more rapid action, is easily repeated and, if unsuccessful, does not preclude other treatment methods.

2. Compression. Compression can be effective in controlling the growth of haemangiomas and the platelet-trapping capacity. However, the head and neck generally do not lend themselves to this form of treatment.

3. Embolization or small percutaneous intralesional injection and compression. Embolization, when performed prior to surgery, reduces the vascularity of the lesion and, thus, can reduce blood loss during surgery (Azzolini et al 1982, Burrows et al 1987). Careful planning with selective angiography is required. Embolic agents in use include polyvinyl alcohol-calibrated particles (Ivalon) or Gelfoam pellets. The risk of migration of the embolic particles to ectopic sites with subsequent infarction and necrosis of tissue is a serious, but infrequent complication.

Direct injection of isobutylcyanoacrylate (super glue) or sodium tetradecyl sulphate, a sclerosing agent, (Anavi et al 1988), is efficacious and should be followed by compression of the injected area for a short period of time.

4. Laser treatment. Laser treatment is indicated for the treatment of superficial vascular lesions, particularly if redness persists after involution of the mass. Various types of lasers are available. The carbon dioxide (CO_2) laser (Levine & Bailin 1982, Ratz & Bailin 1987), argon laser (Apfelberg et al 1982, Hobby 1983) and neodynium:YAG lasers (Landthaler et al 1986) may produce scarring by non-specific thermal destruction of the perivascular dermis. The pulsed dye laser with a wavelength of 577 nm is selectively absorbed by oxyhaemoglobin, and minimal heat radiates into the surrounding tissues. Scarring of the skin is therefore less likely to occur.

5. Surgical excision. Surgical intervention is indicated when important functions are threatened. Examples include, inter alia, potential obstruction of airway or vision. Consideration for the possibility of nerve injury and cosmetic deformity is important. In some patients a reduction in vascularity of the lesion with pre-operative embolization is useful (Schrudde & Petrovivi 1981). Pre-operative intralesional administration of sclerosant may also be helpful (Azzolini et al 1982).

6. Radiotherapy and cryotherapy. The potential for growth retardation and the development of a neoplastic lesion later in life has made radiotherapy for a benign superficial vascular lesion an unpopular treatment option. Zochodyne et al (1984) report a case in which an astrocytoma developed 22 years after radium patches and focal irradiation were used in an infant to treat two scalp haemangiomas. Cryotherapy leads to damage of the epidermis and dermis causing permanent scarring. This treatment option is no longer recommended.

7. Special considerations. Subglottic haemangiomas were traditionally treated with tracheostomy followed by observation until the haemangioma regressed. External radiation therapy, radium implants, systemic steroids, sclerosing agent and cryotherapy have not provided consistent results (Kveton & Pillsbury 1982, Shikhani et al 1986). More recently, treatment with the CO_2 laser to vaporize the lesion has proved successful in opening the airway. Laser treatment within the airway has proved to be safe and has not demonstrated any short- or long-term major complications (Wenig & Abramson 1988).

Orbital haemangiomas which are small, peripheral and not obstructing vision, require careful and constant monitoring. If they enlarge, intralesional or systemic steroid therapy should be given (Pasyk et al 1984). If there is no response to steroids and if the position is such that further enlargement may obstruct vision, then the haemangioma should be excised at an early stage while it is still localized (Thomson et al 1979). Urgent treatment is required if vision is obstructed and is best performed in cooperation with an ophthalmology colleague.

Treatment of the Kasabach–Merritt syndrome requires systemic therapy with steroids in a dose of 2–4 mg/kg/day (Larsen et al 1987, Krafchik 1989). If bleeding is a problem, platelet concentrates, fresh frozen plasma and cryoprecipitate should be used (Straub et al 1972). The literature abounds with other treatment options. Koerper et al (1983) reported on the use of Dipyridamole and aspirin, both inhibitors of platelet function. Heparin (100 mg/kg) given every 4 hours until bleeding ceases, is controversial. Epsilon aminocaproic acid and tranexamic acid, which inhibit fibrinolysis, have been successful (Neidhart & Roach 1982, Warrell & Kempin 1985). Platelet deficiency in the Kasabach–Merritt syndrome has also been shown to respond to treatment with alpha-interferon (Mulliken unpublished). For the most part, these controversial treatment options are not required, but a constant vigil for potential problems is necessary.

Vascular malformations

Characteristics. Vascular malformations result from abnormal development of blood vessels or lymphatic channels (Mulliken & Glowacki 1982). They are usually present at birth, but may not be clinically obvious until later in infancy or early childhood. They grow proportionately with the patient, but may increase in size following trauma, infection, or endocrine changes such as pregnancy and puberty (Kaban & Mulliken 1990). There is no proliferation or involution phase, and spontaneous resolution is rare. They do not respond to steroids. Unlike haemangiomas, vascular malformations are associated with skeletal abnormalities in 35% of cases (Boyd et al 1984). Skeletal changes usually manifest as expansion of bone deep to a cutaneous vascular malformation. At a cellular level, endothelial cells are normal in quantity and mast cells are not prominent (Krafchik 1989).

Vascular malformations are classified anatomically, according to the type of vessel involved (Mulliken 1988). Thus, arterial, venous, capillary or lymphatic malformations can be identified, venous and lymphatic types being more common than arterial or capillary malformations (Krafchik 1989). The classification is as follows:

1. Arterial malformations are ectasias or aneurysms involving arteries or arterioles.

2. Venous malformations, which previously were incorrectly termed 'cavernous haemangiomas', do not involve.

3. An arterio-venous malformation (AVM) typically has increased pulsations, raised temperature, a thrill on palpation and a bruit on auscultation. In the head and neck region, these tend to be symptomatic. If a high flow across the fistula exists, a hyperdynamic circulation develops. Cardiomegaly and congestive cardiac failure may ensue in an infant. As a consequence of the shunt, blood flow distal to the fistula may be decreased. This results in opening of collateral vessels due to ischaemia.

4. Capillary-venous malformations are completely compressible, and they distend on exertion and when dependent. They often have calcified thrombi (phleboliths) within, due to the slow blood flow (Burrows et al 1983). It may be difficult to differentiate this malformation from a lymphatic malformation, and angiography with contrast and/or CT scan may be necessary (Burrows et al 1983). The basic problem is one of outflow of blood. Enlargement is due to venous obstruction, and arterial embolization is therefore of little use since the malformation will continue to fill from adjacent veins or capillaries.

5. A capillary malformation of which the port-wine stain (previously incorrectly termed 'capillary haemangioma') is an example, does not spontaneously regress. In the Sturge–Weber syndrome, a capillary malformation of the face in the distribution of the ophthalmic or maxillary division of the trigeminal nerve is associated with ipsilateral vascular malformations over the cerebral cortex. In the Rendu–Osler–Weber syndrome, hereditary haemorrhagic telangiectasia are associated with arterial aneurysms, and in the Louis–Barr syndrome, telangiectasias of the head or face are associated with central nervous system degeneration leading to ataxia (Mulliken 1988).

6. Lymphatic malformations are divided according to their size into: cystic hygroma, lymphangioma (localized or diffuse) and combined lymphatic and venous types (haemangioa-lymphoma). They are often blue due to haemorrhage into adjacent tissues. Inflammation frequently leads to lymphangitis.

Organs may be involved in disseminated haemangiomatosis. Disseminated haemangiomatosis is present when more than three organ systems are involved (e.g. skin, liver, dura). The liver is the most frequent organ affected, and high-output failure, due to arteriovenous shunting, may complicate the condition. Mortality rates for patients with disseminated haemangiomatoses may reach 30% in spite of intensive treatment (Krafchik 1989).

Radiology. Plain films usually reveal diffuse soft-tissue masses. Phleboliths are frequently noted in capillary–venous malformations and skeletal changes are common. Whether the bone changes are due to direct involvement or are reactive to increased blood flow, is controversial.

Angiography is helpful in determining the haemodynamic nature and extent of malformations (Kaban & Mulliken 1990). Dilated vascular spaces with normal or enlarged feeding arteries and draining veins can be delineated (Burrows et al 1983).

Computerized tomography, when used with contrast, is a useful test. MRI with gadolinium contrast medium provides detailed tissue definition and information on the closeness of neurovascular bundles. On MRI, a flow void is seen on T1 images, but enhancement is seen on T2 images.

Lymphatic malformations can be differentiated from vascular malformations using a radiolabelled red cell 'blood-pool' study and nuclear isotope scanning. Labelled red blood cells will not pool in a pure lymphatic malformation.

Treatment. The differentiation of vascular malformations into low-flow (capillary, venous and most combined malformations) and high-flow (arteriovenous) malformations is important for treatment purposes.

Low-flow vascular malformations are generally not symptomatic. Pain may occur when thrombosis develops in the lesion. This responds to analgesics and anti-inflammatory agents. Discomfort is often improved with compression garments. Injection of sclerosant into venous malformations may be successful in obliterating the channels (Kaban & Mulliken 1990).

If the malformation is well-localized, excision may be feasible. Since the abnormal vessels are likely to extend beyond the visible malformation, complete removal of the abnormal vessels is often not possible. Consequently, adjacent vessels enlarge (Kaban & Mulliken 1990).

High-flow lesions may become symptomatic and may therefore require intervention. Conservative therapy with compression garments should be initiated as soon as the diagnosis is made, if this form of treatment is feasible. If this is inadequate, angiographic delineation of the AVM should be performed. Flow characteristics of the malformation must be determined and feeding vessels identified. Superselective arterial embolization may obliterate or reduce blood flow to an AVM. It has the added advantage of being able to block the feeding vessels, if these are accessible, and can fill the abnormal vascular spaces within the malformation as well. Prevention of reflux of embolic material is achieved with the use of balloon catheters.

Laser therapy is effective in the management of cutaneous capillary malformation such as port-wine stains and is currently the treatment of choice for this condition. Because lymphangiomas do not involute, if they are large and impairing function, they may require surgical excision

(Irving 1990). Repeated aspiration of a large cystic hygroma may promote a reduction in size.

Experience has demonstrated that excision of an AVM is frequently followed by a high recurrence rate (Young 1988). If small and localized, the arteriovenous fistula may be successfully excised. When the AVM is large, feeding vessels may be ligated. Repeated surgery is often necessary. Complications of surgery include haemorrhage, delayed wound healing and progression of a previously quiescent malformation to an enlarging symptomatic problem. Where bony changes are secondary, surgery on the bones is safe. Thorough haematological evaluation for coagulopathy is imperative preoperatively (Kaban & Mulliken 1990).

Vascular malformations are not malignant tumours, and radical extirpation is not justifiable. Removal in stages is acceptable for large lesions.

Congenital epulis

Characteristics

'Epulis' is a descriptive term which describes a soft-tissue tumour arising from the alveolus. 'Congenital epulis', however, describes a congenital granular cell myoblastoma (Irving 1990). Females are affected eight times more frequently than males. The origin of this tumour, although disputed, is postulated to be from mesenchyme tissue (Irving 1990).

Clinically, a benign, lobulated painless mass is attached to the incisor or canine region of the maxilla or mandibular alveolus (Fig. 25.1). The infant may not be able to close his or her mouth.

Treatment

Treatment is early excision along the base of the mass at the alveolar rim. Indications for surgery are functional inability to close the mouth and cosmetic reasons. If left alone it may regress. Being benign, wide excision is not required. The incision on the alveolus will heal rapidly and need not be sutured. Recurrence does not occur, even with incomplete excision. A complication developing in the underlying teeth is rare (Irving 1990).

Mucous cyst and ranula

Characteristics

This is a common oral lesion occurring on the floor of the mouth, but may occur in the buccal mucosa or mucosa of the lip. A mucocele can range from 1 to 20 mm in diameter, is usually asymptomatic and appears as a bulging, translucent, bluish mucosal cyst containing mucoid material. The cyst arises in mucosa containing salivary glands and is postulated to result from obstruction of the excretory duct of a minor salivary gland. Pressure build-up in the duct causes the excretory duct to rupture. Saliva collects in the surrounding tissues and becomes circumscribed with a wall of granulation tissue.

Obstruction and rupture of the larger ducts such as that of the sublingual or submaxillary gland produces a larger mucocele known as a 'ranula' (Fig. 25.2). Apart from its larger size, it is identical to the smaller versions (Rush 1983).

Treatment

Treatment consists of wide surgical unroofing of the lesion followed by suturing the fibrous lining of the cyst to the oral mucosal at its margin. This is termed marsupialization (Rush 1983). Free drainage of secretions reduces the chance of recurrence.

Carbon dioxide laser surgery is an alternative excision

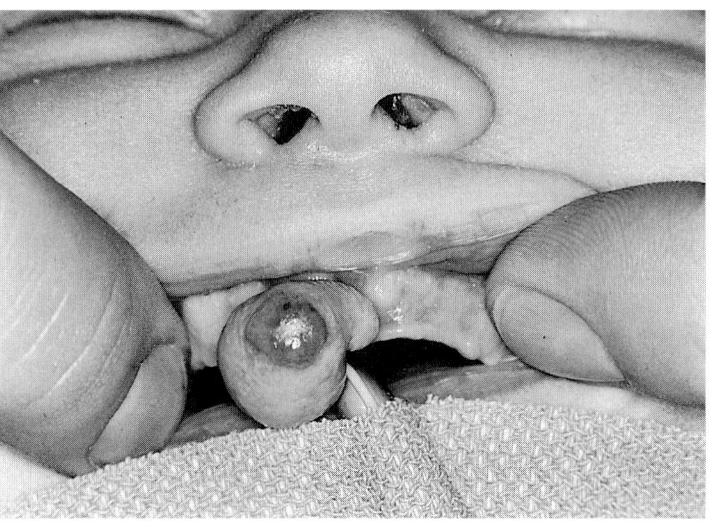

Fig. 25.1 Congenital epulis.

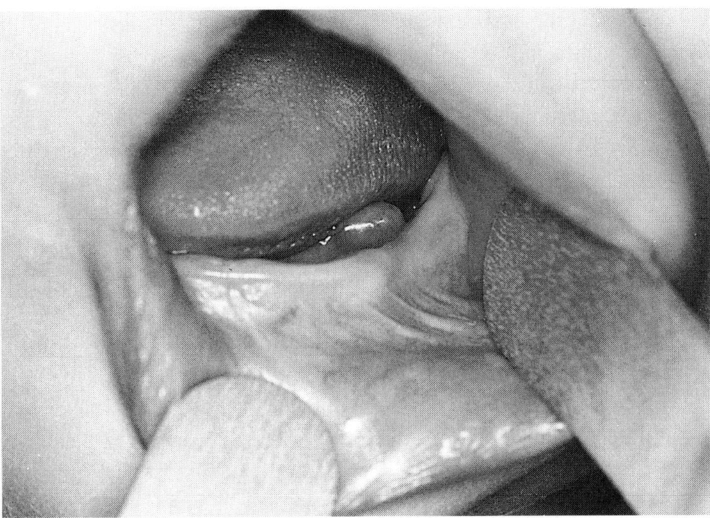

Fig. 25.2 Ranula.

option. It has the reported advantage of reduced pain and swelling following surgery (Kaban & Mulliken 1990).

Benign tumours of the jaws

Tumours of the jaw can be divided into those arising from the epithelial tissue (odontogenic origin) and those arising from the surrounding connective tissue (non-epithelial tissue).

Odontogenic (epithelial) tumours

Odontoma.

1. Characteristics. The mesenchyme of the dental follicle may produce a benign odontogenic tumour. These are common in children and develop most often in the mandible (Kaban & Mulliken 1990). 'Compound' odontomas are considered to be primitive teeth, while 'complex' odontomas have tooth elements but have not differentiated into teeth.

Being asymptomatic, this tumour is often found as an incidental finding on a routine diagnostic X-ray. Radiologically, the cortex around the tumour is normal or thinned (Kaban & Mulliken 1990).

2. Treatment. Enucleation and/or curettage is the treatment of choice. Recurrence is unlikely. Since the defect is small, bone reconstruction is usually not necessary.

Ameloblastoma.

1. Characteristics. This is a rare tumour, accounting for less than 1% of all odontogenic tumours (Kaban & Mulliken 1990). In children, ameloblastomas are generally unicystic and appear clinically and radiographically similar to a dentigerous cyst.

A painless swelling often develops. On X-ray, an area of radiolucency associated with an impacted or displaced molar tooth is generally noted.

2. Treatment. Meticulous enucleation with bone burring of the margins is the recommended treatment (Kaban & Mulliken 1990). Close follow-up is required because of the potential for recurrence.

Non-odontogenic (mesenchymal) tumours

Giant-cell lesions.

1. Characteristics. These lesions present as an asymptomatic, local swelling involving the mandible more frequently than the maxilla. It typically occurs in children between the ages of 10 and 20 years. According to Kaban & Mulliken (1990), giant-cell lesions include central giant-cell granuloma (CGCG), brown tumour of hyperparathyroidism and giant-cell tumour. Because, histologically, these lesions are indistinguishable, brown tumour will be indicated by elevated serum parathyroid hormone, calcium and alkaline phosphatase levels with a low serum phosphorus level. Radiologically, a unilocular or multilocular radiolucent lesion is noted.

2. Hyperparathyroidism should be investigated and, if present, managed appropriately. Parathyroidectomy is usually followed by regression of the lesion. Curettage may be adequate therapy for CGCG lesions. If recurrence occurs, resection of the involved region and reconstruction may be necessary (Posnick et al 1992c).

Fibro-osseous lesions.

1. Fibrous dysplasia

(i) Characteristics. Fibrous dysplasia is an abnormal proliferation of bone-forming mesenchyme. Progressive asymmetrical painless facial deformity develops during the first or second decade of life. Involution often begins when adult life is reached. There is a preponderance in females. Monostotic fibrous dysplasia involves one bone, while in polyostotic fibrous dysplasia many bones may be involved. Polyostotic fibrous dysplasia associated with precocious puberty and café-au-lait skin lesions is known as Albright's syndrome. A hereditary form that involves the jaws is known as cherubism.

In cranio-orbital fibrous dysplasia, lesions are usually progressive and do not involute with time. Apart from cranial vault deformity and dysplasia of the maxilla, irreversible eye damage may occur when the greater wing of the sphenoid adjacent to the optic foramina, is involved (Posnick 1992, Jackson et al 1982). Fibrous dysplasia of the jaws is more often monostotic than polyostotic and pain may be present if growth is rapid (Kaban & Mulliken 1990).

Serum calcium, phosphorus, and alkaline phosphatase levels are normal. Microscopic examination reveals a mixture of fibrous tissue, bone, giant cells and blood vessels (Kaban & Mulliken 1990).

(ii) Radiology. Radiographic findings depend on the amount of bone component present. In the fronto-orbital region, increased density of the bone may be noted. In other areas, fibrous dysplasia may appear as multilocular radiolucent areas.

(iii) Treatment. Treatment depends on the growth pattern of the tumour and must be individualized to the patient. Surgery is indicated to confirm the diagnosis histologically and often for cosmetic reasons (Kaban & Mulliken 1990). When there is a rapid increase in the size of the tumour, pain, paresthesia, or a functional deficit such as proptosis, impaired vision or trismus, surgery should be considered. When function is impaired, surgery is required despite the potential for growth of the residual tumour (Kaban & Mulliken 1990).

Resection and immediate reconstruction with carved cranial bone graft is our method of choice (Posnick et al 1992c). Munro & Chen (1981) described excision of the lesion and replacement with bone grafts. The combination of micro and miniplates, and screws for fixation have been a useful addition to achieve three-dimensional aesthetic reconstruction of miniplate units (Posnick 1992).

Malignant transformation has been reported after radiation therapy. This is no longer an acceptable treatment option. Sudden rapid expansion or the onset of paresthesia should be viewed with suspicion of malignant change (Kaban & Mulliken 1990).

2. Cherubism

(i) Characteristics. A common presentation of cherubism is painless growth of the jaw beginning at 3 or 4 years of age and progressing bilaterally and symmetrically in the jaws until about 10 years of age. Inheritance is via an autosomal dominant trait with 50 to 70% penetrance in females and 100% penetrance in males (Kaban & Mulliken 1990). The

jaw-bones are replaced by fibro-osseous tissue with a variable number of giant cells (Kaban & Mulliken 1990). Diagnosis is based on the family history and the typical symmetric physical findings.

(ii) Radiology. Radiological findings consist of bilateral

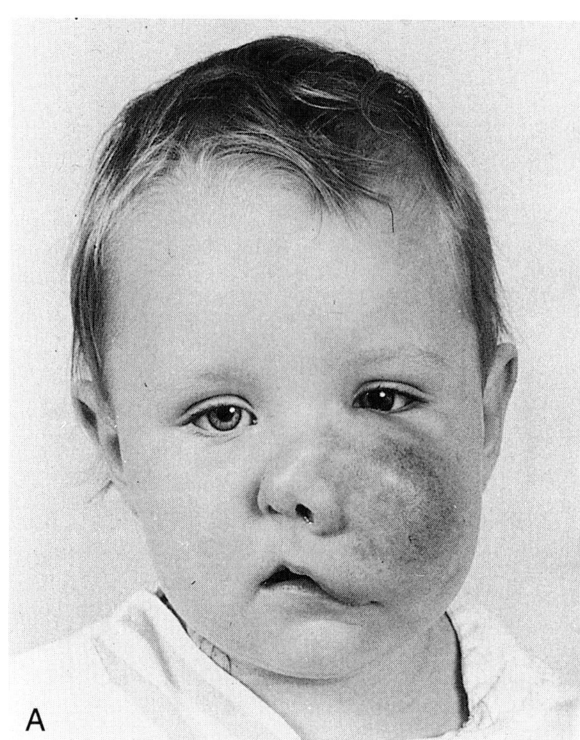

A

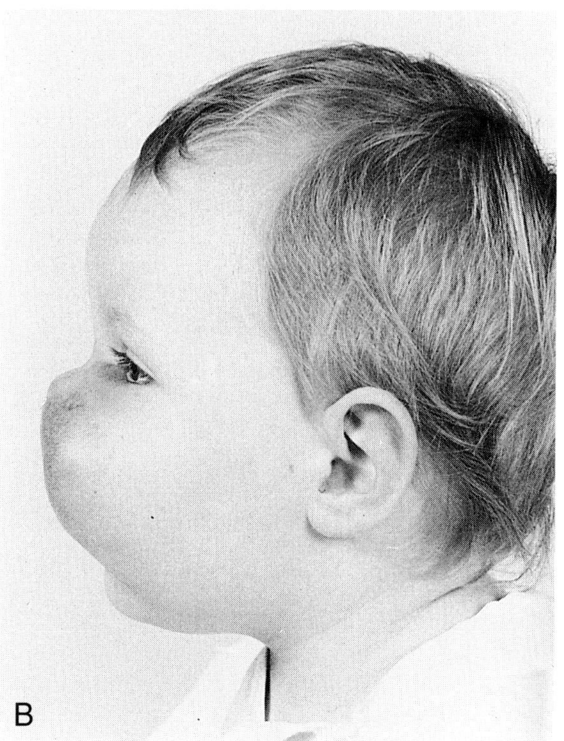

B

Fig. 25.3

symmetric radiolucencies with cortical expansion and thinning (Kaban & Mulliken 1990). The bone density improves as the condition stabilizes.

(iii) Treatment. Treatment is conservative. When the disease becomes stable, surgical contouring can be considered.

3. Osteoblastoma. Although osteoblastoma is most commonly seen in the vertebrae and long bones (80% of cases), the skull and jaws may occasionally be involved in children (Kaban & Mulliken 1990). It may present swelling, and a dull aching pain. If the bone of the glenoid fossa is involved, trismus may be present. A solitary radiolucent lesion is seen on X-ray.

Treatment requires complete resection of the lesion. Recurrence is likely if excision is incomplete (Kaban & Mulliken 1990).

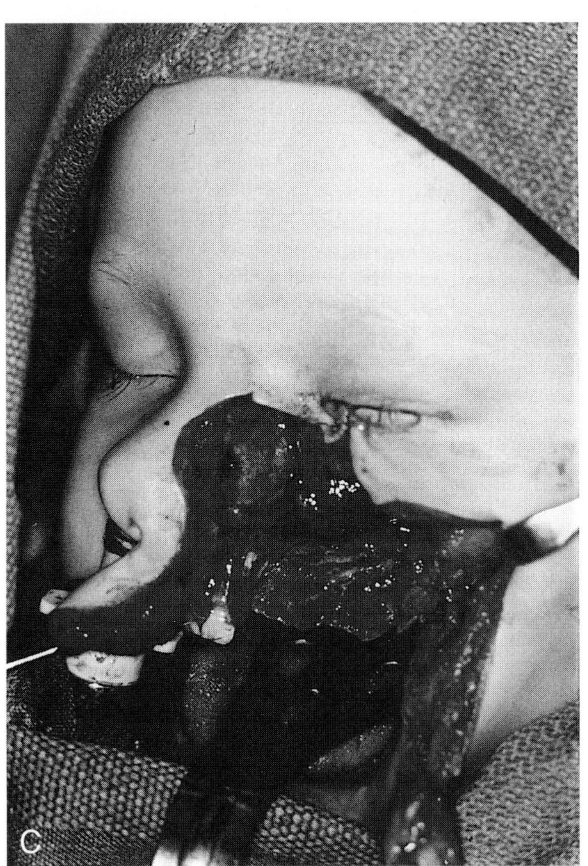

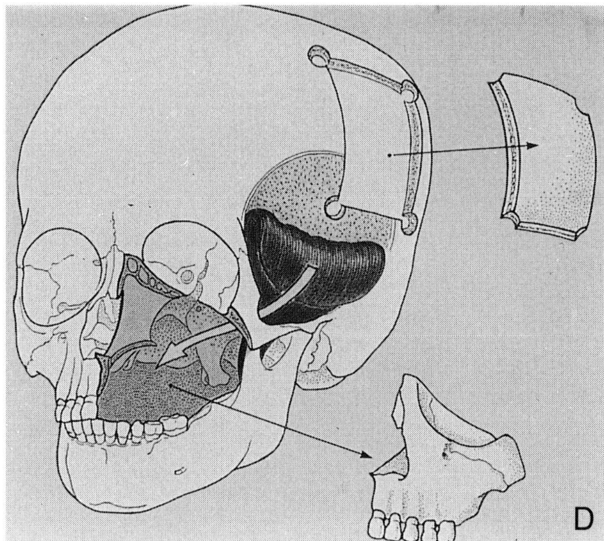

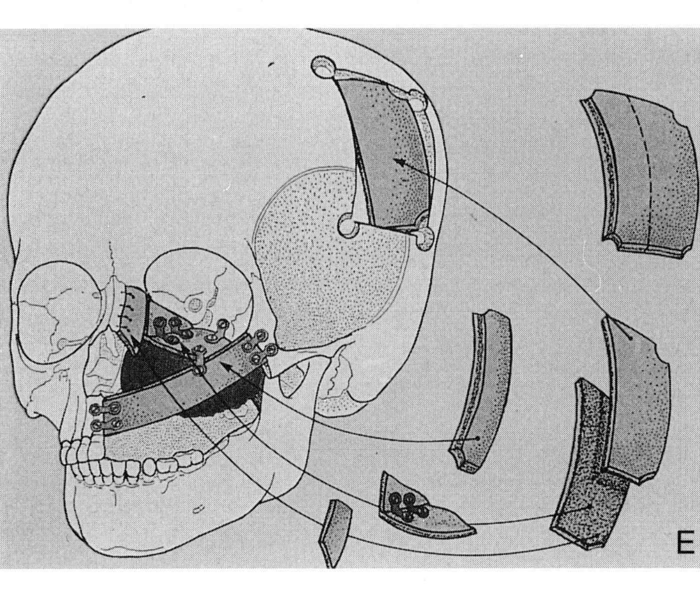

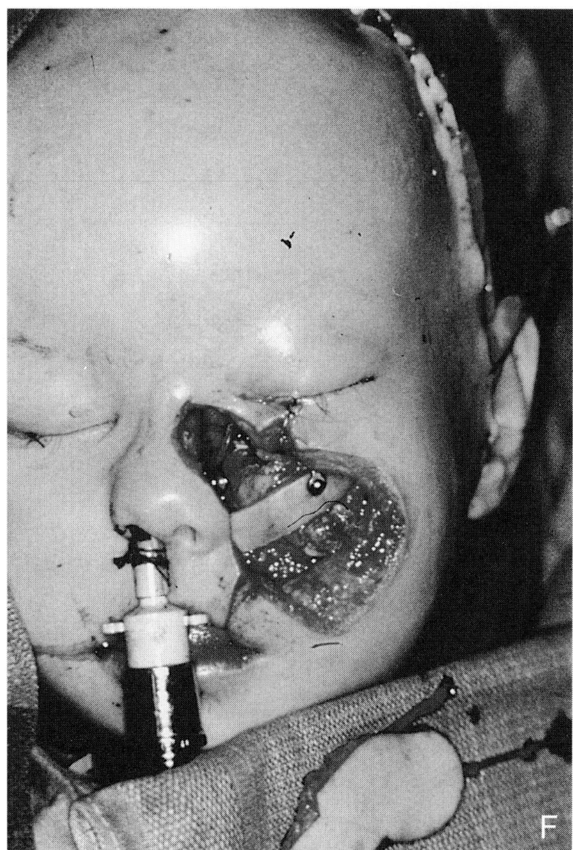

Fig. 25.3

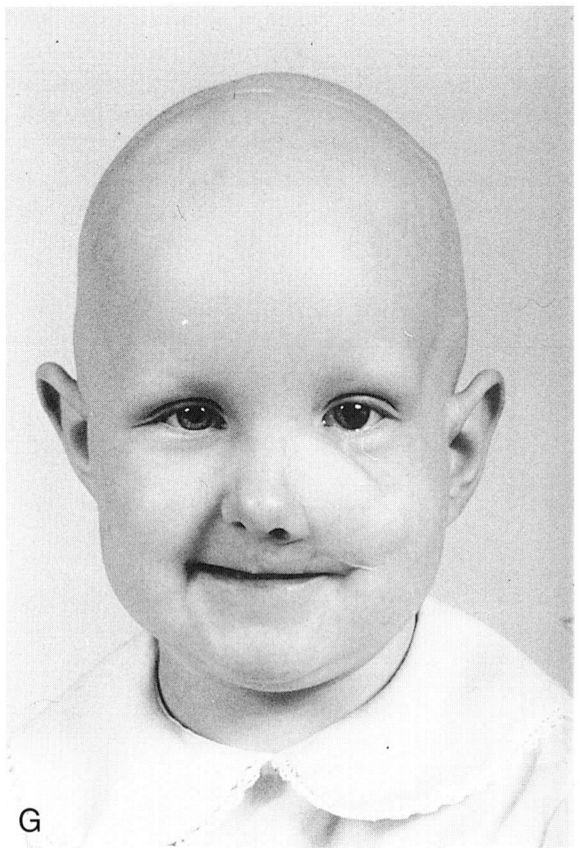

G

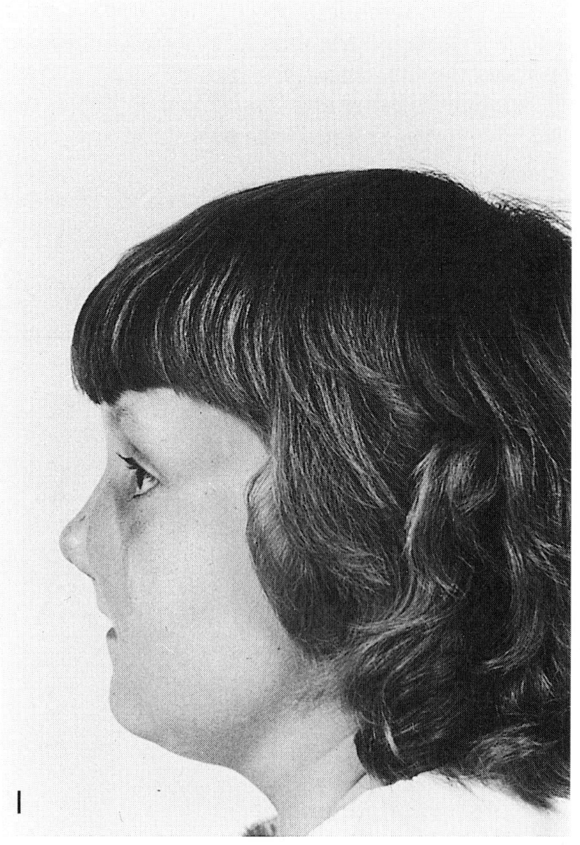

I

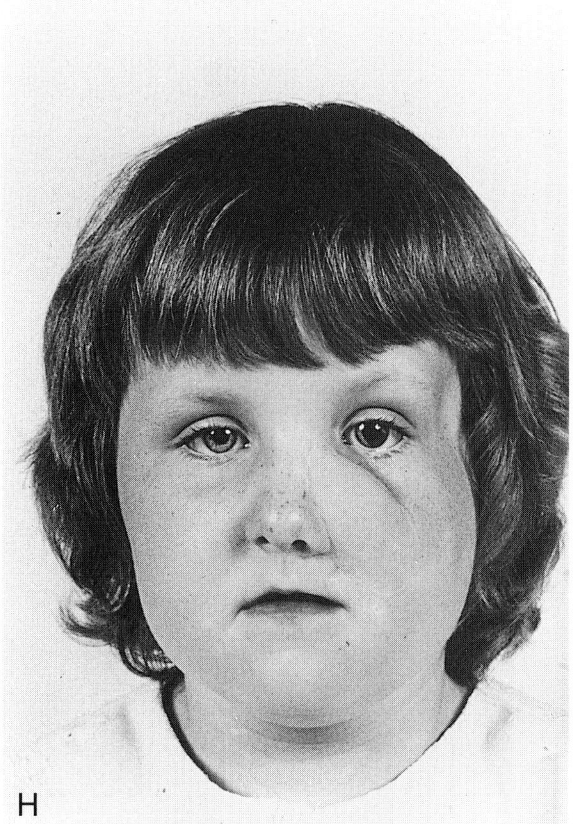

H

Fig. 25.3 A, B. An 18-month old girl with biopsy-proven rhabdomyosarcoma of the left cheek extending into bone. **C.** Surgical resection after chemotherapy. **D, E**. Illustrations demonstrating en bloc resection and reconstruction using calvarial bone grafts. **F.** Bony reconstruction now complete. A free radial forearm flap was used for soft-tissue reconstruction. **G.** Appearance 4 weeks after operation demonstrating good facial nerve function. **H, I.** Appearance 3 years following completion of treatment.

4. Myxoma

(i) Characteristics. Myxomas are generally seen in children under the age of 10 years, commonly in the non-tooth-bearing region of the mandibular angle and ramus (Kaban & Mulliken 1990). The child presents with a rapidly growing, painful swelling of the jaw.

(ii) Treatment. Complete resection of the tumour is required as there is a high recurrence rate after incomplete removal. Reconstruction should be performed after clear margins are confirmed.

MALIGNANT TUMOURS

Leukaemia (31%), central nervous system tumours (18%) and lymphoma (14%) account for more than half of the malignant tumours that occur in children (Altman & Schwartz 1983). Malignant tumours of the head and neck in childhood typically present as a solid mass. Any mass developing in the head and neck region of a child should be regarded with suspicion. Some childhood benign lesions in this region can be easily differentiated from malignant tumours on the basis of position, general characteristics and temporal sequence. These include enlarged inflammatory lymph nodes, haemangiomas, vascular malformations, thyroglossal duct cysts, fat necrosis, dermoid cysts, and the mass of a congenital muscular torticollis (Altman & Schwartz 1983). A malignant tumour may produce local symptoms as a result of its location and rapid progression. Non-specific systemic symptoms, such as failure to thrive, may also be present. Apart from primary malignancies which originate in the head or neck region, malignancies may stem from metastatic spread or direct extension from adjacent areas (Behrman & Vaughan 1987).

Malignant epithelial tumours

These tumours are rare in children—unlike the situation in adults. Kaban & Mulliken reported a muco-epidermoid carcinoma of the anterior maxilla in a 16-year-old girl. Initial symptoms were pain and swelling of the upper lip and maxillary alveolus. Complete resection together with radical neck dissection was recommended as in an adult (Kaban & Mulliken 1990). Parotid malignancies are the subject of another chapter in the book (Ch. 23). In the paediatric population they are rare, but when they do occur, investigation and management are similar to those in the adult population. Malignant skin tumours are rare in children.

Malignant mesenchymal tumours

Rhabdomyosarcoma.

Characteristics. Rhabdomyosarcoma accounts for almost one-third of malignancies of the head and neck in children under 15 years of age (Fig. 25.3). In the USA, the incidence is 4 per million children. The head and neck is the most commonly involved region, and in 30% of cases there is orbital involvement (Posnick et al 1992a). Patients present with a progressive swelling, not present at birth. Progressive growth may lead to facial distortion and functional impairment. A solid fixed, immobile mass is palpated.

Radiology. Plain X-rays and CT scans are required to assess the nature and the extent of the lesion. MRI may provide information as to soft-tissue involvement and tissue planes. These investigations also facilitate planning of the excision and reconstruction.

Treatment. The role of surgery in the treatment of head and neck rhabdomyosarcoma in childhood has undergone a radical transformation in the recent past. With present knowledge in the availability of sophisticated craniofacial surgical techniques, some large parameningeal tumours have become accessible to 'en bloc' surgical resection. Availability of craniofacial reconstructive techniques and composite free vascularized tissue transfer methods allows reconstruction of large resection defects with satisfactory cosmetic results. The devastating long-term side-effects of large-volume radiation to a young child when delivered to the orbit in the mid-face region are becoming increasingly apparent. The dose of radiation needed for adequate treatment of head and neck rhabdomyosarcoma is approximately 5000–6000 cGy administered over a 4–6 week period. With such high doses, acute complications of radiation such as severe mucositis and epidermal desquamation are very likely. Furthermore, there is a considerable long-term risk of chronic radiodermatitis, osteonecrosis, and pituitary and thyroid damage with growth hormone and thyroxin deficiency. There is an increased incidence of radiation-induced second malignancies such as bone and soft-tissue sarcomas and thyroid and skin carcinoma. Some theories report up to 40% severe ocular and retinal damage that required enucleation after orbital irradiation and an even higher incidence development of cataracts. Photophobia is a major life-long problem in these irradiated patients. The adverse effects of high-dose radiation on the normal growth and development of the cranium, orbit, jaw, temporomandibular joint and dentition are severe and well known.

Ewing's sarcoma

Characteristics. This sarcoma accounts for 5–15% of primary bone tumours in paediatric patients. It presents during the first or second decades of life, frequently involving the femur or pelvis. Although rare in facial bones (1–3%) (Fig. 25.4), the mandible is the most commonly involved bone (Posnick et al 1992a).

The patient often presents with a swelling over the involved region which often is painless. Other symptoms such as headaches may be associated and they often reflect associated muscle trismus.

Radiology. No pathognomonic radiological signs are present, but the characteristic radiological features are diffuse, mottled, osteolytic or blastic bone destruction with cortical expansion, periosteal reaction and associated soft-tissue mass. In head and neck cases, bone expansion, cortical erosions and pure lytic bone destruction are more common, whereas periosteal reaction and associated soft-tissue mass are seen less frequently. The goal of treatment is local control by surgical excision or radiation and adjuvant combination chemotherapy to control micrometastatic disease (Posnick et al 1992a).

Radiation therapy for local control, although initially effective has been followed by a 15% incidence of second primaries. The choice of local treatment (i.e. radiation or surgery) should be individualized according to age, site, size, extent and resectability of the primary tumour. The potential early and late morbidity of each treatment modality requires careful consideration.

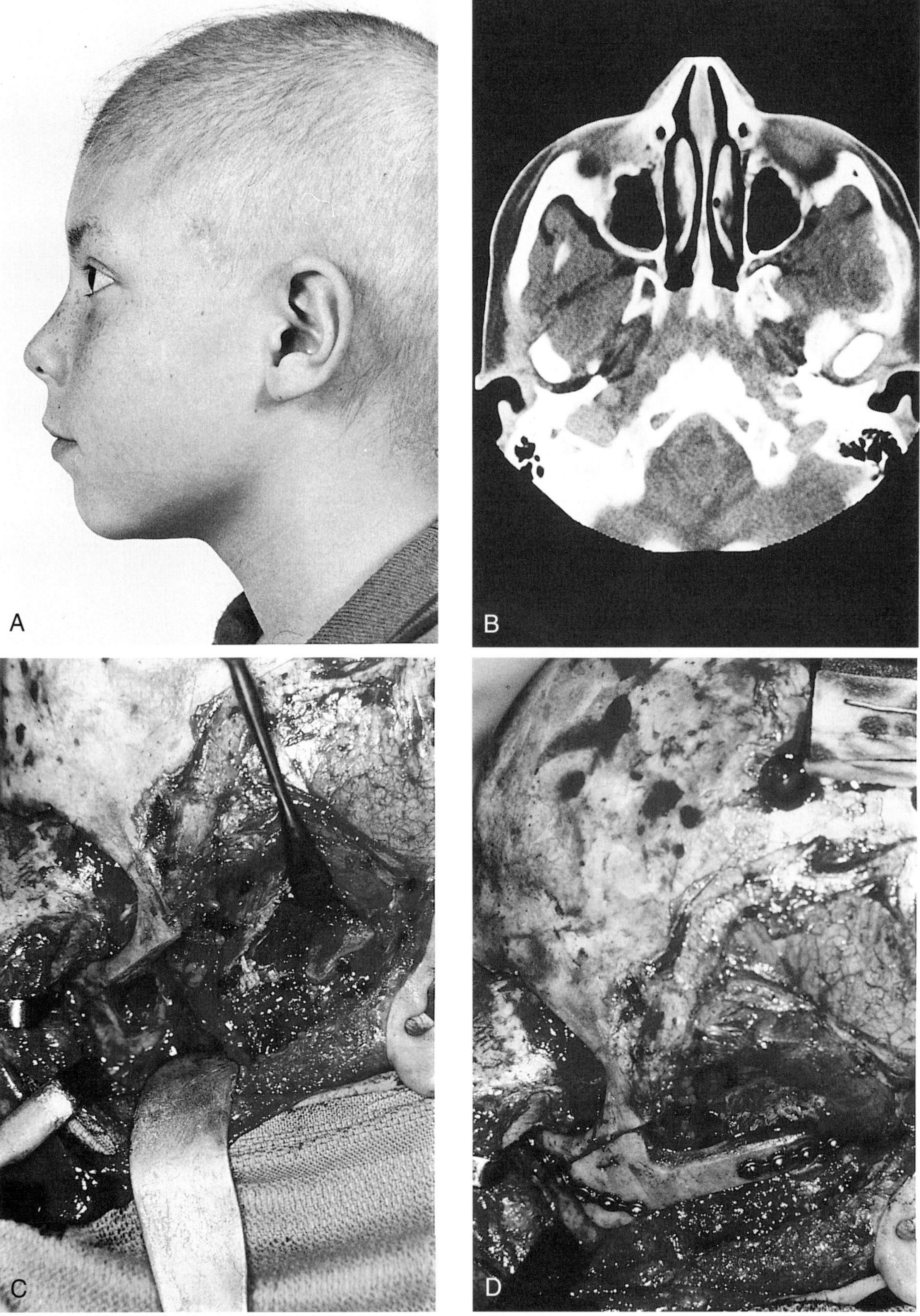

Fig. 25.4

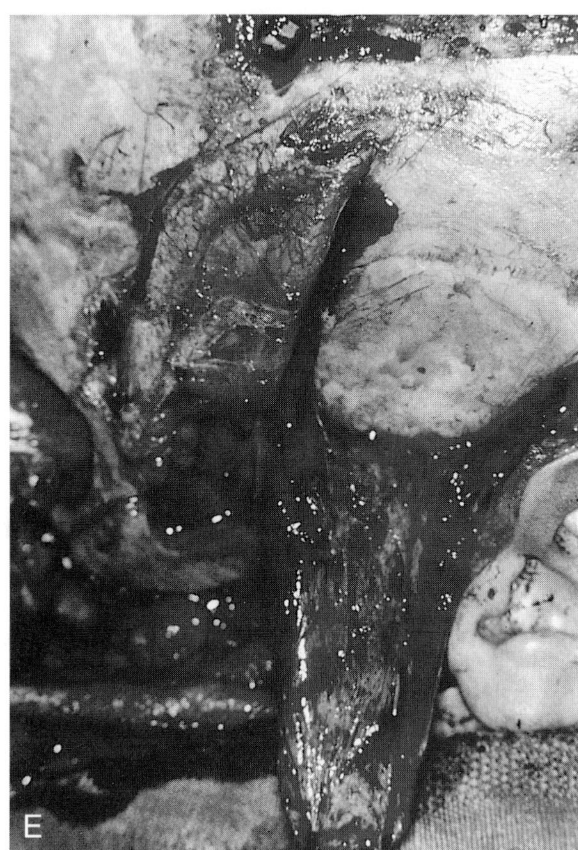

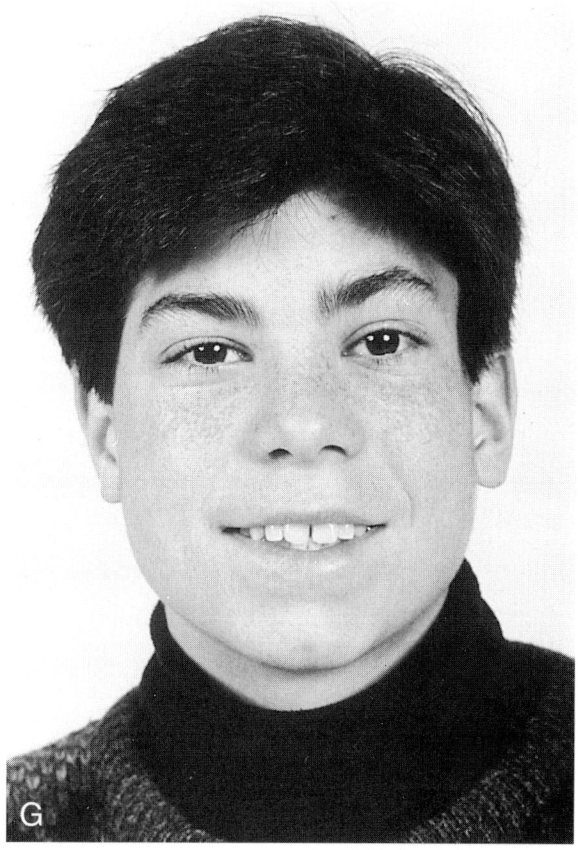

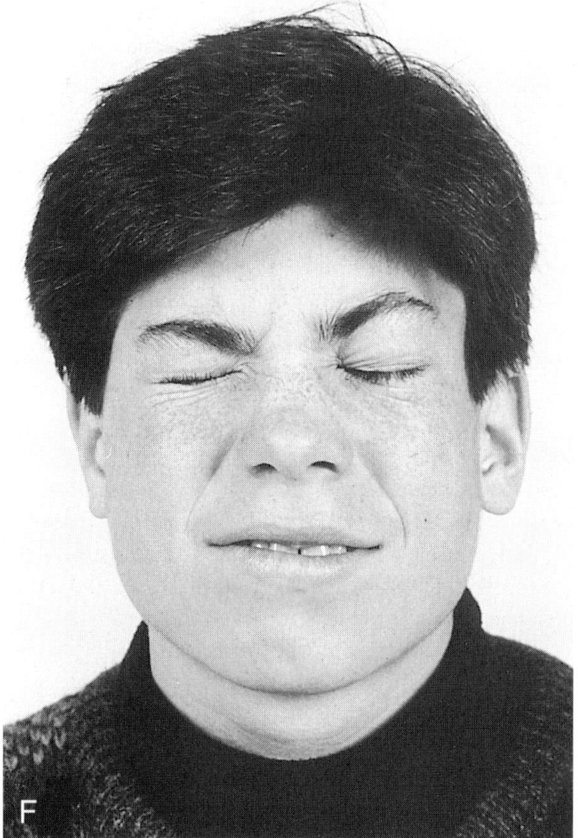

Fig. 25.4

Because radiation therapy has a devastating effect on further growth of the facial bones in the treatment field, it is not used to control local disease. An exception is made when the disease is extensive and surgical free margins cannot be expected.

EXCISION TECHNIQUES FOR MALIGNANT TUMOURS OF THE HEAD AND NECK

Although each patient presents with a unique set of circumstances, when surgical excision is selected for local tumour management a complete excision with free margins must be achieved. Multi-drug adjuvant chemotherapy is used for systemic disease. At the time of the definitive surgery, the biopsy site and tract are also excised 'en bloc' with the tumour. A coronal scalp incision is generally used to provide wide exposure of the calvarium and upper facial structures. Where possible, the facial nerve is preserved or immediately reconstructed.

RECONSTRUCTION TECHNIQUES

Recent advances in craniofacial surgery, microsurgery and free tissue transfer have made extirpation and immediate reconstruction possible. Cranial bone graft can be harvested from unaffected areas and then used to reconstruct bony

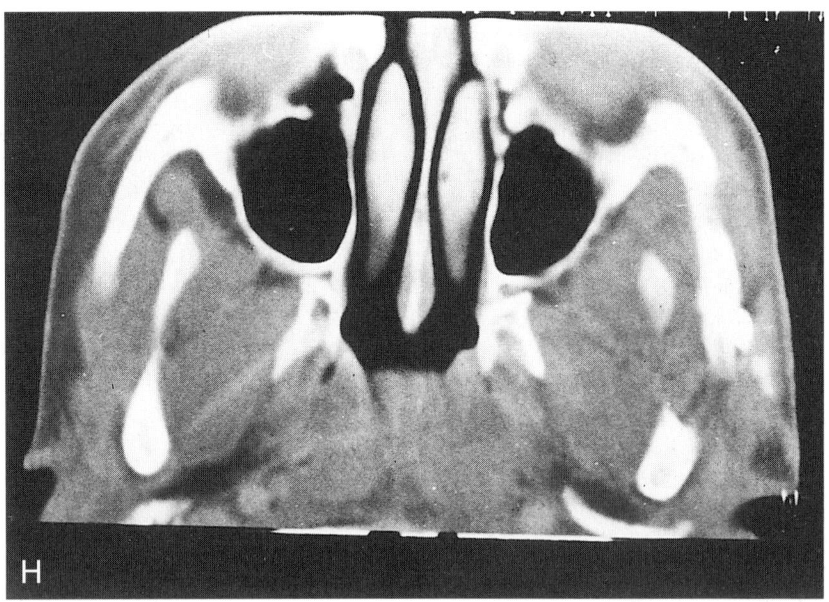

Fig. 25.4 **A.** This 12-year-old boy with a Ewing's sarcoma of the left zygomatic arch underwent chemotherapy. The biopsy site of the temporal region is visible. **B.** Pretreatment CT scan demonstrates a mass in the left zygomatic arch extending into the infratemporal fossa. **C.** The defect following en bloc resection of the tumour mass. **D.** The zygomatic complex is reconstructed with a full thickness cranial bone graft stabilized with titanium plates and screws. **E.** The posterior half of the temporalis muscle is elevated and inset to fill the soft-tissue defect over the reconstructed zygomatic complex. **F.** Two years following completion of treatment there has been a satisfactory return of facial nerve function. **G.** A satisfactory cosmetic appearance has been achieved. **H.** The CT scan at 2 years postoperatively demonstrates the reconstructed zygomatic complex.

defects, fixation being achieved with titanium mini-plates and microplates and screws. When needed, the temporalis muscle can be utilized as a regional vascularized flap to cover the graft and provide a vascularized bed.

To promote early reliable bone healing, rigid fixation of the osteotomized bone fragments not only improves the overall three-dimensional aesthetic results, but also reduces the risk of skeletal relapse and bone graft resorption.

Chemotherapy is resumed 2 weeks after surgical resection with immediate reconstruction. Adjuvant chemotherapy, combined with effective local control, has a cure rate of 70 to 80% for tumours of the head and neck in children when they present without known systemic spread (Posnick et al 1992b).

PROBLEMS AND COMPLICATIONS

Radiation therapy when used as treatment to control head and neck tumours in children may produce problems specific to the organ or tissue irradiated. The eyes develop cataracts and xerophthalmia. Hearing may be affected by a sensory-neural hearing loss. Irradiation of both non-endocrine (salivary) glands and endocrine (pituitary-hypothalamic axis) glands reduces glandular function. Growth disturbances of the craniofacial skeleton, facial soft tissues, and developing dentition, and the risk of TMJ anklyosis, may lead to the late development of severe facial deformity and morbidity in a child (Posnick et al 1992b).

We have been disappointed with the use of cranial bone grafts placed into edentulous tooth-bearing areas as they are so often thin and knife-edged, and the overlying oral mucosa may ulcerate. Heavy reconstruction plates in the mandible have been disappointing because they have resulted in stress-shielding and bone graft resorption. Erosion of overlying tissue and exposure of plate is a constant concern. In these circumstances, composite free tissue transfer has facilitated mandibular reconstruction. Numerous bone donor sites have been used. In children, the fibula provides excellent vascularized tissue which can be osteotomized as needed and fixed with miniplates, and it has minimal donor site morbidity (Posnick et al 1992b). If the craniofacial skeleton is replaced with methylmethacrylate it will be prone to infection and may later require removal.

Once bone has healed, if autogenous bone is selected, there is little concern about infection later in life.

Soft-tissue reconstruction, when indicated, has several advantages to the overall reconstruction: (i) covering bone grafts and fixation devices with well-vascularized tissue to facilitate bony union and limit infection; (ii) providing bulk for contour restoration; (iii) providing skin for improved aesthetics; (iv) lining for nasal and oral cavities; and (v) a secure vascularized barrier to separate and protect the intracranial contents. The needed soft tissue can be achieved with regional muscle flaps, such as the temporalis, if available, regional skin flaps, such as the check rotation flap, or by free tissue transfer when adequate regional flaps are not available. Flap selection will depend on the size and nature of the defect (bulk versus skin versus lining), and donor site availability and morbidity. For example, a soft-tissue defect in the palate can be reconstructed with a free muscle flap such as the rectus abdominis with the raw muscle surface allowed to epithelialize spontaneously. A large facial skin and soft-tissue defect may require a latissimus dorsi musculocutaneous flap. A smaller skin and facial defect may be managed with a free radial forearm flap. Free tissue transfer in children for head and neck defects can, with proper planning and surgical care, be accomplished safely and reliably. With the potential for these reconstructive options, many previously inoperable malignancies can now be handled effectively by surgery.

REFERENCES

Altman A J, Schwartz A D (eds) 1983 Malignant diseases of infancy, childhood and adolescence, 2nd edn. W B Saunders, Toronto, pp 1–21

Anavi Y, Har-El G, Mintz S 1988 The treatment of facial haemangioma by percutaneous injections of sodium tetradecyl sulphate. Journal of Laryngology and Otolaryngology 102: 87

Apfelberg D B, Maser M R, Lash H, Rivers J 1982 The role of the argon laser in the management of haemangiomas. International Journal of Dermatology 21: 579

Argenta L C, Bishop E, Cho K J, Andrew A F et al 1982 Complete resolution of life-threatening haemangiomas by embolisation and corticosteroids. Plastic and Reconstructive Surgery 70: 739

Azzolini A, Bertaini A, Riberti C 1982 Superselective embolisation and immediate surgical treatment. Annals of Plastic Surgery 9: 42

Bartlett J A, Riding K H, Salked L J 1988 Management of haemangiomas of the head and neck in children. Journal of Otolaryngology 17: 111

Bartoshesky L E, Bull M, Feingold M 1978 Corticosteroid treatment of cutaneous haemangiomas: how effective? Clinics in Paediatrics 17: 625

Behrman R E, Vaughan V C III 1987 Neoplasms and neoplasm-like structures. In: Nelson W E (ed) Nelson textbook of paediatrics, 13th edn. W B Saunders, Philadelphia, p 1079

Boyd J B, Mulliken J B, Kaban L B, Upton J III et al 1984 Skeletal changes associated with vascular malformations. Plastic and Reconstructive Surgery 74: 789

Burrows P E, Mulliken B J, Fellows K E, Strand R D 1983 Childhood haemangiomas and vascular malformations: angiographic differentiation. American Journal of Radiology 141: 483

Burrows P E, Lasjaunias P L, TerBrugge K, Floodmark O 1987 Urgent and emergent embolisation of lesions of head and neck in children: indications and results. Paediatrics 80: 386

Campbell E, Colton J 1955 The surgery of theodoric. Appleton-Century-Crofts, New York

Campis L K, Pillemer F G, DeMaso D R 1990 Psychological considerations in the paediatric surgical patient. In: Kaban L B (ed) Paediatric oral and maxillofacial surgery, W B Saunders, Toronto

Edgerton M T 1976 The treatment of haemangioma: with special reference to the role of steroid therapy. Annals of Surgery 183: 517

El-Dessouky M, Azmy A F, Raine P A, Young D G 1988 Kasabach–Merritt syndrome. Journal of Paediatric Surgery 23: 109

Erickson E H 1950 Eight stages of man in childhood and society. Norton, New York, pp 219–234

Garcia R L, Dixon S L 1984 Occlusion amblyopia secondary to a mixed capillary-cavernous haemangioma. Journal of the American Academy of Dermatology 10: 263

Garfinkle T J, Handler S 1980 Haemangiomas of the head and neck in children—a guide to management. Journal of Otolaryngology 9: 439

Hamill P V, Drizd T A, Johnson C L, Reed R B et al 1979 Physical Growth. National Centre for Health Statistics percentiles. American Journal of Clinical Nutrition 32: 607

Hobby L W 1983 Further evaluation of the potential of the argon laser in the treatment of strawberry haemangiomas. Plastic and Reconstructive Surgery 71: 481

Holinger P H, Brown W T 1967 Congenital webs, cysts, laryngoceles and other anomalies of the larynx. Annals of Otology, Rhinology and Laryngology 76: 744

Irving I M 1990 Tumours of the head and neck. In: Lister J, Irving I M (eds) Neonatal surgery, 3rd edn. Butterworths, Toronto, pp 111–121

Izant R J 1987 Paediatric surgery. In: Davis J H (ed) Clinical surgery C V Mosby, Toronto, pp 3067–3080

Jackson I T, Hide A H, Gomuwka P K, Laws E R Jr et al 1982 Treatment of cranio-orbital fibrous dysplasia. Journal of Maxillofacial Surgery 10: 138

Kaban L B, Mulliken J B 1990 Vascular anomalies of the maxillofacial region. In: Kaban L B (ed) Paediatric oral and maxillofacial surgery. W B Saunders, Toronto, pp 399–420

Koerper M A, Addiego J E Jr, deLorimer A A, Lipow H et al 1983 Use of aspirin and dipyridamole in children with platelet trapping syndromes. Journal of Paediatrics 102: 311–314

Krafchik B 1989 Vascular lesions in children. Canadian Journal of Dermatology 1: 71

Kushner B J 1982 Intralesional corticosteroid injection for infantile adnexal haemangioma. American Journal of Ophthalmology 93: 496

Kveton J F, Pillsbury H C 1982 Conservative treatment of infantile subglottic haemangioma with corticosteroids. Archives of Otolaryngology 108: 117

Landthaler M, Haina D, Brunner R, Waidelich W et al 1986 Neodymium–YAG laser therapy for vascular lesions. Journal of the American Academy of Dermatology 14: 107

Larsen E C, Zinkham W H, Eggleston J C, Zitellu B J 1987 Kasabach–Merritt syndrome: therapeutic considerations. Paediatrics 79: 971

Levine H, Bailin P 1982 Carbon dioxide laser treatment of cutaneous haemangiomas and tattoos. Archives of Otolaryngology 108: 236–238

Luce E A 1986 Forward to head and neck surgery. Surgical Clinics of North America 66: 1

Margileth A M, Museles M 1965 Current concepts in diagnosis and management of congenital cutaneous haemangiomas. Paediatrics 36: 410

Martin H E 1940 The history of lingual cancer. American Journal of Surgery 48: 703–716

Melamed B G, Siegel L J 1975 Reduction of anxiety in children facing hospitalisation and surgery by use of filmed modeling. Journal of Consulting and Clinical Psychology 43: 511

Mulliken B J 1988 Classification of vascular birthmarks. In: Mulliken B J, Young A E (eds) Vascular birthmarks: hemangiomas and malformations. W B Saunders, Toronto, pp 24–37

Mulliken J B, Glowacki J 1982 Haemangiomas and vascular malformations in infants and children: a classification based on endothelial characteristics. Plastic and Reconstructive Surgery 69: 412

Munro I T, Chen Y R 1981 Radical treatment for fronto-orbital fibrous dysplasia: the chain link-fence. Plastic and Reconstructive Surgery 67: 719

Neidhart J A, Roach RW 1982 Successful treatment of skeletal haemangiomas and Kasabach–Merritt syndrome with aminocaproic acid. American Journal of Medicine 73: 434

Pasyk K A, Dingman R O, Argenta L C, Sandal G S 1984 The management of haemangiomas of the eyelid and orbit. Head and Neck Surgery 6: 851

Posnick J C 1992 The use of rigid fixation in the management of paediatric head and neck tumours. In: Gruss J S, Manson PM, Yarmachuk M J (eds) Rigid fixation of the craniomaxillofacial skeleton. Butterworth, London

Posnick J C, Louie G, Zuker R M, Weitzman S 1992a Ewing's sarcoma: primary involvement of the zygoma undergoing resection and immediate reconstruction. Plastic and Reconstructive Surgery 89: 956–961

Posnick J C, Polley J W, Zuker R M, Chan H S L 1992b Chemotherapy and surgical resection combined with immediate reconstruction in a 1-year old with rhabdomyosarcoma of the maxilla. Plastic and Reconstructive Surgery 89: 320

Posnick J C, Cleland H J, Zuker R M, Mock D 1992c Recurrent giant cell lesion of the nasomaxillary region in a child: excision and immediate reconstruction with a free rectus abdominus muscle transfer. Journal of Oral and Maxillofacial Surgery 50: 1009–1015

Posnick J C, Polley J W, Zuker R M, Chan H S L 1992d Chemotherapy and surgical resection combined with immediate reconstruction in a 1-year-old with rhabdosarcoma of the maxilla. Plastic and Reconstructive Surgery 89: 320–325

Rapidis A D, Economidis J, Goumas P D et al 1988 Tumours of the head and neck in children. A clinico-pathological analysis of 1007 cases. Journal of Craniomaxillofacial Surgery 16: 279

Ratz J L, Bailin P L 1987 The case for the carbon dioxide laser in the treatment of port wine stains. Archives of Dermatology 123: 74

Robertson J 1958 Young children in hospitals. Basic Books, New York, pp 19–24

Rush B F Jr 1983 Tumours of the head and neck. In: Schwartz S I (ed) Principles of surgery, 4th edn. McGraw-Hill, New York pp 557–601

Schrudde J, Petrovivi V 1981 Surgical treatment of giant haemangiomas of the facial region after arterial embolisation. Plastic and Reconstructive Surgery 68: 878

Shikhani A H, Marsh B R, Jones M M, Holliday M J 1986 Infantile subglottic haemangiomas: an update. Annals of Otology, Rhinology and Laryngology 95: 336

Straub P W, Kessler S, Schreiber A, Frick P G 1972 Chronic intravascular coagulation in Kasabach–Merritt syndrome. Archives of Internal Medicine 129: 475–478

Thomson H G, Ward C M, Crawford J S, Stigmar G 1979 Haemangiomas of the eyelid: visual complications and prophylactic concepts. Plastic and Reconstructive Surgery 63: 641

Warrell R P Jr, Kempin S J 1985 Treatment of severe coagulopathy in the Kasabach–Merritt syndrome with aminocaproic acid and cryoprecipitate. New England Journal of Medicine 313: 309

Wenig B L, Abramson A L 1988 Congenital subglottic haemangiomas: a treatment update. Laryngoscope 98: 190

Williams B H 1980 Vascular neoplasms. Clinics in Plastic Surgery 7: 397

Young A E 1988 Arteriovenous malformations In: Mulliken J B, Young A E (eds) Vascular birthmarks: haemangiomas and malformations. W B Saunders, Philadelphia, pp 228–245

Zak T A, Morin J D 1981 Early local steroid therapy of infantile eyelid haemangiomas. Journal of Paediatric Ophthalmology and Strabismus 18: 25

Zarem H A, Edgerton M T 1967 Induced resolution of cavernous haemangiomas following prednisolone therapy. Plastic and Reconstructive Surgery 36: 76

Zochodyne D W, Cairncross J G, Arce F P, MacDonald J C et al 1984 Astrocytoma following scalp radiotherapy in infancy 11: 475

Zuker R M, Posnick J C 1992 The role of microsurgery in paediatric craniofacial reconstruction. Clinics in Plastic Surgery 19: 833–839

26. Resection and reconstruction of extensive and complex tumours of the head and neck

Neil F. Jones

INTRODUCTION

Even today, patients occasionally develop extensive tumours of the head and neck by the time of their initial presentation. The majority are basal-cell carcinomas or squamous-cell carcinomas of the face and scalp which, in addition to their peripheral extension, may also invade deeper vital structures such as the skull, dura, orbit and maxillary sinus. Less frequently, tumours arising deeply within the oral cavity or maxillary sinus may invade the overlying facial skin, and tumours of the hypopharynx may occasionally spread to involve the overlying neck skin. Many of these tumours rapidly progress to their advanced stage due to the aggressive biological potential of the tumour itself, but others present in such advanced stages due to patient neglect and failure or delay in seeking medical attention. Patients may also occasionally present with extensive tumours due to the development of multiple recurrences following failure of primary surgical or radiotherapy treatment. These tumours are obviously staged as T4 tumours on the TNM system, but they have often been described colloquially in the literature as 'gigantic', 'massive', 'advanced', and even 'horrifying' (Jackson & Adams 1973, Savage 1983, Caldarelli & Regowski 1985).

Definition of whether a defect following tumour resection is 'extensive' or 'complex' remains arbitrary and is dependent on the individual surgeon's previous experience. An 'extensive' defect may be arbitrarily defined as any defect greater than 50 cm^2 following resection. 'Complex' describes a defect involving two or more epithelial surfaces with exposure or segmental resection of the underlying facial or cranial bones and associated with a three-dimensional volume deficit.

In the past, these extensive tumours have been considered inoperable usually because resection would automatically lead to further exposure of vital structures, especially the dura and brain, and secondly because the resultant defect could not be covered by conventional reconstructive techniques such as split-thickness skin grafts or tubed pedicle flaps. Furthermore, before the development of axial pattern and musculocutaneous flaps, a basic tenet of surgical philosophy had been that the defect created following resection of aggressive tumours of the head and neck should only be covered primarily with a split-thickness skin graft so that any subsequent development of a local recurrence would not be hidden beneath a flap and therefore allow early recognition. This left the patient with considerable functional disability and potentially a grotesque appearance until definitive reconstruction could be performed 6 months to a year later. Even this secondary reconstruction usually involved multiple stages and consequently a prolonged hospitalization. With the advent of the deltopectoral flap and the various musculocutaneous flaps such as the latissimus dorsi, pectoralis major, trapezius and sternomastoid flaps, immediate reconstruction of defects of the head and neck has become accepted (Robson 1976) but these techniques are still limited for truly extensive defects by their arc of rotation and area of available tissue. However, microsurgical free tissue transfer can now provide coverage of virtually any size defect, and success rates of greater than 95% have been achieved in centres performing a large volume of microsurgery. Consequently, resection of an extensive tumour of the head and neck is no longer limited by the constraints of conventional reconstructive techniques. With the development of diagnostic radiological imaging, CT and MRI scanning have allowed improved pre-operative evaluation of tumours of the head and neck. The marriage of these parallel developments in radiological imaging and microsurgery have led to a change in philosophy of the surgical management of patients with extensive tumours of the head and neck.

PRE-OPERATIVE ASSESSMENT

This subset of patients with aggressive primary or recurrent tumours should be evaluated pre-operatively to determine the histological type of tumour, the local extent of the tumour and whether metastases have occurred. For primary tumours, a histological diagnosis should be obtained from an initial biopsy. For recurrent tumours, details of the patient's previous treatment should be reviewed—including the histological diagnosis, the extent of previous surgical resection and reconstruction, and details of radiotherapy or chemotherapy dosage. Localization of the extent of the tumour is now routinely obtained from both CT and MRI scans. If the tumour is suspected of involving the common carotid or internal carotid artery systems, carotid angiography is performed. If necessary, a pre-operative balloon occlusion and xenon brain scan will allow the surgeon to determine whether the collateral circulation is adequate to allow resection of the ipsilateral carotid artery. Finally, a metastatic work-up should now include a CT scan of the chest and liver.

Based on the biological behaviour of the specific histological type of tumour, the local extent of the tumour, the results of a metastatic survey and, if necessary, details of previous treatment, a decision can be made as to whether the tumour can be resected with free margins. If so, a radical curative resection can be planned. If this is not possible, surgery may still provide a significant interval of palliation. Palliative surgery is justified to remove a bleeding or fungating tumour so that the patient can be relieved of his pain for a reasonable period of time. These decisions and any eventual surgery should optimally be performed by a multi-disciplinary team consisting of an ENT surgeon, a neurosurgeon and a plastic and reconstructive surgeon with input from a radiotherapist and radiologist. Compared with this team approach, a single surgical team may be tempted to compromise the oncological margins of resection in an attempt to preserve sufficient local tissue for reconstruction. The resection team has complete jurisdiction to excise as much normal tissue surrounding the tumour as is felt necessary to accomplish a three-dimensional tumour-free margin. Incisions and exposure are discussed pre-operatively to avoid compromising the later use of a regional flap or a recipient artery or vein for microsurgical anastomoses.

PRINCIPLES OF RESECTION

Surgical exposure to the various areas of the head and neck has already been covered in many of the previous chapters. Especially for tumours involving the scalp and skull and the middle third of the face and orbit, craniofacial incisions and osteotomies derived from craniofacial surgery greatly facilitate the resection which may therefore require interdisciplinary collaboration between the ENT surgeon and neurosurgeon (Jackson et al 1983). Multiple frozen sections of every margin of the specimen should be examined meticulously by a pathologist present in the operating room. Only if every margin can be confidently assessed as being free of tumour should immediate reconstruction be continued by a separate reconstructive team.

PRINCIPLES OF RECONSTRUCTION

In certain circumstances, radical resection of extensive tumours followed by immediate reconstruction usually by microsurgical free tissue transfer may be indicated for several reasons. First, pre-operative evaluation of these extensive lesions has been revolutionized by developments in radiological imaging. Axial and coronal CT scans and coronal and sagittal MRI scans allow dramatic anatomical definition of the extension of these tumours. Computerized three-dimensional reformatting can even produce a spatial display of the operative resection required to encompass the tumour. Secondly, many patients have failed previous surgery or radiotherapy and a final radical resection may result in such an extensive defect or communication between the dura and nasopharynx or oral cavity that split-thickness skin grafts and other simpler methods of reconstruction cannot be used. Immediate microsurgical reconstruction may therefore allow one final attempt at radical curative resection or at least allow a palliative resection to preclude progressive facial disfigurement and intractable pain or expedite the fitting of a prosthesis (Maillard et al 1976).

When a free flap is used for reconstruction, this usually cannot be elevated simultaneously with the resection in an attempt to reduce the operating time until the precise size and geometry of the defect has been established.

Obviously, the most significant complication inherent with immediate microsurgical reconstruction following resection of these extensive tumours is that positive margins may be discovered several days later when permanent histological sections become available, despite clear margins on initial frozen sections. Furthermore, depending upon the biological behaviour of the primary tumour, the incidence of local recurrence may be high. A recurrence developing beneath a free flap may be difficult to detect clinically. With the resultant delay in diagnosis, such recurrences may become inoperable. However, these potential drawbacks to radical resection and immediate microsurgical reconstruction of primary aggressive tumours may be circumvented by pre-operative three-dimensional computerized planning, intra-operative collaboration with dedicated pathologists, and postoperative serial CT and MRI scanning to detect recurrences.

EXCISION AND RECONSTRUCTIVE TECHNIQUES

The surgical techniques employed vary according to the pathology and also according to the anatomical site within the head and neck.

Scalp and skull

Excision

Extensive involvement of the scalp and underlying skull is usually due to basal-cell or squamous-cell carcinomas.

Depending on the depth of resection, five different types of resultant defect may be encountered:

1. intact periosteum
2. absent periosteum with exposed skull
3. partial resection of the outer table of the calvarium
4. full-thickness resection of the calvarium
5. resection of dura with exposed brain.

Reconstruction will be dictated both by the depth of resection and the surface area of the defect.

Reconstruction

If the periosteum remains intact, even after resection of a large surface area of the scalp, reconstruction can be readily accomplished using split-thickness skin grafts. Once the periosteum has been resected, or if the outer table of the skull has been resected, reconstruction of such extensive scalp defects has conventionally been accomplished using large transposition or rotation scalp flaps with split-thickness skin grafting of the remaining periosteum in the donor defect (Gaisford et al 1958). The pedicled latissimus dorsi and trapezius musculocutaneous flaps can also be used for these defects in which the periosteum or outer table of the calvarium has been resected. However, their limited arc of rotation confines their use to the occipital and parietal regions of the scalp and skull. For other large surface-area defects in which the periosteum or the outer table of the calvarium have been resected, and certainly for extensive

defects in which there has been full-thickness excision of the skull, microsurgical free tissue transfer has become the method of choice.

McLean & Buncke (1972) first described free tissue transfer for scalp reconstruction using free omentum covered with a split-thickness skin graft. In addition to the omentum (Barrow et al 1984), the groin flap (Chater et al 1977, Chavoin et al 1980), the latissimus dorsi musculocutaneous flap (Maxwell et al 1980), the latissimus dorsi muscle and split-thickness skin graft (Jones et al 1988, Pennington et al 1989), the latissimus dorsi combined with either a serratus muscle flap (Harii et al 1982) or a scapular skin flap (Batchelor & Sully 1984), the scapular or parascapular skin flap (Chiu et al 1984), the radial forearm flap (Chicarilli et al 1986, Wei et al 1987) and the extended deep inferior epigastric flap (Miyamoto et al 1986) have all been advocated for microsurgical reconstruction of large scalp defects. Because the scapular flap and radial forearm flap have a fairly defined size of donor defect, they cannot truly be considered as flaps of choice for extensive scalp defects. Free omental transfer requires an abdominal incision with its attendant morbidity. Therefore, the latissimus dorsi muscle with a split-thickness skin graft is probably the optimal choice for reconstruction of extensive scalp defects following tumour excision (Jones et al 1988, Furnas et al 1990) (Fig. 26.1). Furthermore the latissimus dorsi muscle may be thinned on its external (skin) surface and covered with a sheet of split-thickness skin graft to produce excellent cosmetic results (Rowsell et al 1986).

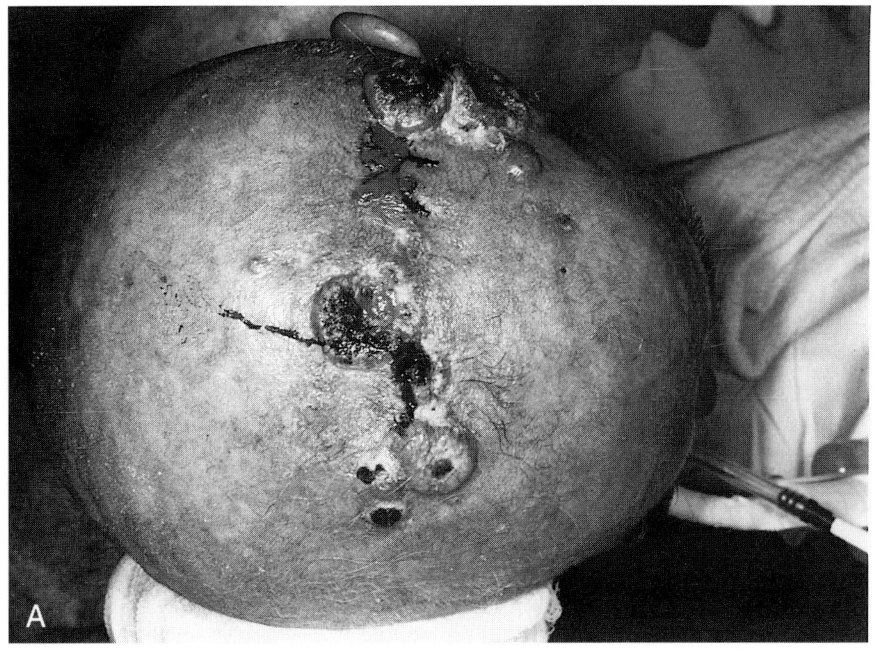

Fig. 26.1

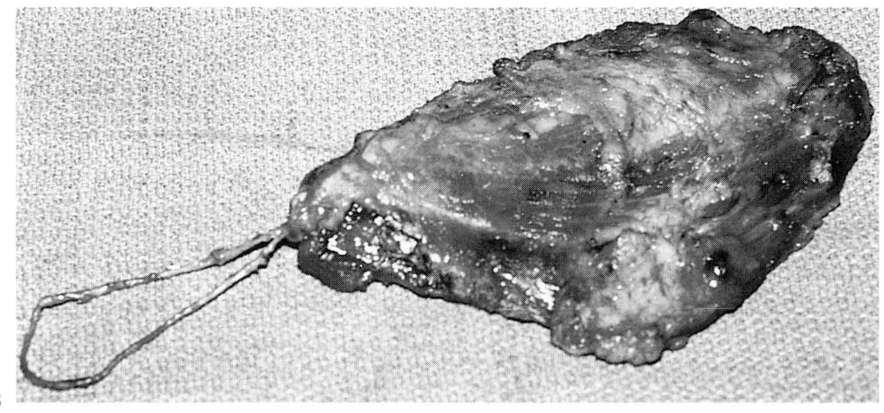

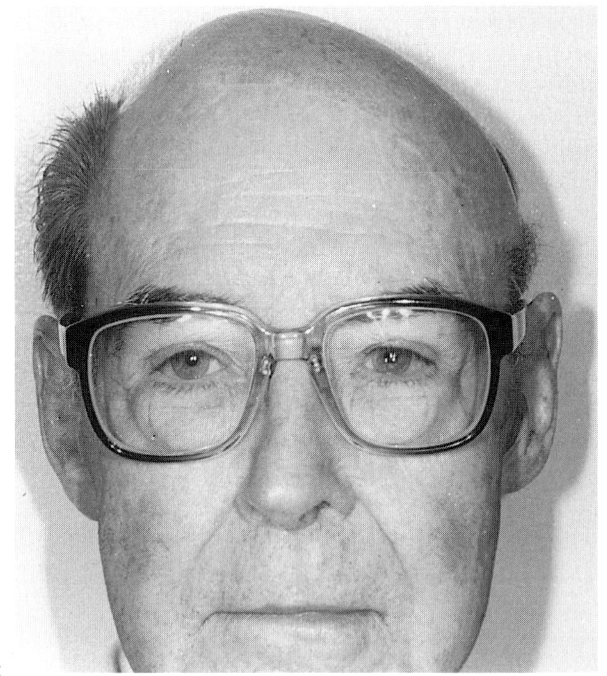

Fig. 26.1   **A.** A 70-year-old man with multiple squamous-cell carcinomas of the scalp previously treated by local excision and radiotherapy. CT scan bone windows revealed involvement of the outer table of the skull. **B.** Wide resection of the left frontal, temporal and parietal scalp and right parietal scalp, periosteum and outer table of the skull resulted in a 20 x 15 cm defect of the scalp and outer table of the skull which was covered with a latissimus dorsi free muscle flap. The latissimus muscle was thinned on its external (skin) surface and covered with sheets of split thickness skin grafts. **C, D.** The patient remains free of disease 4 years postoperatively with a very acceptable cosmetic result.

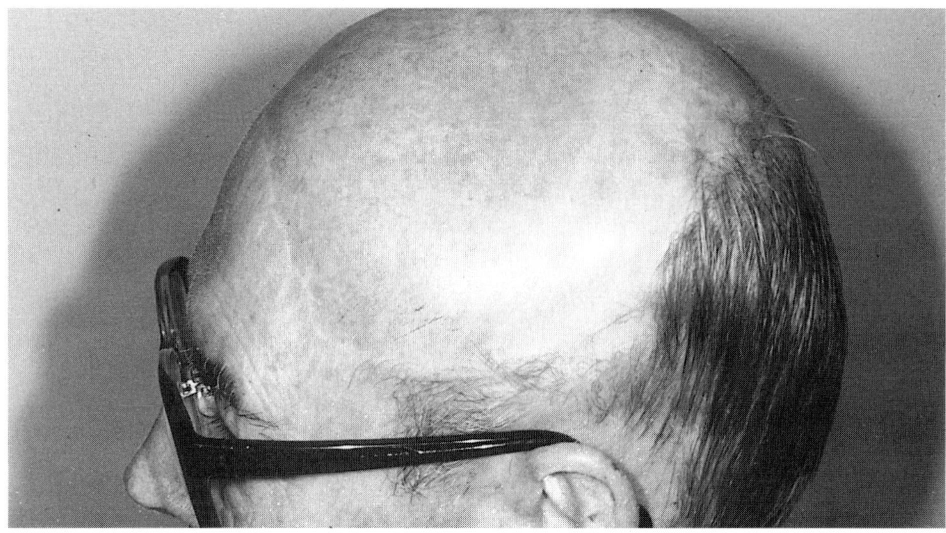

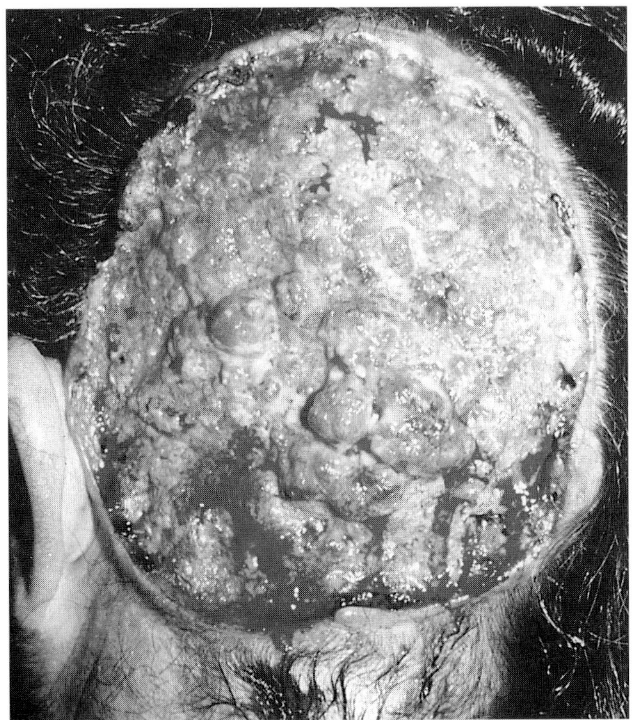

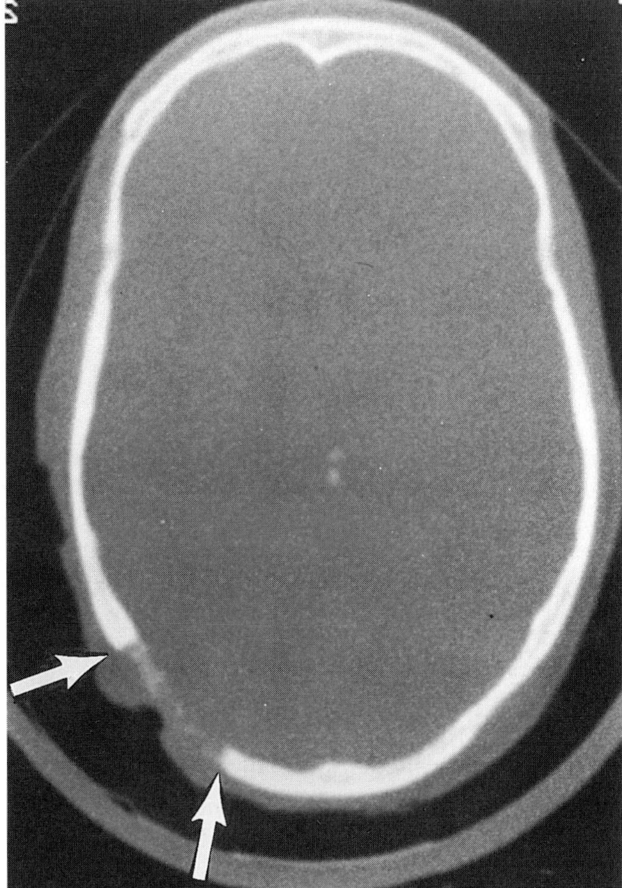

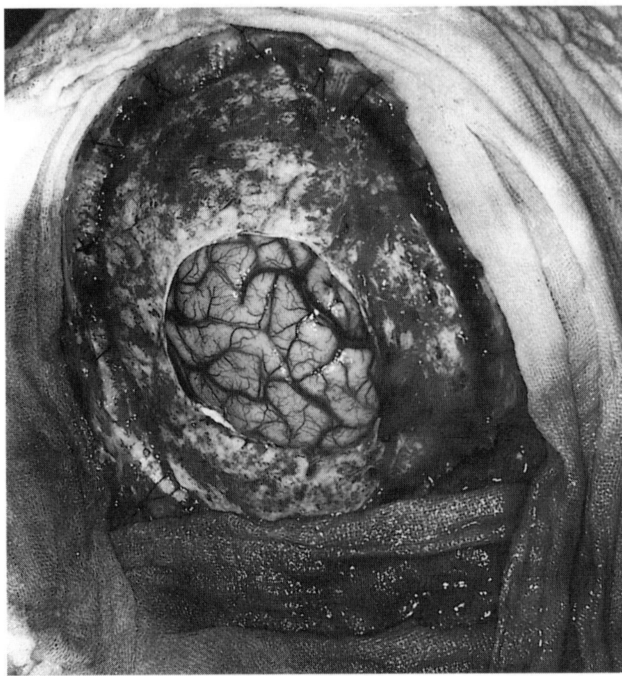

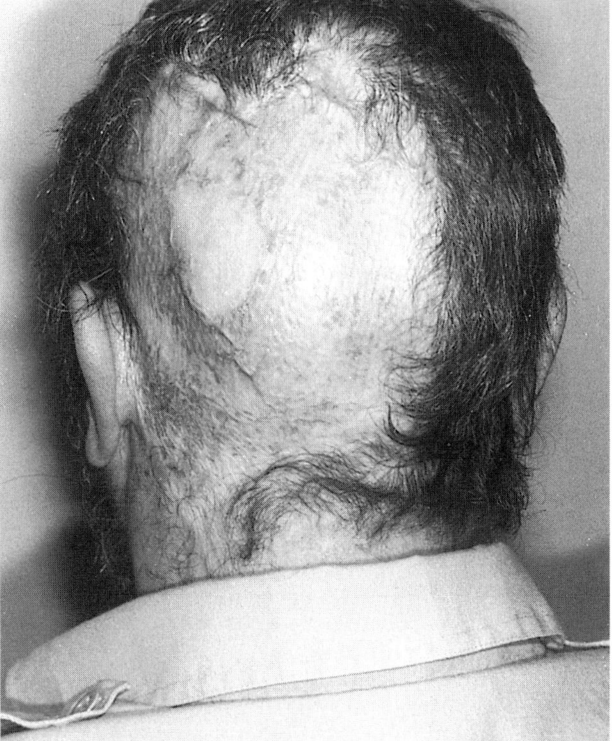

Fig. 26.2 A. A 48-year-old man with a massive basal-cell carcinoma of the posterior scalp present for the previous 20 years. **B.** Bone algorithms from the CT scan revealed full-thickness invasion of both outer and inner tables of the left occipital skull. **C.** After radical resection of the occipital scalp and periosteum, a 12 x 12 cm craniectomy revealed a 2 cm diameter nodule of BCC on the left occipital dura. Following wide excision of the dura, the dural defect was reconstructed with a fascia lata graft and the 21 x 18 cm scalp defect was reconstructed using a free latissimus dorsi muscle flap covered with meshed split-thickness skin graft. **D.** There has been no clinical or radiological evidence of tumour recurrence 5 years postoperatively. The patient has declined secondary reconstruction of the bony defect of the skull.

When full-thickness skull and dura have been resected, reconstruction of the dura and bone have to be addressed in addition to soft-tissue coverage. While it has been advocated that dural defects do not need to be reconstructed but merely covered with a vascularized flap, this is risky, especially when the defect allows dependent drainage of cerebrospinal fluid. An attempt should therefore be made to obtain 'water-tight' closure of the dura using autogenous fascia lata grafts (Fig. 26.2). Simultaneous bony reconstruction of calvarial defects at the time of soft-tissue reconstruction of extensive scalp defects remains controversial. Large skull defects have conventionally been reconstructed using split rib grafts as a secondary procedure (Longacre & Destefano 1957, 1958). Alloplastic material such as methylmethacrylate and titanium metal plates have also been utilized but may be complicated by infection. Smith et al (1983) first reported the simultaneous reconstruction of a large scalp and skull defect using a custom-made titanium plate covered by a latissimus dorsi musculocutaneous free flap. Split rib grafts covered with a latissimus dorsi free muscle flap or musculocutaneous flap is probably the method of choice for reconstruction of large scalp and skull defects, especially when postoperative radiotherapy may be required (Stueber et al 1985). Occasionally, vascularized bone grafts may be used to reconstruct complex full-thickness defects of the scalp and skull using the iliac crest—internal oblique free flap (Shenaq 1988).

Middle third of the face, orbit, maxilla and palate

Excision

Resection of advanced basal-cell and squamous-cell carcinomas of the middle third of the face and T4 carcinomas of the maxillary sinus results in complex three-dimensional volume deficits when compared with the large surface area defects of the scalp. In addition, the resection involves two or more epithelial surfaces, involving combinations of palatal mucosa, buccal mucosa, external facial skin or the lateral nasal cavity. Such resections may be classified into a hierarchy of increasing complexity:

Lateral External skin with parotidectomy
    External skin and orbital exenteration

Central Palate and maxilla
    Palate, maxilla and external skin
    Palate, maxilla, external skin and lateral nose
    Palate, maxilla, external skin and orbital exenteration
    Palate, maxilla, external skin, orbit and anterior cranial base
    Palate, maxilla, external skin, orbit, anterior cranial base and frontal dura

These middle-third facial defects may be divided arbitrarily into central and lateral defects. Lateral defects result from wide excision of skin from the middle third of the face and cheek and are occasionally associated with a parotidectomy or orbital exenteration. These defects are essentially large surface area defects and do not involve a volume deficit. Since they do not involve the palate or oral mucosa, they usually require only one epithelial surface to be reconstructed and therefore the patient is at minimal risk of developing an orocutaneous fistula or a cerebrospinal fluid leak and meningitis. On the other hand, a typical central defect is produced following resections which involve excision of the skin of the middle third of the face communicating with the maxilla. As these resections become more radical, the defect may involve the lateral nose, an orbital exenteration or the anterior cranial base and frontal dura. Consequently, these complex defects not only require the reconstruction of several separate epithelial surfaces to prevent the development of an orocutaneous fistula but they also represent a three-dimensional volume deficit of the maxilla.

Reconstruction

Conventional reconstruction of lateral defects of the middle third of the face has usually been accomplished using cervical or cervicopectoral rotation flaps, the deltopectoral flap (Bakamjian & Poole 1977), and the pedicled musculocutaneous flaps—the pectoralis major (Ariyan & Cuono 1980), the latissimus dorsi (Schuller 1982) and the extended trapezius flaps (Rosen 1985). The cervical and cervicopectoral flaps and the deltopectoral flap provide skin with a good colour and texture match but may be limited by the area of tissue that may be transferred. They still have a place in the armamentarium of the reconstructive surgeon even in this era of free flaps. The pectoralis major musculocutaneous flap will provide a moderately large surface area of skin but its arc of rotation may limit its superior reach. Pedicled latissimus dorsi and extended trapezius musculocutaneous flaps may be compromised by the effect of gravity on the weight of the skin paddle and underlying muscle resulting in flap separation at the superior margin of the defect. Free flaps are occasionally indicated for coverage of these lateral defects, and the groin flap, deltopectoral flap, radial forearm flap, scapular flap and the inferior epigastric artery flap (Maruyama & Osafune 1987) have all been described for microsurgical reconstruction of lateral defects. The free groin flap provides skin of reasonable colour match and texture, but its vascular anatomy may occasionally compromise successful microvascular transfer. The radial forearm flap can provide thin, sometimes hairless skin, but reconstruction of an extensive lateral defect may produce an unacceptable donor site. The latissimus dorsi musculocutaneous flap, scapular flap and deep inferior epigastric artery flap, while not ideal for reconstructing facial skin, do provide large areas of tissue. The latissimus dorsi musculocutaneous free flap and the radial forearm flap have become the preferred choice if microsurgical free flap coverage of large lateral defects of the middle third of the face is necessary (Jones et al 1988).

The typical central defect following hemimaxillectomy and orbital exenteration has normally been reconstructed using a split-thickness skin graft held in position by a stent. After healing of the skin grafts has been achieved, the patient is fitted with an obturator prosthesis. Conventional flap closure of palatal and orbital defects using the tongue flap, forehead flap, deltopectoral flap (Bakamjian & Poole 1977), Tagliacozzi flap and temporalis muscle flap (Bakamjian & Souther 1975) has also been advocated. Small free flaps such as the dorsalis pedis flap, radial forearm flap (MacLeod et al 1987), and vascularized jejunum (Black et al 1971) have been reported for closure of palatal defects when other conventional methods have failed. The scapular osteocutaneous flap can also be used for bony palatal reconstruction by placing a skin graft on the muscle cuff and

periosteum of the blade of the scapula (Swartz et al 1986).

However, extensive basal-cell carcinomas originating in the skin of the middle third of the face may invade along the periosteal planes of the facial and orbital skeleton to involve the periorbita and anterior cranial base. Similarly, T4 tumours of the maxillary sinus may invade superiorly into the orbit and anterior cranial base. Following craniofacial resection of these advanced tumours which extend to involve the anterior cranial base, the dura or dural graft overlying the frontal lobes is in direct communication with the nasopharynx or oral cavity. Consequently, it becomes imperative in these extreme central defects that the dura be separated from the nasopharynx and oral cavity by well-vascularized tissue to prevent cerebrospinal fluid leakage, ascending infection and resultant meningitis. For small defects of the anterior cranial base, the galeal flap or temporalis muscle flap can be reliably used to separate the dura from the nasopharynx. However, if there is extensive communication

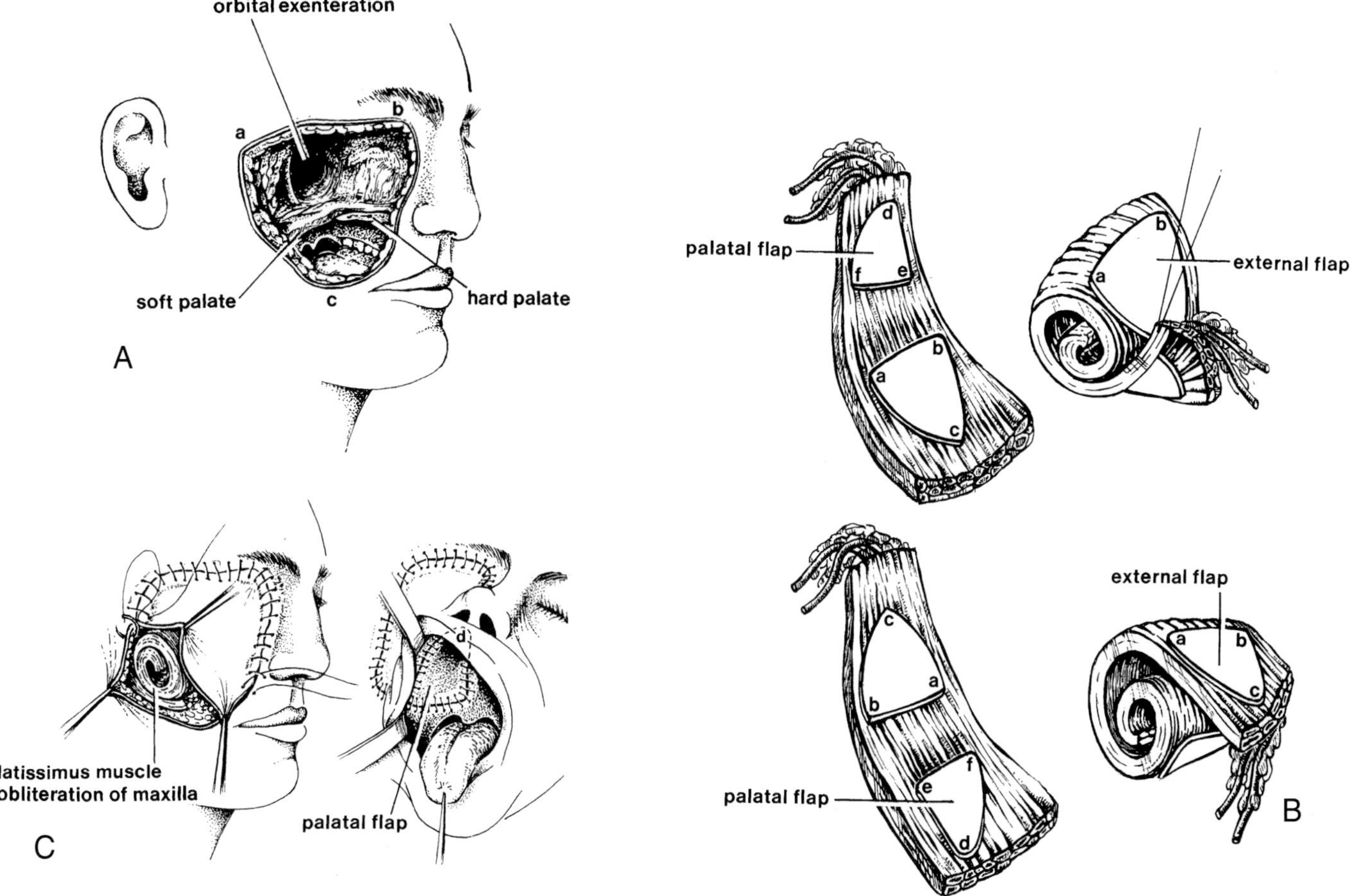

Fig. 26.3 **A.** External facial skin (a, b, c) and palatal defects following radical hemimaxillectomy and orbital exenteration. **B.** The two alternative designs of a 'double paddle' free latissimus dorsi musculocutaneous flap differ in whether the palatal defect is closed first with the proximal skin paddle and the muscle rolled clockwise to fill the maxillary cavity or whether the external facial skin defect is reconstructed first with the proximal skin paddle and the lattissimus muscle rolled counterclockwise. **C.** With either design, one skin paddle is used to reconstruct the hemipalatal defect and one paddle is used to reconstruct the defect in the external facial skin. The intervening muscle and distal latissimus dorsi muscle is used to obliterate the concavity of the maxilla.

between the dura of the anterior cranial fossa and the nasopharynx or oral cavity because of an associated hemimaxillectomy, the complex three-dimensional geometry of this defect cannot be reliably reconstructed using a split-thickness skin graft and obturator prosthesis or even a galeal or temporalis flap.

In these situations, free tissue transfer may be the only available option (Fujino et al 1981, Baker 1984). A 'double paddle' or 'triple paddle' free latissimus dorsi musculocutaneous flap may be helpful in such defects (Jones et al 1988, Shestak et al 1988, Earley 1989). By measuring the exact dimensions of the palatal and external facial skin defects and the distance of the two defects from the recipient vessels, two separate skin paddles can be precisely mapped overlying the latissimus dorsi muscle (Fig. 26.3). One skin paddle is used to reconstruct the hemipalatal or total palatal defect and the second paddle is used to close the defect in the external facial skin. The remaining latissimus muscle is then draped along the undersurface of the dura of the anterior cranial fossa and used to obliterate the hemimaxillectomy or bilateral maxillectomy cavities. A third skin paddle (Fig. 26.4) may be used to provide inner lining for the lateral nasal wall, otherwise mucoperichondrium is stripped from the ipsilateral surface of the nasal septum and either the latissimus dorsi muscle or a de-epithelialized portion of the external skin paddle is sutured to the nasal septum to prevent the future development of a mucocele.

The rectus abdominis musculocutaneous free flap has also been described for reconstruction of similar orbital–maxillectomy defects (Chicarilli & Davey 1987).

Because of the weight of the latissimus dorsi muscle and skin paddle, there is a tendency for gravity to act on the flap leading either to dehiscence of the superior suture line or to ischaemia and subsequent necrosis of the superior inset. Both mechanisms lead to the same result—partial separation of the flap from the superior margin of the defect. This can be prevented by suspending the muscle filling the maxillectomy cavity with non-absorbable sutures placed through drill holes in the remaining bony skeleton. In addition, the palatal skin paddle is made slightly smaller than the defect to suspend it tightly across the roof of the oral cavity. Postoperatively, packs are placed within the oral cavity for several days to prevent downward migration of the free latissimus dorsi musculocutaneous flap. The patient may be nursed in a slight head-down position in the early postoperative period to maintain the muscle component of the flap against the undersurface of the dura, cranial base or orbital floor. These precautions should prevent prolapse of the palatal skin paddle and have allowed early resumption of oral feeding and intelligible speech. However, closure of these large palatal defects with autogenous free flap tissue may be a disadvantage, making it impossible to fit the patient with a dental prosthesis. Secondary osseo-integration may obviate this problem in the future. Finally, because the

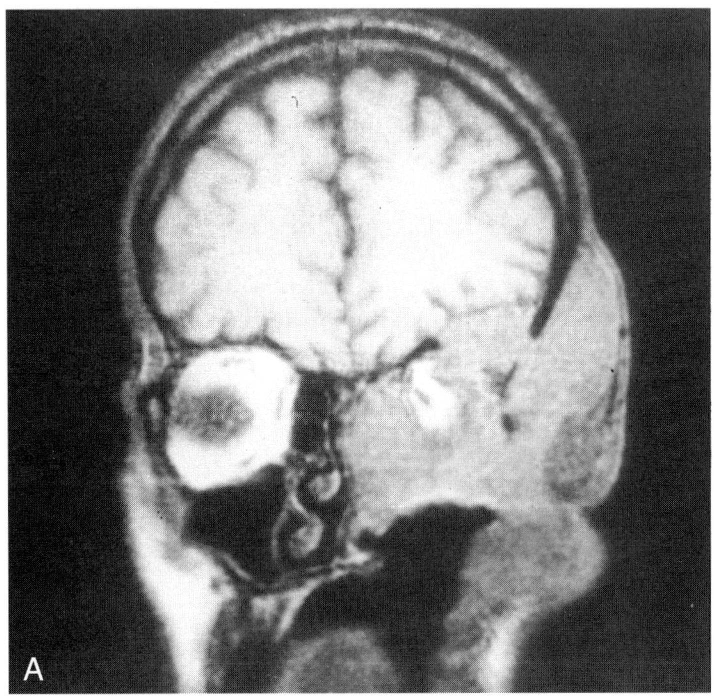
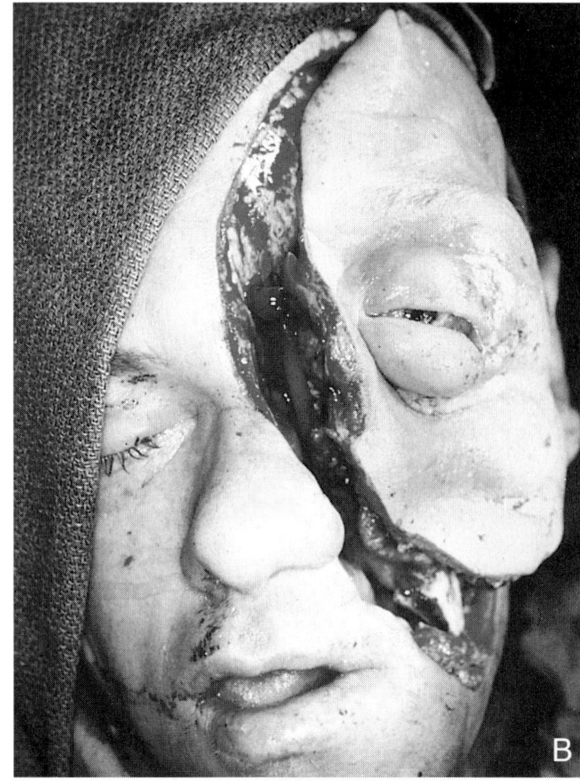

Fig. 26.4

C
D
S
N
O
E
D
dural graft
sphenoid sinus
nasal septum
nasopharynx
hemi-palatal and
oral mucosal defect
triple skin paddles
F

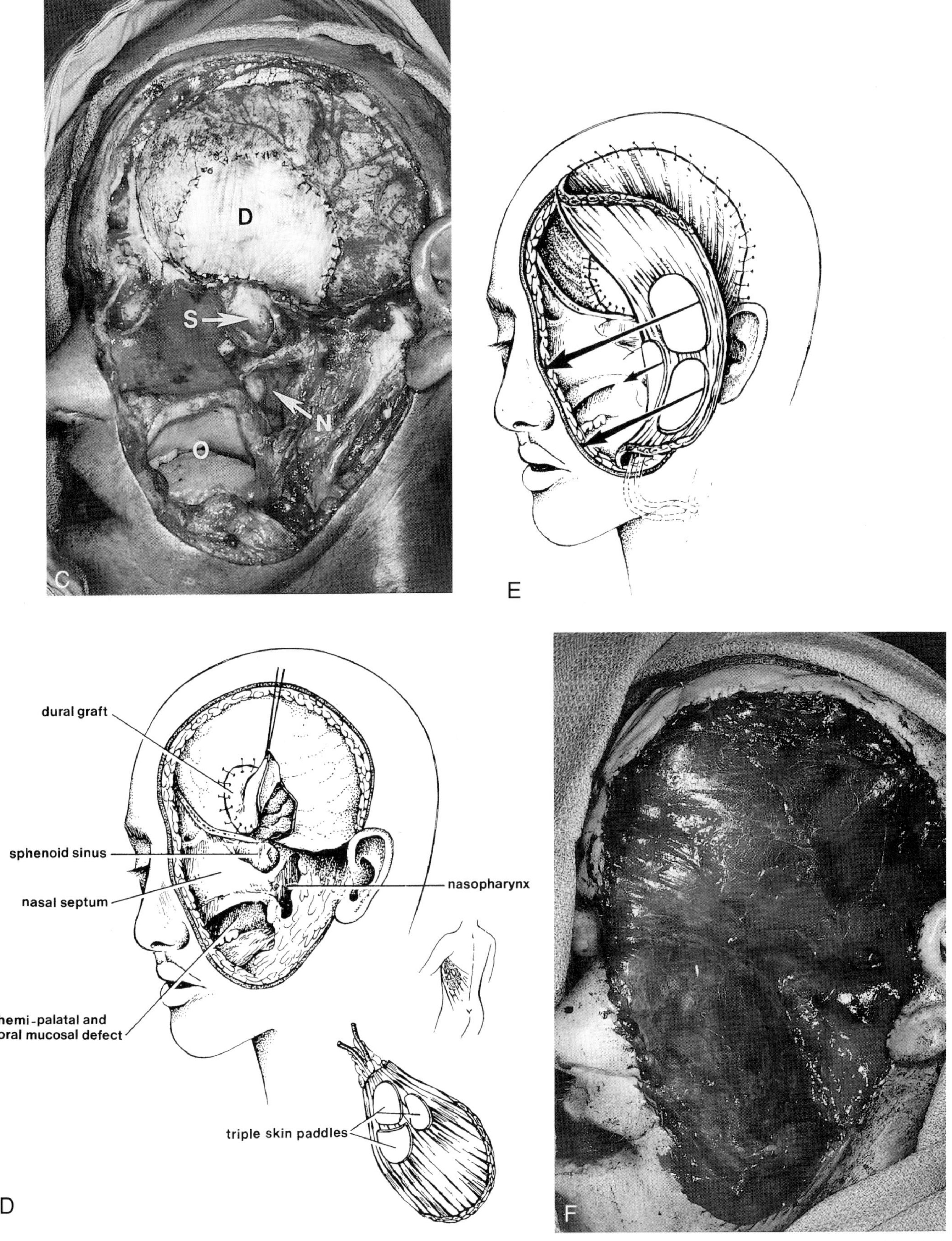

Fig. 26.4

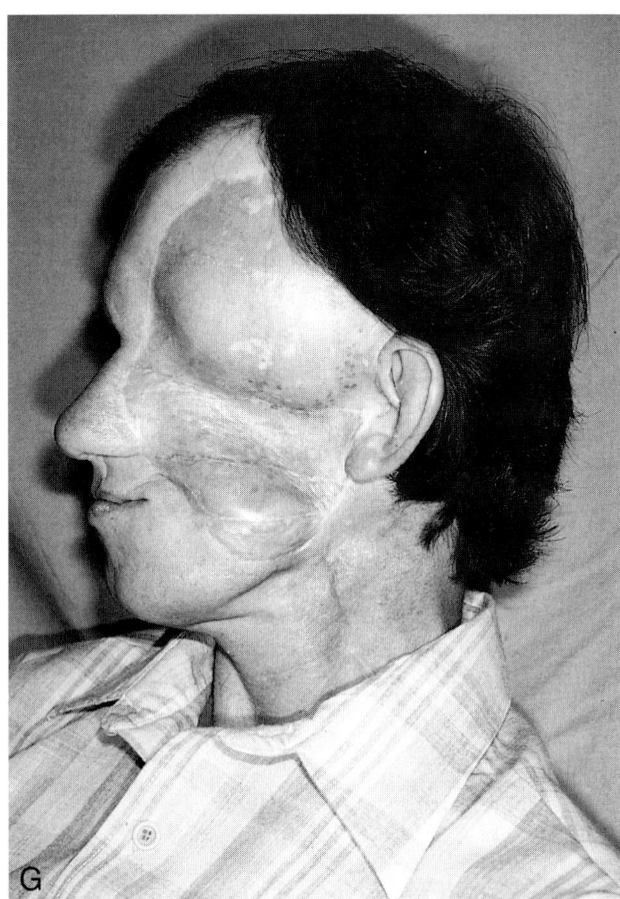
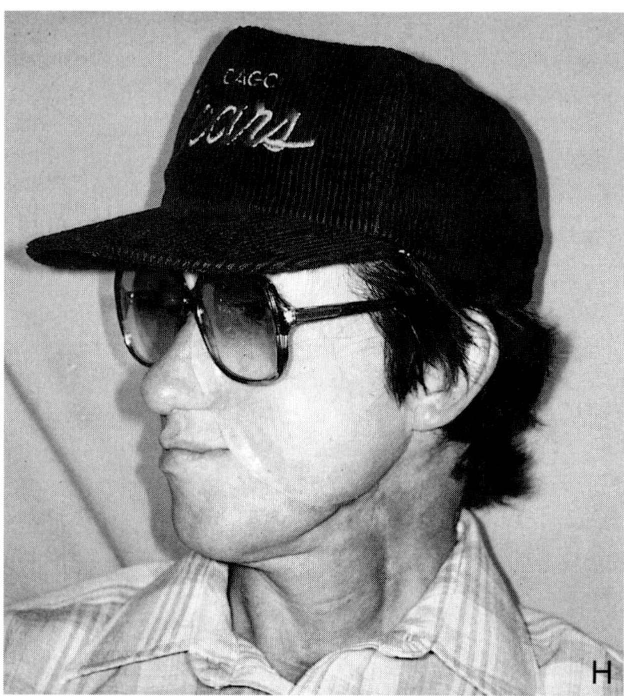

Fig. 26.4 **A.** Coronal MRI scan of a T4 recurrent squamous-cell carcinoma of the left maxillary sinus in a 34-year-old man showing superior extension of the tumour from the orbit into the anterior cranial fossa and posteriorly into the sphenoid sinus. **B.** Metastatic work-up was negative, and a palliative resection of virtually the entire left side of the face, maxilla, orbit, portions of the left frontal, parietal and temporal skull and the left half of the hard and soft palate was performed. **C.** The surgical defect measured 20 x 17 cm with exposure of the dural graft over the frontal and temporal lobes (D), the open sphenoid (S) and frontal sinuses and nasopharynx (N) and a 9 x 6 cm defect encompassing the left hemipalate and oral mucosa (O). **D, E, F.** A free latissimus dorsi flap with three separate skin paddles was used to reconstruct the defect. One skin paddle provided reconstruction of the left hemipalate and closure of the intra-oral defect. The second paddle provided closure of the left lateral wall of the nasopharynx, and the third skin paddle provided reconstruction of the left lateral wall of the nose. The muscle was draped to cover the dural graft of the fontal and temporal lobes and packed into the sphenoid sinus. Split-thickness skin grafts were used to cover the surface of the muscle. **G, H.** The patient was fitted with a facial prosthesis held in position by spectacles and was maintained in pain-free palliation for 2 years postoperatively.

external skin paddle does not have quite the same colour and texture as facial skin, a secondary procedure may be required to remove the skin and subcutaneous tissue of this external skin paddle and replace it with full-thickness skin grafts from the neck to improve the final cosmetic appearance.

Lower third of the face

Excision

The majority of tumours involving the lower third of the face arise intraorally and, depending on their depth of invasion, may extend into the mandible or, occasionally, erode superficially into the overlying external skin. Less frequently, tumours arising in the external facial skin may invade deeply into the mandible and the muscles of mastication. Resection is therefore dependent on the depth of tumour invasion assessed by bi-manual palpation, X-rays of the mandible, and, more reliably, by CT and MRI scans. Resection of such tumours may therefore involve:

1. oral mucosa alone
2. external skin alone
3. full-thickness 'through and through' defect of oral mucosa and external skin
4. oral mucosa and marginal mandibulectomy
5. oral mucosa and segmental mandibulectomy
6. 'through and through' defect of oral mucosa, segmental mandibulectomy and external skin.

Reconstruction

Extensive defects of the lower third of the face, by definition, will consist of full-thickness excision of at least two of the three tissue components—mucosa, bone and skin, either as:

1. 'through and through' defects of oral mucosa and external skin, or
2. 'through and through' defects of oral mucosa and external skin with a segmental mandibulectomy.

Reconstruction is dependent on the length of missing mandible, whether the mandibular defect is lateral or symphyseal and the size of the oral or external skin defect. The longer the bony segmental defect, the more complex the reconstruction since this will require multiple osteotomies in the reconstructed bone graft. Resection and reconstruction of extensive defects of the lower third of the face is essentially similar to those techniques described in Chapters 3 to 8.

Hypopharynx and oesophagus

Excision

Resection of tumours of the larynx, hypopharynx and cervical oesophagus has already been discussed (see Chs 11,12 and 13). However, there are three circumstances which mandate more extensive resection of the hypopharynx and oesophagus and consequently require a more complicated reconstruction:

1. associated resection of overlying cervical skin
2. proximal extension of the superior margin of resection
3. distal extension of the inferior margin of the resection below the sternal inlet or total oesophagectomy.

Patients with primary laryngeal or hypopharyngeal cancer may occasionally present with local spread to the overlying neck skin. Alternatively, patients who have already undergone a laryngectomy may develop a stomal recurrence. In both of these circumstances, wide resection of the involved cervical skin will be necessary in addition to a conventional laryngopharyngectomy or completion pharyngectomy to obtain local control.

Secondly, the superior margin of resection of a laryngopharyngectomy may need to be extended more proximally to the level of the base of the tongue or even into the floor of the mouth to achieve a tumour-free margin. This results in a significant discrepancy between the circumference of the superior pharyngeal defect and the lumen of a conventional jejunal conduit. In the most extreme cases, resection may encompass the entire floor of the mouth and pharynx down to the cervical oesophagus.

Thirdly, the distal margin of resection in the cervical oesophagus may have to be extended below the sternal inlet to achieve a tumour-free margin and, sometimes, if endoscopy reveals multiple foci of tumour within the intrathoracic oesophagus, a total oesophagectomy may be required.

Reconstruction

Patients who undergo wide resection of involved cervical skin in association with a laryngopharyngectomy or completion pharyngectomy will obviously require soft-tissue coverage simultaneously with a conventional free jejunal transfer. Simultaneous soft-tissue coverage is mandatory not to provide coverage of the bowel itself, since split-thickness skin grafts 'take' very satisfactorily on the serosa of a free jejunal transfer, but to cover and reinforce the superior and inferior jejunal anastomoses to prevent subsequent fistulae; secondly to cover and protect the exposed carotid artery following unilateral or bilateral radical neck dissection to prevent carotid artery 'blow-out' and, thirdly, to protect the microsurgical arterial and venous anastomoses to prevent anastomotic rupture. Various options are available to provide this soft-tissue coverage, including:

1. vascularized segment of mesentery and split-thickness skin graft
2. unilateral pectoralis major muscle flap and split-thickness skin graft

3. bilateral pectoralis major muscle flaps with split-thickness skin graft
4. second free flap.

For small to moderate defects of the overlying cervical skin, an additional segment of mesentery can be harvested with a conventional free jejunal transfer (Nahai et al 1984). This vascularized mesentery can then be used to protect the exposed carotid artery, and the arterial and venous microanastomoses and itself can be covered with a split-thickness skin graft (Fig. 26.5). Since split-thickness skin grafts 'take' satisfactorily both on the serosa of the free jejunal transfer and on the mesentery, an added advantage of this technique is that it will allow direct monitoring of the viability of the free jejunal transfer. Moderate sized defects of the overlying cervical skin are best covered by using a pectoralis major muscle flap covered with a split-thickness skin graft (Ariyan & Cuono 1980). The use of the pectoralis major muscle alone covered with a split-thickness skin graft provides better aesthetic definition to the neck rather than using the often bulky skin paddle of a pectoralis major musculocutaneous flap. Occasionally, for very extensive defects of the cervical skin extending from the level of the mandible down to the clavicles, bilateral pectoralis major muscle flaps covered with a split-thickness skin graft, or even a second free flap such as a radial forearm flap or a latissimus dorsi muscle flap covered by a split-thickness skin graft, may be required (Fig. 26.6). To prevent dehiscence of the superior inset of bilateral pectoralis major muscle flaps due to the effect of gravity, the muscle fascia of the pectoralis major may need to be suspended from the inferior border of the mandible using fine-gauge dental wires.

In some patients, the superior margin of resection of a laryngopharyngectomy may need to be extended more proximally to the level of the base of the tongue or even into the floor of the mouth to achieve a tumour-free margin. This results in a discrepancy in circumference between a conventional jejunal transfer and the superior defect, and even a slight discrepancy between the superior pharyngeal defect and the jejunum may explain the higher incidence of post-operative fistulae at the proximal anastomosis. Occasionally, this cannot be overcome either by partially opening the jejunum along its antimesenteric border or by transecting the upper end of the jejunum obliquely rather than transversely. Options to overcome this size discrepancy at the superior pharyngeal defect include:

1. vascularized conduit of colon
2. vascularized gastric antrum
3. double-folded free jejunal transfer
4. inverted J-shaped free jejunal transfer.

The circumference of the transverse or sigmoid colon is obviously greater than the jejunum, but the risk of abdominal sepsis is higher following harvesting of colon (Nakayama et al 1964). Transfer of the inferior border of the gastric antrum may allow prefabrication of a funnel with a larger superior stoma and the added advantage that a flap of vascularized omentum supplied by the gastro-epiploic vessels can be harvested in addition to provide associated soft-tissue coverage of the neck (Mixter et al 1990). However, a potential disadvantage of this technique is that the longitudinal suturing required to fabricate the tube may predispose this technique to a higher incidence of orocutaneous fistula. Harashina et al (1985) described a technique to overcome the dysphagia occasionally due to

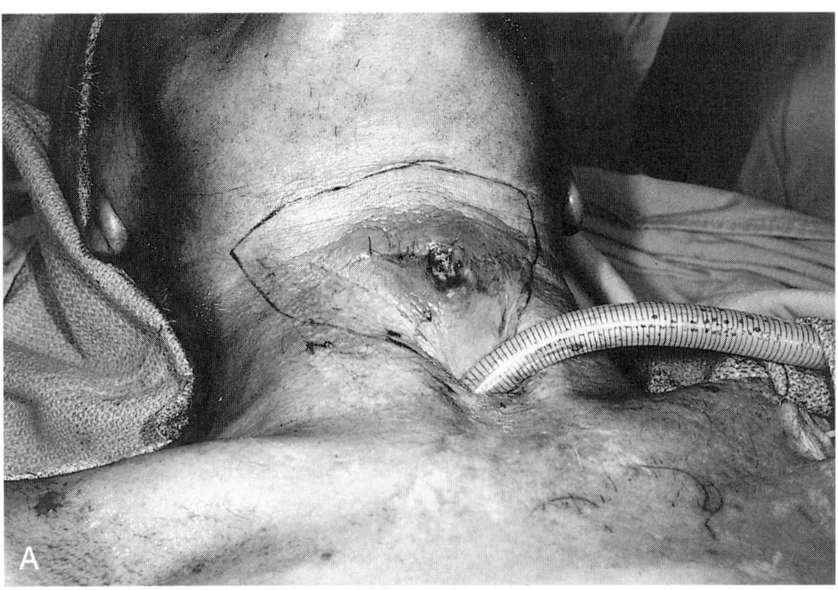

Fig. 26.5

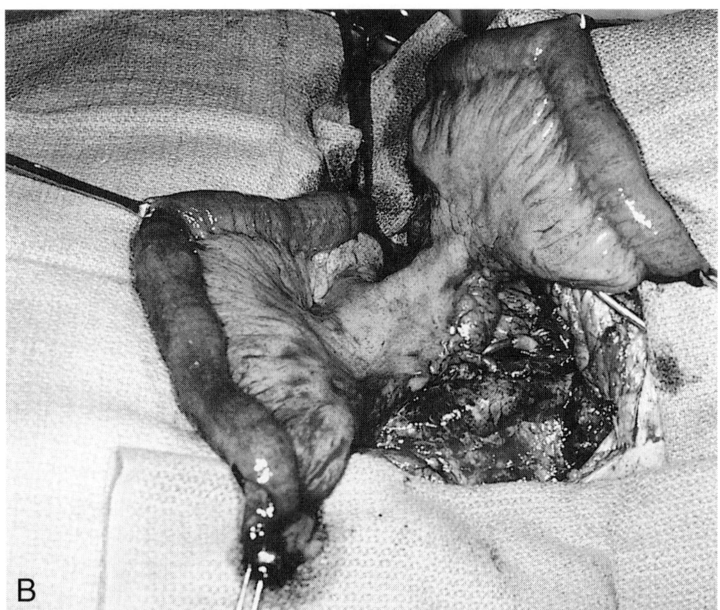

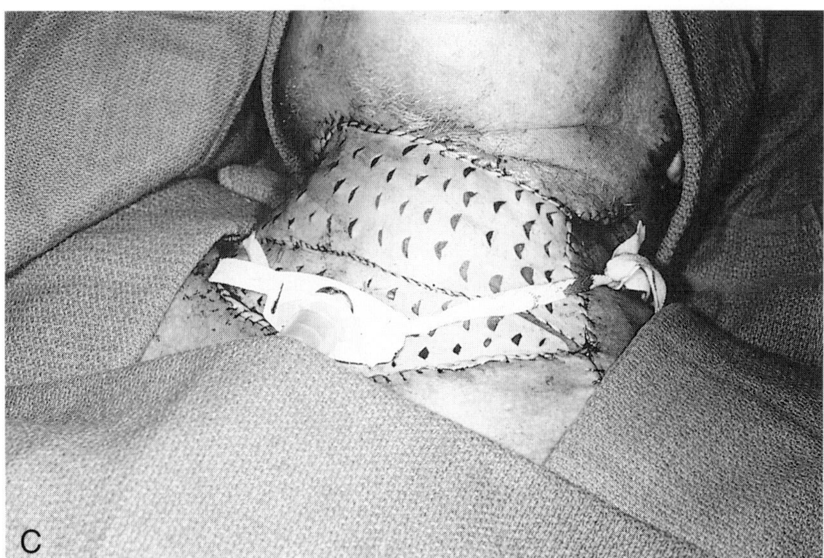

Fig. 26.5 A. Recurrent squamous-cell carcinoma of the pharynx eroding the overlying cervical skin prior to completion pharyngectomy and wide resection of the cervical skin. **B.** Two separate jejunal segments are harvested on a singular vascular arcade. One jejunal segment will be used for reconstruction of the pharyngeal–oesophageal defect. The jejunum will be removed from the second segment leaving a vascularized segment of mesentery to provide coverage of the carotid arteries and the microvascular anastomoses. **C.** Final coverage of the defect in the neck is provided by a quilted split-thickness skin graft applied over the mesentery.

peristalsis in a free jejunal transfer in which the jejunum was incised longitudinally and then folded and sutured to double the size of the lumen. This double-folded free jejunal transfer could conceivably be used in patients with large proximal pharyngeal defects, but, because it is of equal calibre throughout its length, the circumference of the distal lumen then becomes much greater than the cervical oesophagus. For this reason, an inverted J-shaped jejunal funnel can be prefabricated on a back table to enlarge the proximal stoma of a free jejunal transfer to overcome the size discrepancy and in the most extreme case will allow reconstruction of the entire floor of the mouth extending from the symphysis of the mandible anteriorly to the nasopharynx overlying the cervical fascia posteriorly (Jones et al 1991). The prefabricated J-shaped funnel then tapers into the normal lumen of the jejunum which allows end-to-end anastomosis to the remnant of the cervical oesophagus at the sternal inlet.

If the distal margin of resection in the cervical oesophagus has to be extended below the sternal inlet or if a total oesophagectomy is necessary, reconstruction of the hypopharynx and oesophagus is best achieved using a gastric pull-up. Occasionally, total oesophageal reconstruction can be performed using a long segment of jejunum which remains pedicled within the abdomen but with a single arterial and venous anastomosis in the neck. A long segment of jejunum can be mobilized in a Roux-en-Y fashion remaining vascularized on its inferior mesenteric pedicle, then rerouted through the mediastinum and anastomosed end-to-end to the pharyngeal stoma. The superior mesenteric vascular pedicle is then anastomosed to vessels in the neck in the usual microsurgical fashion. Long, skin-lined conduits, fabricated from two radial forearm flaps, or a single medial leg flap, have also been described for total oesophageal reconstruction, but these require microsurgical anastomoses to recipient vessels both in the neck and in the abdomen (Chen et al 1989).

CONCLUSIONS

There is little doubt that radical resection of aggressive primary tumours of the head and neck with immediate reconstruction, usually by microsurgical free tissue transfer and followed by adjuvant radiotherapy or chemotherapy, provides the best possible chance for cure of the cancer and functional and social rehabilitation of the patient. The goals of immediate reconstruction are to obtain a healed wound in the fastest possible time to allow early restoration of oral feeding and, if necessary, speech. Immediate one-stage reconstruction with reliable pedicled or free flaps decreases the length of hospitalization, allowing the patient to return to his home environment much faster than having to undergo multiple staged reconstructions. It also allows an early start to adjuvant radiotherapy within 6 weeks of surgery. Because microsurgical free tissue transfer will provide coverage of virtually any size defect in the head and neck, this technique will allow the oncological surgeon to perform a more radical resection of these aggressive tumours, but whether this will eventually translate to improved patient survival or a decreased incidence of local recurrences remains uncertain. However, there are encouraging reports that radical resection of tumours of the maxillary sinus followed by immediate reconstruction is now being reflected in improved patient survival (Robertson et al 1992).

Once local recurrences develop, survival rates are

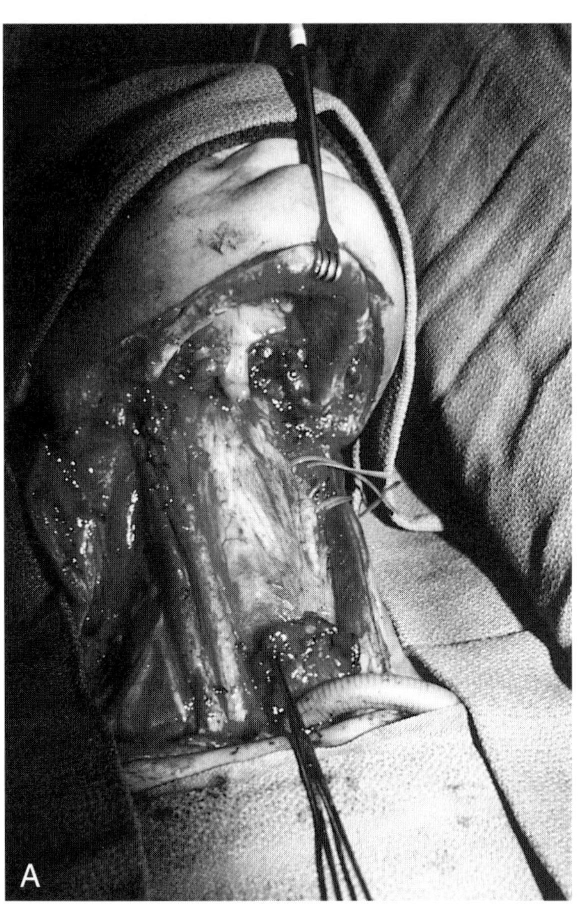

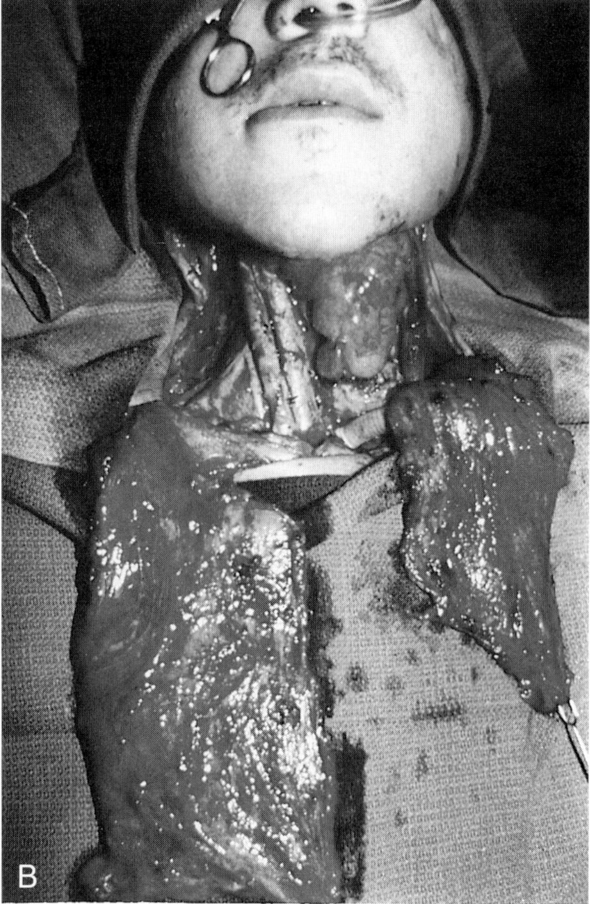

Fig. 26.6

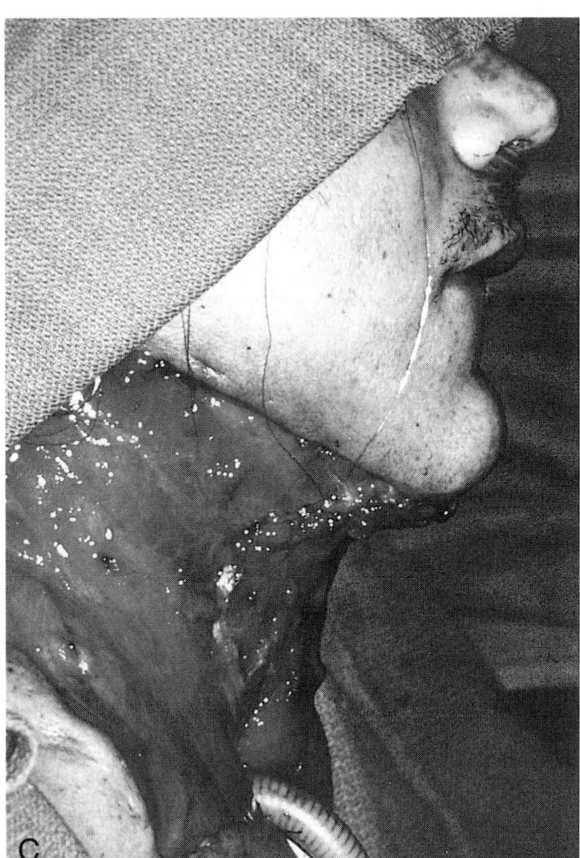
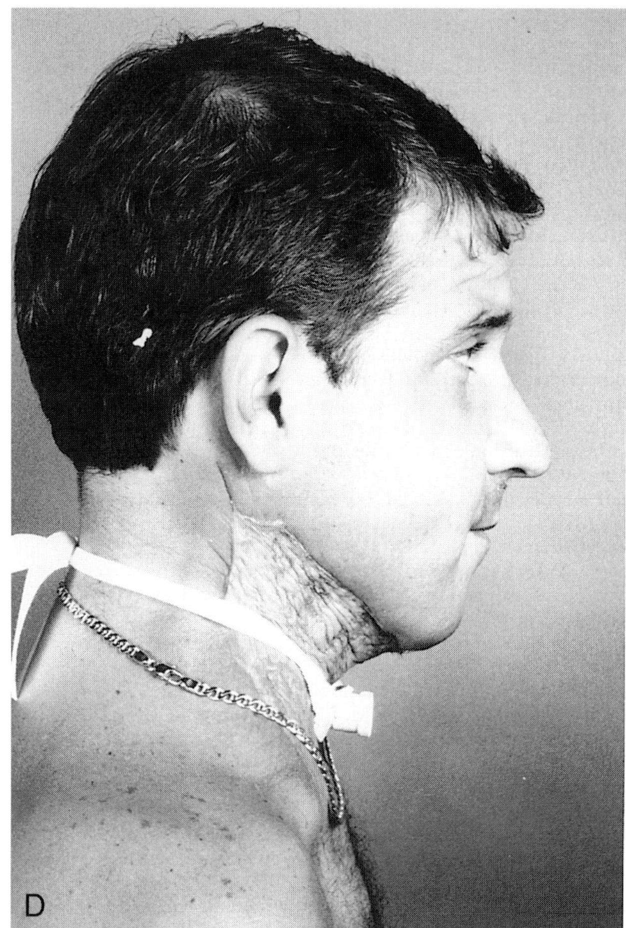

Fig. 26.6 A. In this patient an extensive pharyngo-cutaneous fistula developed following treatment of a T4 squamous-cell carcinoma at the base of the tongue with radiotherapy. Palliative resection involved the entire floor of the mouth from the symphysis of the mandible all the way posteriorly to the cervical fascia and the pharynx and cervical oesophagus down to the sternal inlet together with the entire overlying cervical neck skin from the angles of the mandible superiorly to the clavicles inferiorly. **B.** After reconstruction of the floor of the mouth, pharynx and cervical oesophagus with an inverted J-shaped free jejunal transfer, bilateral pectoralis major muscle flaps were elevated through a mid-line sternal incision and bilateral axillary counter incisions. **C.** The pectoralis muscle flaps were suspended using fine-gauge dental wire passed through drill holes in the inferior border of the mandible and through the muscle fascia, and the muscles were then covered with a quilted split-thickness skin graft. **D.** A satisfactory appearance to the neck was achieved without the development of a flexion contracture.

markedly reduced, but patients with extensive recurrent tumours of the head and neck should still not be dismissed as 'inoperable'. They, too, should be evaluated for a similar wide resection and immediate reconstruction, but as a palliative procedure. The argument for delayed reconstruction is quite inappropriate for recurrent tumours, since, if further recurrences do develop, it is highly unlikely that any other therapeutic modality will improve the patient's survival, and therefore the concern of being unable to detect a recurrence beneath a flap is rather academic. Palliative resection of a fungating or bleeding tumour may provide dramatic relief of pain. Immediate one-stage reconstruction may allow restoration of oral feeding and an acceptable facial appearance so that the patient is not forced to withdraw from society and live as a recluse. Perhaps the most impressive benefit of this approach, however, is that the patient can rapidly return to his home environment and live comfortably with dignity for the remaining few months of his life.

REFERENCES

Ariyan S, Cuono C B 1980 Use of the pectoralis major myocutaneous flap for reconstruction of large cervical, facial or cranial defects. American Journal of Surgery 140: 503

Bakamjian V Y, Poole M 1977 Maxillofacial and palatal reconstructions with the deltopectoral flap. British Journal of Plastic Surgery 30: 17–37

Bakamjian V, Souther S 1975 Use of temporal muscle flap for reconstruction after orbito-maxillary resection for cancer. Plastic and Reconstructive Surgery 56: 171–177

Baker S R 1984 Closure of large orbital-maxillary defects with free latissimus dorsi myocutaneous flaps. Head and Neck Surgery 6: 828–835

Barrow D L, Nahai F, Tindall G 1984 The use of greater omentum vascularized free flaps for neurosurgical disorders requiring reconstruction. Journal of Neurosurgery 60: 305

Batchelor A G G, Sully L 1984 A multiple territory free tissue transfer for reconstruction of a large scalp defect. British Journal of Plastic Surgery 37: 76–87

Black P W, Bevin A G, Arnold P G 1971 One-stage palate reconstruction with a free neo-vascularized jejunal graft. Plastic and Reconstructive Surgery 47: 316–320

Caldarelli D D, Regowski J E 1985 Surgical management of recurrent or advanced squamous cell cancer of the head and neck. Clinics in Plastic Surgery 12 : 505

Chater N L, Buncke H J Jr, Alpert B 1977 Reconstruction of extensive tissue defects of the scalp by microsurgical composite tissue transplantation. Surgical Neurology 7: 343–345

Chavoin J P, Gigaud M, Clouet M, Laffitte F, Costagliola M 1980 The reconstruction of cranial defects involving scalp, bone, and dura following electrical injury: report of two cases treated by homograft, free groin flap, and cranioplasty. British Journal of Plastic Surgery 33: 311–317

Chen H, Tang Y, Noordhoff M S 1989 Reconstruction of the entire esophagus with 'chain flaps' in a patient with severe corrosive injury. Plastic and Reconstructive Surgery 84: 980–984

Chicarilli Z N, Davey L M 1987 Rectus abdominis myocutaneous free flap reconstruction following a cranio-orbital-maxillary resection for neurofibrosarcoma. Plastic and Reconstructive Surgery 80: 726–731

Chicarilli Z N, Ariyan S, Cuono C B 1986 Single stage repair of complex scalp and cranial defects with the free radial forearm flap. Plastic and Reconstructive Surgery 77: 577–585

Chiu D T, Sherman J E, Edgerton B W 1984 Coverage of the calvarium with a free parascapular flap. Annals of Plastic Surgery 12: 60–66

Earley M J 1989 Primary maxillary reconstruction after cancer excision. British Journal of Plastic Surgery 42: 628–637

Fujino T, Maruyama Y, Inuyama I 1981 Double-folded free myocutaneous flap to cover total cheek defect. Journal of Maxillofacial Surgery 9: 96–100

Furnas H, Lineaweaver W C, Alpert B S, Buncke H J 1990 Scalp reconstruction by microvascular free tissue transfer. Annals of Plastic Surgery 24: 431–444

Gaisford J C, Hanna D C, Susen A F 1958 Major resection of scalp and skull for cancer with immediate complete reconstruction: fourteen cases. Plastic and Reconstructive Surgery 21: 335

Harashina T, Inoue T, Andoh T, Sugimoto C, Fujino T 1985 Reconstruction of cervical oesophagus with free double folded intestinal graft. British Journal of Plastic Surgery 38: 483–487

Harii K, Yamada A, Ishisara K et al 1982 A free transfer of both latissimus dorsi and serratus anterior flaps in thoracodorsal anastomoses. Plastic and Reconstructive Surgery 70: 620–629

Jackson R, Adams R H 1973 Horrifying basal cell carcinoma: a study of 33 cases and a comparison with 435 non-horror cases and a report on four metastatic cases. Journal of Surgical Oncology 5: 431

Jackson I T, Laws E R, Martin R D 1983 A craniofacial approach to advanced recurrent cancer of the central face. Head and Neck Surgery 5: 474–488

Jones N F, Hardesty R A, Swartz W M, Ramasastry S S, Heckler F R, Newton E D 1988 Extensive and complex defects of the scalp, middle third of the face, and palate: the role of microsurgical reconstruction. Plastic and Reconstructive Surgery 82: 937–950

Jones N F, Eadie P A, Myers E N 1991 Double lumen free jejunal transfer for reconstruction of the entire floor of mouth, pharynx and cervical oesophagus. British Journal of Plastic Surgery 44: 44–48

Longacre J J, Destefano G A 1957 Further observations on the behavior of autogenous split rib graft in the reconstruction of extensive defects of the cranium and face. Plastic and Reconstructive Surgery 20: 281

Longacre J J, Destefano G A 1958 Experimental observations of the repair of extensive defects of the skull with split rib grafts. Plastic and Reconstructive Surgery 21: 372

McLean D H, Buncke H J Jr 1972 Autotransplant of omentum to a large scalp defect with microsurgical revascularization. Plastic and Reconstructive Surgery 49: 268–274

MacLeod A M, Morrison W A, McCann J J, Thistlethwaite S, Vanderkolk C A, Ryan A D 1987 The free radial forearm flap with and without bone for closure of large palatal fistulae. British Journal of Plastic Surgery 40: 391–395

Maillard G F, Stoiber E, Ochsenbein H 1976 Excision of two thirds of the midface and prosthetic replacement. British Journal of Plastic Surgery 29: 186–190

Maruyama Y, Osafune H 1987 Free vertical abdominal fasciocutaneous flap. British Journal of Plastic Surgery 40: 27–30

Maxwell G P, Leonard L G, Manson P N, Hoopes J E 1980 Craniofacial coverage using the latissimus dorsi myocutaneous island flap. Annals of Plastic Surgery 4: 410

Mixter R C, Rao V K, Katsaros J, Noon J, Tan E 1990 Simultaneous reconstruction of cervical soft tissue and esophagus with a gastro-omental free flap. Plastic and Reconstructive Surgery 86: 905–909

Miyamoto Y, Harada K, Kodama Y, Takahaski H, Okano S 1986 Cranial coverage involving scalp, bone and dura using free inferior epigastric flap. British Journal of Plastic Surgery 39: 483–490

Nahai F, Stahl R S, Hester T R, Clairmont A A 1984 Advanced applications of revascularized free jejunal flaps for difficult wounds of the head and neck. Plastic and Reconstructive Surgery 74: 778–781

Nakayama K, Yamamoto K, Tamiya T, Makino H, Odaka M, Ohwada M, Takahashi H 1964 Experience with free autografts of the bowel with a new venous anastomosis apparatus. Surgery 55: 796

Pennington D G, Stern H S, Lee K K 1989 Free flap reconstruction of large defects of the scalp and calvarium. Plastic and Reconstructive Surgery 83: 655–661

Robertson A G, Rao G S, Al-Sammarie A, Soutar D S 1992 The management of tumours arising in the maxillary antrum. Clinical Oncology 4: 240–243

Robson M C 1976 Resection and immediate reconstruction for patients with 'inoperable' recurrent head and neck cancer. Surgical Clinics of North America 56: 111–123

Rosen H M 1985 The extended trapezius musculocutaneous flap for cranio-orbital facial reconstruction. Plastic and Reconstructive Surgery 75: 318

Rowsell A R, Godfrey A M, Richards M A 1986 The thinned latissimus dorsi free flap. A case report. British Journal of Plastic Surgery 39: 210

Savage R C 1983 Orbital exenteration and reconstruction for massive basal cell and squamous cell carcinoma of cutaneous origin. Annals of Plastic Surgery 10: 458–466

Schuller D E 1982 Latissimus dorsi myocutaneous flap for massive facial defects, Archives of Otolaryngology 108: 414

Shenaq S S M 1988 Reconstruction of complex cranial and craniofacial defects utilizing iliac crest—internal oblique microsurgical free flap. Microsurgery 9: 154

Shestak K C, Schusterman M A, Jones N F, Johnson J T 1988 Immediate microvascular reconstruction of combined palatal and mid facial defects using soft tissue only. Microsurgery 9: 128

Smith P J, Morgan B D G, Crockard H A 1983 Immediate total scalp and skull reconstruction. Microsurgery 4: 23

Stueber K, Salcman M, Spence R J 1985 The combined use of the latissimus dorsi musculocutaneous free flap and split rib grafts for cranial vault reconstruction. Annals of Plastic Surgery 15: 155–160

Swartz W M, Banis J C, Newtown E D, Ramasastry S S, Jones N F,

Acland R 1986 The osteocutaneous scapular flap for mandibular and maxillary reconstruction. Plastic and Reconstructive Surgery 77: 530–545

Wei F C, Tsao S B, Chang C N, Noordhoff M S 1987 Scalp, skull and dura reconstruction on emergency basis. Annals of Plastic Surgery 18: 252–256

Index